PUBLIC HEALTH
Communication
Critical Tools and Strategies

Claudia F. Parvanta, PhD

Professor and Director, Florida Prevention Research Center
Department of Community and Family Health
College of Public Health
University of South Florida
Tampa, Florida
Lead Author and Editor

David E. Nelson, MD, MPH

Director, Cancer Prevention Fellowship Program
National Cancer Institute, National Institutes of Health
Bethesda, Maryland
Editor, Chapter Contributor

Richard N. Harner, MD

Principal, BrainVue Systems
Philadelphia, Pennsylvania
Editor, Chapter Contributor

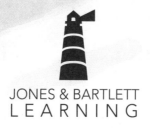

JONES & BARTLETT
LEARNING

World Headquarters
Jones & Bartlett Learning
5 Wall Street
Burlington, MA 01803
978-443-5000
info@jblearning.com
www.jblearning.com

Jones & Bartlett Learning books and products are available through most bookstores and online booksellers. To contact Jones & Bartlett Learning directly, call 800-832-0034, fax 978-443-8000, or visit our website, www.jblearning.com.

Substantial discounts on bulk quantities of Jones & Bartlett Learning publications are available to corporations, professional associations, and other qualified organizations. For details and specific discount information, contact the special sales department at Jones & Bartlett Learning via the above contact information or send an email to specialsales@jblearning.com.

Production Credits

VP, Executive Publisher: David D. Cella
Publisher: Michael Brown
Associate Editor: Lindsey Mawhiney Sousa
Associate Editor: Danielle Bessette
Editorial Assistant: Ashley Puffer
Production Manager: Daniel Stone
Senior Marketing Manager: Sophie Fleck Teague
Composition: Integra Software Services Pvt. Ltd.

Cover Design: Theresa Manley
Director of Rights & Media: Joanna Gallant
Rights & Media Specialist: Merideth Tumasz
Media Development Editor: Shannon Sheehan
Cover Image (Title Page, Part Opener, Chapter Opener):
    © Marilyn Volan/Shutterstock
Printing and Binding: Edwards Brothers Malloy
Cover Printing: Edwards Brothers Malloy

Library of Congress Cataloging-in-Publication Data

Names: Parvanta, Claudia F., editor. | Nelson, David E., M.D., editor. |
  Harner, Richard N., editor.
Title: Public health communication : critical tools and strategies / [edited by]
  Claudia F. Parvanta, David E. Nelson, Richard N. Harner.
Other titles: Public health communication (Parvanta)
Description: Burlington, MA : Jones & Bartlett Learning, [2018] | Includes
  bibliographical references and index.
Identifiers: LCCN 2017009690 | ISBN 9781284065947
Subjects: | MESH: Health Communication—methods | Public Health Practice |
  Communications Media
Classification: LCC RA425 | NLM WA 590 | DDC 362.1—dc23
LC record available at https://lccn.loc.gov/2017009690
978-1-284-06594-7

6048

Printed in the United States of America
21 20 19 18 17   10 9 8 7 6 5 4 3 2 1

Acknowledgments

Many of the people who helped with ideas or materials for this text are credited where their contributions appear. We thank them for providing cutting-edge thinking as well as examples of health communication in action. Their work represents some of the best of the best, and we truly appreciate being able to showcase it in our text.

On the editorial side, Alesha Hruska, MPH, MS, contributed valuable critiques as well as editorial assistance in putting this text book together. It simply would not be here without her work. Patricia Turo, MS, initiated the editorial tracking system, which was then followed by Angela Parvanta, Marina Ghatley, Kristin Raspanti, and Kelly Cuccolo. The University of the Sciences Behavioral and Social Sciences Department Administrator, Lara Schneider, provided usually indispensable and timely help with logistics. Thank you all for your generous help.

The ancillary materials were created by students at the University of the Sciences, including Swana Thomas, Khaleema Major, Leila Kulaib, and Khizra Hydari. Kelly Cuccolo revised and updated the glossary in addition to creating slides.

The Jones & Bartlett Learning crew of Mike Brown, Lindsey Mawhiney Sousa, and Merideth Tumasz all provided great help and support. We thank the *Essentials* series editor, Richard Riegelman, for his insights and gentle prodding.

It really does take a village to write a text! Thank you to everyone.

—*Claudia F. Parvanta, PhD*

Contents

Foreword xi

Prologue xii

About the Editors xiii

Chapter Contributors xiv

Extended Case Study Contributors xv

Appendices xvi

Text Box Contributors xviii

Contributors xx

Chapter 1 Introduction to Public Health Communication 1

Introduction 1
The Fundamentals 2
   Communication 2
   Public Health 2
   The Ecological Model 4
   Determinants of Health 4
   Health Communication as a Lever in the
      Population Health Model 5
What's Old and What's New in Health
   Communication 6
   The Foundation 6
   How Do We Determine the Effectiveness of
      Health Communication Interventions? 6
      Then: Hierarchies and Funnels 6
      Now: The Customer Journey and Touchpoints 7
Public Health Communication as a Career 8
   Entry-Level Competencies in Public Health
      Communication 9
   Credentialing in Health Communication 10
   Organizations That Serve as Health
      Communication Incubators 13
Conclusion: The Scope of Health
   Communication 14

Chapter 2 Population Health: A Primer 17

Introduction 17
Evolution of the Leading Causes of Death 17

The Era of Environmental Disease (Circa 1900) 18
The Era of Expanding Health Care (Circa 1950) 18
The Era of Lifestyle and Health Risk Behaviors
   (Circa 1970) 18
The Era of Social Determinants (Circa 2000) 19
Leading Health Indicators Approach 20
   Healthy People 2020 20
   Health Disparities 23
Health Rankings 23
Gathering Data to Communicate About
   Population Health 25
   Sources of Information 25
      Health Outcomes Data 25
      Health Determinants Data 25
      Comprehensive Population Health Reports 27
   Evidence-Based Policies and Programs 28
Communication Challenges 29
   Confronting Public Perceptions About Risk:
      Perception Versus Reality 29
   The Stigma of Chronic Disease: "It's Your
      Own Darn Fault" 30
Conclusion 30

Appendix 2 Communicating About Infectious Disease 33

Chapter 3 A Public Health Communication Planning Framework 39

Introduction: The Importance of Planning 39
   Approaches to Planning 40
   Health Communication Within the Ecological
      Model 41
Health Communication Planning
   Overview 41
   Subplans 41
      Macro Plan 41
      Strategic Health Communication Plan 41
      Implementation Plan 43
      Evaluation Plan 43
      Partnership Plan 43
      Dissemination and Publication Plan 43
Program Examples 43

Step-by-Step Planning. 44
   Developing the Macro Plan 44
      Step 1: Analyze the Problem and Its Place in the
         Ecological Framework 44
      Step 2: Select a Primary Intervention Based
         on Evidence. 47
      Step 3: Identify Relevant Audiences. 47
      Step 4: Choose a Core Communication Strategy
         for Each Audience. 48
      Step 5: Select an Overall Approach 50
      Step 6: Choose Partners 52
      Step 7: Model the Intervention and Conduct a SWOTE
         Analysis. 53
   Strategic Thinking. 60
      Managing Strengths and Weaknesses 61
      Maximizing Opportunities and Defending
         Against Threats. 62
      "Baking In" Ethics 62
Conclusion 62

**Appendix 3 ATV Safety: You Make the Choice
Case Analysis. 65**

Chapter 4   How to Communicate
About Data. 77

Introduction. 77
Public Health Data Systems 77
   Surveillance Systems. 77
   Where to Find Public Health Data 78
People and Numbers 82
   Numeracy 82
   Tendencies and Biases 82
Data Communication Principles 83
   Assess Audience Numeracy and Level of
      Involvement. 83
   Remember Your Ethical Responsibility. 83
   Minimize the Number of Data Items. 83
   Select Data That Are Familiar and Easy to
      Understand. 84
   Explain Unfamiliar Terms 84
   Consider Framing Effects. 84
   Provide Context. 84
   Integrate Data into an Overall Communication
      and Implementation Plan. 85
Show Me the Data: Presenting Public Health
   Numbers 85
   Presenting Data Using Words. 85
   Presenting Data Visually 86
      Visual Fundamentals 86
      Specific Visual Modalities. 86
      Infographics. 88
Conclusion 91

**Appendix 4 Addressing Chlamydia in a North
Carolina County 93**

Chapter 5   Understanding and Reporting
the Science. 97

Introduction. 97
Evaluating the Quality of Public Health
   Science. 98
   Research Factors 98
      Study Design 98
      Representativeness and Causality 98
   Level of Scientific Consensus 99
      Research Syntheses 99
      Contextual Information 100
   Information Sources 101
How Lay Audiences Assess Science-Based Public
   Health Information 102
   Level of Interest in Health and Extent of
      Scientific Knowledge .102
   Culture and Worldview. 103
   Trust and Belief. 103
   Information Processing and Interpretation. 103
Science Communication Fundamentals. 104
   Content. 104
   Context. 105
   Overload. 105
Putting It All Together 105
   Single Overriding Communication Objective. 105
   Case Study: Communicating Science from
      a Research Study Article 106
   Case Study: Communicating Science from a
      Comprehensive Report 107
   Case Study: Interpreting Science for
      Communication to the Public. 109
Conclusion 109

**Appendix 5 From Research to Patient Education:
Distilling the Science for the Health of the Public 111**

Chapter 6   Communicating for Policy and
Advocacy. 123

Introduction. 123
   How Citizens Shape Public Policy. 124
      Indirect Route: Elections, Political Action Committees,
         and Super PACs 124
      Direct Routes: Lobbying, Advocacy, and Activism 125
   Organizations That Do Extensive Advocacy. 126
Strategic Policy Communication 126
   Communicating with (Public) Policy Makers. 126

The "Cookbook" 128
   1. State What You Want to Accomplish *129*
   2. Define the Audience *131*
   3. Research and Craft the Message *131*
   4. Choose the Spokesperson *133*
   5. Deliver the Message *136*
   6. Evaluate Your Progress *138*
Preparing and Delivering a Policy Presentation 138
   Doing Your Research: The First Step in Tailoring
     a Presentation to the Policy Maker *140*
   Writing the Policy Brief *141*

Advocacy 141
   Community-Based Prevention Marketing for Policy
     Development: A New Planning Framework 141
   Use of New and Traditional Media 142
     New Media Advocacy *142*
     Traditional Media Advocacy *143*
     Media Relations Tools *145*
     Data Collections and Report Cards *145*
   Anticipating Audience Questions 145

Example of a Successful Policy Change
   Communication Campaign 145
Conclusion 149

Chapter 7   Health Literacy and Clear Health
              Communication **151**

Introduction 151
   Modeling Health Literacy 152
   Human Learning and Development 152
   Attention 153
Basic Literacy and Its Components 153
   Types of Literacy 153
   How Literate Is the U.S. Public? 153
Determinants of Health Literacy 154
   Communication Skills 155
   Knowledge 156
   Culture 156
   Local Language Proficiency 157
   Context 157
   Complexity of Health Care 158
Improving Health Literacy Through National
   Policy 160
   Plain Writing Act of 2010 161
   Patient Protection and Affordable Care Act 161
   Healthy People 2020 161
   National Action Plan to Improve Health
     Literacy 161
Assessing Health Literacy 162
   Instruments to Measure Health Literacy 162

     REALM *163*
     TOFHLA *163*
     NVS *163*
     eHEALS *163*
     NUMi *163*
     HLSI *163*
     Health Literacy Tool Shed *163*
   Health Literacy in Clinical Practice 164
   Health Literacy Universal Precautions Toolkit 164
Developing and Assessing Materials 164
   Key Principles 164
   Clear Communication Index 165

Appendix 7A CDC Clear Communication Index Before
     and After Example: NVDRS **169**

Appendix 7B CDC Clear Communication Index Before
     and After Example: Thimerosal **171**

Appendix 7C Case Study – Smokefree.gov **173**

Chapter 8   Behavior Change Communication:
              Theories, Models, and Practice
              Strategies **177**

Introduction: The Power (?) of Persuasion 177
Theory in Health Communication for Behavior
   Change 178
   The Value of Theory in Health
     Communication 178
   Sources of Theory in Health Communication 178
   Behavior Change Theory 180
     Health Belief Model *180*
     Transtheoretical Model *180*
     Social Cognitive Theory *180*
     The Precaution Adoption Process Model *182*
     Integrative Model (Theory of Reasoned Action
       and Theory of Planned Behavior) *182*
     Elaboration Likelihood Model *183*
     Diffusion of Innovations *183*
Theory Derived from Communication
   Studies 184
   Message Framing 184
   Inoculation Theory 185
   Extended Parallel Process Model 192
   (Media) Uses and Gratifications Theory 193
   Message Sensation Value and Sensation
     Seeking 193
   Media Richness Theory 193
Applying Theory to Practice Strategies 193
   Intervention Mapping 194

From Theory-Based Methods to Practice
Strategies......................................194
Participatory Approach 194
Entertainment Education.......................194
Elaboration Likelihood Model Applications 198
Tailoring 205
Social Marketing.................................. 205
Immutable Laws of Social Marketing 206
Customer Orientation...........................206
Behavior.......................................206
Segmentation..................................206
Exchange: Benefits, Barriers, and Competition 213
Examples and Resources 214
Conclusion: What Is Next?..................... 214

**Appendix 8 Programmatic Research in Health
Communication Campaigns 219**

Chapter 9   Formative Research 223

The Scope of Formative Research................ 223
Reviewing and Analyzing Existing
Information...................................224
Exploratory Research Processes 225
Marketing as an Organizing Framework 225
Social Marketing 226
Differentiating Behavioral Doers from Non-Doers:
A Positive Deviance Approach 228
Audience Segments and "Personas"...............232
Profiles to Personas............................232
Customer Journey Mapping.....................233
Research Tools.................................... 234
Quantitative Methods..........................238
Data Mining 238
Developing Surveys.............................239
Qualitative Methods 244
Observation and Participation 244
Reported Behavior 246
Conclusion 248

**Appendix 9 Framing Messages About Sexual Health:
Research for Engaging All Stakeholders 251**

**Chapter 10   Media Vehicles, Platforms,
and Channels................ 265**

Introduction..................................... 265
A Word About Terminology 266
An Overview of Media Use in the United States 266
Sources 266

The Big Picture....................................266
Broadcast Media Channels........................268
Media Channel Selection 269
Theory-Informed Media Selection
Framework 269
Media Richness Theory..........................269
Uses and Gratifications Theory 269
Person-, Place-, and Time-Mediated Touchpoints
in the Customer Journey.......................269
Media Management Framework 270
"Inform Me": The Search for Information.......... 272
Media You Earn: News...........................272
Media You Own: Your Website or Blog 272
Search Engine Optimization 273
Inbound Marketing.............................274
"Engage Me": Social Media...................... 276
Which Social Media Predominate?...............276
Demographic Breakdown........................276
A Sampling of Social Media Tools by Function
and Use 277
Cell Phone Texting 277
Social Networking Sites: Facebook
and Friends.................................284
Twitter: Micro Blogging 287
Using Social Media Effectively in Public Health
Communication 288
"Entertain Me" 290
Cross-Channel or Transmedia Storytelling 290
Virtual Worlds and Gaming......................290
Conclusion 298

**Appendix 10A Harnessing the Power of Radio
to Raise HIV Testing Rates....................... 301**

**Appendix 10B Health Communication Strategies
for Hispanic Enrollment into the Affordable
Care Act Health Insurance Exchanges:
A Case Study.................................305**

**Chapter 11   Implementing a Communication
Intervention 315**

Introduction: Are You Ready? 315
Planning Tools—Again 316
RE-AIM...316
SMART..319
Effect Size.....................................320
The Creative Brief 321
Elements of a Creative Brief 322
Use Feedback from Early Pre-testing...............322

From the Creative Brief to Concepts 326
From Concepts to Messages and Materials 330
Matching Content to Media Channels 332
   Content Management and Strategy 332
     Content-Focused Components 332
     People-Focused Components 333
   Production and Dissemination Factors 333
     Production Value 333
     Reach and Scalability 333
     Sustainability. 333
     Cost-Effectiveness 334
Pre-testing Your Content. 335
   In-Person Pre-testing 335
     Questions for Pre-testing Content 336
   Higher-Tech Pre-testing 341
     Usability Testing 341
     Physiological Effects Testing 341
   Testing the Final Media Package. 346
     In-Situ Testing. 346
     Test Marketing. 346
Preparing the Work Plan, Timetable, and
   Budget 346
   Defining Partner Roles 346
     International Partners 346
     Partnering in the United States 347
   Budget. 350
     Direct Costs 350
     Indirect Costs. 350
     In-Kind Contributions 350
     Total Budget 350
   Timeline 353
     Measurement and Evaluation 353
Summary Implementation Plan. 355
Conclusion 355

Appendix 11 Campaign to Sustain Hand-Washing Behaviors in an Urban Informal Settlement in Kenya **361**

Chapter 12 Evaluating a Health Communication Program. 369

Introduction. 369
Three Central Evaluation Questions 371
   Doing the Right Things? 371
     Is there empirical "proof of concept" from a
      well-conducted prior study? 371
     Does the program plan specify how its objectives
      will be met in a theoretically plausible manner? 372
     Are program procedures acceptable to the local
      community? 372

   Doing the Right Things Right? 372
   Doing Enough of the Right Things to Make a
     Difference? 373
     Making Enough Noise, and Capturing Any
      Difference It Made 373
     Differences That Make a Difference. 373
Capturing the Basics. 374
   Program Exposure 374
     Exposure Complexities 374
     Measuring Exposure by Channel. 375
   Program Outcomes 375
     Goals and Smart(er) Objectives. 375
     Short-Term and Longer-Term Objectives 375
     Measures of Outcomes 375
   Cost-Effectiveness. 376
E-Media Considerations. 376
   New E-Health Sources of Information 376
   E-Health as a Source of New Research
     Questions. 376
   E-Media Advantages and Disadvantages
     for Research 377
Study Designs 377
   Randomized Controlled Trials 377
   Quasi-experiments. 378
   Correlational Studies 378
   Sampling 379
   Evaluation via Indicators 379
Using Qualitative and Quantitative Data 379
Evaluation Frameworks 381
   CDC Evaluation Framework 381
   RE-AIM, PRECEDE–PROCEED, and
     Inform-Persuade 382
   E-Health Frameworks 382
Conclusion 382

Appendix 12 Evaluation of the National GYT (Get Yourself Tested) Campaign. **387**

Chapter 13 Clinician–Patient Communication. 391

Introduction. 391
Conceptual Framework for Effective
   Clinician–Patient Communication 392
   Dichotomies 393
   Goals 394
   Barriers. 394
Getting Started 395
   Levels. 395
   Modes 395

Tools................................396
External Issues 397
Clinician–Patient Encounter.................... 397
Respect.................................397
Preparation in Environment, Body, and Mind 397
Listening................................398
Story.................................399
Physical Examination......................400
Progressive Dialogue.......................400
Review and Summation......................400
Special Cases 400
Language Barriers.........................400
Informed Consent.........................402
The Dying Patient.........................402
Prospects....................................... 403
Conclusion 404

Chapter 14 The Role of Communication in Cancer Prevention and Care..... 409

Introduction................................... 409
Background................................409
Information and Communication 410
Chapter Goals.............................410
The Cancer Control Continuum.................. 410
Prevention...............................410
Detection and Diagnosis......................411
Treatment 411
Palliative Care and End of Life 412
Survivorship 412
The Cancer Information Landscape 413
The Internet..............................413
Television 413
Social Media 414
Peer Groups..............................414
Cancer Communication
in Clinical Settings 414
Patient-Centered Care.......................414
Complexity 415
Health Literacy............................415
Examples...................................... 415
Preventing Cervical Cancer...................415
Shared Treatment Decisions...................415
LIVESTRONG for Survivors 416
Conclusion 416

Appendix 14 Health Literacy in the Context of Cancer Care: Fox Chase Cancer Center 419

Chapter 15 Crisis and Emergency Risk Communication: A Primer 427

Introduction................................... 427
Attack..................................427
Transformations...........................428
Outbreak................................428
Response................................428
A Basic Risk Framework 432
Presenting Risk...........................434
The Psychology of Risk Perception..............434
Presenting a Risk Assessment 436
Report Content 436
The Written Document.......................437
Oral Presentation..........................438
Poster Session............................438
Remote Presentations.......................438
Engaging the Public in Risk Assessment
and Reporting 439
Emergency Risk Communication 439
What Distinguishes ERC from Routine Health
Communication? 439
Channels and Media Choices.....................439
Do Social Media Stand Out? 440
Psychological Needs During a Disaster 441
The Stages of Crisis and Emergency Risk
Communication 445
Pre-event Planning.........................447
Who Is in Charge?..........................447
Message and Audience 453
Topic-Specific Pre-crisis Materials...................453
Message Maps 454
Communicating During an Emergency 461
Seven Recommendations......................461
Conclusion 462

Appendix 15A Liberia Ebola Response Strategic Communication Plan in 2014— Unoffical Draft 467

Appendix 15B Social Media System for Dengue Prevention in Sri Lanka 475

Chapter 16 Health Communication in Resource-Poor Countries 481

Introduction................................... 481
Overview of International Health Communication .. 482
The Millennium Development Goals 482
The Global Burden of Disease 482

x   **Contents**

History of Health Communication in Resource-Poor
Countries..482

The Intersection of Communication and
International Health 483

Health Communication for Development............ *483*

*Theoretical Underpinnings of International Health
Communication* *483*

Health Communication Campaigns in Developing
Countries.................................... 484

Communication Approaches......................484

Interpersonal Communication Approaches........... *484*

Community-Level Approaches.................... *488*

Mediated Communication *490*

Interactive Communication Technologies *491*

Entertainment-Education: An Integrated Approach ... *493*

When More Is Better: Using a Transmedia
Approach 495

SIAGA Campaign.............................. *496*

Soul City *496*

*Ndukaka: Changing Norms Around Female Genital
Mutilation*.................................. *497*

Conclusion 499

Glossary and Common Abbreviations 503

Index 523

Foreword

As you begin browsing this text, we want to prevent you from experiencing a sense of déjà vu. This is not a second edition. The authors and editors of *Essentials of Public Health Communication*, published in 2011, have responded to requests to create a new text for graduate-level students in public health as well as a new text for undergraduate learners. The book you hold in your hands (or are viewing on screen) is designed to meet the needs of master in public health (MPH) or doctoral-level (DrPH or PhD) students in health communication as well as those in the health professions. Given this target audience, it features larger-scale programs, evidence-based interventions, and research. By comparison, the undergraduate text offers more community-based and campus-level examples and somewhat less emphasis on research.

This text is designed to cover the skills emphasized by the National Public Health Information Coalition (NPHIC) in its Certified Communicator in Public Health (CCPH) credentialing program as well as the Certified Health Education Specialist (CHES) exam. We expect that working professionals will find the text to be a useful resource as well.

This edition does include some material that was previously published in *Essentials of Public Health Communication*. But please don't stop reading here! Communication is one of the most rapidly changing fields in public health. Not only have the media channels changed dramatically since *Essentials* was published, but so have the public health challenges and campaigns. We have identified a distinguished group of contributors for this text and given them more space to explore their topics. As a result, you will find new and exciting examples of highly diverse communication programs, ranging from promoting health insurance enrollment in the United States to fighting Ebola in west Africa; from the national "Tips from Former Smokers" campaign to a county-level anti-e-cigarette plan developed by a team of MPH students; from the national "Get Yourself Tested" program (for HIV prevention) to a campus-based vending machine effort to promote healthy snacking; and from communications across the cancer spectrum to a Dutch program to build psychological resilience in school children. We are extremely pleased with the contributed cases from our colleagues in academia, public service, and the private sector. By reading and practicing the "how to" steps in the chapters and referring to these case studies, you will be well on your way to gaining competencies in public health communication.

Claudia F. Parvanta, PhD
David E. Nelson, MD, MPH
Richard N. Harner, MD

Prologue

Public Health Communication: Critical Tools and Strategies is perfectly designed to meet the needs of master in public health (MPH) or doctoral-level (DrPH or PhD) students in health communication as well as those in the clinical and administrative health professions. It builds on the authors' extensive experience and is a text that you will find both solidly grounded in theory and focused on practical applications.

Public health communication has become central to nearly every challenge facing public health. Those who take advantage of this text will acquire skills that will serve them well as they deal with these challenges. There is no doubt in my mind that *Public Health Communication: Critical Tools and Strategies* is poised to become the classic text for public health communications. I'm confident that you will agree.

Richard Riegelman MD, MPH, PhD
Professor and Founding Dean
Milken Institute School of Public Health
The George Washington University

About the Editors

Claudia F. Parvanta, PhD

Professor and Director, Florida Prevention Research Center

Department of Community and Family Health
School of Public Health
University of South Florida
Tampa, Florida
Lead Author and Editor

Claudia Parvanta, PhD, is a Professor in the Department of Community and Family Health, College of Public Health, and Director of the Florida Prevention Research Center, at the University of South Florida, Tampa. In addition to teaching and mentoring students, she leads the Center's efforts to increase colorectal cancer screening through community based prevention marketing. Previously, Dr. Parvanta headed the Department of Behavioral and Social Sciences at the University of the Sciences in Philadelphia (2005–2016). Her research emphasized health literacy and culturally competent health communication. From 2000 to 2005, Dr. Parvanta directed the Division of Health Communication in the Office of Communication at the Centers for Disease Control and Prevention (CDC). She was central to the agency's communication response to the 9/11 attacks, anthrax, and SARS. Before government and academia, Dr. Parvanta worked at Porter Novelli, a global social issues communication company. Dr. Parvanta has designed, managed, or evaluated health and nutrition social marketing programs in more than 20 countries. She is the 2016 recipient of the Public Health Education and Health Promotion Division of APHA's Distinguished Career Award.

David E. Nelson, MD, MPH

Director, Cancer Prevention Fellowship Program
National Cancer Institute, National Institutes of Health
Bethesda, Maryland
Editor and Chapter Contributor

David E. Nelson, MD, MPH, currently heads up the National Cancer Institute's (NCI) Cancer Prevention Fellowship Program. He previously spearheaded efforts to develop the Health Information National Trends Survey (HINTS) for NCI, was the Acting Director of the Bureau of Smoking or Health, and directed the Behavioral Risk Factor Surveillance System (BRFSS) for the CDC. He co-edited *Essentials of Public Health Communication* (Jones and Bartlett, 2011); with B. Hesse, published *Making Data Talk* (Oxford University Press, 2009); and was the lead author (with Brownson, Parvanta, and Remington) of *Communicating Public Health Information Effectively: A Guide for Practitioners* (APHA, 2002).

Richard N. Harner, MD

Principal, BrainVue Systems
Tampa, Florida
Editor, Chapter Contributor

Richard N. Harner, MD, is a clinical neurologist with more than three decades of clinical, teaching, and research experience. He directed the Neurology Department at the Graduate Hospital of the University of Pennsylvania and established the first center for the comprehensive medical and surgical treatment of epilepsy in the eastern United States. After 20 years, he moved to become Professor and Vice Chairman of Neurology at the Medical College of Pennsylvania, where he established a second epilepsy center and directed postgraduate neurology education. He has authored numerous scientific articles, and does private consulting for the biotechnology and pharmaceutical industries.

Chapter Contributors

The authors of chapters not written by the editors are listed below in alphabetical order.

Danielle Blanch-Hartigan, PhD, MPH, is Assistant Professor of Health Studies, Department of Natural and Applied Sciences, Bentley University, in Waltham, Massachusetts. She recently served as a Cancer Prevention Fellow in the Behavioral Research Program and Office of Cancer Survivorship at the National Cancer Institute, National Institutes of Health, Rockville, Maryland. Blanch-Hartigan is a co-author of Chapter 14.

Wen-ying Sylvia Chou, PhD, MPH, is Program Director of the Health Communication and Informatics Research Branch, National Cancer Institute, National Institutes of Health, Rockville, Maryland. Chou is a co-author of Chapter 14.

David W. Cragin, PhD, DABT, is Adjunct Professor, Department of Health Policy and Public Health, University of the Sciences, Philadelphia, Pennsylvania, and Professor of International Pharmaceutical Engineering Management, Peking University, Beijing, China. Cragin is the co-author of Chapter 15.

Carmen Cronin, MPH, recently completed her studies at Drexel University in Philadelphia. During 2015–2016, she pursued a U.S. Student Fulbright grant in Uganda, where she conducted research with adolescent girls and women in urban, rural, and refugee contexts. Cronin is the co-author of Chapter 16.

Jonathan P. DeShazo, PhD, MPH, is Assistant Professor and Masters in Health Administration Program Director, School of Allied Health Professions, Virginia Commonwealth University, Richmond, Virginia. DeShazo is the co-author of Chapter 12.

Erika M. Hedden, PhD, MJ, CMPP, is an Associate Director in U.S. Oncology Global Medical Affairs at Merck Inc., in the greater Philadelphia area. Hedden is also Adjunct Professor, Health Communication, at the University of the Sciences. She is the author of Chapter 7.

May Grabbe Kennedy, PhD, MPH, was formerly Associate Professor and Graduate Studies Director in the Social and Behavioral Health Department, Virginia Commonwealth University, School of Medicine, Richmond, Virginia. Kennedy is the co-author of Chapter 12.

Patrick L. Remington, MD, MPH, is Associate Dean for Public Health and Professor, School of Medicine and Public Health, University of Wisconsin, Madison, Wisconsin. He currently is on the advisory committee for *Healthy People 2020*. Remington is the author of Chapter 2.

Suruchi Sood, PhD, is Associate Professor, Department of Community Health and Prevention, Dornsife School of Public Health, Drexel University in Philadelphia. Sood is the co-author of Chapter 16.

Chan Le Thai, PhD, MPH, is Assistant Professor, Department of Communication, Santa Clara University. She recently served as a Post-Doctoral Fellow in the Health Communication and Informatics Research Branch, National Cancer Institute, National Institutes of Health, Rockville, Maryland. Thai is a co-author of Chapter 14.

Extended Case Study Contributors

Authors of larger case studies that appear in appendices or multiple chapter boxes are listed here in the order in which their case material first appears in the book.

▶ Tips from Former Smokers

Diane Beistle, B.A. (Branch Chief*); **Crystal Bruce**, MPH (Acting Team Lead, Campaign Development Team*); **Kevin C. Davis**, MA (RTI International); **Carol Haney** (Qualtrics); **Michelle Johns**, MA, MPH (Health Communication Specialist*); **Josh Millman** (Vice President, Plowshare Group); **Jane Mitchko**, MEd (Deputy Branch Chief*); **Salimah Mohamed**, MPH (Health Communication Specialist*); **Mark Pajewski** (Plowshare Group); **Deesha Patel**, MPH (Health Communication Specialist*); **Paul Shafer**, MA (Research Economist, RTI International); **Robert Rodes**, MS, MEd, MBA (Team Lead, Research, Evaluation and Technical Assistance Team*); **Maggie Silver**, MPH (Health Communication Specialist*). Authors indicated by* work in the Health Communications Branch, Office on Smoking and Health, CDC/ONDIEH/NCCDPHP.

▶ Proposed Public Health Communications Campaign for Tobacco Free Alachua (TFA)

Natalie Belva, Rachel Hojnacki, Allison Justice, Sherezade Rodriguez, Samantha Susock. The Campaign Plan was presented in partial fulfillment of the requirements for the degree of master of arts in mass communication at the University of Florida, April 2014.

▶ Get Yourself Tested

Framing Case Study (Chapter 8) and GYT National Campaign (Chapter 12)

Allison Friedman, MS (Travelers' Health Branch, Division of Global Migration & Quarantine (DGMQ), National Center for Emerging and Zoonotic Infectious Diseases (NCEZID)); **Jennifer Uhrig**, PhD (RTI International, Research Triangle Park, NC); **Booker Daniels**, MPH (NCHHSTP/Division HIV/AIDS Prevention/ Prevention Communication Branch/National Partnerships Team, CDC, Atlanta, GA); **Carla M. Bann**, PhD (RTI International, Research Triangle Park, NC); **Lisa Gilbert**, PhD (Center for Communication Science, RTI International, Research Triangle Park, NC); **Jon Poehlman**, PhD (RTI International, Research Triangle Park, NC); **Sarah Levine; Melissa Habel; Elizabeth Clark; Rachel Kachur; Kathryn Brookmeyer; Mary McFarlane; and Tina Hoff.**

Appendices

Authors of material used in appendices are listed below in the order in which their material appears in the text, by chapter and title.

Chapter 2   Communicating About Infectious Disease

Amy Jessop, PhD, MPH, University of the Sciences, Philadelphia, Pennsylvania

Chapter 3   ATV Safety: You Make the Choice

Maria Brann, PhD, MPH, Indiana University-Purdue University, Indianapolis, Indiana

Brandi N. Frisby, PhD, University of Kentucky, Lexington, Kentucky

Kerry Byrnes, PhD, Collin College, Plano, Texas

Chapter 4   Addressing Chlamydia in a North Carolina County

Jessica K. Southwell, MPH; **Matthew C. Simon**, MA; **Kasey P. Decosimo**, MPH, University of North Carolina, Chapel Hill, North Carolina

Chapter 5   From Research to Patient Education: Distilling the Science for the Public

Theresa J. Barrett, PhD, New Jersey Academy of Family Physicians, Trenton, New Jersey

Robert Sprague and Frances Reimers, PCI Communications, Arlington, Virginia

Chapter 8   Programmatic Research in Health Communication Campaigns

Nancy Grant Harrington, PhD; **Philip C. Palmgreen**, PhD; **Lewis Donohew**, PhD, University of Kentucky, Lexington, Kentucky

Chapter 9   Framing Messages About Sexual Health: Research to Engage All Stakeholders

Susan D. Kirby, DrPH, CHES, President, Kirby Marketing Solutions

Susan J. Robinson, PhD, Visiting Researcher, Georgia Institute of Technology Institute for People and Technology, Atlanta, Georgia

Chapter 10 A: Harnessing the Power of Radio to Raise HIV Testing Rates

Jeremy Smith (National Director) Incite, Austin, Texas

Matthew Scelza, MA (Director), Incite, Los Angeles, California

B: Health Communication Strategies for Hispanic Enrollment into the Affordable Care Act Health Insurance Exchanges

Dirk G. Schroeder, ScD, MPH (Chief Health Officer and Executive Vice President, *HolaDoctor* Inc. and Associate Professor (Adjunct) of Global Health, Emory University, Atlanta, Georgia

Gloria P. Giraldo, MPH, Program Manager, Latino Health Access, and Lecturer at California State University, Fullerton, California

Brianna Keefe-Oates, MPH, National Program Manager, *HolaDoctor*, Inc., Atlanta, Georgia

Chapter 11   Campaign to Sustain Hand Washing Behaviors in an Urban Informal Settlement in Kenya

Renée A. Botta, PhD; **Leah Scandurra**, MA; **Rina Muasya**, MA candidate, University of Denver, Colorado

Kelly Fenson-Hood, MA, Executive Director, Power of Hope, Kibera, Boulder, Colorado

Chapter 12   Evaluation of the National GYT (Get Yourself Tested) Campaign

Allison Friedman, MS, Travelers' Health Branch, Division of Global Migration & Quarantine (DGMQ), Atlanta, Georgia

Sarah Levine

Melissa Habel

Elizabeth Clark

Rachel Kachur

Kathryn Brookmeyer

Mary McFarlane

Tina Hoff

Chapter 14   Health Literacy in the Context of Cancer Care: Fox Chase Cancer Center

Linda A. Fleischer, PhD, MPH (Associate Research Professor) and **Stephanie Raivitch**, BS (Director Resource Education Center), Fox Chase Cancer Center, Philadelphia, Pennsylvania

Rima Rudd, PhD, Senior Lecturer on Health
Literacy, Education, and Policy, Harvey T. H.
Chan School of Public Health, Harvard University,
Boston, Massachusetts

**Chapter 15 A: Liberia Ebola Response Strategic
Communication Plan**
Ministry of Health and Social Welfare, Liberia
Jana L. Telfer, MA (Associate Director for
Communication Science (Former),

National Center for Immunization and Respiratory
Diseases, Centers for Disease Control and
Prevention, Atlanta, Georgia

B: Social Media System for Dengue Prevention in Sri Lanka
May O. Lwin, PhD (Associate Professor); **Santosh
Vijaykumar**, MA, PhD (Senior Research Fellow);
Karthikayen Jayasundar (Research Assistant), Wee
Kim Wee School of Communication and Information,
Nanyang Technological University, Singapore

Text Box Contributors

Authors who have contributed original material for inclusion in chapter boxes are listed here in the order in which their material appears in the text by chapter and box number.

▶ Chapter 1

Box 2: **Cynthia Baur**, PhD, Senior Advisor, Health Literacy, Office of the Director, Centers for Disease Control and Prevention, Atlanta, Georgia

Box 5: **Moshe Engelberg**, CEO of ResearchWorks, Inc., Oceanside, California

Box 6:- **Kristine A. Smith**, MA, CCPH, Credentialing Manager, National Public Health Information Coalition (NPHIC), Marietta, Georgia

▶ Chapter 3

Box 7: **Ranita Chakrabarti**, MPH. Ms. Chakrabarti was a student at Thomas Jefferson University when she completed the study referred to in the box.

Box 9: **N. Belva, R. Hojnacki, A. Justice, S. Rodriguez, S. Susock.** The Campaign Plan was presented in partial fulfillment of the requirements for the degree of master of arts in mass communication at the University of Florida, April 2014.

▶ Chapter 6

Box 2, Box 8: **Public Health Institute/Health in All Policies and American Public Health Association**

Box 5: **Patricia McLaughlin**, MA, Former AVP, Communications, Legacy Foundation, Merrillville, Indiana

Box 15: **Rosemarie O'Malley Halt**, RPh, MPH, Advocacy Director, Maternity Care Coalition, Philadelphia, Pennsylvania

▶ Chapter 7

Box 5: **Stacy Robison**, MPH, MCHES, President and Co-founder, CommunicateHealth, Inc., Northampton, Massachusetts

▶ Chapter 8

Box 1: **Alesha G. Hruska**, MS, MPH, MCHES, University of the Sciences, Philadelphia, Pennsylvania

Box 3: **Allison Friedman**, MS, Travelers' Health Branch, Division of Global Migration & Quarantine (DGMQ), National Center for Emerging and Zoonotic Infectious Diseases (NCEZID), Atlanta, Georgia; **Jennifer Uhrig**, Director, Social and Behavior Change Research Program, RTI International, Research Triangle Park, North Carolina; **Booker T. Daniels II**, MPH, Health Communication Team Lead, Centers for Disease Control and Prevention, Atlanta, Georgia; **Carla M. Bann**, RTI International; and **Jon Poehlman**, PhD, Health Communication Scientist, RTI International, Research Triangle Park, North Carolina

Box 4: **Ross Shegog**, PhD, Associate Professor, University of Texas School of Public Health, Houston, Texas

Box 7: **Nedra Kline Weinreich**, MS, President, Weinreich Communications, Los Angeles, California

Box 8 and Figures 5-10: **Nikki Spencer**, BA, and **Matthew Kreuter**, PhD, MPH, Health Communication Research Laboratory, Brown School of Social Work, Washington University, St. Louis, Missouri

Box 9 and Figures 14-16: **Jeff Jordan**, President and Executive Creative Director, Rescue Social Change Group, San Diego, California

▶ Chapter 9

Box 1: **Marian Huhman**, PhD, Assistant Professor, University of Illinois at Urbana-Champaign, Urbana, Illinois

Box 3: **Martine Bouman**, PhD (Scientific Director); **Sarah Lubjuhn**, PhD (Research Fellow), Center for Media & Health, Gouda, The Netherlands; **Arvind Singhal**, PhD, Professor of Communication, University of Texas at El Paso, El Paso, Texas

Box 5 and Figure 5: **Jim Tincher**, MBA, Journey-Mapper-in-Chief, Heart of the Customer, Minneapolis, Minnesota

Box 9 and Figure 8: **Sara Bauerle Bass**, PhD, MPH, Director, Risk Communication Laboratory, Temple University Department of Public Health, Philadelphia, Pennsylvania

Box 10 and Figures 9–11: **Ankit Lodaya**, PhD candidate, University of the Sciences, Philadelphia, Pennsylvania

▶ Chapter 10

Box 2: **Matthew Prior**, MPH. Prior was a Communication and Policy Coordinator at the Philadelphia Department of Public Health, Division of Disease Control, STD Control Program, when he completed the study referred to in the box.

Box 3: **Hilary N. Karasz**, PhD, Public Information Officer, Public Health, Seattle & King County, Washington; and Lindsay Bosslet, MPH, Public Health, Seattle & King County, Washington

Box 9: **Nedra Kline Weinreich**, MS, President, Weinreich Communications, Los Angeles, California

Box 10: **Joan E. Cowdery**, PhD, Professor, Health Education, Eastern Michigan University, Ypsilanti, Michigan; **Sun Joo (Grace) Ahn**, PhD, Assistant Professor, University of Georgia, Grady College of Journalism & Mass Media Communication, Department of Advertising and Public Relations, Athens, Georgia

▶ Chapter 11

Box 2: **Renée A. Botta**, PhD, **Leah Scandurra**, MA, and **Rina Muasya**, MA candidate, University of Denver, Colorado; **Kelly Fenson-Hood**, MA Executive Director, Power of Hope, Kibera, Boulder, Colorado

Box 9 and Figure 1: **Andy S. L. Tan,** PhD, MPH, MBA, MBBS, Assistant Professor, Harvard T. H. Chan School of Public Health, Boston, Massachusetts; **Rachel Douglas**, MPH, Fraser Health Authority, Surrey, British Columbia; **Victoria Lee**, MD, MPH, MBA, CCFP, FRCPC, Fraser Health Authority, Surrey, British Columbia; **Ellen Peterson**, MBA, Langley Division of Family Practice, Langley, British Columbia; **Geoffrey Ramler**, BSc, Fraser Health Authority, Surrey, British Columbia; **Jeff Plante**, MD, Langley Division of Family Practice, Langley, British Columbia

Box 12 and Figures 4 and 5: **Sara Bauerle Bass**, PhD, MPH, Associate Professor, Temple University, Philadelphia, Pennsylvania

▶ Chapter 13

Box 3, Box 8: **Sue Checchio**, MS, independent health communication consultant

▶ Chapter 15

Box 1: **Kristen Alley Swain**, PhD, Assistant Professor, The Meek School of Journalism and New Media, University of Mississippi, University, Mississippi

Box 2: **Samuel Dilito Turay**, MPH, President and CEO, Hands for Life, Sierra Leone

Contributors

Sun Joo Ahn, PhD
Assistant Professor
University of Georgia, Grady College of Journalism
    & Mass Communication
Department of Advertising and Public Relations
Athens, Georgia

Shannon Baldwin, BA
Research Area Specialist, The Institute for Health
    Promotion Research
University of Texas Health Science Center
San Antonio, Texas

Carla M. Bann, PhD
RTI International
Research Triangle Park, North Carolina

Theresa J. Barrett, PhD
Deputy Executive Vice President,
New Jersey Academy of Family Physicians
Trenton, New Jersey

Sarah B. Bass, PhD, MPH
Associate Professor of Public Health, College of
    Public Health
Temple University
Philadelphia, Pennsylvania

Cynthia Baur, PhD
Professor and Director
Horowitz Center for Health Literacy
University of Maryland
College Park, Maryland

Natalie Belva
Digital Media Manager
United Cerebral Palsy of New York City
New York, New York

Danielle Blanch-Hartigan
Bentley University
Waltham, Massachusetts

Renée A. Botta, PhD
University of Denver
Denver, Colorado

Martine Bouman, PhD
Scientific Director, Center for Media & Health
Gouda, The Netherlands

Maria Brann, PhD, MPH
Indiana University-Purdue University,
Indianapolis, Indiana

Kerry Byrnes, PhD
Collin College
McKinney, Texas

Susan Checchio, MSc
Princeton, New Jersey

Wen-ying Sylvia Chou, PhD, MPH
Program Director of the Health Communication and
    Informatics Research Branch,
National Cancer Institute,
National Institutes of Health (NIH),
Rockville, Maryland

Joan E. Cowdery, PhD
Professor, Health Education
Eastern Michigan University
Ypsilanti, Michigan

David W. Cragin, PhD, DABT
Professor in International Pharmaceutical
    Engineering Management
Peking University, Beijing
Adjunct Professor of Health Policy & Public Health,
University of the Sciences, Philadelphia,
    Pennsylvania

Carmen Cronin, MPH
Drexel School of Public Health
Department of Community Health and Prevention
Philadelphia, Pennsylvania

Kasey P. Decosimo, MPH
University of North Carolina, Chapel Hill,
    North Carolina

Gini Dietrich
CEO, Ament Dietrich, Inc.
Chicago, Illinois

Lewis Donohew, PhD
College of Communication and Information
University of Kentucky
Lexington, Kentucky

Kelly Fenson-Hood, MA
Executive Director
Power of Hope, Kibera
Boulder, Colorado

Linda Fleisher, PhD, MPH
Senior Scientist, Center for Injury Research and
	Prevention
Children's Hospital of Philadelphia
Philadelphia, Pennsylvania

Allison Friedman, MS
Travelers' Health Branch, Division of Global
	Migration & Quarantine (DGMQ)
National Center for Emerging and Zoonotic
	Infectious Diseases (NCEZID)
Atlanta, Georgia

Brandi N. Frisby, PhD
University of Kentucky,
Lexington, Kentucky

Gloria P. Giraldo, MPH
Program Manager, Latino Health Access, and
	Lecturer
California State University, Fullerton
Orange County, California

May Grabbe Kennedy, PhD, MPH
Department of Health Policy & Public Health
University of the Sciences
Philadelphia, Pennsylvania

Nancy Grant Harrington, PhD
University of Kentucky, Department of
	Communication
Lexington, Kentucky

Sarah Harris
VP & Founder, INCITE
Austin, Texas

Erika M. Hedden, PhD, MJ, CMPP
Associate Director in US Oncology Global Medical
	Affairs, Merck Inc
Adjunct Professor, Health Communication,
University of the Sciences
Philadelphia, Pennsylvania

Rachel Hojnacki, MA
Ohio National Financial Services
Cincinnati, Ohio

Allison J. Hudson, MA
Assistant Director of Development
University of Florida Harn Museum of Art
Gainesville, Florida

Marian Huhman
Assistant Professor,
University of Illinois at Urbana-Champaign
Urbana, Illinois

Karthikayen Jayasundar
Research Assistant Wee Kim Wee School of
	Communication and Information,
Nanyang Technological University
Singapore

Amy B. Jessop, PhD, MPH
Associate Professor of Health Policy and Public
	Health,
University of the Sciences
Philadelphia, Pennsylvania

Jeff Jordan
President & Executive Creative Director, Rescue
	Social Change Group
San Diego, California

Hilary Karasz, PhD
Public Information Officer,
Public Health, Seattle & King County
Seattle, Washington

Brianna Keefe-Oates, MPH
National Program Manager, HolaDoctor, Inc.,
	Atlanta, Georgia

Susan D. Kirby, DrPH, CHES
President, Kirby Marketing Solutions,
Visiting Instructor, UCLA School of Public Health
Del Mar, California

Matthew Kreuter, PhD, MPH
Associate Dean for Public Health & Professor,
Brown School of Social Work,
Washington University, St. Louis
Kahn Family Professor of Public Health
St. Louis, Missouri

Sarah Lubjuhn, PhD
Research Fellow Center for Media & Health,
Gouda, The Netherlands

May O. Lwin, PhD
Associate Professor Wee Kim Wee School of
    Communication and Information,
Nanyang Technological University
Singapore

Edward Maibach, PhD, MPH
George Mason University,
Fairfax, Virginia

Jane Mitchko, MEd
Deputy Branch Chief, Health Communications
    Branch Office on Smokinig and Health, Centers for
    Disease Control and Prevention
Atlanta, Georgia

Rina Muasya, MA
School Sanitation Officer
ECOTAT
Nairobi, Kenya

Rosemarie O'Malley Halt, RPh, MPH
University of the Sciences,
Philadelphia, Pennsylvania

Philip C. Palmgreen, PhD
University of Kentucky,
Lexington, Kentucky

Evan Perrault, PhD
Assistant Professor, University of Wisconsin
Eau Claire Department of Communication and
    Journalism
Eau Claire, Wisconsin

Jon Poehlman
RTI International
Research Triangle Park, North Carolina

Matthew Prior, MPH
State Policy and Communications Manager
National Coalition of STD Directors
Washington, DC

Stephanie Raivitch, BS
Director Resource Education Center,
Fox Chase Cancer Center
Philadelphia, Pennsylvania

Frances Reimers
Principal
Firestarter Communications LLC
Alexandria, Virginia

Patrick L. Remington, MD, MPH
University of Wisconsin-Madison School of Public
    Health
Madison, Wisconsin

Susan J. Robinson, PhD
Visiting Researcher
Georgia Institute of Technology
Institute for People and Technology
Atlanta, Georgia

Stacy Robison, MPH, MCHES
President and Co-Founder,
Communicate Health Inc.
Northampton, Massachusetts

Sherezade Rodriguez, MA
Product Marketing Strategist
352 Inc.
Atlanta, Georgia

Rima Rudd, PhD
Senior Lecturer on Health Literacy, Education, and
    Policy,
Harvey T.H. Chan School of Public Health,
Harvard University, Boston, Massachusetts

Leah Scandurra, MA
University of Denver
Denver, Colorado

Matthew Scelza, MA
Director, INCITE
Los Angeles, California

Dirk G Schroeder, ScD, MPH
Chief Health Officer and Exec VP, HolaDoctor Inc
Associate Professor (Adjunct) of Global Health,
Emory University
Atlanta, Georgia

Ross Shegog, PhD
Associate Professor
University of Texas
Houston, Texas

Matthew C. Simon, MA
University of North Carolina, Chapel Hill
Chapel Hill, North Carolina

Arvind Singhal, PhD
Marston Endowed Professor of Communication,
University of Texas at El Paso
El Paso, Texas

Jeremy Smith
National Director, Incite
Austin, Texas

Suruchi Sood, PhD
Dornsife School of Public Health,
Drexel University, Philadelphia, Pennsylvania

Jessica K. Southwell, MPH
University of North Carolina at Chapel Hill,
North Carolina Institute for Public Health
Chapel Hill, North Carolina

Robert Sprague
PCI- A Communications Company
Alexandria, Virginia

Samantha Susock, MA
Digital Media Editor
Heery International, Inc
Atlanta, Georgia

Kristen Alley Swain, PhD
Assistant Professor, Meek School of Journalism and
    New Media,
University of Mississippi

Andy Tan
Assistant Professor
Department of Social and Behavioral Sciences,
    Harvard School of Public Health
Cambridge, Massachusetts

Jana L. Telfer, MA
Associate Director for Communication Science
    (Former),
National Center for Immunization and Respiratory
    Diseases,
Center for Disease Control
Atlanta, Georgia

Chan Le Thai, PhD, MPH
Assistant Professor
Department of Communication
Santa Clara University
Santa Clara, California

Jim Tincher, MBA
Heart of the Customer
Minneapolis, Minnesota

Samuel Dilito Turay, MPH
President and CEO
Hands for Life, Sierra Leone
Philadelphia, Pennsylvania

Santosh Vijaykumar, MA, PhD
Senior Research Fellow
Wee Kim Wee School of Communication and
    Information,
Nanyang Technological University, Singapore

Nedra Kline Weinreich, MS
President, Weinreich Communications
Los Angeles, California

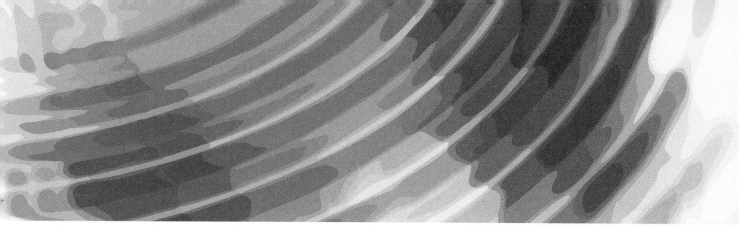

CHAPTER 1

Introduction to Public Health Communication

Claudia Parvanta, PhD

LEARNING OBJECTIVES

By the end of this chapter, the reader will be able to:

- Provide a definition of and rationale for public health communication.
- Describe *Healthy People 2020* objectives for health communication.
- Explain how communication fits into the ecological model of public health and supports other public health objectives.
- Describe new developments in health communication.
- Identify competencies in health communication defined by the Council on Linkages between Academia and Public Health Practice.
- Identify government agencies that serve as research incubators in health communication.
- Describe the job of a professional health communicator as defined by the National Public Health Information Coalition.

▶ Introduction

Public health communication is an interdisciplinary field of scholarship and practice that uses everything we know about communication to improve health among individuals and populations. A public health communication practitioner may specialize in health education and promotion, risk communication, or media relations; concentrate on research in communication, behavioral or social science, or digital technology; follow a path that includes teaching, writing, art, entertainment, or rhetoric; or be the biggest digital or data-crunching nerd you know. Such a professional might have a background in journalism, mass communication, health education, a bench science, healthcare delivery, advertising, or marketing. The diversity of expertise that flows into health communication makes it one of the richest, most creative fields of study and practice. Just as "it takes a village to raise a child," so it takes an interdisciplinary team to communicate effectively about health with the public.

▶ The Fundamentals

Communication

Communication in and of itself is an extremely complex field with centuries of study. The National Communication Association (NCA), a scholarly professional organization, defines the *discipline* of **communication** as focusing "on how people use messages to generate meanings within and across various contexts, and is the discipline that studies all forms, modes, media, and consequences of communication through humanistic, social scientific, and aesthetic inquiry."[a] With many models proposed over the years, the **transactional model of communication**, derived from the burgeoning psychological and information theories of the 1960s and 70s, has stood the test of time. As Barnlund emphasized in his original exposition of the model, communication " … is not a reaction to something, nor an interaction with something, but a transaction in which man invents and attributes meaning to realize his purposes."[1] To simplify greatly, this meaning is generated by a process of encoding and decoding. A communicator encodes (e.g., puts thoughts into words and gestures), then transmits the message via a channel (e.g., speaking, email, text message) to the other communicator(s), who then decodes the message (e.g., take*s* the words and applies meaning to them). The message may be degraded by noise (e.g., any physical, psychological, or physiological distraction or interference), preventing the message from being completely received or fully understood as the sender intended.

This description covers two-thirds of a communication transaction, which ends with comprehension. Ultimately, though, the recipient's *response* is the way we know that a message has been understood as intended. If the response fits our expectations, we believe our communication was successful. Unfortunately, according to the great Finnish communication scholar Osmo A. Wiio, "Communication usually fails, except by accident."[b] Most of the science of health communication exists to reduce this failure rate.

A clear line once separated what worked best in interpersonal communication versus mass communication, but in recent years digital technologies have permanently abolished this distinction. We can, and often do, think of "an audience of one," and concomitantly have conversations with many of these single-person audiences (see **BOX 1-1**).

The responses we seek are conditioned by our social and cultural context, the choice of medium, and what we are trying to accomplish. In health communication, we usually seek to promote a behavior change, or a change in a behavioral antecedent, such as knowledge or attitude.

Public Health

There are numerous definitions of "health," but all include a concept of individual physical and mental well-being that is sustained throughout the full lifecourse, from prenatal development and birth, until what is considered a timely death. Public health is concerned with promoting the conditions that give everyone the chance to have a healthy life. According to the U.S. government's Department of Health and Human Services (HHS), everyone should be able to "[a]ttain high quality, longer lives free of preventable disease, disability, injury, and premature death."[c] The key U.S. government strategy for promoting, planning, and assessing public health activities is known as *Healthy People 2020* (**HP 2020**); it measures progress in population health through large trends, such as increased life expectancy and decreased chronic disease prevalence. HP 2020 contains 26 **Leading Health Indicators** that represent significant threats to public health related to disparities in access, social factors, and physical environments, as well as specified objectives for other areas of public health. **BOX 1-2** discusses the development of objectives in health communication and information technology (IT).

a. NCA (https://www.natcom.org/discipline).

b. Wiio's laws are communication-specific versions of Murphy's laws—for example, "If a message can be interpreted in several ways, it will be interpreted in a manner that maximizes the damage." More can be found at http://www.cs.tut.fi/~jkorpela/wiio.html#who.

c. HP 2020 overarching goal 1 (http://www.healthypeople.gov/2020/About-Healthy-People).

d. See http://www.cdc.gov/mmwr/mmwr_nd/ for *MMWR* summaries.

BOX 1-1 Audience of One, Conversations with Many

Audience of One

"Audience of one" is neither a rock group nor a religious ideal, but rather the data- and social media–enabled phenomenon of being able to understand and communicate with an individual as if that person were the only one who matters. This idea comes from the metaphor of being in a theater and feeling as if the performer is speaking or singing directly to you. (Listen to Roberta Flack's classic song, "Killing Me Softly with His Song.") With sufficient background data and a grasp of context, communicators can tailor messages and media so that each recipient feels as if a personal message were received.

Conversations with Many

Most of us grew up with the idea that a conversation was something you shared with one, or at most, a few individuals. Conversations allow for candid expressions about our thoughts and feelings. In the marketing world, "word of mouth" was the strongest endorsement for a product, as people were more likely to listen to the opinions of friends and family than to the claims made by advertisers. Now, in a world awash with Twitter, blogs, and more immediate social media, we can share with multitudes the thoughts we used to share only with our friends. Corporations use call centers, crowd-sourced Twitter analysis and responses, and more impersonal means to manage the interactive demands of conversational media. However, many professional health communicators, due to other work demands, find it difficult to keep up their end of the conversation.

BOX 1-2 *Healthy People 2020* Objectives: National Priorities in Health Communication and Health Information Technology

Healthy People is a participatory, federally led process for creating national health goals and objectives that reflects available evidence and stakeholders' views on the most important issues in public health. Although the governing body of *Healthy People 2020* is made up of federal agencies, the goals and objectives are developed through collaboration with organizations and individuals in all sectors of society. All objectives for the next decade must be supported by data collected at the end of the previous decade. The U.S. Department of Health and Human Services (HHS) tracks these data over time to establish progress and collaborates with stakeholders to generate multiple, collective actions at different levels—local, state, and national—that improve the public's health. The *Healthy People 2020* objectives, launched in 2010, are based on a determinants of health framework for understanding and addressing the main causes of illness, disability, and premature death.

   Healthy People 2020, and *Healthy People 2010* before it, identified objectives for communication and health information technology. In HP 2010, HHS recognized health communication as a distinct, cross-cutting topic area and included two objectives for Internet access and the quality of health websites. The inclusion of health communication objectives in 2010 confirmed the importance of communication as an intellectual framework, a scientific endeavor, and a set of processes and interventions for health improvement in public health policy making. The topic area expanded in the HP 2020 program to include more objectives for both health communication and health information technology. The added health information technology objectives attest to the increasing importance of digital health as useful not only for clinical and administrative purposes, but also for consumer and patient engagement and provider–patient communication.

   The priorities for the HP 2020 health communication and health information technology objectives emerged from a series of meetings and online discussions, as well as from public comments. The objectives identify communication and information technology activities that can be measured during a decade and available data sources. Ideally, an objective's data source should remain consistent from one decade to the next to allow for longer time trend analyses. More practically, different data sources may have to be used depending on funding availability, new priorities for data collection, and changes in the frequency of data collection. The topics covered in the HP 2020 objectives include health literacy, provider–patient communication, consumer and patient use of digital health resources, health information technology access and diffusion, and the use of social marketing for public health communication. The objectives' full text and most recent data, as well as relevant literature and interventions, are available at www.healthypeople.gov.

(continues)

BOX 1-2 *Healthy People 2020* Objectives: National Priorities in Health Communication and Health Information Technology   *(continued)*

The importance of health communication and health information technology for achieving national health goals will continue to increase as more people use digital technologies to search for health information, track and manage health behaviors and indicators, and engage with health services and providers in a more interactive way. The *Healthy People* objectives will continue to evolve for 2030 and reflect the changing environment and contribution of communication and information technologies to health outcomes.

How Are We Doing?

Each health communication and health information technology objective included in the *Healthy People* framework has baseline data, one or more data updates during the decade, and an end-of-decade target. Here, we highlight three of the objectives, including their baseline numbers, updates, and targets. The latest data are available from www.healthypeople.gov.

- *Health literacy objective*: Increase the proportion of persons who report that their healthcare provider always gives them easy-to-understand instructions about what to do to take care of their illness or health condition.
  - 2011 baseline: 64.1%
  - 2020 target: 70.5%

- *People's use of electronic personal health management tools objective*: Increase the proportion of persons who use the Internet to keep track of personal health information, such as care received, test results, or upcoming medical appointments.
  - 2007 baseline: 14.3%
  - 2014 update: 28.1%
  - 2020 target: 15.7% [Exceeded target; need to revise]

- *Crisis and emergency risk messages that demonstrate best practices objective*: Increase the proportion of crisis and emergency risk messages embedded in print and broadcast news stories that explain what is known about the threat to human health.
  - 2010–2011 baseline: 83.5% of messages
  - 2020 target: 88.9%

Cynthia Bauer, CDC.

The Ecological Model

Inherent in the HP 2020 framework is the **ecological model** of public health (**FIGURE 1-1**). According to Fielding, Teutsch, and Breslow, the ecological model

> emphasizes the importance of the social and physical environments that strongly shape patterns of disease and injury as well as our responses to them over the entire life cycle, providing a broader conceptualization of important determinants of health not easily identifiable or rectifiable within the medical model. Healthy communities, which are defined by having the capacity to allow each individual to be healthy, must address all these components.[2]

Determinants of Health

As suggested by the goals of HP 2020, much public health effort is directed toward creating healthy communities. High-risk environments—such as those with more pollution, fewer green spaces, fewer outlets for

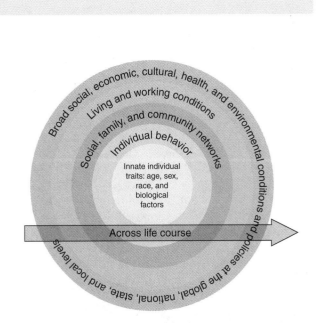

FIGURE 1-1 An ecological model.
Modified from U.S. Department of Health and Human Services, Advisory Committee for HP 2020.

healthy food, more traffic, or more crime—are considered to place an unfair burden on the people living in them. Tremendous human and material resources are required to produce clean air, water, and food;

keep infectious diseases at bay; ensure environmental and worksite safety; and provide affordable health care to all. Our gains in life expectancy in the United States are almost exclusively due to advances in public health on these fronts. While many public health achievements alter our physical world (e.g., reduction in the amounts of environmental lead, fluoridation of drinking water), the majority now rely on societal and individual adoption of recommended behaviors. Some of the disparities that persist in public health are due to lingering inequities in the distribution of resources along social—and often geographic—borders. Others, however, are due to low uptake of healthy behaviors.

In their 2014 working paper, Stewart and Cutler summarize the impact of six behaviors that the U.S. government has tracked in relation to changes in life expectancy (LE) and quality-adjusted life expectancy (QALE) from 1960 to 2010.[3] Overall LE increased by 6.9 years during this period. As shown in **FIGURE 1-2**, the authors estimate that reductions in cigarette smoking and motor vehicle fatalities contributed nearly 2 of these years. At the same time, these gains were partially offset by the negative effect of rising rates of obesity and accidental drug overdoses.

At the population level, we could add even more years to our lifespan if we could only behave in a healthy manner. Data from the Behavioral Risk Factor Surveillance Survey (BRFSS) show that, for example, only 13% of people sampled had the recommended consumption of fruit intake, and 9% had the recommended consumption of vegetables in 2013.[4] These puny rates were found despite the U.S. government's decades-long program promoting "Five a Day" as the minimum number of servings of fruits and vegetables to be consumed each day. For many reasons, it takes a lot of time, and more than just a friendly reminder, to get most people to adopt a new behavior that they find difficult to follow.

Health Communication as a Lever in the Population Health Model

Population health addresses a number of individual health behaviors. Communication is a key public health tool to affect these behaviors. This point was emphasized by Robert Hornik in his 2014 keynote address to a National Academy of Sciences workshop on "Communicating to Advance the Public's Health." According to Hornik:

> Health communication should focus not on population outcomes (such as increased life expectancy) or on categories of behaviors (such as limiting environmental toxins, reducing exposure to tobacco smoke, and safer sex), but rather on individual behaviors.[5]

His examples of using communication to encourage healthy behavior include influencing people to test for radon gas in their homes to reduce environmental toxicity, convincing policy makers to outlaw smoking in public places to reduce population exposure to tobacco toxins, and persuading people to use condoms to reduce sexually transmitted disease.

It is important to note that Hornik includes policy and advocacy as forms of health communication that change behavior—in this case, the behavior of legislators and politicians. This brings health communication in line with the ecological model for public

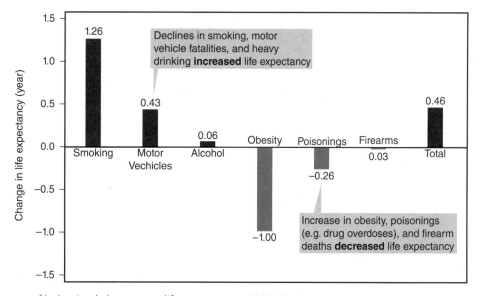

FIGURE 1-2 The impact of behavioral changes on life expectancy, 1960–2010.

health, which favors societal change, and systemic, or "upstream" intervention. **Upstream interventions** are directed at the source of a problem, at the broadest or earliest point of entry. **Downstream interventions** attempt to modify conditions for individuals at the narrowest or latest point of entry.

Health communication alone cannot change some systemic determinants of poor health, such as oil spills, poor social environments, limited health-care resources, or poverty. But even though health communicators are not all-powerful, their responsibilities run deeper than we might think. If those who need critical information to protect their health are not seeking or receiving it, understanding it, or being moved to action, we can use health communication to influence these behaviors. If the policy makers who determine national, state, and local laws, regulations, and public services have not received crucial information or been moved to action, we can use policy communication and advocacy to promote changes in public policy. The ecological approach to public health communication requires that all factors affecting a particular health condition be explored, and in particular that an effort to change the upstream factors accompany efforts to help individuals improve their own health outcomes downstream. This is an ethical and professional principle that many practitioners embrace, even though their ability to conduct upstream advocacy may be constrained by political forces or regulations.

▶ What's Old and What's New in Health Communication

The Foundation

The main activities of scientific public health communication have not changed significantly in the past few decades. They begin and end with health outcomes data in the following cycle:

- Collect and analyze epidemiological data (e.g., National Health and Nutrition Examination Survey, cancer and notifiable disease registries, local statistics) to identify health problems (e.g., childhood obesity, tobacco-related deaths).
- Identify the causes of health problems as well as their behavioral/environmental antecedents. Use local surveys, state surveys (e.g., Behavioral Risk

Factor Surveillance System BRFSS[e]), or national surveys (e.g., Health Information National Trends Survey [HINTS[f]]). Use qualitative research to utilize an existing, or develop a new, strong scientific theory to test in a larger sample.
- Develop communication strategies to modify behavior, behavioral antecedents, or policies for improved environmental conditions (**BOX 1-3**).
- Determine which communication strategies are effective at changing behavior, antecedents, or regulations or programs to improve environmental conditions (**BOX 1-4**).
- Repeat the process, as necessary, until goals are achieved.
- Set up maintenance programs.

How Do We Determine the Effectiveness of Health Communication Interventions?
Then: Hierarchies and Funnels

Health communication has often relied on what McGuire called a **hierarchy of effects** (HOE) to measure the impact of a health communication intervention. It is difficult to say who originated this approach because it was developed in stages. Advertising started using what was called the "attraction–interest–decision–action" model (attributed to Philadelphian E. St. Elmo Lewis) more than 100 years ago, in the early 1900s. In 1961, Lavidge (a marketer) and Steiner

---

BOX 1-3 Behavioral Determinants

According to Robert Hornik, "The process of developing a population health initiative should begin with investigating the hypothesized determinants of the targeted behavior … If you are trying to influence a behavior in a particular population, then the focus needs to be on what influences them, not what influences you" (pp. 3–4). He points out that telling people to eat more fresh produce will not help them change their behavior if no fresh produce is available to them. A better strategy in this case would be to communicate with producers and consumers to improve supply and stimulate demand.

IOM (Institute of Medicine). Communicating to advance the public's health: Workshop summary. Published March 17, 2015. NAS: Prepublication proof. March 17, 2015 http://iom.nationalacademies.org/Reports/2015/Communicate-to-Advance-Publics-Health.aspx. pp. 3–4.

---

e. http://www.cdc.gov/brfss/
f. http://hints.cancer.gov/

BOX 1-4 Broad and Persistent Communication Required to Produce Changes in Health Behavior

Even when population health improvement communication campaigns have promising messages for the target audience, they often fail because they do not have an effective strategy for obtaining the needed exposure strategy. .... The most significant changes in public health behaviors have been associated not with one-time communication efforts, but rather with multifaceted, "all but the kitchen sink" campaigns by multiple entities over long periods of time. (p. 4)

IOM (Institute of Medicine). Communicating to advance the public's health: Workshop summary. Published March 17, 2015. NAS: Prepublication proof. March 17, 2015 http://iom.nationalacademies.org/Reports/2015/Communicate-to-Advance-Publics-Health.aspx. p. 4.

(a psychologist) expanded this model by identifying six steps that a potential customer takes, moving through the cognitive[g] domains of awareness and knowledge, the affective[h] domains of liking and preference, and the decision-to-action "conative" domains of conviction and purchase. Lavidge and Steiner suggested potential advertising vehicles (e.g., skywriting and jingles to create awareness, status and glamour appeals to create preferences, point-of-purchase cues to create desire to purchase) and market research tools appropriate to each step.[6]

In 1984, McGuire further expanded the model and adapted it to public health campaigns, along with the classic communication transfer from source to receiver. The lower effects in the HOE include exposure, attention, interest, and comprehension. By comparison, the higher-order set of effects includes acquisition of skills, changes in attitude, short-term retention of information, long-term retention of information, decision making, one-time performance of a behavior, reinforcement of the behavior, and maintenance of the behavior indefinitely through complex life changes.[7]

Neither the stepwise nature of these effects nor the relative difficulty of producing them has been the subject of definitive research. However, in practice, many communication programs realized their resources were sufficient only to attain the lower-level effects in the HOE. Often there was insufficient exposure to the messages to produce any higher-order effects; in

turn, and unsurprisingly, none of these more desirable effects occurred. Post hoc analysis of these failed communication campaigns has given the HOE considerable credibility. It is worth noting that HOE preceded several of the individual change theories that are now popular in health communication.

Marketing experts modeled the process for group change in the form of a funnel. People at the wide end of the funnel might become aware of a specific product or brand. As the funnel narrowed, fewer dropped through to consider purchasing the offering, fewer still purchased it, and a very few would remain loyal to the brand or even extol its virtues to others. From an individual perspective, the potential customer would consider many brands and narrow down the choices until purchase. Marketing programs count on very large audiences at the awareness creation stage to make this process profitable, which explains why most well-known commercial brands invest heavily in mass-media advertising.

Now: The Customer Journey and Touchpoints

Public health communication professionals have embraced most of the new technology, media, and methods available to their commercial advertising counterparts. Where they might lag slightly behind is in visualization of the "customer" and in mounting multidimensional efforts to engage customers through a time and space journey toward adoption of a health-promoting behavior.

David Court and others writing for *the McKinsey Quarterly*[8] in 2009 coined the term **customer journey** to describe the conversion of the marketing "funnel" into a series of recurrent orbits that a customer enters when considering, evaluating, advocating for, or purchasing a specific product (**FIGURE 1-3**). The order in which these steps are listed here is intentional. According to David Edelman,[i] "The Internet has upended how consumers engage with brands. ... [T]hey connect with myriad brands—through new media channels beyond the manufacturer's and the retailer's control or even knowledge ... [T]hey often expand ... the pool before narrowing it. After purchase these consumers may remain aggressively engaged, publicly promoting or assailing the products ... collaborating in the brand's development, and challenging and shaping their meaning."[9] In other words,

---

g. How you think.
h. How you feel.
i. https://hbr.org/2010/12/branding-in-the-digital-age-youre-spending-your-money-in-all-the-wrong-places. Accessed July 19, 2015.

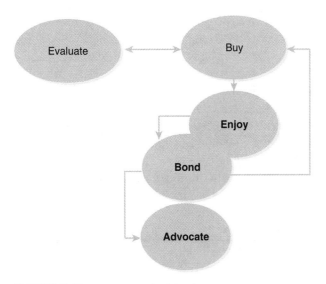

FIGURE 1-3 The customer decision journey.

Based on Edelman DC. Branding in the digital age: You're spending your money in all the wrong places. Harvard Business Review. https://hbr.org/2010/12/branding-in-the-digital-age-youre-spending-your-money-in-all-the-wrong-places. Accessed July 19, 2015.

even though the funnel offered some whirls, it was still a one-way process from awareness to purchase and possibly loyalty. The customer journey, in contrast, includes those consumers who become brand advocates even before they purchase a product, as well as many who bond with a brand and promote it, and others who become publicly disparaging after the purchase of a product or service.

The standard parts of a customer journey include a form of engagement, information, guidance, and support (**BOX 1-5**). Identifying the best way to deliver these encounters requires "customer journey mapping." Today, organizations use various forms of media and outreach to accomplish each specific form of contact. We will come back to customer journey mapping in our discussion of formative research.

▶ Public Health Communication as a Career

A wealth of new strategies, media, and tools have enriched health communication in recent years. In addition, there are numerous ways to acquire training and many places to apply these skills. In the private sector, "medical communication" agencies conduct user research and develop branding and customer experience strategies, along with many media extensions. A background in pharmaceutical marketing or health care combined with health communication or public relations skills can lead to a position in such a firm. Many of the same firms, as well as other types of companies, tend to hire graduates of advanced degree programs to work on government-related programs and activities. Not surprisingly, then, a wide range of communication positions are found within

---

BOX 1-5 Simplified Customer Journey and Touchpoints

M. Engelberg ResearchWorks, Inc.

There are equal parts hype and confusion around creating a world-class customer experience. Start by getting the customer journey right. We designed this three-step process, part of our *CustomerFirst* Framework, to show you how.

1. *Understand the customer journey.* Observe customers as they deal with their challenges and engage with your product and company. Listen to what they want and need. Gain a rich understanding of the problems customers face, their workflow needs and limitations, what they find frustrating and motivating, how they really want their experience to be, and what turns them off.
2. *Map the customer journey.* List all the interactions or "touchpoints" between you and your customers. Visually sequence these touchpoints across three stages—before, during, and after using your product. Color-code key touchpoints to signify which are hotspots that need troubleshooting, which are opportunities for you to provide greater value, and which can differentiate you from competition.
3. *Improve the customer journey.* Set objectives for what you want customers to think, feel, and do (i.e., experience) at each significant touchpoint. For example, when researching product options, you might want customers to think your product is easiest to use, to feel confident in their assessment, and to contact a sales representative. Use these objectives to drive how you optimize the customer journey at each touchpoint.

Once you get the customer journey right, then work backward to design the technology that is needed to bring it to life. Then it is not just your product, but the whole customer experience that sets you apart.

government agencies (the public sector). Increasingly, these positions require special public health communication competencies.

Entry-Level Competencies in Public Health Communication

The role of communication in public health is derived from the "Essential Public Health Services" identified by the **Centers for Disease Control and Prevention (CDC)** (**FIGURE 1-4**). Health communication supports several of the services, but is essential to address the need to "[i]nform, educate, and empower people about health issues."

When developing guidelines for hiring communication experts, public-sector organizations are likely to refer to the "Core Competencies for Public Health Professionals: Communication Skills" adopted in June 2014 by the Council on Linkages Between Academia and Public Health Practice. **TABLE 1-1** lists the entry-level (Tier 1) expectations for these competencies.

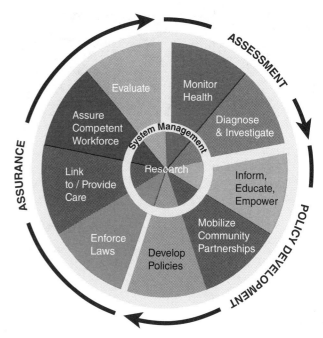

FIGURE 1-4 Ten essential public health services.

The Public Health System and the 10 Essential Public Health Services. Centers for Disease Control and Prevention Web site. http://www.cdc.gov/nphpsp/essentialservices.html. Accessed July 19, 2015.

TABLE 1-1 Council on Linkages' Core Competencies in Communication, 2014		
Communication Skills		
Tier 1	*Tier 2*	*Tier 3*
3A1. Identifies the literacy of populations served (e.g., ability to obtain, interpret, and use health and other information; social media literacy)	3B1. Assesses the literacy of populations served (e.g., ability to obtain, interpret, and use health and other information; social media literacy)	3C1. Ensures that the literacy of populations served (e.g., ability to obtain, interpret, and use health and other information; social media literacy) is reflected in the organization's policies, programs, and services
3A2. Communicates in writing and orally with linguistic and cultural proficiency (e.g., using age-appropriate materials, incorporating images)	3B2. Communicates in writing and orally with linguistic and cultural proficiency (e.g., using age-appropriate materials, incorporating images)	3C2. Communicates in writing and orally with linguistic and cultural proficiency (e.g., using age-appropriate materials, incorporating images)
3A3. Solicits input from individuals and organizations (e.g., chambers of commerce, religious organizations, schools, social service organizations, hospitals, government, community-based organizations, various populations served) for improving the health of a community	3B3. Solicits input from individuals and organizations (e.g., chambers of commerce, religious organizations, schools, social service organizations, hospitals, government, community-based organizations, various populations served) for improving the health of a community	3C3. Ensures that the organization seeks input from other organizations and individuals (e.g., chambers of commerce, religious organizations, schools, social service organizations, hospitals, government, community-based organizations, various populations served) for improving the health of a community

(continues)

TABLE 1-1 Council on Linkages' Core Competencies in Communication, 2014		*(continued)*
Communication Skills		
Tier 1	*Tier 2*	*Tier 3*
3A4. Suggests approaches for disseminating public health data and information (e.g., social media, newspapers, newsletters, journals, town hall meetings, libraries, neighborhood gatherings)	3B4. Selects approaches for disseminating public health data and information (e.g., social media, newspapers, newsletters, journals, town hall meetings, libraries, neighborhood gatherings)	3C4. Evaluates approaches for disseminating public health data and information (e.g., social media, newspapers, newsletters, journals, town hall meetings, libraries, neighborhood gatherings)
3A5. Conveys data and information to professionals and the public using a variety of approaches (e.g., reports, presentations, email, letters)	3B5. Conveys data and information to professionals and the public using a variety of approaches (e.g., reports, presentations, email, letters, press releases)	3C5. Conveys data and information to professionals and the public using a variety of approaches (e.g., reports, presentations, email, letters, testimony, press interviews)
3A6. Communicates information to influence behavior and improve health (e.g., uses social marketing methods, considers behavioral theories such as the Health Belief Model or Stages of Change Model)	3B6. Communicates information to influence behavior and improve health (e.g., uses social marketing methods, considers behavioral theories such as the Health Belief Model or Stages of Change Model)	3C6. Evaluates strategies for communicating information to influence behavior and improve health (e.g., uses social marketing methods, considers behavioral theories such as the Health Belief Model or Stages of Change Model)
3A7. Facilitates communication among individuals, groups, and organizations	3B7. Facilitates communication among individuals, groups, and organizations	3C7. Facilitates communication among individuals, groups, and organizations
3A8. Describes the roles of governmental public health, health care, and other partners in improving the health of a community	3B8. Communicates the roles of governmental public health, health care, and other partners in improving the health of a community	3C8. Communicates the roles of governmental public health, health care, and other partners in improving the health of a community

The Council on Linkages Between Academia and Public Health Practice. Core Competencies for Public Health Professionals. http://www.phf.org/corecompetencies. Accessed July 15, 2015.

To prepare graduates for careers in health communication, most master's and doctoral degrees in public health will use the **competency** models developed by the **Association of Schools of Public Health (ASPH)** in 2012. These competencies appear in **TABLE 1-2**.

Credentialing in Health Communication

While a number of graduate-level degree programs in health communication exist, there is no single credentialing organization for such professionals. Neither academic programs nor individuals are credentialed based on their academic training in health communication. The National Commission for Health Education Credentialing (NCHEC) awards the Certified Health Education Specialist (CHES) credential to individuals who meet required academic preparation qualifications and successfully pass a competency-based exam. Continuing education (through the Society for Public Health Education [SOPHE] and other providers) is required to maintain certification. The Master CHES (M/CHES) credential requires both advanced coursework and professional experience. Health education and health communication overlap in many areas, and

TABLE 1-2 Competencies in Advocacy and Communication Expected of Graduates from Master's and Doctoral-Level Programs in Public Health

Core Competency Area		DrPH Competency		MPH Competency
All		(Subsumed in A2)	F1	Describe how the public health information infrastructure is used to collect, process, maintain, and disseminate data.
		(Subsumed in B8.)	F5	Apply legal and ethical principles to the use of information technology and resources in public health settings.
			F7	Demonstrate effective written and oral skills for communicating with different audiences in the context of professional public health activities.
Advocacy	A1	Present positions on health issues, law, and policy.		(Subsumed in F7 to a lesser degree.)
	A2	Influence health policy and program decision-making based on scientific evidence, stakeholder input, and public opinion data.	F10	Use informatics and communication methods to advocate for community public health programs and policies.
	A3	Utilize consensus-building, negotiation, and conflict avoidance and resolution techniques.		(Subsumed in F7 to a lesser degree.)
	A4	Analyze the impact of legislation, judicial opinions, regulations, and policies on population health.	F8	Use information technology to access, evaluate, and interpret public health data.
	A5	Establish goals, timelines, funding alternatives, and strategies for influencing policy initiatives.		(Subsumed in F6 more generally.)
	A6	Design action plans for building public and political support for programs and policies.		(Subsumed in F10 more generally.)
	A7	Develop evidence-based strategies for changing health law and policy	F9	Use informatics methods and resources as strategic tools to promote public health

(continues)

TABLE 1-2 Competencies in Advocacy and Communication Expected of Graduates from Master's and Doctoral-Level Programs in Public Health *(continued)*

Core Competency Area		DrPH Competency		MPH Competency
Communication	B1	Discuss the interrelationships between health communication and marketing.		(Subsumed in F4.)
	B2	Explain communication program proposals and evaluations to lay, professional, and policy audiences.		(Subsumed in F6.)
	B3	Employ evidence-based communication program models for disseminating research and evaluation outcomes.	F4	Apply theory- and strategy-based communication principles across different settings and audiences.
	B4	Guide and organization in setting communication goals, objectives, and priorities.		
	B5	Create informational and persuasive communications.	F6	Collaborate with communication and informatics specialists in the process of design, implementation, and evaluation of public health programs.
	B6	Integrate health literacy concepts in all communication and marketing initiatives.	F2	Describe how societal, organizational, and individual factors influence and are influenced by public health communications.
	B7	Develop formative and outcome evaluation plans for communication and marketing efforts.		(Subsumed in F6.)
	B8	Prepare dissemination plans for communication programs and evaluations.		
	B9	Propose recommendations for improving communication processes.	F3	Discuss the influences of social, organizational and individual factors on the use of information technology by end users.

Association of Schools and Programs of Public Health.

the M/CHES is worth keeping in mind while selecting coursework in health communication.

For practicing professionals, the **National Public Health Information Coalition (NPHIC)** has created a credentialing process based on an extensive portfolio review. NPHIC awards a "Certified Communicator in Public Health" credential to public health communicators whose portfolios pass a qualifying examination. This organization conducted an extensive job analysis prior to creating its credentialing scheme.

BOX 1-6 provides more information on the NPHIC and its certification process.

Organizations That Serve as Health Communication Incubators

The following paragraphs are replete with acronyms that belong to the *lingua franca* of the public health and health communication communities. Now is a good time to begin to recognize and use them. At the national level, the U.S. Department of Health and Human Services (HHS) has long led efforts to research and disseminate evidence-based practice in health communication through its Office of Disease Prevention and Health Promotion (ODPHP)[j] and its primary public-facing agencies: the National Cancer Institute (NCI)[k] of the National Institutes of Health (NIH), the CDC, and the Agency for Health Research Quality (AHRQ).[l] In addition to ODPHP and CDC, the Office of the National Coordinator (ONC) for health

---

BOX 1-6 National Public Health Information Coalition

Kristine A. Smith, MA, CCPH
Credentialing Program Manager, National Public Health Information Coalition

Job Analysis: Professional Health Communicator

The National Public Health Information Coalition (NPHIC) is a CDC-affiliate organization whose members represent a variety of public health communication specialties, including public information and public affairs, risk communication, health promotion and marketing, community relations, social media, and communications research and evaluation. As part of its Certified Communicator in Public Health (CCPH) credentialing program, NPHIC has developed a job analysis delineating five core competencies and seven related skill sets that are necessary to effectively shape, spread or understand the impact of a public health message.

The CCPH core competencies are:

1. *Communicate with a range of stakeholders and populations by using resources, techniques, and technologies* (messages, messengers, and means). Inherent in this competency is how well an individual can communicate health messages to both internal and external publics while making clear distinctions among stakeholders, partners, and audiences.
2. *Apply interpersonal skills in communication with public health colleagues, partners, and the public.* This competency advances the idea that small-group communication is often an appropriate and effective public health communication channel and that successful communication requires persuasion skills.
3. *Influence individuals and communities by using media, community resources and social marketing techniques.* This competency supports a multichannel, multivehicle approach to public health communication that calls for use of traditional and new media along with community relations and adaptation of the "Five Ps" principle (product, price, place, people, promotion) of social marketing to allow audiences to receive, understand, and act upon a health message.
4. *Provide communication advice to public health leadership* recognizes that health communicators can play an important role in advancing public health policy if given a "seat at the table" among decision makers. While many health communicators may not have this opportunity, it is important to be able to foment and present a strong argument for strategies and tactics that the communicator believes will be essential to the overall efficacy of a health message, campaign, or policy initiative.
5. *Demonstrate proficiency in written communication.* At whatever audience level, the ability to choose the right words, employ economy of language, and use correct punctuation, grammar, and appropriate writing style is essential. Shortcomings in this area will quickly confuse or derail your message.

In addition to having these core competencies, candidates hoping to earn the CCPH credential must be expert in two skill set areas, and have a working knowledge of the others. There are seven skill sets: media relations, social media, health marketing, cross-cultural communication, risk communication, communications research and evaluation, and integrated skills, which encompass knowledge of CDC initiatives such as *Healthy People* goals and Winnable Battles and public health law and ethics issues, among others.

Courtesy of Smith KA, Credentialing Program Manager, NPHIC.

---

j. http://www.health.gov/communication/
k. http://cancercontrol.cancer.gov/brp/hcirb/index.html
l. http://www.ahrq.gov/cpi/centers/ockt/index.html

information technology (HIT)[m] leads the working group responsible for setting goals and objectives in health communication and health IT. Other agencies within HHS, such as the Food and Drug Administration (FDA),[n] the National Institute for Environmental Health (at NIH),[o] and the Substance Abuse and Mental Health Services Administration (SAMHSA),[p] as well as the U.S. Department of Agriculture (USDA)[q] have contributed much to the health communication evidence base and continue to fund positions, research, and consumer-focused programs.

The National Academy of Sciences Institute of Medicine (NAS/IOM) has been recently reorganized as the National Academies of Science, Engineering, and Medicine: National Academy of Medicine.[r] A nongovernmental entity dependent on donor support, the NAM (previously IOM) has supported numerous workshops and efforts to develop consensus reports that have helped define or shape health communication, health literacy, and related areas.

The U.S. Agency for International Development (USAID),[s] which falls under the State Department, is a global leader in using social marketing and health communication in countries where infectious disease, lack of safe and effective birth control, low educational levels, and extreme poverty contribute significantly to poor population health. USAID funds numerous health communication projects that are executed by consortia of university partners and contracted agencies that may be branches of commercial advertising and marketing companies, or not-for-profit agencies, or nonprofit entities, such as CARE,[t] Heifer International,[u] Save the Children,[v] and World Vision,[w] to mention

only a few. USAID collaborates closely with the World Health Organization (WHO),[x] UNICEF,[y] the World Bank,[z] and bilateral partners (e.g., the Canadian International Development Association,[aa] the United Kingdom's Department for International Development).[ab] All of these organizations and others have contributed extensively to what we know about health communication interventions outside of the United States.

In the healthcare communication arena, the European Association for Communication in Healthcare (EACH)[ac] and its U.S. counterpart, the American Academy for Communication in Healthcare (AACH),[ad] have been setting a research and training agenda for the past several years in patient–provider communication. And the newly formed Society for Health Communication[ae] will soon bring members belonging to the health communication sub-chapters of APHA (Public Health Education and Promotion[af]), the National Communication Association (NCA), the International Communication Association (ICA),[ag] the Society for Public Health Education (SOPHE), and anyone else wishing to join, into one virtual community to share resources, promote the field, and develop competency guidelines.

▶ Conclusion: The Scope of Health Communication

Although health communicators tend to think otherwise, most Americans do not walk around thinking about health, much less "health behavior." While we sometimes say that the number of tobacco-related

---

m. http://www.healthit.gov/newsroom/about-onc

n. http://www.fda.gov/aboutfda/centersoffices/officeofmedicalproductsandtobacco/cdrh/ucm115786.htm

o. http://www.niehs.nih.gov/health/index.cfm

p. http://www.samhsa.gov/health-information-technology/samhsas-efforts

q. http://www.usda.gov/wps/portal/usda/usdahome

r. http://nam.edu/

s. http://www.usaid.gov/

t. http://www.care.org/work

u. http://www.heifer.org/ending-hunger/our-impact/index.html#sharing-knowledge

v. http://www.savethechildren.org/site/c.8rKLIXMGIpI4E/b.6146357/k.2755/What_We_Do.htm

w. http://www.worldvision.org/our-impact/health

x. http://www.who.int/about/agenda/en/

y. http://www.unicef.org/cbsc/

z. World Bank, Capacity Development Resource Center: http://web.worldbank.org/WBSITE/EXTERNAL/TOPICS/EXTCDRC/0,,menuPK:64169181~pagePK:64169192~piPK:64169180~theSitePK:489952,00.html

aa. http://www.international.gc.ca/international/index.aspx?lang=eng#

ab. https://www.gov.uk/government/organisations/department-for-international-development/about

ac. http://www.each.eu/tag/health-communication/

ad. http://www.aachonline.org/dnn/default.aspx

ae. http://www.SocietyForHealthCommunication.org

af. http://www.apha.org/apha-communities/member-sections/public-health-education-and-health-promotion

ag. http://www.icahdq.org/

deaths on a daily basis is like two jumbo jets colliding, it is only when a plane actually crashes that anyone pays attention. Thus, part of the challenge of health communication is getting audience members to notice that we are speaking to them. There are so many media outlets, and so many messages, that health communicators need to use precise tools to "cut through the clutter." This same lesson applies to individuals and decisions makers who are setting policy.

Beyond indifference, health communicators need to contend with outright rejection or dismissal of the information that they are providing. It sometimes takes a measles outbreak at a California theme park to remind Americans that their unvaccinated children do not have "herd immunity" and can get communicable diseases. Indeed, polio, which had once been nearly eliminated from the planet, has resurged in Nigeria, Pakistan, and Afghanistan due to political upheaval preventing mass immunization of the populations in those countries. Our challenge is to maintain the public's trust in evidence-based information and dispel myths or conspiracy theories. We need to remember that the arrival of even one patient with Ebola to a U.S. hospital can lead to panic. Being able to communicate effectively with the public in real or potential crises or emergencies requires special skills and techniques.

Finally, well-honed skills are required to communicate effectively with an individual who wants information to deal with a personal health issue. Providers can use empathy and other interpersonal communication skills to strengthen the impact of their persuasion and adherence messages. Helping patients understand decision-making tools or instructions also requires familiarity with best practices and guidelines in health literacy and related areas.

We recognize five key health communication areas that must be addressed by professionals working in this realm:

- Communicating to inform the public and create trust in evidence
- Communicating to motivate and encourage individuals to change behavior
- Communicating with decision makers to affect policy
- Communicating about precautions and risk during emergencies
- Communicating with individuals in healthcare settings

Other key topics related to health communication include evaluation, cancer communication, and examples from international settings.

Wrap-Up

Chapter Questions

1. Using the transactional model of communication, describe the process of message exchange among communicators.
2. What is the goal of communication, and which factors affect the responses we seek?
3. How have new developments in technology influenced the HP 2010 and HP 2020 priorities and objectives in health communication and health information technology?
4. What are the implications of failing to consider the ecological model when shaping the interventions that health communicators consider and choose?
5. How can focusing health communication, policy, and advocacy efforts on individual behaviors influence the health of populations?
6. Given that health communication is an exceedingly interdisciplinary field, what is the importance of having competencies and credentialing for professional health communicators?

References

1. Barnlund DC. A transactional model of communication. In: Akin J, Goldberg A, Myers G, Stewart J, eds. *Language Behavior: A Book of Readings in Communication*. The Hague, Mouton. 1970:49. http://www.degruyter.com/downloadpdf/books/9783110878752/9783110878752.fm/9783110878752.fm.xml#page=45. Accessed September 10, 2016.

2. Fielding JE, Teutsch S, Breslow L. A framework for public health in the United States. *Public Health Rev* 2010;32:174-189.
3. Stewart ST, Cutler DM. *The Contribution of Behavior Change and Public Health to Improved U.S. Population Health*. NBER Working Paper No. 20631. October 2014.
4. Moore LV, Thompson FE. Adults meeting fruit and vegetable intake recommendations — United States, 2013. *MMWR*. July 10, 2015;64(26);709-713.

5. Institute of Medicine. Communicating to advance the public's health: workshop summary. March 17, 2015. http://iom.nationalacademies.org/Reports/2015/Communicate-to-Advance-Publics-Health.aspx.

6. Lavidge RL, Steiner GA. A model for predictive measurements of advertising effectiveness. *J Marketing*. 1961;25:59-62.

7. McGuire WJ. Public communication as a strategy for inducing health promoting behavioural change. *Prev Med*. 1984;13:299-319.

8. Court D, Elzinga D, Mulder S, Vetvik OJ. The consumer decision journey. *McKinsey Qtly*. June 2009. http://www.mckinsey.com/insights/marketing_sales/the_consumer_decision_journey.

9. Edelman DC. Branding in the digital age: you're spending your money in all the wrong places. *Harvard Bus Rev*. December 1, 2010. https://hbr.org/2010/12/branding-in-the-digital-age-youre-spending-your-money-in-all-the-wrong-places. Accessed July 19, 2015

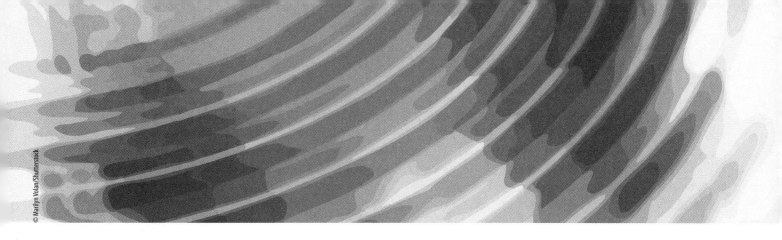

CHAPTER 2

Population Health: A Primer

Patrick L. Remington, MD, MPH

LEARNING OBJECTIVES

By the end of this chapter, the reader will be able to:

- Describe how the leading causes of death in the United States have changed over the past century and discuss the corresponding changes in focus on prevention and control of disease.
- Describe what is meant by health outcomes, determinants, and indicators for chronic disease at the community and population levels.
- Explain how a county-level health ranking is created.
- Identify sources of information on population health outcomes and determinants.
- Describe challenges in communicating about chronic disease.
- Identify difficulties and recommendations for communicating about vaccines and emerging infectious diseases.

▶ Introduction

This chapter provides common ground for health communicators in the science of population health. There are challenges inherent in communicating about chronic and infectious diseases today, given our history, our societal and cultural trends, and the evolution of microbes.

▶ Evolution of the Leading Causes of Death

Over the past century in the United States, advances in public health and health care have led to dramatic changes in the **leading causes of death** and have increased **life expectancy** by an average of 30 years. A white man born in 1900 could have expected to live another 47 years, compared to 75 years in the year 2000. A black woman born in 1900 had a life expectancy of 34 years in 1900, compared to 75 years in 2000; a white woman born in 2000 has a life expectancy of 80 years.[1-3]

Racial and other discrepancies persist and are the subject of much of the discussion in this chapter. Nonetheless, all of us can expect much longer lives than our great grandparents could anticipate. Students of demography know life expectancy calculations rely heavily on surviving our first year of life. In 1900, as many as 30% of infants in some U.S. cities died before reaching their first birthday. Today, fewer than 6 infants per 1000 born alive in the United States die before reaching their first birthday.[4] Most scientists attribute this gain to advances in public health, especially the control of certain infectious diseases.[5] The appendix to this chapter discusses several global infectious disease communication challenges that remain.

What accounts for these large trends in infant or adult death rates? Our understanding evolved over the course of the 20th century. In particular, our views about the factors that affect the public's health can be organized into four distinct historical eras: the era of environmental factors, the era of health care, the era of health behavior, and the era of social and economic factors.

The Era of Environmental Disease (Circa 1900)

In the early 1900s in the United States, the leading causes of disease and death were primarily associated with the unhealthy environments in which people lived. In 1900, pneumonia, influenza, tuberculosis, diarrhea, enteritis, and ulceration of the intestines were the leading causes of death, accounting for nearly one-third of all deaths.[6] These health problems resulted from poor sanitation (e.g., typhoid), an unhealthy food supply (e.g., pellagra and goiter), poor prenatal and infant care, and unsafe workplaces or hazardous occupations.[7]

In response to these health problems, the federal government, state governments, and local departments of public health developed laws and regulations intended to improve public health in the United States. Occupational safety laws, restaurant and food establishment laws, fluoridation and other drinking water laws, and motor vehicle safety laws and regulations emerged as a result.[7,8] These government policies led to dramatic reductions in communicable diseases and maternal and child mortality. As a result, Americans began to live longer and chronic diseases took over as the primary causes of death and disability.

The Era of Expanding Health Care (Circa 1950)

By the middle of the 20th century, heart disease and cancer had become the leading causes of death in the United States. In response, the focus of interventions began to shift from public health approaches to increasing healthcare services, including the delivery of **clinical preventive services** such as the detection and treatment of high blood pressure, vaccines for childhood disease, and improved maternal and prenatal care.

Despite this focus on preventive services, most of the attention of the healthcare system focused on the treatment of diseases. As Evans commented, "[B]y midcentury the providers of health care had gained an extraordinary institutional and even more intellectual dominance, defining both what counted as health and how it was to be pursued."[9] By the early 1970s, the United States had developed extensive and expensive systems of health care, underpinned by health insurance systems that covered most—but not all—children and adults.[9]

The Era of Lifestyle and Health Risk Behaviors (Circa 1970)

As heart disease, cancer, stroke, and lung disease became the leading causes of death during the mid-1900s, public health researchers began to focus on identifying their causes. Large-scale studies such as the Framingham Heart Study, the Seven Countries study, and the British Doctors study began to identify the leading causes of chronic diseases. In turn, researchers began to elucidate the important contributions of cigarette smoking, diet, physical inactivity, and high blood pressure to the leading causes of death.

In 1974, the Canadian government published the *Lalonde Report*, which was recognized as the first modern government report to question the direct link between health care and the public's health.[10] It proposed a new framework suggesting that health be considered along four broad dimensions: human biology, environment, lifestyle, and healthcare organization. In addition, the report emphasized the role of individuals in changing their behaviors to improve their health.[11]

In 1993, the publication of the now-acclaimed paper entitled "Actual Causes of Death" by McGinnis and Foege[12] drew attention to the fact that many deaths were due to preventable causes. Later updated (by Mokdad and colleagues at the Centers for Disease Control and Prevention [CDC][13]), these studies concluded that approximately half of all deaths that occurred in 1990 and 2000 could be attributed to a limited number of preventable factors (**FIGURE 2-1**). Among the highest listed preventable causes of death in order of prevalence are tobacco, poor diet and physical inactivity, and alcohol consumption. These findings, along with escalating healthcare costs and an aging population, argued for the urgent need to establish a more preventive orientation in the U.S. healthcare and public health systems.

Expert opinion at the time suggested that lifestyle factors had the largest and most unambiguously measurable effects on health.[9-15] Behaviors related to diet, exercise, and substance abuse were also factors most readily portrayed as under the control of individuals. The Health Belief Model (HBM, developed by Irwin Rosenstock and colleagues in the Behavioral Sciences Section of the U.S. Public Health Service in

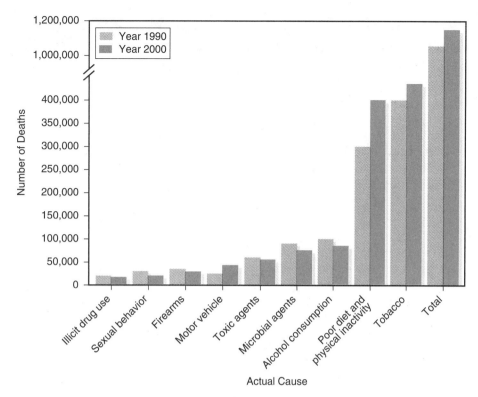

FIGURE 2-1 Actual causes of death in the United States, 1990 and 2000.
Data from Mokdad AH, Marks JS, Stroup DF, Gerberding JL. Actual Causes of Death in the United States, 2000. JAMA. 2004;291(10):1238–1245.

the 1950s) and other psychologically-based models that focused on perceptions of vulnerability, knowledge of an effective course of action, and a sense of behavioral control, became the foundation of public health education. In 1960, Rosenstock briefly suggested that perhaps the pendulum had swung too far toward a belief that health behaviors were the major determinant of health[16] but continued to be a proponent of HBM and went on to found and chair the first Department of Health Behavior and Health Education at the University of Michigan from 1975–1983.

With the recognition that personal behaviors contributed to health, regular collection of such data emerged as a major surveillance and research achievement. In 1984, for example, CDC implemented the first state-wide telephone-based surveillance system for health behaviors.[17] This system, known as the Behavioral Risk Factor Surveillance System (BRFSS),[a] monitors health risk behaviors at the population level and collects information on health risk behaviors, preventive health practices, and healthcare access primarily related to chronic disease and injury. The BRFSS completes more than 400,000 adult interviews each year (more than 506,000 in 2014), making this surveillance system the largest telephone health survey in the world.

The Era of Social Determinants (Circa 2000)

By the beginning of the 21st century, public health research focused farther "upstream"—on factors that increase not only the risk of diseases, but also their environmental and societal causes. Both the public and policy makers had grasped how the physical environment, medical care, and personal health behaviors could have widespread and indiscriminate effects on health. If you smoked cigarettes or lived in an area with a high air pollution level, whether rich or poor, you could succumb to the effects of these unhealthy contaminants. However, public health leaders were about to suggest a more subtle link between access, affordability, and health.

Sir Michael Marmot performed some of the early studies—the so-called Whitehall Studies—showing the link between socially defined categories of "class" and health in Great Britain. The Whitehall Studies, which are some of the longest epidemiological studies of social and economic factors affecting health in the world, are still ongoing.[b] **BOX 2-1** discusses a major finding from one of Marmot's early studies.

The first officially stated U.S. government goals to reduce racial, ethnic, and gender-based health disparities appeared in *Healthy People 2010*. Armed with data, CDC Director Dr. David Satcher fought the prevailing political winds to move the United States

a. http://www.cdc.gov/brfss/
b. https://www.ucl.ac.uk/whitehallII

BOX 2-1 Marmot's Studies of Social Class and Health

One of the most important social epidemiologists of our generation is Sir Michael Marmot, whose studies of British civil servants clearly illustrate the health impact of social class.

The four job categories in **FIGURE 2-2** reflect different education and income profiles among British civil servants. In the figure, we see increased mortality at each occupational level (the social gradient). Taking known modifiable risk factors into account (i.e., statistically controlling for them) explains some, but not all, of this increased risk. The amount of mortality not explained by these risk factors, in a British system where all people have access to medical care, is quite remarkable.

This example highlights individuals' occupational category as a marker of social class and socioeconomic status. Such relationships have also been shown for income, education, and other components of the social determinants of health.

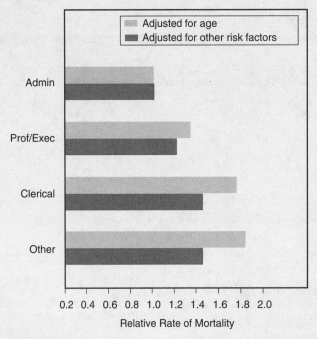

FIGURE 2-2 Whitehall study.

Data from Sreenivasan G. Justice, Inequality, and Health. IN: The Stanford Encyclopedia of Philosophy (Fall 2014 Edition). Edward N. Zalta (ed.). Available at: http://plato.stanford.edu/archives/fall2014/entries/justice-inequality-health/. Assessed July 12, 2015.

in this direction (**BOX 2-2**). For example, one study estimated that eight times more lives would be saved by correcting educational disparities than by medical advances over the same period.[18] Another study estimated a 1% to 3% reduction in mortality rates would occur for each year of additional schooling.[19] **FIGURE 2-3** illustrates the dramatic association of educational attainment with mortality rates for men and women.

In the past 15 years, the role of "social determinants" of health—such as income, education, occupation, and social cohesion—has been more widely acknowledged among public health and healthcare professionals. We have entered the era of making policy based on data derived from leading health indicators.

▶ Leading Health Indicators Approach

Healthy People 2020

Healthy People 2020[c] (HP 2020) provides a comprehensive set of 10-year national goals and objectives for improving the health of all Americans. This initiative tracks the nation's health through more than 1200 objectives organized in 42 distinct public health topic areas. Most objectives provide opportunities for public health professionals to set goals and track progress. At the same time, the size and scope of these health objectives create a challenge for health communicators.

c. http://www.healthypeople.gov.

BOX 2-2 David Satcher and the Health Determinants Approach

According to David Satcher,[1] former CDC Director and U.S. Surgeon General from 1998 to 2002:

> Reducing health disparities, primarily those based on race/ethnicity and gender, has long been a public health priority in the United States. … Recent developments led by the World Health Organization (WHO), however, have accelerated the thinking about the causes of health inequities—i.e., disparities that are systematic, avoidable, and unjust[2]—and how best to address their reduction.[3,4] The WHO Commission on Social Determinants of Health concluded in 2008 that the social conditions in which people are born, live, and work are the single most important determinant of one's health status.[3] Certainly, individual choices are important, but factors in the social environment are what determine access to health services and influence lifestyle choices in the first place. Social determinants are defined by WHO as follows: "… the circumstances in which people are born, grow up, live, work and age, and the systems put in place to deal with illness. These circumstances are in turn shaped by a wider set of forces: economics, social policies, and politics."[5]

References

1. Satcher D. Include a social determinants of health approach to reduce health inequities. *Public Health Rep.* 2010;125(suppl 4):6–7.
2. Braveman P, Gruskin S. Defining equity in health. *J Epidemiol Community Health* 2003;57:254–258.
3. World Health Organization. Closing the gap in a generation: health equity through action on the social determinants of health. *Report from the Commission on Social Determinants of Health.* Geneva: WHO; 2008. http://www.who.int/social_determinants/thecommission/finalreport/en.
4. World Health Organization. World Health Assembly closes with resolutions on public health. 22 May 2009. http://www.who.int/mediacentre/news/releases/2009/world_health_assembly_20090522/en/index.html.
5. World Health Organization. Social determinants of health: key concepts [cited January 18, 2010]. http://www.who.int/social_determinants/thecommission/finalreport/key_concepts/en.

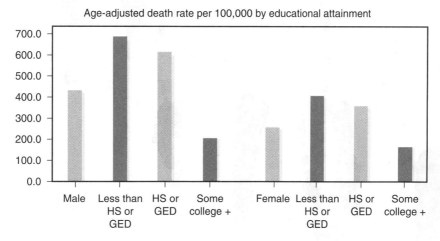

Age-adjusted death rate per 100,000 by educational attainment

FIGURE 2-3 Death rate by educational attainment and sex.
From National Vital Statistics Reports, Vol. 60, No. 3, December 29, 2011. Table 1–8.

The Leading Health Indicators represent a subset of 26 high-priority health issues related to 12 topic areas. The *Healthy People 2020* Federal Interagency Workgroup led the process of selecting the Leading Health Indicators, which are summarized in **TABLE 2-1**.

The federal Office of Health Promotion and Disease Prevention monitors progress for each of the Leading Health Indicators. At last review (2014), it found these results:

- Four leading health indicators (15.4%) met or exceeded targets.
- Ten leading health indicators (38.5%) were improving.
- Eight leading health indicators (30.8%) showed little or no detectable change.

TABLE 2-1 Leading 2020 Health Indicators in the United States

Category	Example	Baseline Value (Year)	Current Value (Year)	Goal
Access to health services	Adults younger than 65 years with medical insurance (percent)	83.2% (2008)	83.1% (2012)	100%
Clinical preventive services	Children aged 19–35 months receiving recommended doses of DTaP, polio, MMR, Hib, hepatitis B, varicella and PCV vaccines (percent)	44% (2009)	68.5% (2011)	80%
Environmental quality	Children aged 3–11 years exposed to secondhand smoke (percent)	52.2% (2005–2008)	41.3% (2009–2011)	47.0%
Injury and violence	Injury deaths (age-adjusted rate per 100,000 population)	59.7 (2007)	57.1 (2010)	53.7
Maternal, infant, and child health	Infant deaths prior to 12 months of age (rate per 1000 live births)	6.7 (2006)	6.1 (2010)	6.0
Mental health	Suicide (age-adjusted rate per 100,000 population)	11.3 (2007)	12.1 (2010)	10.2
Nutrition, physical activity, and obesity	Obesity among adults aged 20 years or older (age-adjusted percent over a 2-year period)	33.9% (2005–2008)	35.3% (2009–2012)	30.5%
Oral health	Persons who visited the dentist in the past year (age-adjusted percent over a 2-year period)	44.5% (2007)	41.8% (2011)	49.0%
Reproductive and sexual health	Knowledge of serostatus among HIV-positive persons aged 13 years or older (percent)	80.9% (2006)	84.2% (2010)	90.0%
Social determinants	Students awarded a high school diploma 4 years after starting ninth grade (percent)	74.9% (2007–2008)	78.2% (2009–2010)	82.4%
Substance abuse	Binge drinking in past 30 days among adults aged 18 years or older (percent)	27.1% (2008)	27.1% (2008)	24.4%
Tobacco	Cigarette smoking among persons aged 18 years or older (age-adjusted percent)	20.6% (2008)	18.2% (2012)	12.0%

U.S. Dept. of Health and Human Services. Healthy People 2020 Leading Health Indicators: Progress Update. http://www.healthypeople.gov/sites/default/files/LHI-progressreport-execsum_0.pdf. Published March 2014.

- Three leading health indicators (11.5%) were getting worse.
- One leading health indicator (3.8%) had only baseline data.

Health Disparities

Over the past three decades, the U.S. government has increased the emphasis on health disparities in the national health goals. In HP 2000, the goal was to *reduce* health disparities among Americans, but HP 2010 seeks to *eliminate* health disparities. The goal in HP 2020 calls on us to *achieve health equity, eliminate disparities, and improve the health of all groups*. To keep on track, HP 2020 reports rates of illness, death, chronic conditions, behaviors, and other types of outcomes in relation to demographic factors that have historically been associated with unequal access and/or illness rates. For example, according to the *Healthy People 2020* data:

- Approximately one-third of the U.S. population identifies themselves as belonging to a racial or ethnic minority population.
- Approximately 12% of the U.S. population not living in nursing homes or other residential care facilities has a disability.
- An estimated 23% of the population lives in rural areas.
- An estimated 4% of the U.S. population aged 18 to 44 years identifies themselves as lesbian, gay, bisexual, or transgender.

In addition, the CDC provides extensive and detailed information about health disparities through reports such as the *CDC Health Disparities and Inequalities Report—United States, 2013.*[d]

Although a vast amount of information about health disparities is available, it is often buried in reports that are read only by public health professionals. Health communicators play a vital role in translating the data into information for the public.

▶ Health Rankings

The idea of ranking states or counties within states using a summary score is based on how the public tends to think about statistics (e.g., sports team rankings). Such scores enable officials to deliver clear communication messages such as "Our state ranks dead last in the national health ranking" or "Our county is the healthiest place to raise children." In 1988, the CDC's *Morbidity and Mortality Weekly Report* (*MMWR*) ranked state-specific death rates from heart disease.[20] This report led to an Associated Press headline that stated, "Midwest, Northeast City Life Hard on Hearts."[21] Subsequent media attention led to heated calls to the CDC from outraged health officials and legislators from the states with the highest death rates, insisting that the CDC refrain from publishing rankings in the *MMWR*.[20]

Since 1990, *America's Health Rankings*[e] has reported on the health of the 50 U.S. states, including measures of health outcomes, health determinants, and programs and policies. This annual report has generated significant interest among the media and among policy makers over the past two decades. Building on this approach, the University of Wisconsin's Population Health Institute measured and ranked the health of its home state's 72 counties. This program led to development of a logic model (**FIGURE 2-4**) positing that health rankings would lead to media attention, engage local community leaders, support the development of evidence-based policies and programs, and eventually improve the health of the community.

An analysis of media coverage from 2004 to 2008 showed that the number of rankings-related stories increased from 23 in 2006 to 47 in 2008.[22] In addition, several news stories made use of accompanying photographs to highlight the determinants of health (e.g., people running and bicycling on paths or exercising in a school exercise facility).

Each year since 2010, the University of Wisconsin's Population Health Institute and the Robert Wood Johnson Foundation have produced the *County Health Rankings*,[f] a "population health checkup" for the United States' more than 3000 counties.[20] The population health of each county is ranked within each state—from the healthiest to the least healthy—using a model that summarizes the overall health outcomes of each county, as well as the factors that contribute to health. Data for each component of the *Rankings* model are selected from a number of national data sources, including the National Center for Health Statistics, BRFSS, and the American Community Survey, among others.

d. http://www.cdc.gov/minorityhealth/CHDIReport.html
e. http://www.americashealthrankings.org/about/annual
f. http://www.countyhealthrankings.org

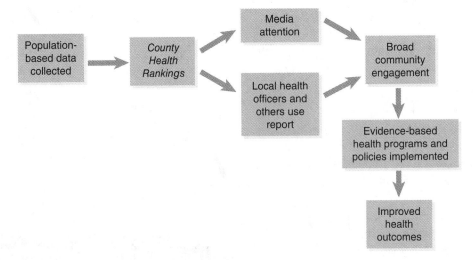

FIGURE 2-4 Logic model for the *County Health Rankings*.

FIGURE 2-5 shows a map of the top five and bottom five counties within each state based on their within-state health outcome ranks. In some states, the healthiest and unhealthiest counties lie far from each other; in other states, the healthiest and unhealthiest counties are adjacent. The five least-healthy counties in each state have premature death rates that are more than twice the rates of the five healthiest counties. These counties with poorer health outcomes also have the highest rates of smoking, teen births, physical inactivity, preventable hospital stays, and children living in poverty.[20]

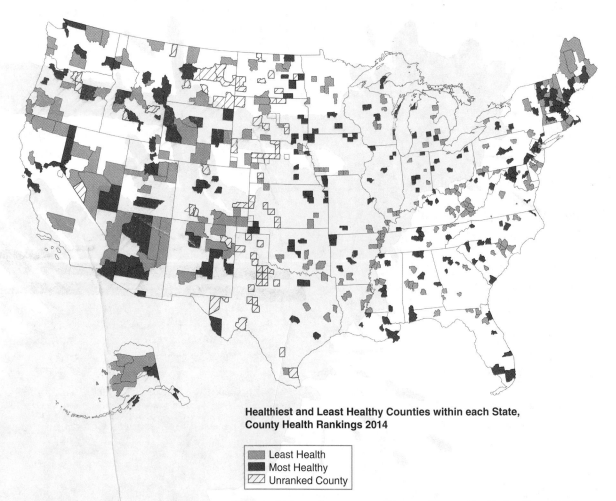

Healthiest and Least Healthy Counties within each State, County Health Rankings 2014

Least Health
Most Healthy
Unranked County

FIGURE 2-5 Healthiest and least healthy counties within each state according to *Country Health Rankings*, 2014.

The *County Health Rankings* have been successful in increasing community dialogue about the factors that make a community healthy for several reasons. First, the model is clear and easy to understand by both the media and the public. The use of summary measures of the health outcomes and health factors translates complex data into a form that policy makers and the public can easily use. It encourages users to "see the forest rather than the trees"—that is, not to place undue emphasis on individual performance measures. In addition, this model demonstrates that multiple factors determine health, ranging from individual health behaviors to the quality of the healthcare and educational systems to the influences of the built environment. This broad definition of health serves as a call to action to create policies and programs that can be linked to improvements or worsening in health outcomes over time.

▶ Gathering Data to Communicate About Population Health

Sources of Information

Numerous sources of information align with the population health model described previously, including health outcomes, health determinants, and evidence-based programs and policies.

Health Outcomes Data

Information about health outcomes (e.g., death and disease) comes from a variety of sources, including vital statistics, healthcare systems, and population-based surveys. Some of the most fundamental information about the health of a community comes from birth and death certificates. These certificates are completed by a physician or medical examiner and reported to the county and state health departments, and ultimately to the CDC's National Center for Health Statistics, where they are made available to public health practitioners and researchers throughout the United States. The CDC provides access to cleaned data sets through CDC Wonder[g] or through finished analytical reports at the National Vital Statistics website.[h]

Disease incidence and prevalence data may be obtained from a number of sources. Cancer incidence data for a sample of residents of the United States have been available since 1974 through the Surveillance, Epidemiology and End Results (SEER) Program at the National Cancer Institute (NCI) and more recently from most state health departments. In addition, administrative data from hospitals and other healthcare providers may provide information about their rates of care for diseases. In addition, data on birth outcomes (e.g., birth weights, prematurity rates) are reported by hospitals to state health departments.

Some information on overall health-related quality of life (**HRQoL**) is collected at the state level and reported to the CDC as part of the BRFSS. Other local initiatives to assess HRQoL tend to be disease specific and are driven by healthcare providers and health services researchers interested in health outcomes that result from particular healthcare treatments. Although these quality of life initiatives generally employ quite detailed self-reported assessments of patient conditions, most have been developed relatively independently.

As an example of health outcomes data, **FIGURE 2-6** shows the leading causes of death overall and for each age group, highlighting those deaths due to injuries. For persons of all ages, four chronic diseases account for 60% of all deaths: heart disease, cancer, stroke, and lung disease. Cancer is the leading cause of death among persons ages 45 to 64, and Alzheimer's disease is now one of the leading causes of death among persons older than age 65. Although unintentional injuries are the fourth-leading cause of death overall, they are the leading cause of death for persons younger than age 45. While some disease rates are increasing, heart disease rates are declining. These rates vary considerably by race, gender, and geographic area.

Health Determinants Data

Health Behaviors CDC's National Health Interview Survey (NHIS) and National Health and Nutrition Examination Survey (NHANES) are primary sources for national data on adult behaviors; at the state and local levels, CDC's BRFSS is the primary source of such data. As noted earlier, BRFSS data are collected monthly in all 50 states, as well as in the District of Columbia, Puerto Rico, the Virgin Islands, and Guam. The questionnaire used in these telephone surveys consists of a fixed core (questions asked every year), rotating core (questions asked every other year), optional modules (standardized sets of questions on specific topics), emerging core (questions for newly arising topics), and state-added modules (questions relevant to the individual state). Items in the BRFSS address smoking, alcohol use, diet, exercise, and other health-related behaviors, such as use of clinical preventive services.

g. http://wonder.cdc.gov
h. http://www.cdc.gov/nchs/nvss.htm

Age Groups

Rank	<1	1–4	5–9	10–14	15–24	25–34	35–44	45–54	55–64	65+	Total
1	Congenital Anomalies 4,758	Unintentional Injury 1,316	Unintentional Injury 746	Unintentional Injury 775	Unintentional Injury 11,619	Unintentional Injury 16,209	Unintentional Injury 15,354	Malignant Neoplasms 46,185	Malignant Neoplasms 113,324	Heart Disease 488,156	Heart Disease 611,105
2	Short Gestation 4,202	Congenital Anomalies 476	Malignant Neoplasms 447	Malignant Neoplasms 448	Suicide 4,878	Suicide 6,348	Malignant Neoplasms 11,349	Heart Disease 35,167	Heart Disease 72,568	Malignant Neoplasms 407,558	Malignant Neoplasms 584,881
3	Maternal Pregnancy Comp. 1,595	Homicide 337	Congenital Anomalies 179	Suicide 386	Homicide 4,329	Homicide 4,236	Heart Disease 10,341	Unintentional Injury 20,357	Unintentional Injury 17,057	Chronic Low. Respiratory Disease 127,194	Chronic Low. Respiratory Disease 149,205
4	SIDS 1,563	Malignant Neoplasms 328	Homicide 125	Congenital Anomalies 161	Malignant Neoplasms 1,496	Malignant Neoplasms 3,673	Suicide 6,551	Liver Disease 8,785	Chronic Low. Respiratory Disease 15,942	Cerebro-vascular 109,602	Unintentional Injury 130,557
5	Unintentional Injury 1,156	Heart Disease 169	Chronic Low. Respiratory Disease 75	Homicide 152	Heart Disease 941	Heart Disease 3,258	Homicide 2,581	Suicide 8,621	Diabetes Mellitus 13,061	Alzheimer's Disease 83,786	Cerebro-vascular 128,978
6	Placenta Cord. Membrane 953	Influenza & Pneumonia 102	Heart Disease 73	Heart Disease 100	Congenital Anomalies 362	Diabetes Mellitus 684	Liver Disease 2,491	Diabetes Mellitus 5,899	Liver Disease 11,951	Diabetes Mellitus 53,751	Alzheimer's Disease 84,767
7	Bacterial Sepsis 578	Chronic Low. Respiratory Disease 64	Influenza & Pneumonia 67	Chronic Low. Respiratory Disease 80	Influenza & Pneumonia 197	Liver Disease 676	Diabetes Mellitus 1,952	Cerebro-vascular 5,425	Cerebro-vascular 11,364	Influenza & Pneumonia 48,031	Diabetes Mellitus 75,578
8	Respiratory Distress 522	Septicemia 53	Cerebro-vascular 41	Influenza & Pneumonia 61	Diabetes Mellitus 193	HIV 631	Cerebro-vascular 1,687	Chronic Low. Respiratory Disease 4,619	Suicide 7,135	Unintentional Injury 45,942	Influenza & Pneumonia 56,979
9	Circulatory System Diseases 458	Benign Neoplasms 47	Septicemia 35	Cerebro-vascular 48	Complicated Pregnancy 178	Cerebro-vascular 508	HIV 1,246	Septicemia 2,445	Septicemia 5,345	Nephritis 39,080	Nephritis 47,112
10	Neonatal Hemorrhage 389	Perinatal Period 45	Benign Neoplasms 34	Benign Neoplasms 31	Chronic Low. Respiratory Disease 155	Influenza & Pneumonia 449	Influenza & Pneumonia 881	HIV 2,378	Nephritis 4,947	Septicemia 28,815	Suicide 41,149

FIGURE 2-6 Leading causes of death by age group, United States, 2013.

Data from National Vital Statistics System, National Center for Health Statistics, CDC. Produced by: National Center for Injury Prevention and Control, CDC using WISQARS™.

Health Care Ideally, comprehensive data on healthcare access, utilization, quality, and costs would be available at the national, state, and local levels. No single repository of such information exists, however. Data on the extent of public and private healthcare insurance coverage is available at the national and state levels—for example, from the Current Population Survey, which is jointly conducted by the U.S. Census Bureau and Department of Labor. Data on healthcare utilization and costs are collected for nearly every individual healthcare encounter between birth and death in administrative and clinical databases within healthcare practices and institutions. Similarly, numerous administrative and regulatory requirements lead to the accumulation of data about the providers of these healthcare services.

Nevertheless, the extent to which all of these data are aggregated and accessible for evaluating utilization, quality, and costs varies widely across the United States, depending on both mandated and voluntary initiatives. Data on health care provided through government programs, such as Medicare, Medicaid, and the Veterans Administration, tend to be relatively accessible. Recent private-sector efforts, such as those led by the National Committee for Quality Assurance (NCQA), HealthGrades, and the Leapfrog group, are increasing the amount of publicly available data on healthcare quality. Other key data sources include the Dartmouth Atlas on Health Care (based on Medicare data), the Commonwealth Fund, the Kaiser Family Foundation, and numerous national- and state-level databases compiled by the Agency for Healthcare Research and Quality (AHRQ).

Social and Economic Factors Data on social and economic factors are available from a number of sources, such as the decennial Census and the more frequently performed American Community Survey, which now provides inter-Census estimates for counties with a population greater than 20,000. Other sources include education data that states are required to collect as part of the federal No Child Left Behind initiative. District- and school-level statistics regarding graduation rates and student performance in reading and math can be accessed online. As well as being available on a national level from the Bureau of Labor Statistics, unemployment data are generally available at the local and state levels from state governments. Information on both violent and property crime are available through the Federal Bureau of Investigation (which collects data on crime reports and arrests from local law enforcement agencies and compiles these data on an annual basis) and from the Bureau of Justice. Notable sources for social phenomena and access data include the Pew Research Center[i] (which conducts its own polls and analyzes national and more geographically focused trends by social topic), the Robert Wood Johnson Foundation,[j] the Rand Corporation,[k] and HP 2020.

Physical Environment Data on environmental factors are available from a variety of sources, of varying availability and quality, across different potential units of analysis—nation, state, county, city, neighborhood, and so forth. For example, data on public water system violations are available in the U.S. Environmental Protection Agency's (EPA) Safe Drinking Water Information System, but the quality of these data varies by state. Alternatively, data may be obtained directly from municipal water departments that publish annual reports of water quality. Data on air quality and toxic releases are available from the EPA, and food contamination data are collected on a national scale by the Food and Drug Administration (FDA) and the U.S. Department of Agriculture (USDA). Selected measures about the built environment are also available for some geographic units of analysis (e.g., neighborhood "walkability," access to healthy foods in a ZIP code) through spatial analytical centers at many universities.

Comprehensive Population Health Reports

Many sources of information about the health of populations exist at the local, state, and national level. One of the most comprehensive sources of information is published annually by CDC's National Center for Health Statistics, entitled simply "Health, United States."[l] The report for 2015 is the 39th report in this series, and includes a comprehensive compilation of health data from a number of sources within the federal government and in the private sector. In addition, each year the report contains a special section focused on a particular aspect of public health, such as the focus on racial and ethnic health disparities in 2015. The 2015 report also features 123 tables that cover a range of topics, including birth rates and reproductive

---

i. http://www.pewresearch.org
j. http://www.rwjf.org
k. http://www.rand.org
l. http://www.cdc.gov/nchs/hus.htm

health, life expectancy and leading causes of death, health risk behaviors, healthcare utilization and insurance coverage, and health expenditures. Highlights from the 2015 report include the following:

- Between 2004 and 2014, the birth rate among teenagers aged 15-19 fell to a historic low of 24.2 per 1,000 females overall.
- In 2014, 17.0% of non-institutionalized adults aged 18 and older were current cigarette smokers, a decline from the rate of 23.2% in 2000.
- Between 2003 and 2013, the age-adjusted heart disease death rate decreased 28%, from 236.3 to 169.8 deaths per 100,000 population.
- Between 2003 and 2013, the age-adjusted drug poisoning death rate involving opioid analgesics increased from 2.9 to 5.1 deaths per 100,000 population.

Evidence-Based Policies and Programs

William Foege, a former CDC Director, introduced the term "consequential epidemiology"[23] to emphasize that, to be effective, epidemiological research must be effectively translated into public behavior change. Health communication is the leading strategy to this end.

The volume of research published about the effectiveness of individual programs and policies far exceeds the ability of any one person to read, summarize, and synthesize on an ongoing basis. To address this problem, researchers conduct evidence-based **systematic reviews** to consolidate all the information from studies addressing a single clinical or public health question. Systematic reviews use explicit and comprehensive methods to identify, select, and critically assess all relevant research on the issue under consideration. To avoid bias, the reviews use standard protocols for searching for literature and appraising and combining study data. Over the past two decades, systematic reviews have increasingly relied on meta-analysis to calculate effect sizes based on the findings of individual studies. Among the questions answered by systematic reviews are the following:

- Which interventions have and have not worked?
- In which populations and settings has the intervention worked?
- What might the intervention cost? What should the individual expect for his or her investment?
- Does the intervention lead to any other benefits or harms?
- Which interventions need more research before we can know whether they truly work?

Finding information about effective programs and policies is easier today than ever before thanks to the advent of online resources. For example, the Cochrane Collaboration is one of the most respected sources of systematic reviews of healthcare interventions; reports are available on the Cochrane.org website. The PubMed Systematic Review filter is available through the National Library of Medicine. This resource specializes in PubMed searches to retrieve citations identified as systematic reviews, meta-analyses, reviews of clinical trials, evidence-based medicine, consensus development conferences, and guidelines. Additional resources for evidence-based reviews of programs and policies are shown in **TABLE 2-2**.

TABLE 2-2 U.S. Sources of Information About Evidence-Based Policies and Programs	
The Guide to Community Preventive Services http://www.thecommunityguide.org/	Contains comprehensive systematic reviews and recommendations on community-based programs and policies.
The Guide to Clinical Preventive Services http://www.uspreventiveservicestaskforce.org/	Contains comprehensive reviews and recommendations by the U.S. Preventive Services Task Force assessing the merits of clinical preventive measures (e.g., screening tests, counseling, chemopreventive agents).
MMWR Recommendations and Reports http://www.cdc.gov/mmwr/indrr_2015.html	Contain in-depth articles that provide program and policy recommendations for prevention and treatment (e.g., recommendations from the Advisory Committee on Immunization Practices).
The National Guideline Clearinghouse http://www.guideline.gov/	A public resource for evidence-based clinical practice guidelines from many sources. It is an initiative of the Agency for Healthcare Research and Quality, U.S. Department of Health and Human Services, and America's Health Insurance Plans.

Reprinted from U.S. Census Bureau, International Population.

The University of Wisconsin's Population Health Institute developed *What Works for Health*, which is included in the *County Health Rankings and Roadmaps.** First developed for the state of Wisconsin, this resource provides a menu of policies and programs for possible implementation in communities corresponding to each of the health determinants in the *Rankings* model for population health. The evidence supporting each intervention is rated based on the quantity, quality, and findings of relevant research. Ratings range from "scientifically supported" to "some evidence," "expert opinion," "insufficient evidence," "mixed evidence," and finally "evidence of ineffectiveness." In addition to determining the effectiveness of the interventions, the Population Health Institute assesses each intervention's likely effect on racial/ethnic, socioeconomic, geographic, or other disparities based on its characteristics (e.g., target audience, mode of delivery) and the best available evidence related to health disparities; the resulting ratings range from "likely to decrease disparities," to "no impact on disparities likely," to "likely to increase disparities."

*http://www.countyhealthrankings.org/roadmaps/what-works-for-health.

To take one example, the Task Force on Community Preventive Services oversees the Guide to Community Preventive Services. The Guide provides evidence-based reviews and recommendations concerning community prevention interventions, hoping to see greater use of interventions shown to work, less use of interventions shown not to work, and more evaluation research on interventions for which there is inadequate evidence to determine whether they work.[24] **BOX 2-3** provides an example of how this kind of information has been used in Wisconsin.

▶ Communication Challenges

Several challenges arise when sharing information with communities about chiefly chronic illness and its causes. Despite overwhelming evidence about the leading causes of disease, the public still pays the most attention to immediate health risks rather than those that affect population health. The failure to heed warnings about chronic health risks may reflect the reality that messages about the causes of health problems are often complex and difficult to assimilate. In addition,

the health information communication pipelines may become clogged by competing messages from multiple sources (e.g., political figures, news media spokespeople) offering opinions and anecdotes about "causes" and "solutions."

Confronting Public Perceptions About Risk: Perception Versus Reality

When communicating risk information to the public or policy makers, scientists have discovered that the "actual" health risk may have little or no relationship to people's **risk perception**—that is, what people believe about the level of risk. For example, the health risks from some environmental exposures, such as chemical toxins, pesticides, and electromagnetic fields, are often difficult to detect when those exposures occur at low levels. The public or policy makers might mistake undetectable risks for undisclosed risks, however, and greatly magnify their importance. This path can lead to demands for costly interventions that may have little real impact on population health. Conversely, the public may sometimes greatly underestimate a risk and ignore recommendations that could have a substantial impact on their health. Either extreme may arise given that reactions often have a strong emotional component (especially fear and anger) and that some members of the public may distrust institutions, organizations, or scientists.

The role of media in shaping public understanding of risk is substantial. Hans Rosling highlighted the difference between media interest and actual risk of disease during the 2009 swine flu epidemic. During a 13-day period in 2009, the World Health Organization (WHO) confirmed that 25 countries reported cases of swine flu, and 31 persons died from this cause. During the same period, approximately 60,000 persons died from tuberculosis (TB), according to WHO data. By comparing the number of news reports found through a Google news search, Rosling calculated a *news/death ratio* of 8176 news stories for each death from swine flu but only 0.1 news story per death for TB. He issued an alert for "media hype" on swine flu and a neglect of tuberculosis.[m]

We can see a similar pattern with Ebola and lung cancer deaths. During 2014, there were 8235 deaths from Ebola worldwide,[25] including one death in the United States, and extensive media coverage of this outbreak. A Google search for "Ebola" returned more than 6 million news stories—about

540 news stories per death from Ebola. By comparison, there were 1.6 million deaths from lung cancer worldwide in 2012,[26] but a Google search returned only 473,000 news stories on this topic, giving a *news/death ratio* of only 0.3. (For more on communicating about infectious disease, see the appendix to this chapter.)

The Stigma of Chronic Disease: "It's Your Own Darn Fault"

Communicating information about the causes of disease can be challenging and complex. People can relate to personal stories about suffering from—or better yet, coping with—cancer, heart disease, or the premature death of a loved one. In contrast, stories about the "determinants of health" are a hard sell. Phrases such as "social determinants," "risk factors," and "upstream causes" have little salience for the U.S. public, which prizes independence and personal responsibility about all else. The phenomena of "fat shaming," the stigmas associated with sexually transmitted diseases and mental health, and even reactions to the Patient Protection and Affordable Care Act suggest that U.S. citizens are more likely than not to believe that everyone should enjoy the ability to make their own lifestyle choices.

A study by Robert and Booske examined factors that the public thinks are important determinants of health by conducting a national telephone survey of nearly 3000 U.S. adults.[27] Respondents said that health behaviors and access to health care have very strong effects on health, but were less likely to report a very strong role for other social and economic factors. Respondents who recognized a stronger role for social determinants of health and who saw social policy as health policy were more likely to be older, female, non-white, and politically liberal and to have less education, income, and quality of health. The conclusion we can draw from this study is that a public education campaign is necessary to broaden the acceptance of a "determinants of health" approach. Widespread embrace of this perspective is not likely to be accomplished by showing great programming[n] on "public" television alone.

▶ Conclusion

Advances in public health have led to changes in the leading health problems—as well as to changes in our understanding of the contributions made by the various factors that influence health. Health communicators can use population health models when designing communication strategies and focus on three major areas along the continuum: health outcomes and the leading causes of death and disability, multiple determinants of health (behaviors, health care, social and economic factors, and the physical environment), and effective programs and policies. For the most part, persuasive behavior-change communication programs have the greatest impact on individual- and community-level actions to improve health, whereas advocacy efforts have the greatest impact on health policy. Threats such as infectious disease require ongoing vigilance and risk communication strategies. The appendix to this chapter describes some of these challenges.

Wrap-Up

Chapter Questions

1. Why is it important to have a national health behavior surveillance system, such as the Behavioral Risk Factor Surveillance System?
2. Describe one of the most important determinants of population health according to the *County Health Rankings* model.
3. What are the four criteria making up health determinant rankings within and among populations? How does the health of your county compare with other counties in your state? How can we communicate the findings from *Rankings* to the public?
4. Name several of the key data sources of health factors, including those for health behaviors, social factors, and economic health determinants.
5. How are evidence-based strategies for public health interventions derived?
6. Explain how you would update one of the following databases of evidence-based health

n. http://www.pbs.org/unnaturalcauses/about_the_series.htm

research: The Community Guide (CDC) or What Works for Health (*County Health Rankings and Roadmaps*).

7. What should be the overarching goals of *Healthy People 2030*?

8. Why is it so difficult to communicate about vaccines?

9. Explain the role of antimicrobial resistance in newly emerging infectious disease. Which kind of health communication program could address this threat?

References

1. Minino AM, Smith BL. Deaths: preliminary data for 2000. *National Vital Statistics Reports.* Hyattsville, MD: National Center for Health Statistics; 2001:49(12).

2. Murphy SL, Kochanek KD, Xu JQ, Heron M. Deaths: final data for 2012. *National Vital Statistics Reports.* Hyattsville, MD: National Center for Health Statistics; 2015:63(9).

3. Anderson RN, DeTurk PB. United States life tables, 1999. *National Vital Statistics Reports.* Hyattsville, MD: National Center for Health Statistics. 2002:50(6).

4. Centers for Disease Control and Prevention. Achievements in public health, 1900-1999: healthier mothers and babies. *MMWR.* 1999;48(38):849–858.

5. Bunker JP, Frazier HS, Mosteller F. Improving health: measuring effects of medical care. *Milbank Qtly.* 1994;72:225–258.

6. Centers for Disease Control and Prevention. Leading causes of death, 1900-1998. http://www.cdc.gov/nchs/data/dvs/lead1900_98.pdf. Accessed September 24, 2015.

7. Centers for Disease Control and Prevention. Ten great public health achievements—United States, 1900–1999. *MMWR.* 1999;48(12):241–243. http://www.cdc.gov/mmwr/preview/mmwrhtml/mm4850a1.htm. Accessed March 16, 2015.

8. Centers for Disease Control and Prevention. Achievements in public health, 1900–1999: changes in the public health system. *MMWR.* 1999;48(50):1141–1147. http://www.cdc.gov/mmwr/preview/mmwrhtml/mm4850a1.htm. Accessed March 16, 2015.

9. Evans RG, Stoddart GL. Models for population health: consuming research, producing policy? *Am J Public Health.* 2003;93(3):371–379.

10. Lalonde M. *A New Perspective on the Health of Canadians: A Working Document.* Ottawa, Canada: Government of Canada; 1974.

11. Minkler M. Health education, health promotion and the open society: an historical perspective. *Health Educ Q.* 1989;16(1):17–30.

12. McGinnis JM, Foege WH. Actual causes of death in the United States. *JAMA.* 1993;270:2207–2212.

13. Mokdad AH, Marks JS, Stroup DF, Gerberding JL. Actual causes of death in the United States, 2000. *JAMA.* 2004;291(10):1238–1245.

14. Evans RG, Stoddart GL. Producing health, consuming health care. *Soc Sci Med.* 1990;31:1347–1363.

15. Mokdad AH,Bowman BA, Ford ES, Vinicor F, Marks JS, Koplan JP. The continuing epidemics of obesity and diabetes in the US. *JAMA.* 2001;286:1195–1200.

16. Rosenstock IM. What research in motivation suggests for public health. *Am J Public Health.* 1960;50(3): 295–302.

17. Remington PL, Smith MY, Williamson DF, Anda RF, Gentry EM, Hogelin GC. Design, characteristics, and usefulness of state-based risk factor surveillance 1981–1986. *Public Health Rep.* 1988;103(4):366–375.

18. Woolf SH, Johnson RE, Philips Jr. RL, Philipsen M. Giving everyone the health of the educated: an examination of whether social change would save more lives than medical advances. *Am J Public Health.* 2007;97:679–683.

19. Elo I, Preson S. Educational differences in mortality. *Soc Sci Med.* 1996;42:47–57.

20. Remington PL, Catlin BB, Gennuso KP. The *County Health Rankings*: rationale and methods. *Population Health Metrics.* 2015;13(11):1–12.

21. Byrd R. Midwest, Northeast city life hard on hearts. Atlanta, GA: Associated Press; 1988.

22. Rohan AM, Booske BC, Remington PL. Using the Wisconsin *County Health Rankings* to catalyze community health improvement. *J Public Health Man.* 2009; 15(1):24–32.

23. Marks JS. Epidemiology, public health, and public policy. *Prev Chronic Dis.* 2009;6(4). http://www.cdc.gov/pcd/issues/2009/oct/09_0110.htm. Accessed July 12, 2015.

24. Brownson RC, Allen P, Jacob RR, et al. Understanding mis-implementation in public health practice. *Am J Prev Med.* 2015;48(5):543–551.

25. World Health Organization. Ebola situation reports. January 7, 2015. http://www.who.int/csr/disease/ebola/situation-reports/en/?m=20150107. Accessed July 21, 2015.

26. World Health Organization, International Agency for Research on Cancer. GLOBOCAN 2012: estimated cancer incidence, mortality and prevalence worldwide in 2012. http://globocan.iarc.fr/Pages/fact_sheets_cancer.aspx?cancer=lung. Accessed July 20, 2015.

27. Robert SA, Booske BC. US opinions on health determinants and social policy as health policy. *Am J Public Health.* 2011;101(9):1655–1663.

Appendix 2

Communicating About Infectious Disease

Amy Jessop, PhD, MPH

▶ Introduction

While chronic diseases are leading causes of morbidity and mortality in the United States, infectious diseases remain a significant concern. Despite the tremendous advances in prevention and control, familiar infections such as influenza and pertussis persist. In addition, new and newly identified infectious diseases such as severe acute respiratory syndrome (SARS) and methicillin-resistant *Staphylococcus aureus* (**MRSA**) emerge periodically. As medical care practices, the environment, infectious agents, and attitudes and beliefs change and adapt, our ability to prevent and treat infections fluctuates.

No one can predict where or when a new infectious disease will emerge or which changes may affect control measures. With increased globalization in business, travel, and food supplies, infectious agents can quickly disperse into diverse populations and threaten large proportions of the globe within days. To respond promptly and effectively to such threats, public health systems must learn from historical events and employ new communication methods to reach at-risk populations.

▶ Vaccines and Vaccine-Preventable Diseases of Childhood

Vaccination is among the most impactful of public health achievements.[1] The world entered the 20th century with infant mortality rates greater than 20%. Of those children who survived infancy, another 20% died before their fifth birthday, largely due to measles, diphtheria, smallpox, pertussis, and other infectious diseases.[2-5] As the 20th century progressed, new vaccines and more extensive public health programs to distribute and administer them helped eradicate smallpox, eliminate poliomyelitis (caused by wild-type viruses), and make death from infectious disease in childhood a rare event.[6]

While vaccines produce strong biological responses, they also elicit strong social and cultural reactions. Concerns about ethics and vaccine safety surrounded early immunization efforts and persist today.[7] Added to these issues are newer challenges related to the increasing number of vaccines, complexity of the immunization schedule, school and workplace mandates, and increasing costs.[8] In an ironic twist, the most challenging issues actually result from the impressive success of vaccines and immunization programs in the United States and other developed countries. The most recent generations of parents have not seen or experienced what were once common childhood infections. Without direct reinforcement from experience, these parents often question whether the benefits of vaccines outweigh the perceived risks and challenges. However, when parents withhold vaccines from their children, both the individual and community benefits of vaccines are threatened.

Communicating About Vaccine-Preventable Diseases

Communication about vaccine-preventable diseases can serve to remind the public and healthcare providers about the threats from infections and the potential costs of under-immunization, help parents and guardians as they approach immunization decision points and influence the development of policies and programs that facilitate the desired immunization actions.

Sources of Data on Vaccine-Preventable Diseases and Vaccination

Communities have counted, monitored, and reported causes of death for centuries. Systematic collection of data regarding infectious conditions in the United States dates back almost 150 years. In 1878, Congress authorized the U.S. Marine Services Hospital to collect and report morbidity reports on contagious conditions including cholera, yellow fever, and smallpox.[9] This collection and reporting of infection data developed into systematic surveillance systems employed by health authorities to enumerate which conditions are present in given populations, locations, and time. A variety of local, state, and national health authorities may request or mandate reporting by hospitals and healthcare providers, laboratories, schools, and others regarding health conditions or symptoms. While each state and locale may have its own set of reportable conditions, they also compile and report a standard set of conditions to the CDC (**TABLE 2A-1**).[10] Transmission of surveillance data among health authorities is facilitated by the National Electronic Disease Surveillance System (NEDSS).[a]

Examples

Morbidity and Mortality Weekly Report *Morbidity and Mortality Weekly Report* (*MMWR*), which is published weekly by the CDC, presents a compilation of the surveillance data collected through NEDSS and other surveillance systems. This accurate and timely reporting of diseases assists authorities in determining the magnitude of health problems (incidence and prevalence), identifying individuals and population groups at risk for infection, and alerting healthcare providers to inform evaluation and delivery of care.

National Immunization Survey The National Immunization Survey (NIS)[b] first implemented in 1994, is performed annually by NCIRD and the CDC, and monitors immunization coverage for children 35 months to 19 years of age. Through telephone surveys conducted with a sample of U.S. households and questionnaires mailed to healthcare providers, NIS determines immunization rates for diphtheria and tetanus toxoids and acellular pertussis vaccine (DTaP), poliovirus vaccine (polio), measles-containing vaccine (MCV), *Haemophilus influenzae* type b vaccine (Hib),

TABLE 2A-1 National Notifiable Infectious Conditions, 2015			
Anthrax	*Haemophilus influenzae*	Novel influenza A virus	Syphilis
Arboviral diseases	Hansen's disease	Pertussis	Tetanus
Babesiosis	Hantavirus	Plague	Toxic shock syndrome (non-streptococcal)
Botulism	Hemolytic uremic syndrome	Poliomyelitis	Trichinellosis
Brucellosis	Hepatitis A	Poliovirus infection	Tuberculosis
Campylobacterosis	Hepatitis B	Psittacosis	Tularemia
Chancroid	Hepatitis C	Q fever	Typhoid fever
Chlamydia trachomatis	Human immunodeficiency virus (HIV) infection	Rabies, animal	Vancomycin-resistant *Staphylococcus aureus*
Cholera	Influenza-associated pediatric mortality	Rabies, human	Varicella

a. http://wwwn.cdc.gov/nndss/nedss.html
b. http://www.cdc.gov/nchs/nis.htm

Coccidioidomycosis	Invasive pneumococcal disease	Rubella	Vibriosis
Cryptosporidiosis	Legionellosis	Salmonellosis	Viral hemorrhagic fever
Dengue virus infection	Listeriosis	Severe acute respiratory syndrome (SARS)	Crimean–Congo hemorrhagic fever
Diphtheria	Lyme disease	*Escherichia coli* (Shiga toxin)	Lassa virus
Ebola virus	Malaria	Shigellosis	Lujo virus
Erlichiosis and anaplasmosis	Measles	Smallpox	Marburg virus
Giardiasis	Meningococcal disease	Spotted fever rickettsiosis	New World arenavirus
Gonorrhea	Mumps	Streptococcal toxic-shock syndrome	Yellow fever

Adapted from 2015 National Notifiable Infectious Diseases, Centers for Disease Control and Prevention website. http://wwwn.cdc.gov/nndss/conditions/notifiable/2015/infectious-diseases/. Accessed October 7, 2015.

hepatitis B vaccine (Hep B), varicella zoster vaccine, pneumococcal conjugate vaccine (PCV), hepatitis A vaccine (Hep A), and influenza vaccine (FLU). Data are used to report official vaccination estimates for the United States and its major geopolitical regions. Additional NIS programs include NIS-Teen, NIS-Adult, 2009 H1N1 Flu Survey, and the National Flu Survey.

Communicating About Vaccine Benefits And Safety

Despite overwhelming evidence pointing to the safety of today's vaccines, negative aspects of vaccination, based largely on erroneous reports of hazards such as autism, often dominate communication about vaccines.[10,11] In a 2008 WHO publication, researchers reported that in the five previous years, Medline recorded five times as many hits for the keyword "vaccine risks" as for the keyword "vaccine benefits."[12] All too often, public health messages about the benefits of protection and scientific support for vaccines must compete with messages of fear. Explaining the risks and benefits of vaccines requires effective communication skills and familiarity with local cultures. Several public health and community-based agencies have developed programs and campaigns to inform the public about the benefits of vaccines and to provide guidance to help overcome hesitancy and fear.

Example: Vaccine Safety Basics

WHO's Vaccine Safety Basics,[c] an e-learning course, was developed to help health educators and healthcare professionals communicate about the safety and benefits of vaccines. The course modules express the need for critical evaluation and assessment of information about vaccines; recognition of target audiences, including their knowledge about vaccines and their perceptions of vaccine risk; outlining fears and concerns of groups to be affected by an immunization program; design of simple, clear, and tailored messages to communicate information about vaccine safety to target audiences; identification of the most suitable means and channels of communication; and alliance with media outlets.

Communicating Effectively About Vaccines: New Communication Resources for Health Officials

In 2009, in response to requests for assistance with messaging to counter vaccine safety and benefit concerns, the Association of State and Territorial Health Officials (ASTHO) interviewed parents and guardians to gather information and develop effective messages and materials for clear and accurate promotion of the benefits of vaccines and informed decision making.

c. http://vaccine-safety-training.org/

The resultant publication, "Communicating Effectively About Vaccines: New Communication Resources for Health Officials,"[d] includes key messages for parents and stakeholders and communication tools designed to help local health officials develop their own vaccine campaigns.

▶ Emerging Infectious Diseases

Approximately 50 years ago, the Nobel laureate Sir MacFarlane Burnett wrote, "One can think of the middle of the twentieth century as the end of one of the most important social revolutions in history, the virtual elimination of the infectious disease as a significant factor in social life."[13] Obviously, this prediction was not realized. Familiar microbial threats remain, and new challenges continue to emerge. The term "emerging infectious disease" (EID) typically applies to infectious diseases for which the incidence has increased in the past two decades or those for which the incidence threatens to increase in the near future. Diseases in this category include (1) new and newly identified infections, such as severe acute respiratory syndrome (SARS); (2) known infections affecting new regions or population groups, such as hepatitis C in young U.S. adults; and (3) known infections that are newly resistant to treatment or public health actions such as multidrug-resistant tuberculosis (MDR-TB) and methicillin-resistant *Staphylococcus aureus* (MRSA).[14]

EIDs affect all regions of the globe. International concern about the threat posed by EIDs led the Institute of Medicine (IOM) to examine the situation and issue the pivotal 1992 report *Emerging Infections: Microbial Threats to Health in the United States* and the follow-up 2003 report *Microbial Threats to Health*, which identified 13 factors accounting for the emergence of EIDs (**TABLE 2A-2**).[15,16] These factors, acting alone or in concert, affect change in infectious organisms and their environments and human contact with, susceptibility to, or response to them.

Communicating About Emerging Infectious Diseases

Real and perceived threats from EIDs can elicit fear. Fear, in turn, may lead to exclusion of or discrimination toward infected persons, especially when infections are associated with stigmatizing health behaviors, as in the case of HIV.[17,18] Fear of discrimination may lead

TABLE 2A-2 Factors Impacting the Development of Emerging Infectious Diseases

- Adaptation and change of microorganisms
- Human susceptibility to infection
- Human demographics and behavior
- Climate and weather
- Changing ecosystems
- Poverty and social inequality
- Economic development and land use
- International travel and commerce
- War and famine
- Lack of political will
- Breakdown of public health measures
- Technology and industry
- Intent to harm

Excerpted from Institute of Medicine. Microbial Threats to Health: Emergence, Detection and Response. Washington, DC: The National Academies Press; 2003.

people to reject or delay screening or diagnosis and result in preventable exposures and worsened health outcomes. Communication designed to reduce exposure and foster screening and treatment must instill trust, allay fear and move people to desired action.

Sources of Data About EID

Collection, verification, and dissemination of data about EIDs are complicated by the factors affecting development and distribution of EIDs noted earlier. Fear of judgment or the stigma associated with health behaviors such as injection drug use or sexual activity may prevent people from seeking care. Additionally, lack of financial and medical resources may limit identification and reporting of infections. Despite these limitations, systems to identify and monitor EIDs operate in the United States and around the globe.

Within its various divisions, CDC operates or authorizes dozens of surveillance systems capturing data about new and potentially EIDs.[e] Among them are the National Malaria Surveillance System (NMSS, overseen by the Division of Parasitic Diseases and Malaria), the Cholera and Other Vibrio Illness Surveillance System (COVIS, overseen by the Division of Foodborne, Waterborne, and Environmental Diseases), and the Emerging Infections Network (EIN, operated under cooperative agreement by the Infectious Disease Society of America). The sheer number, range, and distribution of oversight of surveillance efforts pose major communication challenges.

---

d. http://www.astho.org/WorkArea/DownloadAsset.aspx?id=5464

Example

In the 1940s, agents that inhibit the replication of microorganisms were discovered and processed into antibiotic medications. The promise of the antibiotics, along with documented success of vaccines, is what led Sir MacFarlane Burnett and others to predict the elimination of infectious diseases in our lifetime. However, microorganisms can harbor innate resistance to specific antimicrobial agents that limits the therapeutic potential of antibiotics. Since these agents were first introduced, overuse or misuse of antibiotics in humans and animals has contributed to the spread of antimicrobial resistance and added undue burden and cost to the healthcare system.[19] Each year, an estimated 2 million Americans acquire serious infections that are resistant to one or more antibiotics and 23,000 people die as a direct result of these infections.[20]

National Antimicrobial Resistance Monitoring System for Enteric Bacteria[f]

The National Antimicrobial Resistance Monitoring System (NARMS), established in 1996, is a collaborative effort among state and local public health departments, the CDC, the Food and Drug Administration, and the U.S. Department of Agriculture. NARMS collects data about susceptibility of certain human infections, livestock infections, and microorganisms present in meats processed for retail sale. The system provides information about emerging bacterial resistance, means by which resistance spreads, and ways in which resistant infections differ from susceptible infections.

▶ Conclusion

Advances in public health led to changes in the leading health problems and to changes in our understanding of the contributions of various factors that influence health. Health communicators can use population health models when designing communication strategies, and can focus on the three major areas of the continuum: health outcomes and the leading causes of death and disability, the multiple determinants of health (behaviors, health care, social and economic factors, and the physical environment), and effective programs and policies.

References

1. Centers for Disease Control and Prevention. Ten great public health achievements—United States, 2001-2010. *MMWR*. 2011;60(19):619–623.

2. Meckel RA. Levels and trends of death and disease in childhood, 1620 to the present. In Golden J, Meckel RA, Prescott HM, eds. *Children and Youth in Sickness and Health: A Handbook and Guide*. Westport, CT: Greenwood Press; 2004:3–24.

3. Fenner F, Henderson DA, Arita I, Jezek Z, Ladnyi ID. *Smallpox and Its Eradication*. Geneva, Switzerland: World Health Organization; 1988.

4. U.S. Department of Health, Education, and Welfare. *Vital Statistics: Special Report, National Summaries: Reported Incidence of Selected Notifiable Diseases, United States, Each Division and State, 1920-50*. Washington, DC: U.S. Department of Health, Education, and Welfare, Public Health Service, National Office of Vital Statistics; 1953:37.

5. U.S. Department of Health, Education, and Welfare. *Vital Statistics Rates in the United States, 1940-1960*. Washington, DC: U.S. Department of Health, Education, and Welfare, Public Health Service, National Center for Health Statistics; 1968.

6. Malone, KM, Hinman AR. Vaccination mandates: the public health imperative and individual rights. In *Law in Public Health Practice*. New York, NY: Oxford University Press; 2003:262–284.

7. Kaufman M. The American anti-vaccinationists and their arguments. *Bull Hist Med*. 1967;41(5):463–478.

8. Kimmel SR, Burns IT, Wolfe RM, Zimmerman RK. Addressing immunization barriers, benefits, and risks. *J Fam Pract*. 2007;56(2 suppl vaccines): S61–S69.

9. Legislative hearing on H.R. 1490, "Veterans' Privacy Act;" H.R. 1792, "Infectious Disease Reporting Act;" and H.R. 1804, "Foreign Travel Accountability Act." June 19, 2013. Government Printing Office. http://www.gpo.gov/fdsys/pkg /CHRG-113hhrg82239/html/CHRG-113hhrg82239.htm.

10. MacIntyre CR, Leask J. Immunisation myths and realities: responding to arguments against immunisation. *J Paediatr Child Health*. 2003;39:487–491.

11. Folb PI, Bernastowska E, Chen R, et al. A global perspective on vaccine safety and public health: the Global Advisory Committee on Vaccine Safety. *Am J Public Health*. 2004;94: 1926–1931.

12. Andre FE, Booy R, Bock HL, et al. Vaccination greatly reduces disease, disability, death and inequity worldwide. *Bull World Health Org*. 2008;86(2):140–146.

13. Burnet M. *Natural History of Infectious Disease*. Cambridge, UK: Cambridge University Press; 1962.

e. http://www.cdc.gov/surveillancepractice/stlts.html
f. http://www.cdc.gov/narms/reports/index.html

14. Centers for Disease Control and Prevention. National Center for Emerging and Zoonotic Infectious Diseases (NCEZID). http://www.cdc.gov/ncezid/who-we-are/about-our-name.html. Accessed December 14, 2014.

15. Institute of Medicine. *Emerging Infections: Microbial Threats to Health in the United States.* Washington, DC: National Academy Press; 1992.

16. Institute of Medicine. *Microbial Threats to Health: Emergence, Detection, and Response.* Washington, DC: National Academies Press; 2003.

17. Baral S, Karki D, Newell J. Causes of stigma and discrimination associated with tuberculosis in Nepal: a qualitative study. *BMC Public Health.* 2007;7:211.

18. Herek GM, Gillis JR, Cogan J. Psychological sequelae of hate crime victimization among lesbian, gay, and bisexual adults. *J Consult Clin Psychol.* 1999;67(6):945–951.

19. Roberts RR, Hota B, Ahmad I, et al. Hospital and societal costs of antimicrobial-resistant infections in a Chicago teaching hospital: implications for antibiotic stewardship. *Clin Infect Dis.* 2009;49(8):1175–1184.

20. Centers for Disease Control and Prevention. Antibiotic resistance threats in the United States, 2013. http://www.cdc.gov/drugresistance/pdf/ar-threats-2013-508.pdf. Accessed December 15, 2014.

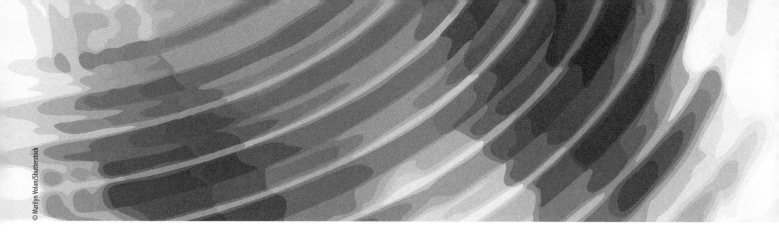

CHAPTER 3

A Public Health Communication Planning Framework

Claudia Parvanta

Claudia Parvanta

LEARNING OBJECTIVES

By the end of this chapter, the reader will be able to:

- Understand the importance of planning.
- Describe the components of a communication plan.
- Select an engagement, information, or persuasion approach.
- Identify the key elements of each core strategy based on best practices.
- Identify stakeholder partnerships that support a communication intervention.
- Create a logic model for a health communication intervention.
- Conduct an assessment of strengths, weaknesses, opportunities, threats, and ethical considerations (SWOTE) for an intervention.
- Apply basic principles to a case study on ATV safety.

▶ Introduction: The Importance of Planning

In health communication, the flurry of new media options gives a breathless feeling to the design of an intervention. But, while we *Tweeted* yesterday and use *Instagram* today (or whatever is trending now), our basic human psychology (like our DNA) has not changed as rapidly. We still take more time to ponder difficult decisions (e.g., buying a car, having prostate cancer surgery) than easy ones (e.g., buying shampoo). The more difficult the decision, or the more complicated or continuous the behavior change, the more ways we need to be convinced of its merits. "Ways" can be translated into messages, channels, sources (experts, friends), economic incentives, ease of performance, regulations and laws, and so on. The surest way to fail in health communication is to not determine which combination of "ways" works best for a particular audience and a particular behavior.

BOX 3-1 provides a sobering example of what can be considered an *unplanned* communication intervention: Angelina Jolie Pitt's 2013 announcement of her preventive double mastectomy (a decision that she based on her high genetic probability of developing breast cancer). While she received record amounts of media attention and there was a surge of interest in the topic, social and commercial media interest subsided after one week.[1,2] A personal and somewhat spontaneous decision, her announcement was not part of a planned communication strategy to direct others to breast cancer prevention resources. We really do not know how many people have been affected by her decision, but like an astronomical star, she might shed light on women's cancer prevention for decades to come. In addition, her case provides a dramatic lesson on what can happen when the equivalent of millions of dollars in advertising and public relations is let loose without a plan—namely, a "big bang" that fizzles out too quickly.

A communication plan is necessary to make the most of available resources so that a program can achieve its goals. Furthermore, a plan is often required to garner sufficient support for an intervention within one's organization. It can be used to attract partners who will help execute the intervention over a sustained period of time. Ultimately, the goals and objectives of a plan are used to measure success—whether the anticipated change does or does not takes place—and to determine which elements of the program should be continued.

Approaches to Planning

Health communication plans vary in their complexity. As the Public Health Foundation has stated, "Strategic communication is based on a simple premise: Deliver the right message, in the right place, at the right time, to the intended target audience."[4]

A stripped-down version of how to do this is described by Noar in his "audience, channel, message, and evaluation" (ACME) framework.[5] The CDC's *CDCynergy* offers a comprehensive approach to planning, managing, and evaluating an intervention. Other useful approaches lie in between these extremes.[6] **BOX 3-2** highlights several of the best free tools for planning public health communication interventions for domestic or global projects. In this text, we work with a slight modification of the *CDCynergy* approach.

While planning requires a systematic approach, it is equally important to enlist the participation of stakeholders in planning, be they community members or patients. In a framework such as community-based prevention marketing (CBPM),[3] community members take the lead in prioritizing problems and reviewing possible interventions.

BOX 3-1 A Sobering Thought About Unplanned Interventions

When acclaimed actress (and United Nations ambassador) Angelina Jolie Pitt disclosed her prophylactic surgery to prevent breast cancer, she made headline news. Among other media coverage, her revelations became the cover story for *Time* (May 27, 2013). There was a dramatic surge in online information seeking about breast cancer the day of, and for a while after, her announcement. For example, the "National Cancer Institute's *Preventive Mastectomy* fact sheet received 69,225 page views on May 14, representing a 795-fold increase as compared with the previous Tuesday. A fivefold increase in page views was observed for the PDQ *Genetics of Breast and Ovarian Cancer* summary in the same time frame. A substantial increase, from 0 to 49%, was seen in referrals from news outlets to four resources from 7 May to 14 May."[2]

All of these rates quickly returned to their preannouncement levels—after only one week. While online information seeking is just one indication of public awareness, this "bump and slump" pattern suggests that even a huge celebrity, an important and frightening topic, and massive media coverage do not generate more than a short-term reaction. There might be millions more who are *thinking* about breast cancer as a result of Jolie Pitt's disclosure, but they are not behaving in ways that are registering as behavior change. It has been left for others to incorporate Ms. Jolie Pitt's brave disclosure into a more comprehensive and sustainable campaign, if they see fit.

References

1. Juthe RH, Zaharchuk A, Wang C. Celebrity disclosures and information seeking: the case of Angelina Jolie. *Genetics Med.* 2015;17:545–553.

2. Noar SM, Althouse BM, Ayers JW, Francis DB, Ribisl KM. Cancer information seeking in the digital age: effects of Angelina Jolie's prophylactic mastectomy announcement. *Med Decis Making* 2015;35(1):16–21. doi: 10.1177/0272989X14556130.

Health Communication Within the Ecological Model

We have learned that health communication is most effective when it is delivered at several levels of the ecological model, taking into account individual, interpersonal, institutional, and community-wide audiences. Effectiveness improves when we match the media channels used to the audiences, or provide a product tie-in.[7,8] A good example of working across the levels of the ecological model is presented in **BOX 3-3**, which fits strategies presented by the CDC to promote physical activity into levels of the ecological model.

TABLE 3-1 outlines another version of the ecological model and shows examples of communication tools to create or support health promotion at each level.

▶ Health Communication Planning Overview

Health communication planning, execution, and evaluation are often represented by a circle to emphasize the ongoing nature of program improvement. The National Cancer Institute uses the format shown in **FIGURE 3-1**.[9] The complex planning process can be divided into several subplans, each with an inherent research task.

Subplans
Macro Plan

The macro plan includes analysis of the problem, the ecological setting, the target population(s), the core intervention strategy, and the partnership mix. This stage of planning is normally undertaken after epidemiological data indicate there is a health problem that affects specific groups of people. If evidence shows that a specific intervention has worked to reduce this problem elsewhere, feasibility testing might be conducted to adapt the intervention to the new population. The less we know about the problem, its potential solution, or the intended audience, the more formative research we must do before taking the next planning steps.

Strategic Health Communication Plan

With audience and behavior change goals identified, this stage of planning focuses on testing specific concepts, messages, materials, and media against these objectives. Such "pretesting" is sometimes referred to as formative research, and at times is considered "process" research. It precedes finalization of the implementation plan.

BOX 3-3 Strategies to Increase Physical Activity in the Community

This CDC resource offers tested interventions for almost every level of the ecological model.

Individual behavior	Individually adapted health behavior change programs
Social, family, and community networks	Social support interventions in community settings
	Enhanced school-based physical education
	Active transport (walking, biking) to school
Living and working conditions	Point-of-decision prompts to encourage use of stairs
	Enhanced access to places for physical activity combined with informational outreach activities
Broad social, economic, and environmental policies	Street-scale urban design and land-use policies
	Community-scale urban design and land-use policies
	Transportation and travel policies and practices

Based on: Centers for Disease Control and Prevention. Strategies to Prevent Obesity and Other Chronic Diseases: The CDC Guide to Strategies to Increase Physical Activity in the Community. Atlanta: U.S. Department of Health and Human Services; 2011. Available at: http://www.cdc.gov/obesity/.

TABLE 3-1 Alternative Version of the Ecological Model with Examples of Communication Tools

Ecological Model Level	Primary Intervention	Communication Support
State, national, global	Policies, laws, treaties, "movements," emergencies. Examples: U.S. seat belt laws; food fortification or enrichment regulations; smallpox and polio vaccination programs; border closing or quarantine to control epidemiological outbreaks.	Advocacy to create or maintain policy or law; national and state-specific reinforcement advertising; incentive programs; package warnings and labels; government educational campaigns; social mobilization (e.g., national immunization days); multimedia emergency information campaign to advise and calm the public.
Living and working conditions	Environmental conditions; hours; policies. Examples: worker safety; time off and vacation policies; creation of walking paths; elimination of lead from gasoline and paint; availability of healthy food choices and healthcare services.	Citizen or worker advocacy (multimedia) to improve conditions; awareness and promotion campaigns for improved facilities and services; state or local lead education campaigns; private-sector advertising for healthy food choices and healthcare services.
Social, community, family	Social norms; elimination of social disparities; provision of community health and social services; cultural "rules" for group behavior. Examples: Community Watch, day care, church ministries of health, volunteers.	Grassroots campaigns; social media, radio, TV, Internet, print or local-based (e.g., church, bar) social marketing or promotional campaigns; opinion leaders and role models; public service announcements (PSAs); health fairs, small-media educational materials; reinforcement of norms through group processes.

Ecological Model Level	Primary Intervention	Communication Support
Individual behavior	Acquisition of beliefs, attitudes, motivation, self-efficacy, products, and services through social marketing, behavior change communications, paid advertising, or psychological counseling.	Social media; multimedia decision aids; educational materials; guidelines; promotional advertising; reinforcement through home, healthcare providers, and community.
Individual biology, physiology	Prevention or treatment of illness; healthcare provider visits; screening tests.	Behavior change communication to maintain or establish good health habits; reminders for screening; healthcare provider communication during office visits; texts or tweets as *aide memoires*.

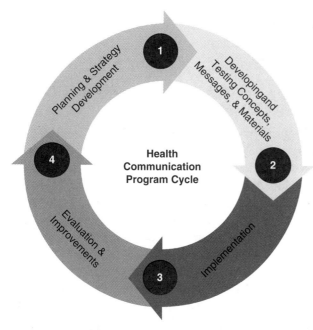

FIGURE 3-1 Health communication planning cycle.

Redrawn from: National Cancer Institute. Making Health Communication Programs Work, p. 11. (DHHS, 2004.)

Implementation Plan

This tactical plan describes what will be done, when, where, how, and with what money, and who is responsible for each piece of the program. Process research is often conducted shortly after the launch of a program to ensure that all operations are running smoothly and messages are getting out and being interpreted as planned. Corrections can be made if this assessment is done early enough.

Evaluation Plan

The evaluation plan defines which aspects of the intervention will be monitored or evaluated to determine the intervention's worth to key stakeholders. Given that most programs want to achieve measurable objectives, baseline data often need to be collected before a program is launched. Therefore evaluation planning must begin in the first days of program development.

Partnership Plan

Planning for continuation and/or expansion of partnerships might also be initiated at the outset of a program to ensure a broader reach, to spread expenses over a longer period, and to provide continuity of leadership and ownership.

Dissemination and Publication Plan

A health communication program can take more than a year to develop, particularly if a great deal of formative research is necessary. Most interventions run for several months to several years and are followed by evaluations that may also extend from days to years. A health communicator can anticipate dedicating five or more years of his or her work life to such an effort! A plan to distribute materials and publish results provides motivation, brings periodic closure, and helps ensure coherent messaging over such long periods of time.

▶ Program Examples

Some health communicators have graciously shared complete case studies of their planning and implementation efforts with us. Highlights of these cases appear in this text where they are most relevant.

Two continuing examples are revisited throughout the text:

- "Tips from Former Smokers" (Tips) was the CDC's first-ever paid national tobacco education campaign. In this unique program, which was launched in March 2012, individuals share their personal experiences related to smoking, including their loss of health, life, and limb. This campaign encourages smokers to seek information about how to quit from informed sources, such as 1-800-QUIT-NOW, government websites, and healthcare providers. Nonsmokers are informed about the harmful effects of secondhand smoke and are encouraged to help their loved ones quit smoking. Messages are disseminated across multiple channels, including television, radio, print, and digital venues, to reach as many people as possible. The primary target audience for the campaign is adult smokers. This case was contributed by a team from the CDC.

- The "Smoke Free Alachua" case was contributed by former University of Florida graduate students in mass communication, who prepared a comprehensive plan in conjunction with their county health department in Florida to discourage use of electronic cigarettes (e-cigarettes).

Other examples illustrate specific concepts and skills and appear in their entirety in other chapters. For health communication planning, the appendix to this chapter offers one such example. In this case study, Brann shows step-by-step (using the *CDCynergy* process) how she and her colleagues developed a plan to promote safety among adolescents using all-terrain vehicles (ATVs) in West Virginia. This state bears the unfortunate distinction of having the highest prevalence of deaths and injuries from ATV use in the United States.

In the case studies presented here, the national-level program "Tips," the state-specific program to promote ATV safety, and the county-level antismoking program have one thing in common: They use the same health communication planning framework. The basic steps are discussed next.

▶ Step-by-Step Planning

Developing the Macro Plan

To develop the macro plan, the health communicator would focus on the following steps:

1. Analyze the problem and the level(s) of the ecological model where the desired change will occur. Based on that analysis, determine what needs to change and where the change must take place.
2. Examine the evidence and select the most effective intervention for bringing about this change.

3. Identify the people whose behavior is the focus of change—that is, the "audience."
4. Identify the primary form of interaction for each audience: engagement, information, or persuasion.
5. Select a process for executing this form of interaction: education, empowerment, marketing, or political action.
6. Identify and recruit partners to accomplish these tasks.
7. Model the intervention and conduct a SWOTE analysis: an assessment of strengths, weaknesses, opportunities, threats, and ethical considerations.

At this level of planning, we do not worry about specific media channels or messages. These considerations will be addressed later, as part of the strategic health communication plan.

Step 1: Analyze the Problem and Its Place in the Ecological Framework

Diagnosing the Problem: The PRECEDE–PROCEED Model
The PRECEDE–PROCEED model has been used to guide countless public health interventions. Developed by Green, Kreuter, and associates in the 1970s,[10] the model works backward from a desired state of health and quality of life, asking which environment, behavior, individual motivation, or administrative policy is necessary to create that healthy state. **FIGURE 3-2** shows the basic precede–proceed model.[11]

PRECEDE–PROCEED divides the process into needs assessment and implementation phases. The needs assessment phase examines the predisposing, reinforcing, and enabling constructs in educational/environmental diagnosis and evaluation (PRECEDE). The implementation phase addresses policy, regulatory, and organizational constructs in educational and environmental development (PROCEED). Predisposing factors include existing beliefs, attitudes, and values (e.g., cultural or ethical norms) that influence whether a person will adopt a behavior. Enabling factors are largely structural, such as the availability of resources, time, or skills to perform a behavior. Reinforcing factors include family and community approval or discouragement. The PRECEDE–PROCEED model has been discussed extensively by Edberg.[12]

A comprehensive diagnosis of a problem often reveals that more than one population and more than one level of the ecological model are involved in creating a problem. All of these inputs should be addressed when planning a successful health communication intervention for that problem.

PRECEDE

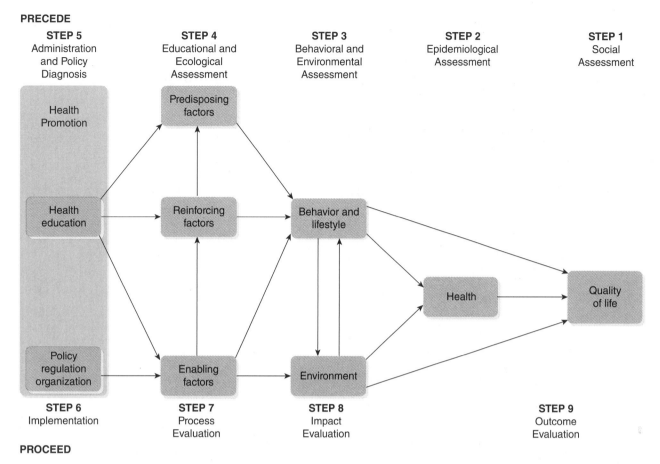

FIGURE 3-2 PRECEDE–PROCEED model.

Reproduced from National Cancer Institute. Theory at a Glance, A Guide for Health Promotion Practice, 2nd Edition. NIH Publication No. 05-3896; 2005.

For example, when families share meals, changing the foods served in those meals often requires agreement by several family members (predisposing factors: beliefs about taste and nutrition, food customs and traditions). Food availability can be limited by season of the year, location of markets, and food purchasing power (enabling factors). In addition, if family members criticize the food (e.g., not tasty), the food preparer is unlikely to repeat the performance (reinforcing factors). As another example, many individuals living in the inner city are too afraid of crime to walk around their neighborhood or to send their children outside to play. All the desire in the world to start an exercise program, and even the offer of free athletic shoes, may not overcome these fears. Thus, a "simple" problem in reality often comprises a complex set of antecedent factors that predispose a belief set, enable or prevent choice, reinforce the status quo, or facilitate change. These factors must be addressed on multiple levels to achieve the desired behavioral change.

The People and Places Framework Maibach, Abroms, and Marosits have developed a framework to

diagram the processes of communication and marketing in terms of their potential for social impact, which they call the **People and Places Model of Social Change** (**FIGURE 3-3**).[13] The People and Places Framework (PPF) asks, "What about the people, and what about the places, needs to be happening for all to be healthy?" Forces that affect people at the individual, social network, or community/population level are referred to as "people fields of influence." Forces that are linked inextricably to a local level or higher administrative level (state, nation, world) are referred to as "place fields of influence."

The PPF suggests that organization marketing and business-to-business approaches and policy (legislative, corporate) advocacy mainly affect place fields of influence. In contrast, social marketing and health communication promote voluntary behavior change based on information, motivation, and self-efficacy, among other psychological processes, and are more effective at changing people fields. A public health planner can use this information to develop an overarching intervention strategy that will target the desired ecological level(s).

BOX 3-4 demonstrates how Tobacco Free Alachua (TFA), a community health partnership in Alachua

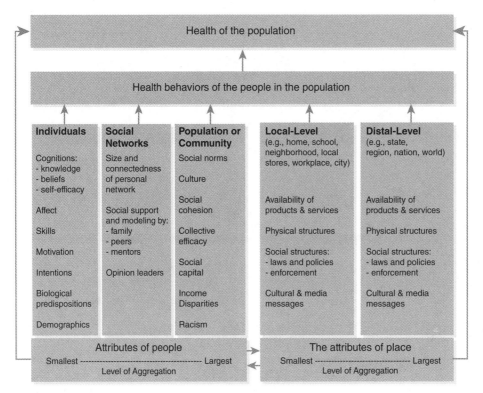

FIGURE 3-3 People and Places Model of Social Change.

Reproduced from Maibach EW, Abroms LC, Marosits M. Communication and marketing as tools to cultivate the public's health: a proposed "people and places" framework. BMC Public Health. 2007; 7.

BOX 3-4 Tobacco Free Alachua Problem Statement

In striving for a tobacco-free future, Tobacco Free Alachua is dedicated to building community support and advocating for the establishment of tobacco-control policies in Alachua County. Accordingly, Tobacco Free Alachua unites members of the local community in its policy work regarding tobacco prevention and reducing exposure to secondhand smoke. Most recently, e-cigarettes have quickly become an issue raising similar concerns as major tobacco products; however, faced with restrictions on funding, Tobacco Free Alachua is restricted from utilizing its grant money to study e-cigarettes in depth. Due to the fact that nicotine poses a potential health threat to the community, including adolescents, a nationwide increase in e-cigarette use is concerning to Tobacco Free Alachua because it limits the organization's ability to fulfill its mission of reducing the use and effects of tobacco at a local level.

Another mounting concern for Tobacco Free Alachua is the fear that e-cigarette advertising is utilizing the same manipulative techniques seen historically in major tobacco advertising. In the past, tobacco companies have specifically marketed cigarettes and smokeless tobacco to teens for generations, through advertising that appealed specifically to teens' ideas of rebellion, freedom, and independence.[1] Furthermore, the marketing of e-cigarettes in candy-like flavors warrants concern, as young people are more likely to use flavored tobacco products than are adults.[2] Consequently, Tobacco Free Alachua's apprehension about the messages being presented in e-cigarette advertising and the targets of those messages prompted a study of online e-cigarette advertisements.

A content analysis examined 61 online video advertisements found on 14 e-cigarette companies' YouTube channels. To determine the validity of the study, intercoder reliability testing using Krippendorf's alpha was conducted, achieving reliability coefficients of 0.82 and 0.91. Researchers determined that the themes commonly observed in traditional cigarette advertising are also present in today's e-cigarette advertisements. Additionally, the major themes identified in e-cigarette advertisements online present appeals aimed at the psychological needs of adolescents—another similarity to traditional tobacco advertisements. Lastly, research found that more than half of the observed advertisements presented e-cigarettes as a safer healthier alternative to traditional cigarettes.

These findings coupled with the aforementioned concerns are significant to Tobacco Free Alachua and warrant immediate attention. As such, an opportunity for a strategic, public health communications plan regarding e-cigarettes exists for Tobacco Free Alachua.

Belva N, Hojnacki R, Justice A., Rodriguez S, Susock S. 2014. Proposed public health communications campaign for tobacco free Alachua. Presented in partial fulfillment of the requirements for the degree of Master of Arts in Mass Communication, University of Florida.

County, Florida, succinctly stated the problem of e-cigarette use in this county. While TFA is a distinct entity separate from the local health department (Florida Department of Health in Alachua County [FDOH-Alachua]), it is supported by the health department's Health Policy Program. By working with the FDOH-Alachua staff, the TFA program is able to incorporate both policy and individual behavior components.

Step 2: Select a Primary Intervention Based on Evidence

The intervention is the "action word" in a program's mission. It could be hand washing, immunization, using condoms, walking to work, eating more vegetables, or something else. Unless the intervention has never been tried, it is better to adapt an existing **evidence-based intervention** than to develop a new intervention from scratch. Doing so has financial implications for the program: It is almost impossible to acquire grant-based funding without referencing evidence-based interventions (EBIs) in the grant application.

Remington discusses how to consult an evidence base for public health interventions, such as *The Community Guide*s or *Cochrane Reviews*.[a] These **systematic reviews** of programs and clinical research studies, taken together, provide an estimate of how effective a particular intervention might be in a particular population. Of course, some interventions may not have generated sufficient evidence yet to warrant such systematic reviews. Their omission from the evidence base does not mean the interventions do not work, but simply signals there have been an insufficient number of studies with appropriate criteria (e.g., sample size, external validity controls) to be included in a meta-analysis. Even when systematic reviews are lacking, however, it is important to read the primary literature in reputable journals to understand the prior approaches used and the outcomes of those interventions.

In addition to these research sources, health communication planners need to consult with representatives from the target population. Interaction with community leaders, either before or after opinion polling, will help merge what the scientific literature suggests is best with what the target community desires. At the conclusion of this stage, determine whether communication will be the primary intervention, or whether it will be developed in support of another intervention such as a new product or service.

The TFA team proposed the following intervention (following an extensive review of the evidence base not shown here):

- Use the Health Belief Model, which has been used extensively in antitobacco campaigns for years).
- Expose the discovered message strategies of e-cigarette advertising (similar to the "truth" campaign),
- Advance the mission of TFA through active education and engagement efforts with parents, educators, and legislators.

Step 3: Identify Relevant Audiences

The behavior of a primary audience is often influenced directly or indirectly by other groups. Identification and targeting of such secondary and tertiary audiences can improve program outcomes.

In health communication planning, the group of people who are most affected by a problem and whose behavior needs to be modified is defined as the **primary audience**. (Sometimes the term "target" is included, as in "primary target audience.") For example, when trying to get mothers in a developing country to use a more nutritious complementary food for their infants, one strategy might be to speak directly to these mothers (the primary audience) and tell them the benefits of nutrition.

Reaching out to the **secondary audience** may also have a great deal of influence on the behavior of the primary audience. For example, research in a developing country community may show that young mothers have very little control over what happens in the household. They may live in their husband's home, and their mother-in-law might actually make most of the decisions. Thus, rather trying to communicate with mothers, it may be more effective to persuade the mothers-in-law that their grandchildren can benefit from improved nutrition.

Continuing this example, to produce change in the behaviors of the mothers and mothers-in-law, the health workers and other influential people in the community may need to be contacted and convinced of the benefits of improved infant nutrition. This group represents a **tertiary audience**, or an audience that can affect the behavior of the secondary and primary audiences.

Sometimes the term "primary audience" is used differently—that is, to refer to the group of people whom you want to *reach first* in a sequence, rather

---

a. http://www.thecommunityguide.org, http://www.cochrane.org

than the primary target of the intervention. That type of audience might be the health workers and community leaders in this example. In fact, if is necessary to conduct a training program for the health workers to bring them up-to-date with new infant nutrition concepts and empower them to be more effective communicators themselves, then the health workers really do become the primary audience for this specific intervention. After the health workers are trained, they can then address the mothers and mothers-in-law as primary and secondary audiences, respectively.

For our purposes, the primary audience is always defined as the group whose behavior is targeted for change. For example, in planning a teenage anti-smoking campaign in the United States, the help of musicians and celebrities who appeal to a younger group might be enlisted. While initial efforts may be directed to the "stars"—the secondary audience—to get them "with the program," the reason for selecting them is to help reach the primary audience—the teenagers. **BOX 3-5** provides TFA's initial description of its audience segments.

BOX 3-5 Tobacco Free Alachua Audiences

Individual Audiences

Tobacco Free Florida focuses on educating all Floridians about the dangers of tobacco, but Tobacco Free Alachua, in particular, focuses on the following target publics within Alachua County:

- Children ages 11–17
- Adults ages 18–24
- Individuals with chronic disease
- Pregnant women
- Low-income households
- Parents
- Small businesses

These audiences are targeted by using "messages that elicit strong emotional response, such as personal testimonials and strong viscerally negative content."*

Secondary Publics

Additionally, Tobacco Free Alachua is concerned with the following groups:

- Public policy influencers and lawmakers
- Educators and school boards
- Tobacco and e-cigarette companies

---

*Tobacco Free Florida. 2014. http://www.tobaccofreeflorida.com/. Accessed January 27, 2014.

Belva N, Hojnacki R, Justice A., Rodriguez S, Susock S. 2014. Proposed public health communications campaign for tobacco free Alachua. Presented in partial fulfillment of the requirements for the degree of Master of Arts in Mass Communication, University of Florida.

Step 4: Choose a Core Communication Strategy for Each Audience

Health communicators have to decide whether they plan to **engage, inform**, or **persuade** as the foundation of their communication strategy.

Engagement Engagement is interactive communication with the expectation of *timely* give-and-take from all parties. In a recent article, three CDC authors make the point that community engagement is not a new concept in public health. But, when "moved online to social media channels, [it] is characterized by interaction with multiple, self-selected communities. These online communities are non-traditional in that they are not defined by space, time, or geography. Rather, online communities are formed by individuals who organize themselves around a given issue."[14] Thus, social media engagement can be used to "build and sustain networks, build trust, [and] mobilize communities, … among other benefits."[14]

The CDC authors offer seven principles of social media engagement based on their considerable experience and review of the literature; these appear in **BOX 3-6**. Research on the actual use of pure engagement strategies within public health communication, and its measurable impact, is sparse.[15] The staffing required to manage online interaction, the decision whether to promote and endorse user-generated content, and the extent to which individuals are "themselves" or represent their organizations online (e.g., is clearance required before posting?) are all challenges to many organizations. CDC's policy to guide these and related areas is available at http://www.cdc.gov/socialmedia/tools/guidelines/pdf/social-media-policy.pdf.[16]

Ethically, it is worth considering whether a public health professional can ever be just another "friend" in an online community. Consider the motivations of such a professional. Unless we are engaged as private individuals, why are we reading posts or using social media tools to gather data? Why are we trying to build up trust or respect in a community? Why are we giving encouragement and support, or disagreeing with what others say? Why do we care about the number of followers or friends we have? And if we generate content, where does it come from? Ultimately, and potentially years down the line, we will use whatever information we gather, whatever relationships we have formed, and whatever trust or respect we have earned to develop and disseminate informative or persuasive messages that we believe will help the community in which we are engaged. Therein lies the difference between using social media as a personal channel for communication and using social media as a tool for

---

BOX 3-6 Principles of Social Media Engagement for Public Health Communication

The following list presents some goals and objectives that maximize the power of social media in public health communication. Note that it is not an exhaustive list.

- *Listen to social media conversations.* This goal involves outright participation in socially mediated dialogues as well as use of media monitoring tools to identify priority topics and information needs.
- *Engage with influencers and their conversations.* "Influencers can include both organizations and individuals and exhibit the characteristics of credibility, persistence in convincing others, and ability to drive conversations so that others take notice of the topic or idea and show support. For example, conducting outreach to bloggers who discuss public health topics that align with an organization's priorities could be an effective way to engage on Twitter."
- *Respond to questions or comments received via social media channels.*
- *Create opportunities for users to engage with your organization, and for your users to engage with each other.* These encounters can range from scheduled social media events such as Twitter chats to simply asking users to comment on posts or materials.
- *Welcome and solicit user-generated content.*
- *Create opportunities to integrate online and offline engagement.* These events can be fun "meet and greet" events, or be driven by disaster response, where social media teams are engaged as volunteers.
- *Leveraging social media for community engagement.*

Each of these strategies requires different levels of staffing, financial resources, and infrastructure.

Modified from: Heldman AB, Schindelar J, Weaver JB. Social Media Engagement and Public Health Communication: Implications for Public Health Organizations Being Truly "Social". Public Health Reviews. 2013;35(1): Epub:6–8.

---

health communication. If health communicators use social media as a tool for obtaining information and effecting change, then a high level of self-awareness is required to avoid privacy issues in data collection and misrepresentations in communication. (Interestingly, the private sector seems to have no qualms about the use of social media as a deliberate part of marketing strategy.)

Informing As is discussed elsewhere, most of the population needs to have raw data and scientific findings decoded into a language they can understand before making an informed decision. The difference between data and information is that data are straightforward facts, whereas information answers questions. The same basic fact can be presented in different ways to make it meaningful to whoever is asking the question.

A variety of theories and techniques can be used to transform data into information that is helpful for different users. For example, individuals who are making decisions might have difficulties reading, using arithmetic functions, or contextualizing information so that it makes sense. Tools to enhance health literacy, numeracy, and cultural competency can be employed to make health information more understandable and meaningful to these consumers. Advocacy and informatics tools make numbers more eloquent for

upstream decision makers. The essential public health service[b] of "inform, educate, and empower" uses all of these kinds of tools. Recent studies of how individuals seek out health information on the Internet have provided new ways for health communicators to present information offline as well.

Persuasion The more strongly the health communicator is vested in the response to his or her information, the further he or she is venturing into the zone of persuasion. As mentioned later in the chapter, marketing approaches can heighten the desirability of certain choices to a potential adopter. These approaches can include many of the same factors that make units of information meaningful and understandable, such as cultural cues and references. Persuasive communication takes the next step by employing theories about how individuals or groups make decisions to change behavior. Most of these theories come from the fields of social or health psychology, where they have been used extensively to persuade individuals to adopt healthier lifestyles. Their application to group dynamics is relatively new, but at least 30 years of practice has shown good results from their use.

We will discuss the ethics of persuasion in our exploration of step 7, which includes conducting a SWOTE analysis of the intervention, introduced

---

b. http://www.cdc.gov/od/ocphp/nphpsp/EssentialPublicHealthServices.htm#es3

earlier. The science, the situation, the society, and the standards of the public health practitioner are all included in the ethical calculus of using persuasive approaches.

Step 5: Select an Overall Approach

According to Rothschild's Behavior Management Model,[18] and to economists at large, when a rational individual is asked to adopt a new behavior, he or she evaluates that behavior in terms of its costs and benefits, as well as the individual's motivations and opportunities to act. The motivation behind this change, and the strategy for best facilitation, are depicted in **FIGURE 3-4**. Estimating the cost/benefit ratio associated with individual adoption of a particular behavior is a good way to select an overall approach.

Educational Approaches If individuals believe that they have much more to gain than to lose from a behavior change (i.e., benefits are obvious and costs are low), then merely providing information or educational approaches might be all that is necessary to prompt a change. Educational approaches work best in the following circumstances:

- The recipient of the information has expressed an interest in, or commitment to, the desired behavior.
- The recipient needs answers to factual questions—that is, What? Who? Where? How?
- The information is simple, clear, and unambiguous.

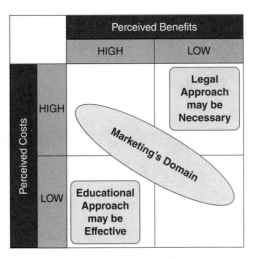

FIGURE 3-4 Interpretation of Rothschild's behavioral management model.

A long-term nationwide example of an educational approach is the ongoing "Safe to Sleep" campaign (launched by the National Institute of Child Health and Development in 1994 as "Back to Sleep"), in which simple informational materials are given to new parents explaining that placing healthy babies on their backs to sleep reduces the risk of sudden infant death syndrome (SIDS).[c] It does not take a lot of persuasion to convince parents to adopt this easily accomplished, no-cost, high-return behavior. In **BOX 3-7**, Chakrabati shares another educational intervention—one that puts pertinent information at the "point of purchase" in vending machines to guide

---

BOX 3-7 Choose Healthier: A Vending Machine Intervention for Better Nutrition

Ranita Chakrabarti

Background

Thomas Jefferson University (TJU) is a leading medical and health sciences educational institution, with the affiliated Thomas Jefferson University Hospital (TJUH) sharing its urban Philadelphia campus. Many of the students, faculty, and hospital employees find themselves hungry when only vending machines are available as a source of nourishment. As a public health student research project, the author developed the Choose Healthier Initiative (CHI) to reduce consumption of unhealthy foods and beverages purchased through vending machines at the TJU/TJUH campus.

The Intervention

Working in collaboration with Tri State Vending (the company that operated the machines), we set up the Choose Healthier program in seven pilot vending locations at both TJU and TJUH. The locations were selected to ensure that all members of the Jefferson community (i.e., healthcare professionals, students, researchers, and other employees) would have access to the pilot machines. Tri State Vending provided a list of all items sold through the machines, which we evaluated for their calories, fat, and sodium content by package size—not serving size.

With the input of registered dieticians, we used a color-coding scheme to provide advice about choices based on our estimation of an item's nutritional value, or lack thereof. The healthier snacks (less sugar, salt, or fat) were named "Better

c. http://www.nichd.nih.gov/sids/

Picks" and were color-coded green; those with more caloric density, sugar, or salt but still offering some benefits were labeled "Limit Picks" and were color-coded yellow; the least healthy snacks were called "Worst Picks" and were color-coded red. Nuts and seeds were placed in a different category of green because, although they offer some important nutrients, they are relatively high in fat calories and salt. Healthier beverages were named "Drink Plenty" and were color-coded green, less-healthy beverages were named "Drink Less" and were color-coded yellow, and least-healthy beverages were named "Drink Rarely" and were color-coded red.

We pretested the color-coding system to ensure that vending machine users understood the criteria and were able to use the system. We were able to label price tags and item "pushers" as well as beverage cans with the color scheme. Only color-coded items were allowed in the pilot vending machines. Promotional materials (e.g., flyers and signs for the vending machines) were posted at different locations in the hospital and university buildings. Detailed program information regarding CHI was posted on the Jefferson Dining Services website, and advertisements were run on LCD monitors throughout the TJU/TJUH center-city campus. A booklet containing the detailed CHI information was created to train the stockers for the initiative. By January 2013. we were ready to go live with the pilot.

Results

Vending Machine Sales

We used sales data as a concrete measure of the intervention's impact. Sales data from November–December 2012 served as the baseline; data from January–February 2013 reflected the intervention. We saw a statistically significant decrease in the purchase of the unhealthiest snacks ("Worst Picks") at the TJU and TJUH vending machines. Sales data also reflected an increase in the sales of healthy snacks ("Better Picks") and an increase in sales of "Limit Picks" as well. For beverages, there was an approximately 6% decrease in sales of "Drink Less" choices and a 1% decrease in "Drink Rarely" options. Concomitantly, there was an increase in sales of "Drink Plenty" options.

Survey

We conducted an intercept survey one month into the intervention to assess the relationship between the color-coding system on the users' choices of snacks and beverages. Apart from demographic information, we asked respondents questions such as "Which kinds of food do you usually purchase at the vending machine?", "Have you used color codes to choose your snack or beverage?", and "What would make you more likely to use the color codes?" While this study used a convenience sample, we did cover all hospital shift schedules and locations where the pilot machines were operating. We did not include persons who said they had not used the machines during the intervention.

Our survey results revealed that a majority of the users used the color codes to make their choice of snacks and beverages. Among these users, a very large percentage agreed that color codes were helpful. Survey results further showed that a significant number of users were very satisfied with the color-coding system. Users' comments and quotes indicate that color-coding the vending machines is a quick and easy way to communicate which snacks or beverages are healthy and which are not. The results of our survey support the results of a previously published study by the University of Auckland,[1] which found that a worksite wellness initiative based on nutritional guidelines is both feasible and acceptable. These findings add to the mounting evidence that color-coded labeling at point of purchase can influence users to make healthier food choices.

Reference

1. Gorton D, Carter J, Cvjetan B, Mhurchu CN. Healthier vending machines in workplaces: both possible and effective. *NZ Med J.* 2010;123(1311):43-52.

hungry hospital personnel and students to healthier snack options.

Policy Approaches At the opposite end of the spectrum, behaviors that appear to offer the individual few personal benefits, are perceived as difficult to maintain, or are costly might require policy—that is, laws or regulations—as a means to enforce change. Most public health hygiene laws, smoke-free restaurant regulations, and requirements to strap children into rear safety seats in motor vehicles fall into this category.

For new laws or regulations to be developed, organizations (e.g., government agencies, concerned citizen groups) must collect data to demonstrate the harm being done, propose solutions to mitigate the problem, and begin an advocacy effort to convince a policy maker (federal, state, or local) to take up the issue in the public policy forum.

Social Marketing Between education and compulsion is a gray zone where cost and benefit are a matter of negotiated exchange. This is the domain of marketing. **Social marketing** can be defined as the "design, implementation, and control of programs aimed at increasing the acceptability of a social idea, practice, [or product] in one or more groups of target adopters. The process actively involves the target population, who voluntarily exchange their time and attention for help in meeting their health needs as they perceive them."[19]

In the world of commercial marketing, people are "consumers" who are trying to solve problems. Sometimes the problems are obvious to them; at other times their needs are latent. A **latent need** is one of which the person is blissfully unaware. Famous examples include lack of body odor, sweet-smelling breath, and sparkling white teeth. If a product can be developed to solve such a latent need, and if the price and convenience factors associated with that solution are reasonable, the marketer who develops the product should realize a profit. Hence, we have Crest whitening strips, Colgate optic white toothpaste, Listerine Whitening Rinse, and scores of other products and brands geared toward meeting latent needs such as a brilliantly white smile.

Social marketing has adapted this approach to address problems of public health. Unlike commercial marketing, social marketing usually does not focus on achieving an adequate profit margin, although more recent efforts seek to build a **sustainability** margin into a product's price. Like traditional marketing, social marketing uses many dimensions to "position" a product, including the product's image, its price, where it is available, and how it is promoted. The Four Ps—product, price, place, and promotion—form the basis for the marketing strategy. Thus, social marketing involves more dimensions than health communication alone. Social marketing has also been used to promote intangible "products"—that is, behaviors. In this case, the dimensions of price, place, and product image are metaphorical.

In summary, depending on whether the change that is proposed is easy or difficult, and whether the benefits are obvious or need to be emphasized, a public health planner might choose education, marketing, or legislative routes as a core strategy.

Step 6: Choose Partners

No one organization has enough time, energy, and resources to make a very large impact on a community, and certainly not on a statewide or national level. Consequently, working with partners[19] has been an essential aspect of health communication planning for at least three decades, if not longer. The term **coalition** is often used to refer to a group of different organizations working together for a common cause or campaign. Such coalitions may be formal or informal, with operational rules and governance depending on the group's mission and resources. Numerous advantages can be realized by establishing coalitions to aid in reaching programmatic goals. Before inviting organizations to join a coalition, however, the lead agency must commit to support such a partnership. Partners selected for a health communication intervention must be connected to, focus their attention on, and have a high level of credibility with the target audience. Committed partners are needed to achieve objectives and sustain interest in a long-term program. The following sections describe two effective ways to select partners.

Audience-Oriented Approach The health communication program identifies groups to receive program messages and services—for example, pregnant women, adolescents, household heads, or isolated geographic groups. With an audience-oriented approach, the lead agency endeavors to find out which groups already work most effectively with the intended audience. Partners also may be chosen on the basis of their connection with the intended beneficiaries (e.g., children of the target families). Having found partners, the next step is for the lead agency to work with those partners to develop a plan of action to reach each target audience.

Task-Oriented, Problem-Solving Approach A health communication program may be developed to accomplish certain tasks—for example, delivering vitamin supplements to all health posts in the United States, or getting all municipalities to draft ordinances for bike paths. Which groups can help get the job done? Partners are selected on the basis of what they have to offer, such as resources, influence, power, logistical support, or access to key individuals or groups.

BOX 3-8 lists the numerous benefits as well as the barriers to be considered before involving partners in a project.

Once again, a SWOTE analysis (discussed below) can help, in this case to assess gaps in personal and organizational qualities and to suggest improvements. Try to select partners that have knowledge, skills, resources, or connections that may be underrepresented in the lead agency. Partners may be working in the same field as your organization or in other fields, including those from the private sector. In sum, you should strive to find partners who have the following characteristics:

- Shared vision
- Experience in the community or with an approach
- Skills that complement your agency's own skills

BOX 3-8 Benefits and Barriers of Health Communication Coalitions

There are several possible benefits to forming coalitions. Such partnerships can offer the following advantages:

■ Provide the knowledge, expertise, perspective, resources, or credibility needed to bridge gaps in your overall program.
■ Conserve resources by avoiding duplication of services, combining resources, and decreasing costs through collective resource-saving opportunities.
■ Increase the visibility and credibility of your program with decision and policy makers, funders, and the media.
■ Use the partners' relationship with the community to mobilize community members toward action through collective advocacy.
■ Combine the forces of leaders, agencies, gatekeepers, and influential people who may be needed to reach your program's goals.
■ Reach specific subgroups within the total population or reach more people within the target audience.
■ Broaden community support and strengthen the community's trust in your program.
■ Identify gaps in current services, so that the coalition members can then work together to create programs to eliminate those gaps.
■ Make a bigger impact.

Consider these potential problems when deciding if a coalition is the best way to accomplish your goal:

■ Coalitions are a time-consuming effort that may take your time away from other projects.
■ Potential members of your coalition must be identified, pursuaded to join, approved internally and possibly trained—all before you can plan the details of your program.
■ Coalition members may require significant alterations in your program ideas.
■ Coalitions may result in a loss of your "ownership" and control for your program.
■ The coalition, or individual members, may take credit for the program's results.

You also will need to handle the difficulties that occur when groups work together. Among these obstacles are the following potential challenges:

■ Historical or ideological differences
■ Institutional disincentives to collaboration or partnering
■ Competition for resources
■ Lack of leadership and a clear sense of direction
■ Domination by one organization or individual
■ Inadequate participation by important groups
■ Unrealistic expectations about partners' roles, responsibilities, or required time commitments
■ Disagreements among partners regarding values, vision, goals, or actions
■ Inability or unwillingness to negotiate or compromise on important issues

Centers for Disease Control and Prevention, Division of Nutrition and Physical Activity. Guide to Working with Coalitions. Unpublished; 1993.

Most critically, the partners in a coalition should be "stakeholders." They should have something "at stake" (their lives, health, reputation, or funding) that depends on the success of the program. Stakeholders might include the following groups, among others:

■ Representatives of the primary, or "target" audience for behavioral change
■ Secondary audience members—for example, gatekeepers to the target audience, who control access to communicating with the target audience (e.g., religious leaders, block captains, organizational leaders)
■ Tertiary audience members (influencers) who have earned the respect and admiration of the target audience (e.g., local personalities such as local

news anchors, respected politicians, other opinion leaders, national figures such as health authorities or celebrities who have a reason to be involved)

Step 7: Model the Intervention and Conduct a SWOTE Analysis

Preparing a Logic Model Logic model gurus (e.g., Goodstadt[21] and Knowlton and Phillips[22]) have written extensively about this program management tool. The W. K. Kellogg Foundation, which funds many public health activities, has produced a *Logic Model Development Guide* that defines a logic model as "a picture of how an organization does its work—the theory and assumptions underlying the program."[23] This Foundation's logic model is shown in **FIGURE 3-5**. In addition,

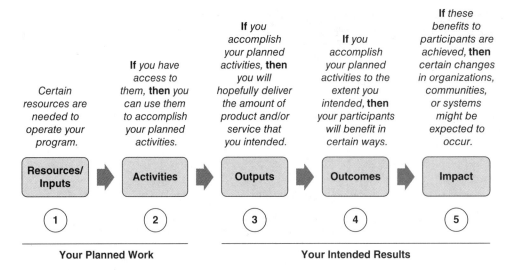

FIGURE 3-5 Basic logic model.

W.K. Kellogg Foundation, The Logic Model Development Guide; Figure 2. p.3. www.wkkf.org.

the University of Wisconsin's Extension Service offers an online course in developing logic models for program management.[d]

Logic models for health programs generally include the following components:

- Planned work: inputs and activities
- Results: outputs, outcomes, and impact
- Some logic models include a situation analysis as part of the document. We handle that a bit later, as a SWOTE analysis.

Logic models are often used to plan a program evaluation. While it would be unwise to fully develop the model without conducting formative research, it can be roughed out before such results are available. In fact, this exercise is one way to determine what you still need to research.

While there is no one right way to create a logic model, we recommend working backward from results to planned work—that is, from impact back to inputs. This strategy prevents "the shoe from telling the foot how big to grow." If the desired results cannot be obtained with the available resources, find partners who can bring more resources, lower your expectations, or find another project.

We also recommend working with the partners to develop a logic model as a group exercise. Ideas can be written on cards, stuck on the wall under basic headings, and then moved around as ideas develop. Once the model is complete, it should be able to fit on one printed page. It can be a big page—computers and apps can help with the graphics and construction. Your colleagues, stakeholders, and partners will use this "big picture" of the program throughout the project and project evaluation.

In the logic model, **resources and inputs** range from tangible items such as money, paid staff or volunteer hours, facilities, data, and equipment, to more intangible items such as expertise, research, or the involvement of collaborators at the local, state, national or global level. Each partner in a coalition may play a part in contributing resources to the program.

Activities are what the program will do. A health communication program often includes the following activities:

- Mass-media activities, such as paid advertising, public service announcements, entertainment education events (e.g., plays, television program scripts, radio soap operas), blogs, YouTube videos, Facebook pages, and student classroom materials
- Patient decision aids, such as computer animations, decision software, pencil-and-paper flipbooks, kits, and worksheets
- Training workshops for healthcare providers, teachers, coaches, or clergy that teach them how to use media effectively
- Outreach and education activities, such as health fairs, speaking engagements, trade shows, and grocery store or drugstore promotional activities

Numbers are associated with activities in terms of what is anticipated and budgeted. For example, the logic model document might specify that the program will conduct 10 teacher training workshops or distribute 10,000 patient decision aids.

Outputs measure the execution of activities, which cannot be determined until a process evaluation is conducted. Nevertheless, goals can be set in advance. For example:

- How many student workbooks need to be delivered to how many sites?
- When, where, and how often should radio spots air? How large an audience will hear these messages?
- How many "page views," downloads, or forms completed are expected from your website?
- If the coalition is contributing to a soap opera or prime-time drama television script, when and where will the episode air? What is the audience size?
- How many people are needed to become "friends" on Facebook? How many times does a YouTube video need to be downloaded?
- How many health facilities, practices, or individual healthcare providers have agreed to use the patient decision aids? How many patients need to receive them?
- For intermediaries (people using the health communications materials to work with others):
    - How many workshops were implemented?
    - How many participants completed pre- and post-tests?
    - How many materials were ordered post training?
    - How many feedback cards or website entries were posted?
- For outreach:
    - How many public appearances, speaking engagements, or health fairs are planned? Where and when?
    - How many grocery stores, pharmacies, or other commercial establishments will run events with the program's materials and speakers?
    - How many trade or industry shows will be attended? Where and when?

Outcomes are normally divided into immediate, intermediate, and long-term ranges. **Immediate outcomes** for mass media might include:

- Next-day recall of the message
- Awareness of the issue
- Change in attitude or motivation to try something

These responses would be determined through survey research. Interactive media allow recipients to respond to website invitations, purchase, donate, or post information immediately.

Intermediate outcomes generally include changes in individual behaviors, enactment of policies, or uptake of technology or strategies by organizations. **Long-term outcomes** could include permanent changes in health behavior, statutes and laws, or environmental quality.

Long-term outcomes may be identical to impact, although the former refers more to individuals (long-term outcome: an individual quits smoking and his life is extended) and the latter to population (impact: the death rate from tobacco goes down). That is, impact is generally measured in terms of population-level health or socioeconomic improvements, such as reductions in age-specific mortality rates, prevalence of disease, and disease-specific mortality rates, or improvements in population measures of quality of life.

SWOTE Analysis A **SWOT analysis** is a standard business tool for reviewing program strengths, weaknesses, opportunities, and threats. We have added an "E" to SWOT, indicating an ethical assessment is part of the health communication program analysis. Strengths and weaknesses refer to conditions that can be controlled, or at least are inherent an organization's ability to implement the program. Opportunities and threats are beyond the organization's control; that is, with or without planning, they will happen on their own. Ethical considerations exist at various levels. It is important to assess whether, either intentionally or inadvertently, the program intervention might harm someone, limit someone's rights, or promise something that cannot be delivered.

As with development of the logic model, a SWOTE exercise is best conducted with partners or stakeholders. Their multiple perspectives will broaden the assessment of total assets and provide a 360-degree picture of opportunities and threats. Again, work with cards, stick them up on the wall under the big headings, and move them around as thinking is refined.

Strengths. There are two ways to consider strengths:

- Strengths as the attributes within the organization, including personnel capabilities, experiences, material resources, organizational commitment, time allotted, and budget.

■ Strengths as the attributes of the intervention/communication campaign, including the positioning of a product or service, its cost, its attractiveness or reputation, and so on. If the product or service is highly desirable (e.g., a "free pizza" night on a college campus), that is a program strength. If the idea is unpopular or hard to sell (e.g., an increase in tuition), this can be a weakness.

Weaknesses. As with strengths, there are two ways to consider weaknesses:

■ Gaps within the organization, such as a lack of knowledge, skills, experience, or material resources. Weaknesses may also be less tangible, such as leaders' lack of commitment to the intervention, a nonexistent or poor reputation in the community, or lack of credibility within a government or other bureaucracy. Of course, insufficient funding and a rushed timeline are also program weaknesses.

■ Weaknesses of the actual intervention. These may include limited availability (e.g., flu vaccine), production costs, distribution hurdles, or basic lack of attractiveness to consumers (e.g., a fecal blood test or colonoscopy for colon cancer screening).

Opportunities. Opportunities are positive factors co-occurring with the time and place for the planned intervention. Partners and stakeholders may provide critical insights into opportunities (as well as threats) that have not yet been discovered. Examples of opportunities include the following:

■ A favorable political climate. (The political climate is more often a threat, however. For example, funding for international family planning programs usually diminishes during Republican presidential administrations and increases under Democratic administrations.) At state and local levels, the governor and congressional leaders can play important roles in supporting or thwarting health promotion activities within the state or congressional district.

■ Funding. Some health promotion programs have benefited from federal stimulus funding. National Institutes of Health (NIH) research funding opportunities, for example, have cyclical deadlines as well as limited duration. Private foundations also issue time-limited calls for proposals. Funding opportunities are something of a two-edged sword, because coalitions that come together solely in response to the availability of funding are often difficult maintain.

■ Technology development and innovation. In the health communication area, continuing development of new technologies, new applications, and major cost reductions favor mass communication as never before.

■ Seasonal, entertainment, and style trends. There are always trends (e.g., in food, clothing, and skin tone) that may support (or threaten) an intervention. For example, interventions to sell sunscreen or warn about skin cancer are likely to be most effective in the summer, unless spots are aimed at the travel channel and target vacationers traveling to sunny climes.

■ Big events that draw a lot of attention. Many, many health promotion programs (as well as commercial advertisers) have linked their efforts to the Olympics, for example. While the Olympics and other major sporting events, (e.g., the World Cup for global interventions and the Super Bowl or World Series for U.S. interventions) draw huge audiences, these events are focused on making the athletes and the sport the "single overriding communication objective," rather than your communication objective. Whatever time they do not manage to fill is given to the event's major commercial sponsors. It is not effective to spend a small fortune to run a small 15-second spot in such a big venue. What can work well is developing a local angle, such as an athlete or Olympic competitor from the community or state. This person can become a spokesperson and can enhance and extend the health communication impact before and after the event itself.

■ Celebrity endorsements. While certainly sympathetic, professionals working in health promotion have a somewhat ghoulish reaction when celebrities announce that they or their loved ones have a health problem. If the person is well known and can be seen as a positive role model, efforts are made to attract the celebrity as a spokesperson. Well-known examples include Cindy Crawford (whose younger brother died of leukemia), Nicole Kidman and Patrick Dempsey (whose mothers died of breast cancer), and, after the fact, Angelina Jolie Pitt. In the early days of the disease, Earvin "Magic" Johnson transformed the national dialogue around human immunodeficiency virus (HIV) and acquired immunodeficiency syndrome (AIDS) with his disclosure of his positive HIV status. Because so many celebrities seem to seek meaning beyond their media careers, services have sprung up to match them up with agencies or issues for which they feel an affinity. Thus, a personal tragedy for a celebrity also represents an "opportunity" to engage with that person with a targeted health issue. Many celebrities find that working for a cause helps them to deal with their loss in a constructive manner.

Threats. Threats are factors that could potentially delay or prevent achieving program objectives but are outside program control. In some ways, all of the factors mentioned previously, if turned around, can be threats. For example:

- Political instability. International work is frequently threatened by clashing political parties, including uprisings, strikes, and localized conflicts. War is the biggest threat—not just to the work of public health practitioners, but (obviously) to the entire planet.
- Environmental catastrophe. Powerful weather systems (e.g., hurricanes, floods), earthquakes, and agricultural conditions (such as droughts) all jeopardize international health communication efforts. Explosions in mines (or oil/gas drilling rigs) not only focus local or national attention for months, but also drain resources from other public health programs. Thus they are tragedies on several levels.
- Activity linked to risky funding, or dependent on personalities. In the United States, organizations, academic institutions, or even small groups can all suffer externally created losses in funding or other resources. Also, the actions of one individual may threaten the reputation of an entire organization or institution. Although celebrities' endorsements may be welcome opportunities, all too often they are risky business. In a notorious example, Tour de France champion Lance Armstrong lost

his credibility as a sportsman following a doping scandal and, in turn, became a much less effective spokesperson for cancer screening. Tabloid exposure can make celebrities unreliable participants in health promotion campaigns. If a celebrity is carefully matched to the target audience and is are willing to work with the program, then his or her risk-taking behavior—and negative consequences—might send the right message. For example, Magic Johnson admitted to unprotected sexual encounters outside of his marriage as the cause of his HIV. Likewise, musicians or actors who were long-time "stoners" have admitted to regretting the drugs they did in their youth, but their mea culpas seem to be less convincing to young people.

How many of these factors can be predicted based on your current situation analysis? Whatever is done at the outset should be remembered, written down, and reevaluated as the program develops. As an example, **BOX 3-9** shows the SWOT developed for the TFA project.

Ethical Dimensions. Ethical dimensions in public health are derived from conflicts of philosophical and moral (i.e., cultural) principles and values. Four stand out:

- Utilitarianism. Defined as the "the greatest good for the greatest number of people," **utilitarianism** is central to public health, and much of public policy, in the United States. Utilitarianism requires forecasting results and presents the possibility that the "ends justify the means." An example of a highly utilitarian public health policy is quarantine and travel restrictions for infectious outbreaks. In this case, the rights of a few are restricted to protect the health of the many.

BOX 3-9 Tobacco Free Alachua's SWOT Analysis

It has been more than 60 years since we learned about the deadly effects of tobacco use; today, the emergence of electronic cigarettes (also known as e-cigarettes, vapors, vaporizers, or nicotine vaporizers), coupled with their increasing use among youth, has inspired considerable debate within the U.S. public health community and is raising concerns similar to those seen historically with major tobacco.[1] Recent discussion regarding the safety of e-cigarettes, the product's ability to help smokers quit, and the risks they pose to children and teens are all significant issues that organizations like Tobacco Free Alachua are facing locally in 2014. Tobacco Free Alachua is also concerned with e-cigarette advertising; more specifically, the messages being presented in advertising and who those messages are targeting.

Furthermore, public health organizations and media have speculated that:

- In advertising, e-cigarettes are presented as a healthy alternative to cigarettes.
- There is uncertainty as to the safety of e-cigarettes and their long-term effects.
- E-cigarette advertisements are utilizing tailored messaging and images that specifically appeal to youth markets, a tactic once used extensively by the U.S. tobacco industry.

(continues)

BOX 3-9 Tobacco Free Alachua's SWOT Analysis *(continued)*

The concern with e-cigarettes is that their effects are unknown, advertisers are focusing on youth markets, and youth users in particular may become addicted to nicotine and eventually seeks out tobacco cigarettes. Due to the lack of research, there is an opportunity to investigate e-cigarette advertisements. If the messages are similar to those once utilized in tobacco campaigns targeting youth markets, it is crucial to understand the dominant themes and appeals in developing future anti-tobacco campaigns and preventing youth initiation and progression of e-cigarette smoking to traditional cigarette smoking.

SWOT Analysis

Strengths of Tobacco Free Alachua:

- Tobacco Free Alachua receives administrative support from Tobacco Free Florida and has access to its parent organization's research and marketing materials.
- Tobacco Free Alachua has strong community ties, including partnerships with the Alachua County School Board, the University of Florida, the Alachua County Board of County Commissioners, University of Florida Health, and other public health and policy organizations.
- Alachua County supports the mission of Tobacco Free Alachua by implementing tobacco-free policies in public schools and parks, in the workplace, and at restaurants and local businesses.
- Alachua County passed an ordinance in 2013 that places restriction on the sale of e-cigarettes and bans the use of the devices in places where traditional tobacco is currently banned under the Florida Clean Indoor Air Act.

Weaknesses of Tobacco Free Alachua:

- A lack of funding from Tobacco Free Florida inhibits Tobacco Free Alachua from conducting research on e-cigarettes in Alachua County.
- Tobacco Free Alachua is prohibited from utilizing Florida Department of Health funding for e-cigarette research. *(Editor's note: Ethical consideration)*
- Tobacco Free Alachua has only four full-time staff members.
- Tobacco Free Alachua is not allowed to lobby directly for policy change. *(Editor's note: Ethical consideration)*

Opportunities for Tobacco Free Alachua:

- Strong community partners can lobby for policy change on behalf of Tobacco Free Alachua.
- Of the five most populous states (California, Florida, Illinois, New York, and Texas), Florida boasts the largest change in smoking prevalence since 2006[2]; this decline presents favorable opportunities for Tobacco Free Alachua to advocate for policy change regarding smoking.
- More than half of adults in Florida are never-smokers[2]; thus, garnering support from parents is a viable opportunity.
- Prevalence of smoking decreases sharply with increasing education[2]; thus, by educating Alachua County citizens, consumption is likely to decrease.

Threats to Tobacco Free Alachua:

- E-cigarette consumption in the United States is on the rise,[3] especially among youth.
- Young people are more likely to use flavored tobacco products than adults,[4] and e-cigarettes are available in candy-like flavors.
- Although not yet proven, e-cigarettes are being marketed as a safer and healthier alternative to tobacco smoking.
- The average smoker attempts to quit 8 to 11 times before succeeding.[5] E-cigarettes present current smokers with an alternative to smoking cessation.
- The federal government has not taken a stance on the sale of e-cigarettes, and these products are currently regulated only at the state and municipal levels.
- E-cigarettes are sold and marketed online, making them easily accessible to adolescents and free from advertising regulations established by the Federal Trade Commission.

References

1. U.S. Department of Health and Human Services. *The Health Consequences of Smoking—50 Years of Progress: A Report of the Surgeon General.* Atlanta, GA: U.S. Department of Health and Human Services, Centers for Disease Control and Prevention, National Center for Chronic Disease Prevention and Health Promotion, Office on Smoking and Health, 2014:1–22.
2. Centers for Disease Control and Prevention. *Behavioral Risk Factor Surveillance System Survey Data.* Atlanta, GA: U.S. Department of Health and Human Services, Centers for Disease Control and Prevention;2010.

3. Centers for Disease Control and Prevention. E-cigarette use more than doubles among U.S. middle and high school students from 2011–2012. 2013. http://www.cdc.gov/media/releases/2013/p0905-ecigarette-use.html. Accessed January 15, 2014.

4. U.S. Food and Drug Administration. FDA parental advisory on flavored tobacco products: what you need to know. March 7, 2011. http://www.fda.gov/downloads/TobaccoProducts/ProtectingKidsfromTobacco/FlavoredTobacco/UCM183262.pdf. Accessed January 27, 2014.

5. DiClemente CC. *Addiction and Change: How Addictions Develop and Addicted People Recover.* New York, NY: Guilford Press; 2003.

Belva N, Hojnacki R, Justice A., Rodriguez S, Susock S. 2014. Proposed public health communications campaign for tobacco free Alachua. Presented in partial fulfillment of the requirements for the degree of Master of Arts in Mass Communication, University of Florida.

■ Deontological principles. Much of public health is also based on **deontological** (duty-based) **principles**, such as "Stick to honorable principles, and the outcomes will take care of themselves." Many in public health believe a just outcome (or end) cannot be achieved through unjust means. A public health program that requires participants to demonstrate economic or nutritional need is an example of a deontological system, as it uses rules—and not privilege (or bribery)—to distribute resources.

■ The Golden Rule. This is probably the first ethical principle that anyone learns. In the Judeo-Christian tradition, it first appears in the Bible in Leviticus, where it is roughly translated as "Love thy neighbor as thyself." The Golden Rule eventually was popularized as "Do unto others as you would have them do unto you." Almost every religion and society recognize the concept of putting oneself in another's place before doing something, for good or for bad. Most public health organizations, but particularly those run by charitable organizations, put "caring" for individuals and their rights and feelings at the top of their core values.

■ Other rights and privileges. From the Declaration of Independence, we remember this statement: "We hold these truths to be self-evident, that all men are created equal, that they are endowed by their Creator with certain unalienable Rights, that among these are Life, Liberty and the pursuit of Happiness." Just how far an individual's right to liberty in the pursuit of happiness may go is often described, in common speech, is as far as the end of someone else's nose—a utilitarian interpretation of life, liberty, and the pursuit of happiness.

In public health, these principles are often pitted against one another. For example, those who suggest that street drugs should be legalized might argue, "In a free country, people should be allowed to harm themselves, as long as they do not hurt anyone else in the process." This is a complicated argument that might wind up comparing the damage to society from crime associated with drug dealing with the individual harm caused by drug ingestion. But what about the healthcare issues associated with drugs—should society bear these costs? Where do harm-reduction strategies, such as a needle exchange programs to offset the additional risks for HIV and hepatitis infection associated with injectable drug use, fall on the moral compass?

Compared with these difficult ethical dilemmas, the ones associated with health communication might seem relatively straightforward. Some will be discussed later in the context of audience research and pretesting, such as "The content will not stigmatize any groups" (e.g., children with birth defects, or persons with HIV) or "We will refrain from using messages that present people who engage in certain behavior in a negative way." There is no absolute way to resolve these dilemmas, because different communities and different cultures will apply their own values and principles in developing solutions. Moreover, as mentioned previously, different political parties in the United States are associated with allowing or disallowing government-sponsored mass-media messages pertaining to, for example, risks of tobacco, risks associated with private ownership of firearms, and use of condoms for prevention of sexually transmitted disease and birth control. Likewise, these values and associated moral codes will vary widely in international settings.

The choice of informing versus persuading may pose an ethical dilemma in some circumstances. One might think, "If I feel strongly that this harms you, or this may help you, shouldn't I use every means at my disposal to convince you of my position?" The very act of selecting a population as the target of a health communication campaign, as well as prioritizing an issue, means that some people and some issues are left out. **BOX 3-10** features a list of ethical issues identified by CDC in *CDCynergy* as most relevant to conducting a SWOTE analysis for a health communications program. It is based on the framework developed by Guttman and Salmon.[23]

Strategic Thinking

Once the logic model and SWOTE analysis are in place, how are they used? To understand their role, we must think about the SWOTE in terms of when and how it might affect the process described in the logical framework.

BOX 3-10   Ethical Considerations in Public Health Communication

Bioethics[e]

Bioethics is the branch of ethics, philosophy, and social commentary that discusses the life sciences and their potential impact on our society. A set of principles or guidelines that are based on bioethics can articulate and assess ethical and moral dilemmas. These ethical guidelines may include the following:

- The obligation to avoid doing harm through the actions of trying to help.
- The obligation to do good by doing one's utmost to better the health of the intended populations.
- Respect for the freedom of every person and community to make their own decisions according to what they think would be best for them.
- Ensuring adherence to justice, equity, and fairness in the distribution of resources, and providing for those who are particularly vulnerable or who have special needs.
- Maximizing the greatest utility from the health promotion efforts, especially when resources are limited and are publicly funded, and considering the good of the public as a whole.

Ethical Considerations Through the Stages of Program Design and Implementation

Each facet of the intervention needs to be examined to determine whether it meets these precepts. The questions provided here can facilitate the application of the precepts to each stage or facet of the intervention and the identification of ethical issues.

Goal-Setting Stage

- Who decides what the goals of the intervention should be?
- Who is targeted by the intervention, and who is excluded?
  - Why was the targeted population chosen?
  - Were populations with the greatest needs targeted or those who were more likely to adopt the recommendations?
- Are representatives of the intervention's target population involved in goal setting?
- How will consent be obtained from the intervention's targeted populations? Are issues that are more relevant to mainstream populations given higher priority?

Designing and Implementation

- Collaboration:
  - Could collaboration with community or other voluntary organizations, with the idea of advancing participation and empowerment, actually serve to exploit these organizations by consuming their limited resources?
  - Are particular organizations made to feel forced to participate in the intervention's activities?
- Use of persuasive strategies and message design:
  - Which kinds of persuasive appeals are used, and to what extent might they be considered to be manipulative?
  - Are the messages persuasive enough?
  - Do they unduly exploit cultural themes or symbols?

---

e. Which ethical principles underlie these decisions?

- Messages on responsibility:
  - Do the messages imply that if people get an adverse medical condition, it is their fault because they did not do enough to prevent it? Such messages might be viewed as potentially harmful because they may literally blame people and make them feel guilty when various circumstances prevent them from adopting the recommended practices.
  - Do the messages make it appear that one person is responsible for preventing others from taking health risks (e.g., spouse, friend, employee)? That is, how much is one person responsible for others?
- Messages that may stigmatize or make people overly anxious:
  - Do messages that try to get people to avoid unwanted health conditions (e.g., AIDS, stroke, smoking) portray those who have the conditions in a negative light?
  - Does the intervention raise the level of anxiety, fear, or guilt among target populations?
- Messages that may make people feel deprived:
  - Does the intervention tell people to avoid doing certain things that give them pleasure, but not provide them with affordable and rewarding alternatives?
  - Does the campaign tell people to avoid cultural practices that are of particular significance to them?
- Messages that make promises that cannot be fulfilled:
  - Does the intervention make promises for good health when it urges people to adopt particular practices, even though those promises might not be fulfilled?
  - Does the intervention contribute to increased demands on the healthcare system, which may not be able to meet the demands?
- Messages that turn health into an ultimate value:
  - Do the messages stress that health is an important value that should be vigorously pursued, and does the intervention make it sound as if those who do not pursue good health are less virtuous or have vices?
  - Does the intervention contribute to making health an ideal or a super value that people need to pursue resolutely?
- Messages that may distract:
  - Does the intervention focus on specific health topics, thereby possibly distracting people from thinking about and pursuing activities related to other important issues?
  - Does the intervention focus on individual behavior changes, and, by so doing, distract people from thinking about the importance of social factors that influence health? That is, are downstream behaviors being blamed before upstream problems for population health?
- Control of people in work organizations:
  - Do interventions that take place in work organizations, although they may be efficient, present opportunities for employers to control the private lives of their employees?

Evaluation Stage

- Who decides the evaluation criteria and the success of the intervention?
- Are the targeted populations and the intervention practitioners involved in the assessment process?

Modified from CDCynergy, http://www.cdc.gov/dhdsp/cdcynergy_training/Content/phase2/phase2step5content.htm. CDCynergy, developed by the Division of Health Communication of CDC.

Managing Strengths and Weaknesses

The strengths and weaknesses identified through the SWOTE analysis are most likely to affect the program inputs.

- Is the program based on the organizational strengths and those of the intervention?
- If not, how can these strengths feature more prominently in the intervention?
- How can the program fix each weakness?

- Do the strengths and weaknesses of the partners balance each other out? This can be a critical question when deciding on partner arrangements.
- Is the proposed program too far from the core business of the organization? (If the mission of the university is to educate students, can a health communication campaign be conducted in the community?)
- Should the program be rethought before the investment in it is too great?

Maximizing Opportunities and Defending Against Threats

Here are the questions that need to be asked (and answered!) about opportunities and threats to achieve the desired outputs and outcomes:

- How can the program exploit each opportunity?
- What must be changed to exploit an opportunity?
- Which does the program maximize: achievement of outputs or achievement of outcomes?
- Are additional alliances needed to take advantage of an opportunity?
- How can the program defend against each threat?
- How realistic are the threats, and how great a risk do they pose?
- When are threats to be accounted for—between inputs and outputs or between outputs and outcomes?
- Are additional alliances necessary to defend against these threats?

"Baking In" Ethics

How can the program and/or organization be fair and conduct the intervention in the most ethical manner possible?

- What are the bases of these decisions?
- What needs to be changed, if anything, to prioritize human rights, gender equity, or other ethical issues over short-term programmatic gains?
- Are more partners needed to accomplish these changes?

As mentioned earlier, the SWOTE analysis is best done with partners and stakeholders. Define the S, W, O, T, and E factors and rank-order them. In most cases, the greatest amount of attention is devoted to the top five items in each of the SWOTE lists. The other items should not be ignored, but they will probably not need to be addressed at the launch of the intervention. Compare the strengths and opportunities for the program against the weaknesses and threats, and use the results of this comparison to make a "go/no-go" decision. Perhaps the program needs to be postponed to allow for an opportunity to emerge, to wait out a threat, or to form a stronger alliance and attract more resources. Alternatively, perhaps the deadline may need to be moved up, for some of the same reasons. These strategic decisions are part of the final plan.

▶ Conclusion

The first stage of health communication planning involves forgetting about communication details and focusing on the major goals and the best ways to reach them. This is the macro plan—that is, the big picture, an overall view of the projects and its components. The macro plan is often developed in consultation with organizational partners, each of whom will have a topical focus, a methodological expertise, and a constituency base. The appendix to this chapter illustrates the application of this principle in a well-developed communication plan to promote all-terrain vehicle (ATV) safety in the United States.

Wrap-Up

Chapter Questions

1. What are the key steps to developing a macro plan for a health communication intervention?
2. Sketch out the basics of the PRECEDE–PROCEED model.
3. What are the differences between informing and persuading your intended audience?
4. Define social marketing. Do you think it is an appropriate approach to use in health communication?
5. What are some criteria for choosing partners for a health communication intervention?
6. Using the ecological model, describe when health communication is most effective and give an example of at least one communication tool at each level.
7. Which information would you need to have to create a logic model for your intervention?

References

1. Noar SM, Althouse BM, Ayers JW, Francis DB, Ribisl KM. Cancer information seeking in the digital age: effects of Angelina Jolie's prophylactic mastectomy announcement. *Med Decis Making* 2015;35(1):16–21. doi: 10.1177/0272989X14556130.

2. Juthe RH, Zaharchuk A, Wang C. Celebrity disclosures and information seeking the case of Angelina Jolie. *Genetics Med.* 2015;17(7): 45–53.

3. Bryant CA, Brown KR, McDermott R, et al. Community-based prevention marketing: organizing a community for health behavior intervention. *Health Promot Pract.* 2007;8:154–163.

4. Public Health Foundation. Planning before you communicate tool. http://www.phf.org/resourcestools/Pages/Planning_Before_You_Communicate_Tool.aspx. Accessed August 16, 2015.

5. Noar SM. An audience-channel-message-evaluation (ACME) framework for health communication campaigns. *Health Promot Pract.* 2012;13(4):481–488. doi: 10.1177/1524839910386901.

6. Institute of Medicine. Communicating to advance the public's health: workshop summary. March 17, 2015. http://iom.nationalacademies.org/Reports/2015/Communicate-to-Advance-Publics-Health.aspx. Accessed August 16, 2015.

7. Wakefield MA, Loken B, Hornik RC. Use of mass media campaigns of change health behavior. *Lancet.* 2010;376(9748):1261–1271. doi: 10.1016/S0140-6736(10)60809-4.

8. Robinson MN, Tansil KA, Elder RW, et al. Mass media health communication campaigns combined with health-related product distribution: a community guide systematic review. *Am J Prev Med.* 2014;47(3):360–371. doi:10.1016/j.amepre.2014.05.034.

9. U.S. Department of Health and Human Services, National Institutes of Health, National Cancer Institute. Making health communication programs work. NIH Publication No. 04-5145. 2004. http://pinkbook.cancer.gov. or http://www.cancer.gov/publications/health-communication/pink-book.pdf accessed September 8, 2016.

10. Green LW, Kreuter MW. *Health Promotion Planning: An Educational and Ecological Approach* (3rd ed.). New York, NY: McGraw-Hill; 1999.

11. National Cancer Institute. Theory at a glance: a guide for health promotion practice (2nd ed.). NIH Publication No. 05-3896. 2005. http://cancercontrol.cancer.gov/brp/research/theories_project/theory.pdf accessed September 8, 2016.

12. Edberg M. *Essentials of Health Behavior. Social and Behavioral Theory in Public Health.* Sudbury, MA: Jones and Bartlett; 2007.

13. Maibach EW, Abroms LC, Marosits M. Communication and marketing as tools to cultivate the public's health: a proposed "people and places" framework. *BMC Public Health.* 2007;7. doi: 10.1186/1471-2458-7-88.

14. Heldman AB, Schindelar J, Weaver JB III. Social media engagement and public health communication: implications for public health organizations being truly "social." *Public Health Rev.* 2013;35. http://www.publichealthreviews.eu/show/i/13 Accessed September 8, 2016.

15. Moorhead SA, Hazlett DE, Harrison L, Carroll JK, Irwin A, Hoving C. A new dimension of health care: systematic review of the uses, benefits, and limitations of social media for health communication. *J Med Internet Res.* 2013;15(4):e85.

16. Centers for Disease Control and Prevention. CDC enterprise social media policy. Issued September 14, 2011; updated January 8, 2015. http://www.cdc.gov/socialmedia/tools/guidelines/pdf/social-media-policy.pdf. Accessed August 16, 2015.

17. Parvanta C, Maibach E, Arkin E, Nelson DE, Woodward J. Public health communication: a planning framework. In: Nelson DE, Brownson RC, Remington PL, Parvanta C, eds. *Communicating Public Health Information Effectively: A Guide for Practitioners.* Washington, DC: American Public Health Association; 2002:4–15.

18. Rothschild, ML. Carrots, sticks, and promises: a conceptual framework for the management of public health and social issue behaviors. *J Marketing.* 1999;63:24–37.

19. Lefebvre RC, Flora JA. Social marketing and public health intervention. *Health Educ Qtly.* 1988;15:299–315.

20. Goodstadt M. The use of logic models in health promotion practice. February 2005. http://logicmodel.weebly.com/uploads/1/7/0/1/17017646/the_use_of_logic_models_in_health_promotion.pdf. Accessed September 8, 2016.

21. Knowlton LW, Phillips CC. *The Logic Model Guidebook: Better Strategies for Great Results.* Thousand Oaks, CA: Sage; 2009.

22. W.K. Kellogg Foundation logic model development guide. 2001. http://www.wkkf.org/resource-directory/resource/2006/02/wk-kellogg-foundation-logic-model-development-guide.

23. Guttman N, Salmon CT. Guilt, fear, stigma and knowledge gaps: ethical issues in public health communication interventions. *Bioethics.* 2004;18(6):1467–8519.

Appendix 3

ATV Safety: You Make the Choice Case Analysis

Maria Brann, PhD, MPH, and **Brandi N. Frisby**, PhD

Step	Information
TABLE 3A-1 Macro Plan Template	
1	Analyze the problem and its place in the ecological framework.
1.1	Health problem statement: What is occurring? Who is affected, and to what degree? What should be occurring? What could happen if problem is not resolved?
1.2	What needs to change? Individual behavior, policies, environmental conditions?
2	*Primary intervention*: What is it? What is the evidence base? What are its advantages and disadvantages?
	What needs to happen for this intervention to solve the problem? Which role will communication play: primary or support?
3	Identify the primary, secondary, and other audiences.
4	For each audience, will you inform, empower, or persuade them?
5	Which core strategy will you use (education, marketing, advocacy/law)?
6	Who needs to be a partner in your coalition? What is their overall partnering role? (Access to people, task specific.)
7	Logic model and SWOT analysis

▶ Phase 1: Describe Problem

Write a Problem Statement

Approximately 25 million Americans ride all-terrain vehicles (ATVs),[1] and ATV popularity has contributed to an increase in injuries and fatalities. The estimated number of ATV injuries that required emergency room treatment increased 33% over a 5-year period, from 110,100 injuries in 2001 to 146,600 injuries in 2006.[2] Nationally, between 2007 and 2011, 1701 people died in ATV accidents.[3] The problem is most alarming in West Virginia, which reported the third highest number of deaths and ranked first in terms of the ATV-injury death rate based on population.[3]

Assess the Problem's Relevance to Your Program

Public research universities have a responsibility to conduct research that can benefit the community in which the university is situated. Given the health communication focus of the academic program, it is vital that as academicians we research the most pressing issues affecting our community. West Virginia has been recognized as one of the most dangerous places to ride an ATV.[4] Despite the danger, an estimated 460,000 ATVs are owned in West Virginia, with another 16,000 being purchased yearly.[5] West Virginia ATV injuries and fatalities have been well documented, with 15% of all ATV literature in the United States focusing solely on West Virginia.[6]

Explore Who Should Be on the Planning Team and How Team Members Will Interact

Original stakeholders who were considered to be on the research team included:

- University researchers
- Researchers-in-training
- ATV riders
- Local business owners (e.g., ATV retailers)

Examine and/or Conduct Necessary Research to Describe the Problem

The university researchers and researchers-in-training consulted a number of sources to understand the scope of the problem. Research from peer-reviewed journals and popular press news stories were used.

Despite the small population in West Virginia, the number of reported ATV deaths per capita is eight times higher than the national average,[5] and crashes have been reported in all but four counties of the state. For nearly 20 years, West Virginia has had the highest population-based ATV-injury death rates.[6] On average, 26 ATV-related deaths occurred annually in West Virginia between 2000 and 2004; since the enactment of ATV safety legislation, West Virginia has averaged 45 deaths annually.[6] In 2006, at least 53 people were killed in ATV crashes—a state record and the highest per capita death toll in the United States.[7] Data from 2007–2011 (the most current data available) identified West Virginia as the top state for ATV deaths, with 104.9 fatalities from

this cause per 10 million.[3] Crashes that go unreported could add significantly to these already high numbers, providing additional support for the need for a safety intervention.

Determine and Describe Distinct Subgroups Affected by the Problem

The high rates of morbidity and mortality for children younger than 16 years of age is especially alarming. One-third of all fatal ATV accidents involve a child younger than age 16.[2] Injuries have increased substantially across every ATV driver age group, including an increase of 76% for children ages 12 to 15, 23% for children ages 6 to 11, and a staggering increase of 233% for children 5 and younger.[8] Further, 26% of all fatal ATV crashes involve a child younger than age 16 and 44% involve a child younger than age 12.[2] Thus, the current risk levels related to ATV use are high for the pediatric population.

Because of the drastic increase in injuries in the pre-teen population and this age group's ability to make their own decisions (as compared to a child who is younger than age 5), we chose to target adolescent ATV riders.

Write a Problem Statement for Each Subgroup You Plan to Consider Further

Adolescent ATV riders (i.e., between the ages of 11 and 15) are not consistently following safe riding practices, which could save their lives. Additionally, this group is under pressure from their social network, including friends and family, to participate in ATV riding, as it is a culturally salient activity. This pressure includes the desire to appear confident, skilled, and courageous when riding, which encourages risky behaviors and avoidance of safety precautions.

Gather Information Necessary to Describe Each Subproblem Defined in the New Problem Statement

Formative focus group data and existing research indicate that ATV riders establish unsafe practices before turning 16 years old. Many focus group participants described riding as a passenger on ATVs as small children and subsequently driving ATVs when in middle school. The majority of individuals involved in ATV crashes are between the ages of 11 and 15 years.[9,10]

Assess Factors and Variables That Can Affect the Project's Direction
Strengths

- ATV campaigns with adolescents have shown to be effective in some areas.[11,12]
- Adolescent campaigns appealing to decision making are most effective.[13]

Weaknesses

- Funding for the project was limited.
- Getting institutional review board (IRB) approval for a project involving children is difficult.
- The campaign designers were non-ATV riders and not native to West Virginia.

Opportunities

- West Virginia has one of the highest morbidity rates for ATV crashes, and a local adolescent was recently killed making the topic, and timing, salient to many people.
- Safety legislation has not been effective,[14] so a new approach is needed.

Threats

- Lack of perceived risk among the target audience
- Lack of control by the target audience (e.g., adolescents had no purchasing power for safety equipment)
- Intervention viewed as adversarial against a culturally ingrained activity

▶ Phase 2: Analyze Problem

List the Direct and Indirect Causes of Each Subproblem That May Require Intervention

According to focus group research data, adolescent ATV riders are not practicing safe riding practices for the following reasons:

- Low knowledge of safe riding practices, such as appropriate-sized machines, necessary gear, and legal restrictions
- Lack of control (e.g., they are unable to purchase safety equipment)
- Apathetic attitude toward safety

- Unsafe riding norms
- Inability to use safety measures (e.g., cost of equipment, unavailability of equipment)
- Invincible attitudes
- Lack of enforcement of laws

Prioritize and Select Subproblems That Need Intervention

For this intervention, the following subproblems were selected:

- ATV riders' knowledge
- ATV riders' attitudes
- ATV riders' norms
- ATV riders' perceived behavioral control
- ATV riders' intentions

Write Goals for Each Subproblem

To address these safety problems, the following goals were established:

- Increase adolescent ATV riders' knowledge of safe riding practices
- Improve adolescent ATV riders' attitudes toward safety behaviors
- Change adolescent ATV riders' normative riding behaviors
- Increase adolescent ATV riders' perceived behavioral control about safety practices
- Increase adolescent ATV riders' intentions to practice safe riding behaviors

Examine Relevant Theories and Best Practices for Potential Intervention
Relevant Theoretical Frameworks

The Theory of Planned Behavior (TPB)[15,16] is one widely used theoretical lens for understanding behaviors and developing messages.[17] TPB argues that attitudes (i.e., evaluation of performing behavior), subjective norms (i.e., perception of social reaction), behavioral control (i.e., performing behavior under one's control), and intentions (i.e., likelihood of performing behavior) are important factors to consider when predicting behaviors.

The Health Belief Model (HBM)[18] is one of the most widely used models for explaining health-related behaviors.[19] This guiding framework assesses perceived threats (i.e., severity and susceptibility), outcome expectations (i.e., perceived benefits and barriers), self-efficacy (i.e., capability of alleviating threat), and cues to action to engage in a desired behavior.

Social marketing[20] is a consumer-oriented process that works through a series of steps to identify and describe a problem and then develop, implement, and evaluate messages to promote behavior change.

Health Communication/Education Best Practices

Scholars and practitioners have argued that targeted educational interventions are vital for decreasing the ATV death and injury rates among children.[21] The educational intervention followed several pedagogical best practices to enhance its message design and participant outcomes, including best practices related to message relevance, clarity, memorable messages, immediacy, and addressing all learning styles. Specifically, scholars have declared it imperative that health behavior messages be relevant,[22] clear,[11] memorable,[23] and credible,[24] so as to increase the intervention's effects on primary target learning and behavioral change.

Consider SWOT and the Ethics of the Intervention Options

Strengths

- Positive association between safety training and always wearing helmets, never riding with/as passengers, and never riding on paved roads[12]
- Training in educational settings, showing a realistic understanding of current ATV practices, and emphasizing consequences exert the most influence over riders[25]
- Relationships found between knowledge about unsafe behaviors and attitudes toward behaviors[26]

Weaknesses

- Large-scale health communication interventions require funding, which is limited.
- Communication cannot overcome some tangible barriers such as the cost of safety equipment.
- Only some middle schools provided access, assistance, and support.

Opportunities

- The research team has expertise in developing health communication messages.

Threats

- Competing normative messages for unsafe behaviors coming from influential others (e.g., family, friends)

Ethics

- Campaign materials had to be developed to be sensitive so as not to offend families who promote—knowingly or unknowingly—this unsafe lifestyle.
- Implementing a campaign in school can generate criticism about the school's role and responsibility in outside behaviors.
- Unable to provide campaign to all students who are potentially affected (due to time, geography, school and parental permissions).
- Need to be sensitive to the development of age-appropriate materials.

For Each Subproblem, Select the Intervention You Plan to Use

An educational health communication intervention with adolescent ATV riders was selected as the focus. When implemented sufficiently and continuously throughout planning, development, delivery, and assessment, health communication messages that are grounded in data and theory can be especially successful in addressing each of the subproblems. Specifically, the health communication strategies can address awareness, knowledge, control, responses to social norms, attitudes, and behaviors.

Explore Additional Resources and New Partners

With a focus on adolescents, and the data supporting interventions in educational settings, it was agreed that schools might be the best site of intervention given that all adolescents are legally required to attend school until the age of 16. With this resource, additional partners included:

- School administrators
- School teachers

Acquire Funding and Solidify Partnerships

Each county's Board of Education (BOE) was contacted. After hearing a persuasive presentation from the researchers, which included information about the design of the project and sample curriculum students would receive, the BOEs agreed to partner on this project. Their support provided the necessary incentive for middle school administrators to partner with the project as well. Health and physical education teachers then joined the project to facilitate its promotion through the use of the health and/or physical education class time and locations. These partners further assisted with disseminating, collecting, and returning permission forms and pre-test data collection.

▶ Phase 3: Plan Intervention

For Each Subproblem, Determine if the Intervention Is Dominant

A health communication education intervention delivered in middle schools was selected as the dominant target to address all subproblems (i.e., knowledge, attitudes, norms, perceived behavioral control, and intentions).

Determine Whether Potential Audiences Contain Any Subgroups (Audience Segments)

Adolescent ATV riders were selected as primary targets for this intervention. Peers of this target audience group were selected as a secondary target, with the goal of educating them so that they could influence their friends' safe riding behaviors.

Finalize Intended Audiences

Adolescents between the ages of 11 and 15 who are ATV riders in north-central West Virginia were selected as primary targets for this intervention.

Write Communication Goals for Each Audience Segment

The long-term goal for the target audience was to have all pre-teen ATV riders practice safe riding behaviors. To achieve this ultimate goal, short-term goals included increased knowledge of safe riding practices, more pro-safety attitudes, perceived safe riding normative behaviors, heightened self-efficacy, and increased intentions to perform safe riding practices.

The goal for the secondary audience was to communicate safe-riding practices to ATV riders.

Examine and Decide on Communication-Relevant Theories and Models

Social marketing principles were used throughout the process to conduct formative research, determine the marketing mix, implement the intervention, and evaluate the campaign. The Theory of Planned Behavior was also used to frame the formative research, message design, and evaluation of the intervention.

Undertake Formative Research

Thirteen focus group discussions and two interviews were held with 79 ATV riders. Of the participants, 65 students (42 males, 23 females) participated in 10 face-to-face focus groups (with an average of 6 participants per focus group) and one face-to-face interview; 8 community members (2 males, 6 females) participated in two online focus groups (with 4 and 3 participants, respectively) and one online interview; and 6 male employees of an ATV dealership participated in one face-to-face focus group. Diverse groups of ATV riders (e.g., varying ages, both sexes, differing riding experience levels) were chosen in an attempt to elicit multiple perspectives on ATV riding behaviors. The adult participants reported retrospectively on their ATV riding as adolescents, and some reported on their children's riding habits.

Write Profiles for Each Audience Segment
Primary Target Audience: Adolescent ATV Riders

To summarize some of the key findings of the research, the data revealed that ATV riders were aware of safe and legal riding behaviors; however, they predominately engaged in unsafe behaviors. For example, many participants claimed that they did not wear helmets primarily due to discomfort or inconvenience. They also saw members of their riding networks engaging in the same unsafe behaviors, which reinforced the contention that they are influenced to engage in similar unsafe behaviors practiced by their friends, siblings, and parents. Some participants noted that traumatic events had the potential to change their unsafe behaviors, as did ATV safety training. Behavioral changes that resulted from traumatic events, however, were short-lived. In other words, the riders possessed knowledge about ATV safety, but there was a disconnect between using this knowledge to engage in safer behaviors; this disconnect could be explained by negative attitudes toward safety, poor demonstration of behavioral control, and negative influences from family and friends who were fellow ATV riders.

Rewrite Goals as Measurable Communication Objectives

- Within five months post intervention, increase adolescent ATV riders' knowledge scores of safe riding practices.
- Within five months post intervention, improve adolescent ATV riders' attitudes toward safety behaviors.
- Within five months post intervention, positively change adolescent ATV riders' normative riding behaviors.
- Within five months post intervention, increase adolescent ATV riders' perceived behavioral control about safety practices.
- Within five months post intervention, increase the number of adolescent ATV riders who intend to practice safe riding behaviors.
- Within five months post intervention, increase the number of adolescent ATV riders who engage in safe riding practices.

Write Creative Briefs

Intended Audience

The target audience included adolescents, ages 11 to 15, who live in north-central West Virginia and ride ATVs.

Objectives

Persuade adolescent ATV riders to practice safe riding behaviors every time they are on an ATV.

Obstacles

- Adolescent ATV riders have already developed unsafe riding habits that are difficult to change.
- The social norms surrounding ATV riding encourage unsafe riding practices.
- A lackadaisical attitude toward safe riding behaviors exists in the ATV riding community.
- Adolescents do not have the funds to purchase safety equipment and must depend on others to provide it for them.

Key Promise

If I practice safe riding behaviors, I will reduce my chance of serious injury or death.

Support Statements/Reasons Why

- As many as 92% of injuries and deaths are attributed to controllable behaviors and can be prevented by wearing proper safety gear and/or riding the appropriate-sized machine.[2]

Tone

To reach the target audience, the communication had to be engaging and not condescending. The presentation also needed to be fun, yet still convey the seriousness of the topic.

Media

The messages were distributed via educational in-person presentations, posters, brochures, activity packets, and branded promotional items (e.g., pencils, bracelets).

Openings

The best opportunity to research the target audience was during the school day while the students were at school. Presenting information in health and physical education classes reached the target audience in a comfortable and relevant setting. The intervention was also delivered in early spring before the primary riding season began in April.

Creative Considerations

Activity packets were created with fun activities (e.g., crossword puzzles, word searches, drawing pages) to engage the participants and give them something to do after the presentation to keep the message salient.

Confirm Plans with Stakeholders

School teachers and administrators were given copies of the curriculum and supplemental items to ensure that everyone was aware of, and provided teaching consistent with, the messages presented. It was agreed that evaluation results would be shared with school officials, participants, and participants' parents.

▸ Phase 4: Develop Intervention

Draft Timetable, Budget, and Plan for Developing and Testing Communication Mix

A working plan was developed, which included a proposed timeline and budget for development, implementation, and evaluation.

Develop and Test Creative Concepts

During several brainstorming sessions with campaign developers and a small group of students (approximately 12), creative concepts were developed for testing. Several different ideas were explored before determining the exact focus of the messages. Tagline ideas generated included Pass on Passengers, S.A.D.D. Riding: Students Against Destructive Decisions when Riding, Master the Machine, Get the Gear, Explore Your Environment, Learn Your Limits, and Make a Choice, among others. Through discussions with campaign designers, teachers, and ATV riders, it was determined that the message needed to include factual, legal information that was all-encompassing because there are several different safety behaviors that should be—but are not currently—being enacted. Additionally, it was determined that the message needed to recognize the budding autonomy of this age group so that it would not sound "preachy."

Develop and Pre-test Messages

A tagline was selected: *ATV Safety: You Make the CHOICE*. A contest was then held, allowing students (who were not necessarily part of the intervention) to produce a logo to be used with the tagline. A panel of researchers reviewed their submissions and selected the logo believed to be the most appealing and relevant. Materials were developed using the tagline and logo and shown to 35 students to assess. Through an open-ended survey and focus group discussion, the following ideas were explored:

- Perception of the main point of the materials
- Appeal
- Readability
- Comprehension
- Suggestions for improvements

Pre-test and Select Settings

The target audience consisted of adolescents, and the only place where all adolescents are required to be is school. Therefore, the health and physical education classrooms in middle schools were the setting for the intervention.

Select, Integrate, and Test Channel-Specific Communication Activities

Working with the available resources, an in-person presentation was selected as the most viable communication channel. After speaking with target audience members, it was determined that a hands-on approach would be best.

Identify and/or Develop, Pre-test, and Select Materials

Materials included a curriculum, posters announcing the presentation, brochures, activity packets, and branded products.

Based on previous research, all of the final materials were branded with the tagline *ATV Safety: You Make the CHOICE*. The message was consistent that adolescents had autonomy to make a choice, and the best choice would be a safe one. Specific messages included how to be safe. Students were encouraged to Check their gear, Handle the machine appropriately, Observe the riding environment, Ignore negative peer pressure, Coach others about safe behaviors, and Enjoy the ride.

Decide on Roles and Responsibilities of Staff and Partners

The three principal researchers were responsible for developing, testing, delivering, and evaluating the messages. The school partners—that is, the teachers and administrators—were responsible for promoting consistent messages and providing access to the target audience.

Produce Materials for Dissemination

Posters were printed to be placed at each middle school to preview the presentation, brochures and activity packets were printed for each student to take home, and products were ordered for each student (i.e., pencils, bracelets). All materials were packaged together in a branded bag for students.

Finalize and Briefly Summarize the Communication Plan

Background
Intended Audiences
Objectives
Concept and Messages
Settings and Channels
Activities

Share and Confirm the Communication Plan with the Appropriate Stakeholders

The researchers confirmed the intervention plan with the educational partners, who promoted the intervention in their schools.

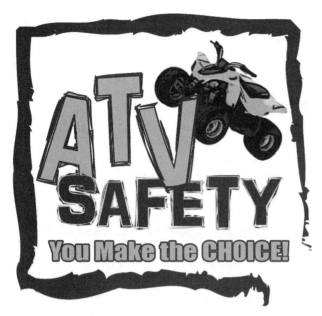

FIGURE 3A-1 ATV logo.

Courtesy of Byrnes K, Frisby BN, Brann M. Using social marketing processes to develop and pilot-test an intervention for pre-teen all-terrain vehicle (ATV) riders. Cases in Public Health Communication & Marketing. 2012;6:45-64. Available from:www.casesjournal .org/volume6.

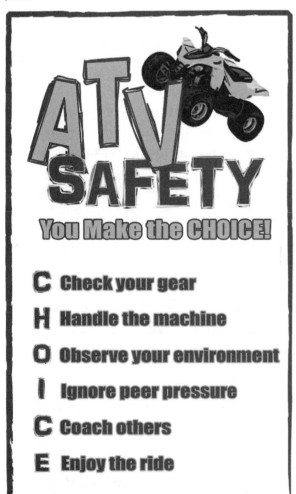

FIGURE 3A-2 ATV brochure.

Courtesy of Byrnes K, Frisby BN, Brann M. Using social marketing processes to develop and pilot-test an intervention for pre-teen all-terrain vehicle (ATV) riders. Cases in Public Health Communication & Marketing. 2012;6:45-64. Available from: www.casesjournal .org/volume6.

▶ Phase 5: Plan Evaluation

Identify and Engage Stakeholders

Stakeholders included the academic researchers and school administrators. The students who participated in the intervention had an interest in improving their safety, and other health communication scholars and public health professionals have an interest in effective messaging strategies.

Describe the Program

The *ATV Safety: You Make the CHOICE* campaign is an ATV safety intervention that:

- Used formative research to develop messages for adolescent ATV riders
- Provided adolescent ATV riders with theoretically framed, evidence-based messages to improve safety
- Evaluated the efficacy of health communication messages to affect knowledge, attitudes, norms, perceived behavioral control, and intentions

Determine Which Information Stakeholders Need and When They Need It

The Board of Education needed to evaluate the curriculum's appropriateness in terms of content and format for the students before granting us permission to visit their schools and implement the intervention. The school administrators and teachers needed the curriculum concepts and schedule before implementation to evaluate the program's relevance and timeliness. All stakeholders needed the summative evaluation upon completion to assess the intervention's effectiveness in reaching the audience with the appropriate message.

Write Intervention Standards That Correspond with the Different Types of Evaluation

The campaign's objectives were chosen as the intervention standards for evaluation purposes:

- Within five months post intervention, increase adolescent ATV riders' knowledge scores of safe riding practices.
- Within five months post intervention, improve adolescent ATV riders' attitudes toward safety behaviors.

- Within five months post intervention, positively change adolescent ATV riders' normative riding behaviors.
- Within five months post intervention, increase adolescent ATV riders' perceived behavioral control about safety practices.
- Within five months post intervention, increase the number of adolescent ATV riders who intend to practice safe riding behaviors.
- Within five months post intervention, increase the number of adolescent ATV riders who engage in safe riding practices.

These objectives were assessed with a pre-test, two-post test survey design.

Determine Sources and Methods That Will Be Used to Gather Data

To evaluate the intervention, surveys were administered to the participants.

Develop an Evaluation Design

After the development and approval of the messages, a baseline survey was administered in February to assess prevailing knowledge, attitudes, norms, perceived behavioral control, intentions, and behaviors related to ATVs. The messages were then delivered in April to (1) align with the beginning of the riding season and (2) work with the schools' request to implement the program prior to standardized testing. In April, students completed a post-assessment survey immediately after exposure to the campaign message; the goal was to evaluate the message's effectiveness in relation to knowledge, attitudes, norms, perceived behavioral control, and intentions as well as to assess the intervention itself. Subsequently, a second post-assessment survey was conducted in September to assess message retention and behavior change following the conclusion of the primary riding season to allow students to integrate what they had learned from the intervention throughout the riding season. According to the Insurance Institute for Highway Safety (2012),[27] most ATV fatalities occur between April and September, the peak riding season, which also supports our time frame for conducting the intervention and evaluation.

Develop a Data Analysis and Reporting Plan

To assess changes in knowledge, attitude, norms, behavioral control, intentions, and behaviors, a series of paired samples t-tests were used to test each of the

items. Once the evaluation was complete, results were disseminated in a report to the educational partners, in a newsletter to participants and participants' parents, and in manuscripts published in academic journals.

Formalize Agreements and Develop Internal and External Communication Plans

Communication of project information occurred via email. This agreed-upon method of communication allowed for a written documentation of communication and was convenient for all partners.

Develop an Evaluation Timetable and Budget

- Baseline data collected: beginning of spring semester (February 2010)
- Immediate post-test data collected: following the intervention toward the end of the spring semester (April 2010)
- Delayed post-test data collected: beginning of the fall semester and end of the peak riding season (September 2010)

Summarize the Evaluation Implementation Plan and Share It with the Staff and Stakeholders

The evaluation plan was agreed upon by the researchers and the dissemination of the evaluation was agreed upon with the partners.

▶ Phase 6: Implement Plan

Integrate Communication and Evaluation Plans

Once everyone agreed upon the plans, they were integrated to ensure the activities were implemented and evaluated.

Execute Communication and Evaluation Plans

Working with individual school systems, dates were selected to present the intervention and timelines were developed around those selected dates. Evaluation surveys and the interactive presentation were implemented in accordance with the agreed-upon timeline.

Manage the Communication and Evaluation Activities

Because the educational partners deferred to the researchers on the project, the campaign was primarily managed through regular communication among the research team members. The partners were kept informed of the progression of the steps through regular communication.

Document Feedback and Lessons Learned

Notes were taken at each meeting, and communication among the researchers occurred at every stage. The research team discussed issues concerning participant involvement (i.e., should parents also be exposed to the workshop) and the timeline of the project (i.e., should the time between assessments be altered). The

project did not move forward until all researchers were in agreement.

Modify Program Components Based on Evaluation Feedback

Responses to communication about the results and procedures have been noted and considered for future development of the campaign.

Disseminate Lessons Learned and Evaluation Findings

Results and process information have been shared in presentation format at professional meetings and in written publications. Additionally, the results of the campaign were shared in newsletter form with each school and each family who participated in the program.

References

1. Helmkamp JC. Family fun—family tragedy: ATV-related deaths involving family members. *Injury Prevent.* 2007;13:426–428.
2. U.S. Consumer Product Safety Commission. 2010 annual report of ATV-related deaths and injuries. December 2011. https://www.cpsc.gov//PageFiles/108609/atv2010.pdf.
3. Williams AF, Oesch SL, McCartt AT, Teoh ER, Sims LB. On-road all terrain-vehicle (ATV) fatalities in the United States. 2013. https://www.adirondackcouncil.org/uploads/pdf/1402318157_ATVfatalitiesinUS_Report.pdf.
4. Helmkamp J. *Stricter legislation could decrease ATV death rate.* 2009. http://www.herald-dispatch.com/opinion/jim-helmkamp-stricter-legislation-could-decrease-atv-death-rate/article_c2d84aa8-05d1-58dc-ad68-26a5d0833153.html.
5. Helmkamp J, Bixler D, Kaplan J, Hall A. All-terrain vehicle fatalities—West Virginia, 1999-2006. *MMWR.* 2008;57:312–315.
6. Helmkamp JC, Ramsey WD, Haas SD, Holmes M. (2008, February). *All-Terrain Vehicle (ATV) Deaths and Injuries in West Virginia: A Summary of Surveillance and Data Sources.* Charleston, WV: Criminal Justice Statistical Analysis Center, West Virginia Division of Criminal Justice Services; February 2008. http://www.dcjs.wv.gov/SAC/Documents/CJSAC_ATVReportFinal.pdf.
7. Associated Press. *State ATV fatalities decrease in 2007. Charleston Gazette.* December 26, 2007. https://www.highbeam.com/doc/1P2-15039586.html. Accessed September 16, 2008.
8. Consumer Federation of America. *ATV safety crisis: America's children still at risk.* 2003. http://www.consumerfed.org/pdfs/atv-safety-crisis-2003-final-all.pdf.
9. Brown RL, Koepplinger ME, Mehlman CT, Gittelman M, Garcia VF. All-terrain vehicle and bicycle crashes in children: epidemiology and comparison of injury severity. *J Pediatr Surg.* 2003;37:375–380.
10. Cvijanovich NZ, Cook LJ, Mann NC, Dean JM. A population-based assessment of all-terrain vehicle injuries. *Pediatrics.* 2001;108:631–635.
11. Atkin CK. Theory and principles of media health campaigns. In: Rice RE, Atkin CK, eds. *Public Communication Campaigns* (3rd ed.). Thousand Oaks, CA: Sage; 2001:49–68.
12. Burgus SK, Madsen MD, Sanderson WT, Rautainen RH. Youths operating all-terrain vehicles: implications for safety education. *J Agromed.* 2009;14:97–104.
13. Austin EW. Reaching young audiences: developmental considerations in designing health messages. In: Maibach E, Parrott RL, eds. *Designing Health Messages: Approaches from Communication Theory and Public Health Practice.* Thousand Oaks, CA: Sage; 1995:114–144.
14. Ross RT, Stuart LK, Davis FE. All-terrain vehicle injuries in children: industry-regulated failure. *Am Surgeon.* 1999;65:870–873.
15. Ajzen I. From intentions to actions: a theory of planned behavior. In: Kuhl J, Beckman J, eds. *Action Control: From Cognition to Behavior.* Heidelberg, Germany: Springer; 1985:11–39.
16. Ajzen I. The theory of planned behavior. *Org Behav Hum Decision Proc.* 1991;50:179–211.
17. Wang X. Integrating the theory of planned behavior and attitude functions: implications for health campaign design. *Health Comm.* 2009;24(5):426–434. doi:10.1080/10410230903023477.
18. Rosenstock IM. Why people use health services. *Milbank Mem Fund Qtly.* 1966;44:94–127.
19. Champion VL, Skinner CS. The health belief model. In: Glanz K, Rimer BK, Viswanath K, eds. *Health Behavior and Health Education. Theory, Research, and Practice* (4th ed.). San Francisco, CA: Jossey-Bass; 2009:45–65.

20. Lee NR, Kotler P. *Social Marketing: Influencing Behaviors for Good* (4th ed.). Thousand Oaks, CA: Sage; 2011.

21. Gadomski A, Ackerman S, Burdick P, Jenkins P. Efficacy of the North American guidelines for children's agricultural tasks in reducing childhood agricultural injuries. *Am J Public Health.* 2006;96:722–727.

22. Rothman AJ, Bartels RD, Wlaschin J, Salovey P. The strategic use of gain- and loss-framed messages to promote healthy behavior: how theory can inform practice. *J Comm.* 2006;56:S202–S220.

23. Daly JA, Vangelisti AL. Skillfully instructing learners: how communicators effectively convey messages. In: Greene JO, Burleson BR, eds. *Handbook of Communication and Social Interaction Skills.* Mahwah, NJ: Lawrence Erlbaum Associates; 2003:871–908.

24. Jones LW, Sinclair RC, Courneya KS. The effects of source credibility and message framing on exercise intentions, behaviors and attitudes: an integration of the elaboration likelihood model and prospect theory. *J Appl Soc Psychol.* 2003;33:179–196.

25. Aitken ME, Graham CJ, Killingsworth JB, Mullins SH, Parnell DN, Dick RM. (2004). All-terrain vehicle injury in children: strategies for prevention. *Injury Prevent.* 2004;10:303–307.

26. Weber K, Martin MM, Members of Comm 401, Corrigan M. Creating persuasive messages advocating organ donation. *Comm Qtly.* 2006;54:67–87.

27. Insurance Institute for Highway Safety. *Motorcycles and ATVs fatality facts.* 2012. http://www.iihs.org/iihs/topics/t/motorcycles/fatalityfacts/motorcycles/2012. Accessed September 12, 2016.

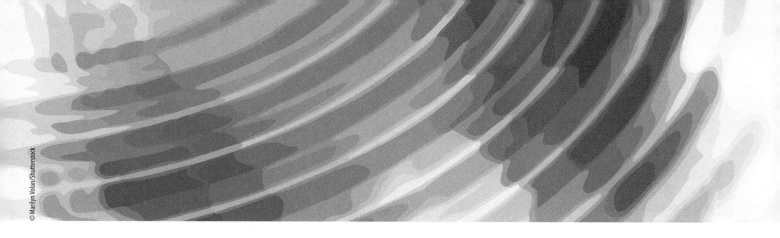

CHAPTER 4

How to Communicate About Data

David E. Nelson

▸ Introduction

The field of public health is based in science, and science is based upon data. Public health practitioners, scientists, researchers, and others need to communicate numerical information, ranging from simple statements ("There were seven new cases of tuberculosis in Pennsylvania last week") to more complicated research findings ("Persons who consume red meat two or more times per week have a 1.3-fold greater risk of developing colon cancer"). The challenge often comes when presenting numerically complex ideas to a public not versed in biostatistics, let alone basic mathematics. This chapter covers the general principles and practice of communicating numerical data to lay audiences; science communication is addressed elsewhere in this text.

▸ Public Health Data Systems

Surveillance Systems

Often considered the cornerstone of public health practice, public health surveillance systems provide a bulk of the data used to assess population health.[1] These systems provide "systematic, ongoing collection, management, analysis, and interpretation of data (e.g., for certain diseases or other health conditions), followed by the dissemination of these data to stimulate public health action."[1,2] Smallpox, tuberculosis, cholera, and other communicable infectious diseases provided the initial stimulus for collecting and monitoring data at the local, state, and finally federal levels in the United States.[1] These initial efforts were meant to pinpoint and respond to outbreaks of illness before they spread. **BOX 4-1** describes two examples of major national surveillance systems that are used extensively to report on notifiable infectious diseases and detect bioterrorist events based on unusual symptoms. **BOX 4-2** provides examples of how surveillance systems were mobilized to inform the public of important health problems.

Where to Find Public Health Data

Public health surveillance data systems also have been added to assess risks and conditions to allow for prevention of illness as well as outbreaks.[14] Although it is not feasible to list all trusted public health data sources, particularly for specific health conditions, injuries, and demographic groups, several websites regularly report current data, show trends over time, or allow users to obtain data for specific population groups (e.g., women aged 18–34 years). **TABLE 4-1**

BOX 4-1 Surveillance and Monitoring Systems Used Extensively in Public Health

National Notifiable Diseases Surveillance System (NNDSS)

NNDSS is a nationwide collaboration that enables agencies at all levels of public health—local, state, territorial, federal, and international—to share notifiable disease-related health information. Public health agencies use this information to monitor, control, and prevent the occurrence and spread of infectious and noninfectious diseases and conditions. The Centers for Disease Control and Prevention (CDC) works in partnership with 57 state, local, and territorial health departments to improve NNDSS. Although disease reporting is mandated by legislation or regulation at the state and local levels, state reporting to the CDC is voluntary. NNDSS staff and health departments also work closely with the Council of State and Territorial Epidemiologists (CSTE).

The list of nationally notifiable infectious diseases is revised periodically. A disease might be added to the list as a new pathogen emerges, or a disease might be deleted as its incidence declines. The list of diseases considered notifiable varies by state and by year. In 2015, there were 107 notifiable conditions, beginning, in alphabetical order, with *Anaplasma phagocytophilum* and ending with yellow fever.[1]

National Syndromic Surveillance Program (NSSP)

A syndrome is a collection of symptoms and findings that may suggest or define a particular disease or disorder. The NSSP emphasizes the use of near "real-time" patient data, primarily from emergency departments, and statistical tools to detect and characterize unusual activity for further public health investigation or response. Syndromic surveillance has now become a routine component of the larger public health surveillance effort and is used for disease or hazardous event detection, situation awareness for mass gatherings and public health emergencies, and ad hoc and population health trend analyses.

For more than a decade, BioSense has been a driver of syndromic surveillance nationwide. The CDC is now evolving BioSense into a National Syndromic Surveillance Program (NSSP) that will build upon the lessons already learned and harness syndromic surveillance expertise at all levels of the public health enterprise. The vision of NSSP is that of a collaboration among local, state, and national public health programs that supports timely exchange of syndromic data and information for nationwide situational awareness and enhanced response to hazardous events and disease outbreaks.[2]

National Vital Statistics System (NVSS)

The NVSS provides the United States' official vital statistics data based on the collection and registration of birth and death events at the state and local levels. The CDC's National Center for Health Statistics (NCHS) works in partnership with the vital registration systems in each jurisdiction to produce critical information on such topics as teenage births and birth rates, prenatal care and birth weight, risk factors for adverse pregnancy outcomes, infant mortality rates, leading causes of death, and life expectancy.[3]

References

1. Centers for Disease Control and Prevention, National Notifiable Diseases Surveillance System. https://wwwn.cdc.gov/nndss/conditions/notifiable/2016/.

2. Centers for Disease Control and Prevention, National Syndromic Surveillance Program. http://www.cdc.gov/nssp/index.html.

3. Centers for Disease Control and Prevention, National Vital Statistics System. http://www.cdc.gov/nchs/nvss.htm.

BOX 4-2 Public Health Data in Action: Two Examples

Salmonella Outbreak Related to Frozen Meals

Infections linked to food represent a major problem both in the United States and worldwide. An estimated 48 million Americans contract, and 3,000 die from, foodborne illnesses each year.[3,4] With the increased centralization of food production, foodborne outbreaks often occur in multiple states.

As shown in **FIGURE 4-1**, one such episode occurred in 18 states in 2010 that was caused by a strain of the *Salmonella* bacterium.[5] The outbreak was identified using DNA fingerprinting through PulseNet in May 2010, which indicated there was a cluster of disease cases with the same DNA pattern. PulseNet is a national network that subtypes bacteria molecular patterns to help identify the cause of suspected foodborne illnesses.

A total of 44 cases were identified between April and June 2010 (**FIGURE 4-2**); of the 43 individuals with available information, 16 were hospitalized (37%). A study conducted in June 2010 compared a small number of ill individuals to those who were not ill but had similar demographic characteristics (i.e., a control group). All study participants were given an extensive survey about recent food consumption. Individuals who consumed Company A's brand of a microwaveable frozen meal consisting of cheesy chicken and rice were 30 times more likely to have developed a *Salmonella* infection compared with those who had not done so. Shortly afterward, the CDC informed Company A about the likely association between its product and the infection, and the U.S. Department of Agriculture convened a meeting of its Recall Committee. Company A issued a recall for all its cheesy chicken and rice frozen meals. Further investigation suggested the contaminated chicken came from a single poultry farm and was the likely source for the bacteria linked to the disease outbreak.

Increased Deaths and Hospital Emergency Department Visits from Illegal or Misused Drugs

In recent years, there have been widespread news media reports about the growing epidemic of deaths and hospital emergency department (ED) visits related to both illegal and legal drug use in the United States.[6] How do we know this problem increased? Because of mortality data regularly collected and reported using the National Vital Statistics System,[7] and because the Drug Abuse Warning Network (DAWN) routinely collects and reports data about drug-related ED visits based on a representative sample of hospital EDs throughout the United States.[8]

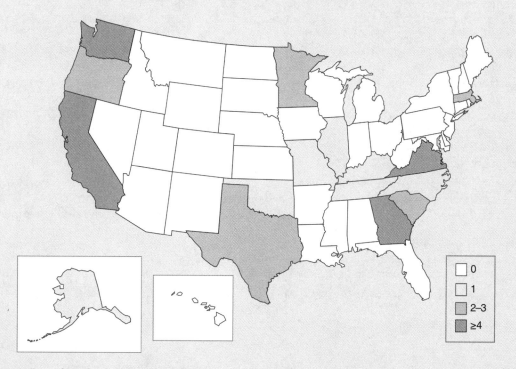

☐	0
☐	1
▨	2–3
▦	≥4

FIGURE 4-1 Number of confirmed cases (*N* = 44) of *Salmonella chester* infection in outbreak associated with frozen meals—18 states, April 4–June 19, 2010.

Reference 5, p. 980: http://www.cdc.gov/mmwr/preview/mmwrhtml/mm6248a2.htm?s_cid=mm6248a2_w#Fig2.

(continues)

BOX 4-2 Public Health Data in Action: Two Examples   *(continued)*

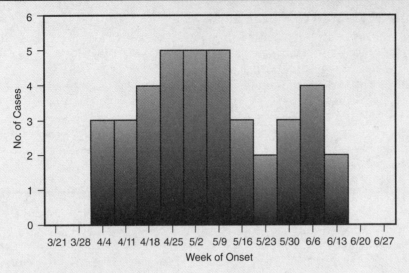

FIGURE 4-2 Number of confirmed cases (*N* = 44) of infection with the outbreak strain of *Salmonella chester*, by week of illness onset—18 states, April 4–June 19, 2010.

Reference 5, p. 980: http://www.cdc.gov/mmwr/preview/mmwrhtml/mm6248a2.htm?s_cid=mm6248a2_w#Fig1

The following list provides examples of key public health data from these surveillance systems that clearly demonstrate the growing extent of the drug overdose problem in the United States[9–12]:

- Drug overdoses kill more than 40,000 people per year in the United States, which is greater than the number of deaths from motor vehicle crashes.
- Drug overdose deaths increased by 117% from 1999 to 2012.
- In the 28 states for which data are available, the number of deaths from heroin overdose doubled between 2010 and 2012 alone.
- Each day, 46 people die from overdoses of prescription painkillers such as Vicodin (hydrocodone) and OxyContin (oxycodone).
- Between 1999 and 2010, the number of deaths from prescription painkillers increased by 400% among women and by 265% among men.
- More than 5 times as many women died from prescription painkiller overdoses in 2010 compared with 1999.
- Drug use and misuse caused approximately 2.5 million emergency department visits in 2011.
- For every 1 woman who dies from a prescription painkiller overdose, 30 women are seen in emergency departments for drug use or misuse.

In addition to raising our awareness of prescription and nonprescription drug overdosing, surveillance data are useful for evaluating the effectiveness of interventions to reduce drug-related problems. Between 2010 and 2012, for instance, the state of Florida enacted new public policy laws and regulations to reduce the problem of drug overdose, especially for prescription pain medications.[13] These measures included mandatory registration of pain clinics, limitations on physician dispensing of certain classes of painkillers from their offices, creation of a statewide drug monitoring program, increased regulation of wholesale drug distributors, and increased law enforcement activities. The overall number of drug overdose deaths in Florida declined by 17% from 2010 to 2012, with the decline being even larger (23%) for overdose deaths from prescription drugs.

contains a selected list of websites that offer users rapid access to current health data, or provide a gateway to a wide range of additional data sources. Strictly speaking, U.S. Census data are not public health data, but are included here because demographic and other types of data available from the Census are increasingly seen as important determinants of health behavior.

Partners in Information Access for the Public Health Workforce—a collaboration among U.S. government agencies, public health organizations, and health sciences libraries—has an especially helpful

TABLE 4-1 Selected Websites for Public Health Data

Website	URL
Gateway Sites to Data Sources	
Health Data (U.S. Department of Health and Human Services)	http://www.healthdata.gov/
CDC Data and Statistics	http://www.cdc.gov/DataStatistics/
Office on Women's Health Quick Data Online	www.healthstatus2010.com
Local Data Sources	
County Health Rankings & Roadmaps	http://www.countyhealthrankings.org/
America's Health Rankings	https://www.apha.org/publications-and-periodicals/reports-and-issue-briefs/americas-health-rankings
Selected Metropolitan/Micropolitan Area Risk Trends (SMART)	http://www.cdc.gov/brfss/smart/smart_data.htm
State Data Sources	
Centers for Disease Control and Prevention (CDC), Sortable Risk Factors and Health Indicators	http://sortablestats.cdc.gov/#/
Agency for Healthcare Research and Quality, National Healthcare Quality and Disparities Reports[a]	http://nhqrnet.ahrq.gov/inhqrdr/state/select
Behavioral Risk Surveillance System Prevalence and Trends Data[a]	http://www.cdc.gov/brfss/brfssprevalence/
Youth Risk Behavioral Surveillance System[a]	http://www.cdc.gov/HealthyYouth/yrbs/index.htm
National Data Sources	
Centers for Disease Control and Prevention (CDC), FastStats A–Z	http://www.cdc.gov/nchs/fastats/Default.htm
Health, United States, 2015 (updated annually)	http://www.cdc.gov/nchs/hus.htm
National Health Interview Survey	http://www.cdc.gov/nchs/nhis/nhis_products.htm
International Data Sources	
World Bank, Health, Nutrition and Population Data and Statistics	http://datatopics.worldbank.org/hnp/
World Health Organization (WHO), Global Health Observatory	http://www.who.int/gho/en/
Census Data	http://factfinder.census.gov/faces/nav/jsf/pages/index.xhtml or http://www.census.gov

[a]National or nationwide data also available.

"Health Data Tools and Statistics" website[a] that is worth exploring. Most state health department websites (and some city or county health department websites) are also excellent sources of state or local health data. Some public health professionals prefer local or state data over national data because they find it more relevant.

▶ People and Numbers

Prior to planning and developing communication materials with public health data, one must first estimate the audience's proficiency with numbers and the biases that influence how they interpret and understand data.

Numeracy

Numeracy, sometimes referred to as quantitative literacy, is the ability to understand and work with numbers. Studies of numeracy among adults in 2013[15] and of mathematical ability among eighth-grade students in 2011[16] paint a grim picture of this ability in the United States. U.S. adults ranked 21st out of 23 countries in numeracy ability, with only 9% of students scoring in the top proficiency level. Eighth-grade students fared a little better, ranking 9th out of 42 countries in mathematical ability. Unfortunately, the United States lags behind other developed countries in mathematical education. This fact may explain why so many people in the United States find numerical data to be overwhelming, as individuals with fewer years of formal education have the most difficulty with numeracy.[15]

A particular problem is the communication of risk (probability) estimates to lay audiences. In one study, for example, when people were asked whether a risk of "5%" or "1 in 20" sounded bigger in the context of prenatal diagnosis of chromosome abnormalities, 81% reported that "1 in 20" sounded bigger.[17] Many people misinterpret probability estimates, believing, for example, that a risk of 1 in 300 for developing a disease is higher than a risk of 1 in 15. Not surprisingly, then, the magnitude of difference between 1 in 1000 and 1 in 10,000,000 can easily be missed.

The implications of low numeracy are clear. Few people are likely to understand the meaning of numbers and concepts commonly used in public health, such as *mean* or *median, confidence intervals,* or $p = 0.005$ versus $p = 0.05$, let alone terms such as *parts per million* or *relative risk*. The vast majority of Americans do not use, remember, or ever learn these terms, which can be overwhelming and difficult to explain in common language. For these reasons, it is necessary to decide whether to share numerical data with the public, choose which data to present, and "style" them appropriately for presentation.[18]

Tendencies and Biases

People's understanding and interpretation of data are strongly influenced by certain tendencies and biases that often lead them to reach incorrect conclusions.[18] People tend to draw conclusions by using shortcut approaches (the "representative heuristic") based on past experience and limited evidence. Examples include believing that one's own experience is widely generalizable to everybody; that a vivid anecdote from someone is more valid than scientific consensus based on years of study; or that a new treatment for multiple sclerosis will be effective in humans because a news story reported promising results with the drug in mice. Anchoring and adjustment bias is the tendency of most people to "anchor" their understanding about data based on the initial number that is presented to them or that they already have in their minds. Because initial impressions tend to be long-lasting, it is important that data communicated to lay audiences are accurate the first time.

Belief that correlation equals causation and failure to consider random effects are two other tendencies that strongly affect how people interpret and explain findings. The belief that correlation equals causation is the logical error of seeing two types of data tending to vary together and concluding that one type of data is causing the other. While this may be true, too often correlations are just correlations. For example, just because ice cream sales and the rate of drowning deaths both increase during the summer months, it does not mean that ice cream *causes* drowning.

People rarely consider that chance alone might explain some scientific findings. Instead, they tend to assume that some type of "discoverable" cause exists, and create unfounded causal explanations. Research has shown, in fact, that people find patterns in data generated completely at random.[19] The failure to consider randomness in public health happens commonly whenever a cluster of disease cases or other adverse

---

a. http://phpartners.org/health_stats.html

health event occurs, such as birth defects, in a local area. These alleged clusters usually lead to speculation and conclusions about the cause, such as an environmental exposure or vaccine. Even when research demonstrates the absence of a causal relationship, many people may refuse to accept chance as the explanation.

▶ Data Communication Principles

In the remainder of this chapter, we provide practical guidance for communicating data to lay audiences, which include the public, policy makers, and news media representatives (journalists). Communicating public health data is much more difficult than implied by the statement that "the numbers speak for themselves."

Decisions about whether to use data at all, which data to select, and how to present data are every bit as complex as decisions about which words to use in public health messages. For starters, keep in mind the single overarching communication objective (SOCO) when deciding whether data belong in the messages. In acute public health situations (e.g., natural disasters), data are not usually helpful, because messages should emphasize specific actions that people can take to reduce their risks.

The following major data communication principles should be considered when deciding whether data should be used and which data to use:

- Assess audience numeracy and level of involvement.
- Remember your ethical responsibility.
- Minimize the number of data items.
- Select familiar and easily understood data.
- Explain unfamiliar terms.
- Consider framing effects.
- Provide context.
- Integrate data into the overall communication and implementation plan.

Assess Audience Numeracy and Level of Involvement

An essential step in audience analysis and formative research is to consider the audience's level of motivation and ability to interpret public health data. Some people will not be persuaded by data-oriented messages, whether due to low numeracy, cultural preference, distrust or dislike of numbers, or other reasons.

In such instances, data should not be used at all. Conversely, if audiences are highly involved in the public health issue and if communicators have sufficient time to effectively explain what the data mean and how they are derived, then even individuals with low numeracy can increase their comprehension of data messages.[18]

Data messages usually resonate better with persons with the following characteristics:[18]

- Those with lower levels of emotional involvement (e.g., fear, anger)
- Those with higher levels of education
- Those who are less familiar with the topic or situation
- Those whose (advocacy) position is supported by the data

Remember Your Ethical Responsibility

The decisions made when selecting and presenting data to audiences can influence audiences' interpretation and understanding of those data.[18] Especially when communication in public health has a persuasive aspect, communicators must make ethical choices about which data or other information to include or exclude. Much more is involved in such decision making than simply crunching numbers for data tables and graphs.[20] Public health professionals are usually seen by lay audiences as highly credible health information sources, so communicators have an important ethical responsibility to be honest and maintain the trust of their audiences. If conclusions based on public health surveillance or research findings are uncertain, it is better to say so rather than to communicate certainty that does not exist.

Ethical responsibility means not selecting and presenting data that are potentially misleading or manipulative so as to support a particular interpretation. Unfortunately, many people in business and politics intentionally and strategically communicate or suppress data as a means to support their own positions. Even scientists and other public health professionals, because of strongly held beliefs, are vulnerable to the same temptation as business people and politicians. Although their intentions may be good, such bias can lead to "cherry picking" data that support a biased position, and not reporting "less favorable" results.

Minimize the Number of Data Items

Regardless of their level of numeracy, people have limited ability to process and understand complex information provided to them. This constraint is referred to as cognitive burden or, when it comes to numbers, as "data overload." Many scientists, unfortunately, are guilty of creating data overload for their lay audiences. They make the mistake of trying to show many numbers to help prove their points, while failing to realize that most audiences are not adept with numbers or scientific concepts.

Most people typically want public health experts (and experts in other fields, too) to communicate their main conclusion(s) and recommendations quickly so they can discern the gist, or main point, of the message. The "more is better" approach, when it comes to communicating health data, is an especially *ineffective* communication strategy and is often counterproductive.[18] For lay audience persuasion, the implication is clear: use data sparingly.[21] When numbers are essential to the message, a good rule of thumb is to use only one or two numbers and start with the more compelling number.

Select Data That Are Familiar and Easy to Understand

It is best to use numbers that nonscientific audiences encounter more commonly. Frequencies (counts) using whole numbers such as 25 or 2000 are likely to be easily understood. Percentages are usually good choices, *except* for conveying personal health risk information, such as the probability of a smoker getting lung cancer.[22] (In that case, describing the denominator and numerator is preferable, as explained later.) However, fractional percentages, such as 0.8% or 0.002%, should be avoided because they are easily misunderstood. Indeed, using whole numbers (without decimal points—that is, 74% instead of 74.3%, or a relative risk of 3 rather than 3.2) is likely to facilitate understanding,[23] as does rounding of large numbers (e.g., 115,000 rather than 115,491). If proportions are used, such as 1 in *X*, use the lowest possible denominator (4 in 10 rather than 40 in 100).

Explain Unfamiliar Terms

Public health communicators often mistakenly believe statistical or epidemiologic terms are understood by others. In reality, statistical significance, probability, relative risk, and similar concepts are not familiar to most lay people. Terms such as these need to be defined in plain language, and additional background material made available through websites or other means for those who may be interested in learning more. Care should always be taken to explain the meaning of numeric representations and to remind the audience

of how to put the data into the proper context. Even the most commonly used public health statistics may be misunderstood without supporting explanation.[18]

Consider Framing Effects

For messages involving health behaviors, data can often be presented in one of two ways, to emphasize positive effects (gain) or to focus on negative effects (loss). The deliberate selection of either perspective is referred to as message framing.[24,25] A gain-frame message for physical activity, for example, would be "Regular exercise can make you feel better physically and mentally, and it can help keep off unwanted pounds." In contrast, a loss-frame message would be "Not exercising regularly increases your chance of gaining weight and feeling depressed."

Research consistently shows that gain-framed messages are more effective than loss-framed messages at encouraging individual behavior changes, such as smoking cessation, skin cancer prevention, and increased physical activity.[25] In these instances, you should use data to demonstrate the benefits of healthier behaviors, such as "Regular use of birth control reduces your risk of an unplanned pregnancy by as much as 99%." In contrast, for disease detection (e.g., early identification of diabetes, screening for cancer), loss-framed messages are more effective than gain-framed messages[26,27]—for example, "People who do not receive colorectal cancer screening tests on a regular basis are at more than double the risk of developing metastatic colon cancer."

Provide Context

To understand what data mean, people need appropriate contextual information. Public health communicators play a crucial role in interpreting and communicating public health findings in their full context and in full light of any prior research. Any numerical data without sufficient background information are meaningless unless they can be placed in their proper perspective. For example, simply reporting there were *Y* cases of influenza in New Mexico in February 2015 provides little value unless further details are given about the number of influenza cases in past months or years so audiences can see whether the current number represents an increase, a decrease, or no change over time.

Understanding probability data (i.e., statistical estimates of risk or benefit) is especially challenging for lay and even health professional audiences.[28] Sometimes a familiar analogy may help with these data's interpretation: "This medication has helped about 50% of those who have taken it—we can hope you win the coin toss, but that's all it is."

Relative risk estimates are good ways to help raise awareness about a health topic,[18] as demonstrated by a common type of news media health story—one that proclaims, "A new study shows food A cuts your risk of heart disease in half." Nevertheless, such information is often misleading when presented without the absolute risk numbers. "Doubling the risk" of cancer, for example, might mean that the absolute risk increased from 1 in 100,000 to 2 in 100,000; that is not a very big effect from an individual's standpoint. A substantial body of evidence indicates that presenting probability data as absolute risk estimates, especially in clinical settings, improves people's understanding.[28-30]

Integrate Data into an Overall Communication and Implementation Plan

Decisions and choices about which data to select and communicate to lay audiences, practitioners, or others should be considered within the "big picture" of public health practice planning, implementation, and evaluation. Although not possible to tailor in every situation, it is important to understand that the means of communicating data depends upon which data were collected and why they were collected in the first place. The case study from a local North Carolina health department presented in this chapter's appendix is an excellent example of how data collection and communication were integral to overall communication planning and implementation. In this case study, notice particularly that (1) surveillance data were used both to identify *Chlamydia* infections as a problem and for evaluation purposes; (2) careful planning was needed to decide which data to collect and communicate for evaluation (pertinent issues included ease of data collection, sustainability, and replicability); (3) ethical issues were prominent; and (4) the selection and presentation of findings relied heavily on the use of mapping software (maps are covered later in this chapter).

▶ Show Me the Data: Presenting Public Health Numbers

Providing extensive details about how to present data is beyond the scope of this chapter, but we will give some suggestions and approaches that will enhance a

presentation and improve the audience's understanding of its message. Paying careful attention to data presentation details—words alone, visual displays, or some combination of the two—can pay major dividends when translating complex data and concepts into simple and clear communication messages.

Presenting Data Using Words

Although data are usually presented in the form of some type of visual display, they can be communicated to audiences simply through the use of words alone. One way to do so is through the use of data metaphors.[31] By *metaphor*, we are referring to the use of text (words) to provide a numeric analogy such that "X is similar to Y."[32] For example, to raise awareness about the impact of the tobacco problem, advocates for many years pointed out that the annual number of deaths from smoking in the United States was equivalent to two jumbo jets crashing every day for a year with no survivors. Here are two other memorable public health data metaphors[33-35]:

- Think of the twin towers of the World Trade Center in New York City falling from terrorist attacks each day—that's the number of deaths from cancer.
- College students consume enough alcohol each year to fill an Olympic-sized swimming pool on each of 3500 campuses in the United States.

Of course, metaphors will not be effective if the analogy used is unfamiliar to the audience. The Olympic pool metaphor for college drinking, although widely quoted, might be such an example. And remember, any metaphor is more effective when heard (not read), when used early during a communication activity, and when it is the only one used.[18]

An alternative way to communicate data through words is to use a short narrative. Larger than a metaphor, a narrative is a vignette, anecdote, or other short text description designed to illustrate a key point. A narrative can be a highly effective way to present data or other types of health information to people because it has the ability to "draw people in" (transport them) to a particular story, often with the additional benefit of evoking emotions.[35] **BOX 4-3** contains a narrative about the impact on parents of the high cost of treatment for an ill child.

One final caution about using words: Avoid substituting everyday language to describe data.[18] It may be tempting to use expressions such as "much higher," "most of the time," "low risk," "frequent," or "minimal risk" when referring to numbers. But doing

BOX 4-3 Example of a Public Health Data-Oriented Narrative

Medical Bills Bankrupt Families of Mentally Ill Children

A 2013 ABC News story highlighted the challenges of high medical bills for parents of children with mental health disorders. One example was the Morrisseys, a Nebraska couple with what is considered a good health insurance policy for their family, who have a teenage daughter, Jaimie [her real name is not used for privacy protection] with Tourette Syndrome, severe anxiety, and anorexia. Ted Morrissey, Jaimie's father, notes that "We've been battling, doing nothing more than jumping hurdles and falling into pits for 11 years."

Requests for financial assistance from governmental programs such as Medicaid and Social Security were not accepted. Although the family's insurance policy covers 80% of costs, nonetheless they have experienced large out-of-pocket expenses related to Jaimie's care. "If you have a $200,000 bill, you have to come up with $40,000 and try to pay that," said her father.

Needless to say, the impact of medical expenses related to Jaimie's care has caused many other difficulties for the family. "We pride [ourselves] in paying our bills, but you end up buying the groceries on credit," reports Morrissey. "We have nothing. Now I am worried about losing my home. This has been devastating."

James SD. Medical bills bankrupt families of mentally ill children. ABC News. February 18, 2013. http://abcnews.go.com/Health/medical-bills-bankrupt-families-children-mentally-ill/story?id=18515291. Accessed January 26, 2015.

so is problematic because people have widely different understandings and interpretations of the meaning of these terms. Stick with the actual numbers.

Presenting Data Visually

Data are most often presented to audiences through visual displays such as graphs, tables, figures, dashboards, and maps. With the rapid advances in information technology, many visual options have been introduced that create new communication possibilities, such as the ability to easily and rapidly create and upload videos to YouTube or other websites.

Keep in mind, though, that more choices and enhanced "bells and whistles" do not necessarily result in improved communication. In this section, we review the essentials of selecting displays and designing them to enhance communication of public health data.

Visual Fundamentals

When considering which visual display to use, choose one that is likely to be familiar and, therefore, easily understood by the audience whenever possible. For example, a "1 to 5 stars" rating system or a simple pie chart may not visually fancy, but will be familiar to and understood by most audiences. Similarly, the color red in the United States is often used to denote danger or high risk, whereas green often indicates "normal" or "safe." Except for persons unable to make this visual distinction, green, yellow, and red are good color choices to convey data values that range from normal to abnormal.

As mentioned earlier in this chapter, cognitive overload is a challenge when interpreting data, and should be minimized in visual data presentations. One approach to eliminate this complication is to limit the number of visuals; rarely is more than one needed except with highly involved audiences. Use short and simple titles, labels, and legends, and consider including a few words that stress the key message (e.g., "the number of infections declined by 95% after vaccine use became widespread"). Key data points should be highlighted using arrows or boldfaced text—these visual signposts are referred to as contextual cues. Finally, avoid clutter by including sufficient "white space" to allow people to readily identify the major point(s). For example, whenever possible use only a small number of bars, lines, or pie slices (e.g., 2–4) in a graph, and eliminate extraneous items such as lines indicating 95% confidence limits.

Specific Visual Modalities

There are many potential visual modalities for presenting health data—and fortunately, some recent research to help guide choices among them. For example, the Visualizing Health project, led by researchers at the University of Michigan and supported by the Robert Wood Johnson Foundation, has identified several visual modalities, some of which are especially valuable for helping people better understand the risks and benefits of disease screening or treatment.[36]

Despite the development of newer approaches, the most common visual ways to present data remain the old standbys: bar charts, line graphs, and pie charts. Except for short lists (**FIGURE 4-3**), tables are not a good choice and should be avoided. Bar charts are likely to be used most often because of their versatility, and because they do an excellent job of displaying the relative magnitude (size) of numbers, such as counts, percentages, or relative risks (**FIGURE 4-4** and **FIGURE 4-5**).[18,29,36]

The Top 10 Leading Causes of Death in The World in 2012

Cause of Death	Number (Millions)
1. Ischemic Heart Disease	7.4
2. Stroke	6.7
3. Chronic Obstructive Pulmomary Disease	3.1
4. Lower Respiratory Infections	3.1
5. Lung Cancer	1.6
6. HIV/AIDS	1.5
7. Diarrheal Diseases	1.5
8. Diabetes	1.5
9. Road Injury	1.3
10. Hypertensive Heart Disease	1.1

FIGURE 4-3 Example of a data table. Legend: Note the use of a short title and shading of alternate rows to facilitate easier reading.

Data from The top 10 causes of death. World Health Organization Web site. http://www.who.int/mediacentre/factsheets/fs310/en/. Accessed January 7, 2015.

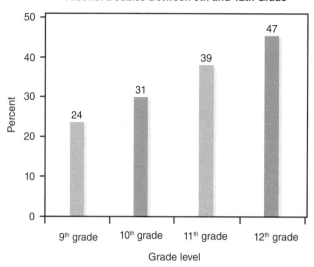

The Percentage of High School Students Using Alcohol Doubles Between 9th and 12th Grade

FIGURE 4-4 Example of a bar chart. Legend: Note how the title contains the key message about how alcohol use increases across grades.

Data from Kann L, Kinchen S, Shanklin SL, et al. Youth risk behavioral surveillance—United States, 2013. Morb Mort Week Rep Surv Summ. 2014; 63(SS-04): 18.

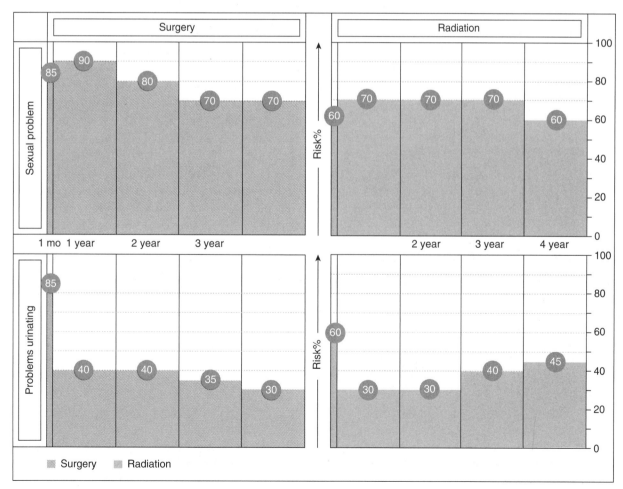

FIGURE 4-5 Bar chart designed to communicate data about the risk of prostate cancer treatment side effects.

Visualizing Health. University of Michigan and the Robert Wood Johnson Foundation Web site. http://www.vizhealth.org/. Accessed January 6, 2015.

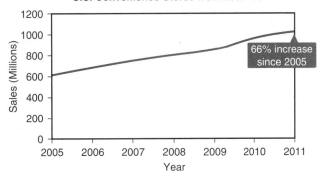

FIGURE 4-6 Example of a line graph.

Data from Delnevo CD, Wackowski OA, Giovenco DP, Manderski MTB, Hrywna M, Ling PM. Examining market trends in United States on smokeless tobacco use: 2005-2011. Tob Control. 2014; 23: 109.

Line graphs are excellent choices for showing data patterns, especially trends over time. Note in **FIGURE 4-6** how the title, and the use of an arrow, help viewers rapidly identify the key message and data point. Pie charts are also familiar images for most audiences; they are useful for demonstrating the relative size of proportions (percentages) totaling 100% and should be strongly considered whenever appropriate (**FIGURE 4-7**).

Dashboards represent a type of visual scale that can be used to reduce a substantial amount of data

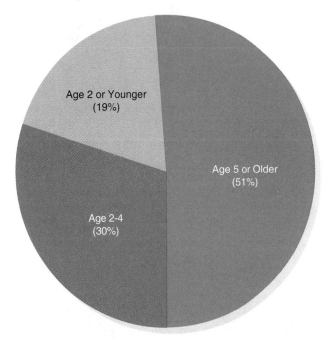

FIGURE 4-7 Example of a pie chart. Note the placement of data labels within the pie slices.

Data from Pringle BA, Colpe LJ, Blumberg SJ, Avila RM, Kogan MD. Diagnostic history and treatment of school-aged children with autism spectrum disorder and special health care needs. NCHS Data Brief No. 97. Hyattsville, MD: Centers for Disease Control and Prevention, National Center for Health Statistics; 2012.

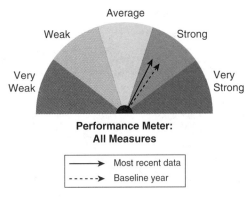

FIGURE 4-8 Example of a state dashboard on health measures from the Agency for Healthcare Quality Research (overall health care quality in Wisconsin). Legend: Note how the text box and arrow indicate the key data communication point.

Data from Agency for Healthcare Quality and Research. National Healthcare Quality and Disparities Reports: Wisconsin state dashboard. http://nhqrnet.ahrq.gov/inhqrdr/Wisconsin /dashboard. Accessed January 27, 2015.

to one or more simple messages. The dashboard in **FIGURE 4-8** was developed by the U.S. Agency for Healthcare Quality. It is based on more than 100 measures, which are nicely condensed into an overall assessment rating of a state's healthcare quality and also indicate change over time.[37]

A substantial body of research shows that icon arrays, also known as pictographs, are excellent choices for helping individuals better understand probabilities, such as the risks or benefits associated with genetic inheritance, disease screening, or treatment choices (**FIGURE 4-9**). They effectively depict the relationship between numerators and denominators in a way not easily done through other visual means.[29,38]

The widespread availability of data sets, coupled with advancements in mapping software, led to the creation of geographic information systems (GIS). GIS mapping has become very important for data visualization research and practice in public health over the past two decades.[39] **FIGURE 4-10** is an example of an isopleth (contour line) map created using GIS software; it shows levels of airborne fine particles.[40] These particles can cause several types of adverse health effects because they are readily inhaled and deposited in the lungs. In the figure, note the especially high concentrations of particulate matter in China, Northern Africa, and Southwest Asia.

Infographics

The advent of more powerful and readily accessible computer software has spawned new ways to visually present data using infographics. An infographic is a visual representation of complex data that is often contextualized to help the reader understand and

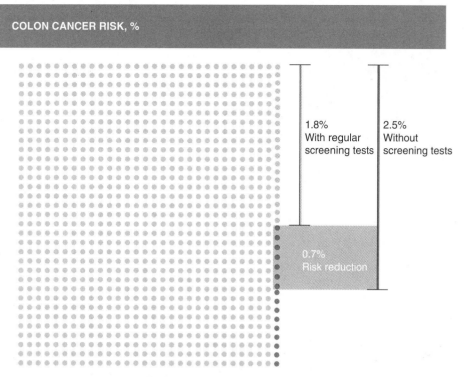

COLON CANCER RISK, %

1.8%
With regular
screening tests

2.5%
Without
screening tests

0.7%
Risk reduction

FIGURE 4-9 Example of an icon array designed to communicate the benefits of colon cancer screening.

Visualizing Health. University of Michigan and the Robert Wood Johnson Foundation Web site. http://www.vizhealth.org/. Accessed January 6, 2015.

Airborne Fine Particulate Matter Levels

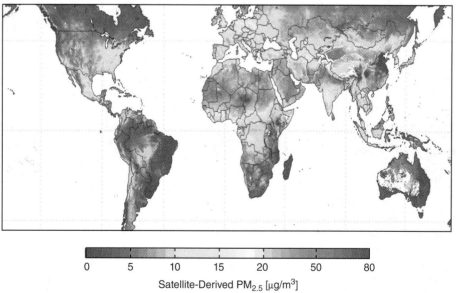

0   5   10   15   20   50   80

Satellite-Derived $PM_{2.5}$ [μg/m³]

FIGURE 4-10 Example of a GIS-generated map.

PM is an abbreviation for particulate matter in the air, such as dust, dirt, liquid, soot, smoke. Particles of less than 2.5 micrometers in diameter ($PM_{2.5}$) are referred to as fine particles.

Courtesy of van Donkelaar, A., R.V. Martin, M. Brauer, R. Kahn, R. Levy, C. Verduzco, and P.J. Villeneuve, Global Estimates of Ambient Fine Particulate Matter Concentrations from Satellite-Based Aerosol Optical Depth: Development and Application, Environ. Health Perspec., doi:10.1289/ehp.0901623, 118(6), 2010.

relate to the numbers. **FIGURES 4-11** to **4-14** from the Visualizing Data Project[36] provide relatively simple examples of infographics that can be used to help raise awareness, describe health risks, or assist people with individual decision making. More elaborate graphics can also be created to help convey a storyline to audiences.[41,42] Guidelines for developing infographics are provided in **BOX 4-4**. In addition, a special

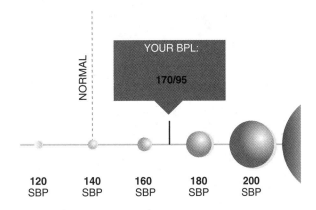

> INCREASED RISK

FIGURE 4-11 Infographic designed to translate a medical test result into a risk estimate for an individual.

Visualizing Health. University of Michigan and the Robert Wood Johnson Foundation Web site. http://www.vizhealth.org/. Accessed January 6, 2015.

RATES OF COLORECTAL CANCER

White Americans	African Americans
89.7	113.5*
PER 100,000	PER 100,000

*23.8 more people per 100,000

FIGURE 4-12 Infographic designed to communicate racial disparities and raise awareness.

Visualizing Health. University of Michigan and the Robert Wood Johnson Foundation Web site. http://www.vizhealth.org/. Accessed January 6, 2015.

CASES OF MEASLES IN THE LAST YEAR

58	58 cases occurred in just two Brooklyn, NY neighborhoods
	Population: 250,000
200	There were 200 total cases of measles in the United States
	Population: 317,000,000

FIGURE 4-13 Infographic designed to raise awareness and put disease outbreak results in context.

Visualizing Health. University of Michigan and the Robert Wood Johnson Foundation Web site. http://www.vizhealth.org/. Accessed January 6, 2015.

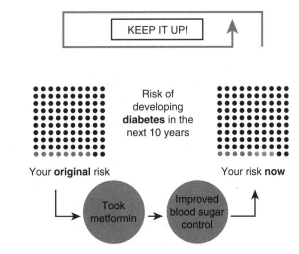

FIGURE 4-14 Infographic designed to communicate data about the benefits of positive behavior change.

Visualizing Health. University of Michigan and the Robert Wood Johnson Foundation Web site. http://www.vizhealth.org/. Accessed January 6, 2015.

BOX 4-4 Infographic Development Guidelines

General Recommendations

- Decide on the storyline (single overriding communication objective [SOCO]) and outline the story.
- Understand the intended audience and communication purpose.
- Let data (carefully reviewed for accuracy) lead the story, but provide contextual information.
- Organize information from left to right, and from top to bottom.
- Keep it simple: Show audiences new information, and combine simple visuals with ample white space.
- Test (formative evaluation) infographics with individuals from the intended audience, and make changes as necessary to ensure rapid and accurate comprehension.

Specific Recommendations

- Use titles and subtitles to set up the story or provide contextual information.
- State the main message in simple language and early in the infographic.
- Break up into sections from top to bottom (more complex infographics).
- Use simple visual images, such as data bar charts or easily understood images or photos.
- Highlight key data using text boxes, arrows, larger font sizes, or text bolding.

Centers for Disease Control and Prevention Social Media. Infographics. Available at http://www.cdc.gov/socialmedia/tools/infographics.html. Accessed July 31, 2015.

set of infographics is available for communicating about the leading health indicators at http://www.healthypeople.gov/2020/leading-health-indicators/LHI-Infographic-Gallery; these infographics may be used free of charge in any communication materials with proper attribution.

▶ Conclusion

Communicating scientific data to members of the public, policy makers, and news media representatives is one of the biggest challenges in public health communication. Most people have limited numeracy and quickly become overwhelmed by the statistics and other numerical data found in public health messages. Nevertheless, with careful attention to decisions about whether to use data, which data to use, and how to present numbers to audiences using words, visual displays, or some combination of the two, data can be communicated more effectively to lay audiences. Doing so serves to increase the knowledge of audiences, and it can result in improved decision making, and better health, at the individual and societal levels.

Wrap-Up

Chapter Questions

1. Why should you use local public health surveillance data whenever possible?
2. What are the implications of low numeracy for communication?
3. How do audiences' tendencies and biases influence their interpretation of data?
4. Describe better approaches to communicate data to people with low numeracy.
5. Why is it that "less is more" when selecting and presenting data to audiences?
6. What are two ways to communicate data using words only?
7. How can cognitive burden be minimized in visual data displays?

References

1. Thacker SB, Qualters JR, Lee, LM. Public health surveillance in the United States: evolution and challenges. *MMWR*. 2012;61(suppl)S3–S9.
2. Porta M, ed. *Dictionary of Epidemiology*. 5th ed. New York, NY: Oxford University Press; 2008.
3. Gould HL, Walsh KA, Vieira AR, et al. Surveillance for foodborne disease outbreaks—United States, 1998-2008. *MMWR Surv Summ*. 2013;62(SS02):1–34.
4. Centers for Disease Control and Prevention. CDC and food safety. March 2014. http://www.cdc.gov/foodborneburden/PDFs/CDC-and-Food-Safety.pdf. Accessed January 5, 2015.
5. Centers for Disease Control and Prevention. Multistate outbreak of *Salmonella chester* infections associated with frozen meals—18 states, 2010. *MMWR*. 2013;62: 979–982.
6. Koba M. Deadly epidemic: prescription drug overdoses. *USA Today*. July 28, 2013. http://www.usatoday.com/story/money/business/2013/07/28/deadly-epidemic-prescription-drug-overdoses/2584117/. Accessed January 5, 2015.
7. Centers for Disease Control and Prevention. Mortality data. http://www.cdc.gov/nchs/deaths.htm. Accessed January 5, 2015.
8. Substance Abuse and Mental Health Services Administration. Emergency department data/Drug Abuse Warning Network (DAWN). http://www.samhsa.gov/data/emergency-department-data-dawn. Accessed January 5, 2015.
9. Paulozzi LJ. Prescription drug overdoses: a review. *J Safety Res*. 2012;43:283–289.
10. Centers for Disease Control and Prevention. Prescription painkiller overdoses: a growing epidemic, especially among women. July 2013. http://www.cdc.gov/vitalsigns/pdf/2013-07-vitalsigns.pdf. Accessed January 5, 2015.
11. Rudd RA, Paulozzi LJ, Bauer MJ, et al. Increases in heroin overdose deaths—28 states, 2010 to 2012. *MMWR*. 2014;63:849–854.
12. Centers for Disease Control and Prevention. Prescription drug overdose in the United States: fact sheet. https://www.cdc.gov/drugoverdose/. Accessed January 5, 2015.
13. Johnson H, Paulozzi L, Porucznik C, Mack K, Herter B. Decline in drug overdose deaths after state policy changes—Florida, 2010-2012. *MMWR*. 2014;63:569–574.
14. Lee LM, Teutsch SM, Thacker SB, St. Louis ME, eds. *Principles and Practice of Public Health Surveillance*. 3rd ed. New York, NY: Oxford University Press; 2010.
15. Goodman M, Finnegan R, Mohadjer L, Krenzke T, Hogan J. *Literacy, Numeracy, and Problem Solving -n Technology-Rich Environments Among U.S. Adults: Results from the Program for the International Assessment of Adult Competencies 2012. First Look*. NCES Pub. No. 2014-008. Washington, DC: U.S. Department of Education, National Center for Education Statistics; 2013.
16. Provasnik S, Kastberg D, Ferraro D, Lemanski N, Roey S, Jenkins, F. *Highlights from TIMSS 2011: Mathematics and Science Achievement of U.S. Fourth- and Eighth-Grade Students in an International Context*. NCES Pub. No. 2013-009 (revised). Washington, DC: National Center for

Education Statistics, Institute of Education Sciences, U.S. Department of Education; 2012.

17. Abramsky L, Fletcher O. Interpreting information: what is said, what is heard—a questionnaire study of health professionals and members of the public. *Prenat Diagn.* 2002;22:1188–1194.

18. Nelson DE, Hesse B, Croyle R. *Making Data Talk.* New York, NY: Oxford University Press; 2009.

19. Hastie R, Dawes RM. *Rational Choice in an Uncertain World: The Psychology of Judgment and Decision Making.* Thousand Oaks, CA: Sage; 2001.

20. Alonso W, Starr A, eds. *The Politics of Numbers.* New York, NY: Russell Sage Foundation; 1987.

21. Zikmund-Fisher BJ, Fagerlin A, Ubel PA. A demonstration that "less can be more" in risk graphics. *Med Decis Making.* 2010;30:661–671.

22. Fagerlin A, Zikmund-Fisher BJ, Ubel PA. Helping patients decide: ten steps to better risk communication. *J Nat Cancer Inst.* 2011;103:1436–1443.

23. Witteman HO, Zikmund-Fisher BJ, Waters EA, Gavaruzzi T, Fagerlin A. Risk estimates from an online calculator are more believable wand recalled better when expressed as integers. *J Med Internet Res.* 2011;13(3);e54. **doi:**10.2196/jmir.1656.

24. Rothman AJ, Salovey P. Shaping perceptions to motivate healthy behavior: the role of message framing. *Psychol Bull.* 1997;121:3–19.

25. Gallagher KM, Updegraff JA. Health message framing effects on attitudes, intentions, and behavior: a meta-analytic review. *Ann Behav Med.* 2012;43:101–116.

26. O'Keefe DJ, Jensen JD. The relative persuasiveness of gain-framed and loss-framed messages for encouraging disease detection behaviors: a meta-analytic review. *J Comm.* 2009;59:296–316.

27. Ferrer RA, Klein WMP, Zajac LE, Land SR, Ling BS. An affective booster moderates the effect of gain- and loss-framed messages on behavioral intentions for colorectal cancer screening. *J Behav Med.* 2012;35:452–461.

28. Gigerenzer G. *Risk Savvy: How to Make Good Decisions.* New York, NY: Viking Penguin; 2014.

29. Zipkin DA, Umscheid CA, Keating NL, et al. Evidence-based risk communication: a systematic review. *Ann Intern Med.* 2014;161:270–280.

30. Akl EA, Oxman AD, Herrin J, et al. Using alternative statistical formats for presenting risks and risk reductions. *Cochrane Rev.* 2011;3:CD006776.

31. Scherer AM, Scherer LD, Fagerlin A. Getting ahead of illness: using metaphors to influence medical decision making. *Med Decis Making.* 2015;35:37–45.

32. Galesic M, Garcia-Retamero R. Using analogies to communicate information about health risks. *Appl Cognit Psychol.* 2013;27:33–42.

33. Rose C. A discussion about cancer in America. In: *The Charlie Rose [Television] Show Transcript*; episode aired April 29, 2004.

34. Wallack LM, Woodruff K, Dorfman L, Diaz I. *News for a Change: An Advocate's Guide to Working with the Media.* Thousand Oaks, CA: Sage; 1999.

35. Scharf BF, Harter LM, Yamasaki J, Haider P. Narrative turns epic: continuing developments in health narrative scholarship. In: Thompson TL, Parrott R, Nussbaum JF. Eds. *Routledge Handbook of Health Communication.* 2nd ed. New York, NY: Routledge; 2011:36–51.

36. University of Michigan, Robert Wood Johnson Foundation. Visualizing Health. http://www.vizhealth.org/. Accessed January 6, 2015.

37. Agency for Healthcare Quality and Research. National Healthcare Quality and Disparities Reports: Wisconsin state dashboard. http://nhqrnet.ahrq.gov/inhqrdr/Wisconsin/dashboard. Accessed January 27, 2015.

38. Garcia-Retamero R, Cokely ET. Communicating health risks with visual aids. *Curr Direct Psychol Sci.* 2013;22:392–399.

39. Cromley EK, McLafferty SL. *GIS and Public Health.* 2nd ed. New York, NY: Guilford; 2011.

40. Centers for Disease Control and Prevention, Division of Heart Disease and Stroke Prevention. Types of thematic maps. http://www.cdc.gov/dhdsp/maps/gisx/resources/maps4.html. Accessed January 21, 2015.

41. Centers for Disease Control and Prevention. Social media: infographics. http://www.cdc.gov/socialmedia/tools/infographics.html. Accessed July 31, 2015.

42. United Kingdom Office for National Statistics. Infographic guidelines. 2013. https://theidpblog.files.wordpress.com/2013/10/infographic-guidelines-v1-0.pdf. Accessed July 31, 2015.

Appendix 4

Addressing Chlamydia in a North Carolina County

Jessica Southwell, Matt Simon, and Kasey Decosimo

▶ Project Overview

In 2013, the Greater-Valley (a pseudonym) District Health Department (GVDHD) recognized that chlamydia incidence in the county represented a major concern. Through a community health assessment, county officials identified that the sexually transmitted disease represented an area of concern relative to other diseases that had received attention in recent years. Other health conditions such as HIV infection and adolescent pregnancy actually appeared to be declining, yet chlamydia prevalence in the county remained high relative to other counties in the state, with Valley County ranking in the top five in the state on that dimension. The Health Department saw a need to address resident sexual behavior and screening behavior, as prevention and detection of the disease are important steps toward reducing future incidence. Given the limited resources of the Health Department for work beyond service provision and surveillance, however, officials also realized they would need to partner with outside organizations to develop and implement a communication campaign and to evaluate that effort.

To secure funds through a grant from a local foundation, county staff needed to identify a partner with communication experience and a partner with social science evaluation experience. They selected a local marketing group and a university-based evaluation team. Opportunities to do formative research and collect summative evaluation data were limited by resources and time available for project implementation—factors that also shaped the project experience.

▶ Planning

Campaign Development

Health Department officials selected a local organization called PeopleDesigns to conduct focus groups with area residents for formative research insights. Based on that work, PeopleDesigns worked in conjunction with the Health Department to create and implement a campaign using radio, print, and other communication channels, such as social media outreach.

Evaluation Planning

Perhaps equally as compelling as the campaign development effort was the strategy devised to evaluate the effort. Development of a method to evaluate the efficacy of the campaign proved challenging, as county officials spent a considerable part of their available budget to develop and implement the campaign. As a result, funds were not available for large-scale surveys that could have assessed resident perceptions, nor did county officials think that an experimental design with random assignment to campaign exposure was appropriate. In light of those constraints, the evaluation partner for the effort, the North Carolina Institute for Public Health at the University of North Carolina at Chapel Hill (UNC), developed a time-based approach to assessing change.

Managing Project Expectations Among Three Partners

A key aspect of the planning process was the ability of each organization to offer a concrete assessment of what could be achieved during the one-year total time period available for the effort. The marketing partner set realistic expectations about the rapid formative research and materials development required for a one-year project schedule (which was tied to project funding). The evaluation team, in turn, recognized that they would need to work with administrative data (i.e., county testing data), rather than seek to collect additional survey data given the time and money constraints; as a consequence, they concentrated on finding appropriate ways to transform administrative records into quantitative outcomes.

During the initial months of the project, the three organizational partners drafted a project charter outlining everyone's role and responsibility, as well as a timeline for activities. The group also committed to a conference call schedule to stay connected throughout the project period and used biweekly calls to share updates and ask questions that proved quite valuable.

▶ Replicable Informatics

One noteworthy aspect of the present chlamydia project is its ability to be replicated in any county in the country collecting surveillance data. A core piece of information for the formative evaluation, and potentially for future summative evaluation, was North Carolina Electronic Disease Surveillance System (NC EDSS) data, which tracks positive communicable disease cases. Our partnership with the North Carolina State Public Health Laboratory also gave us the total number of people who were tested. This statistic is not tracked directly in county NC EDSS reports, or currently by the Health Department. We also used GIS mapping technology, which offered the advantage of placing a low burden on Health Department staff.

Another reason why using surveillance systems worked for this evaluation is that local health departments in North Carolina have well-established screening programs for young women attending public clinics that, through NC EDSS reporting, provide relatively good data about the prevalence of disease in this subpopulation. Chlamydia screening and reporting does have limitations, however. Notably, chlamydia is often asymptomatic in both males and females. It is also a major cause of pelvic inflammatory disease (PID) in females. For this reason, the North Carolina Department of Public Health (NCDPH) recommends that all sexually active young women should be screened for chlamydia during any pelvic exam. Originally, this screening recommendation included only

women aged 22 years or younger. However, beginning in 2008, screening was expanded to include women aged 25 years or younger. It is also recommended that all pregnant women should be tested for chlamydia as part of standard prenatal care. There are no comparable screening programs for young men. Consequently, chlamydia case reports are always highly biased with respect to gender. Public clinics and health departments may do a better job of conducting such screening programs and reporting cases, though they are biased toward young women attending public clinics.

Despite these limitations of obtaining accurate and timely data on chlamydia prevalence, the evaluation team was able to use NC EDSS data to provide baseline maps of confirmed chlamydia cases throughout Valley County. Significant clusters were identified, as the majority of persons with chlamydia lived in a few neighborhoods within one of the county's largest towns. This finding confirmed that the Health Department's priorities were well targeted. In a time when resources (both financial and personnel) are stretched so thin, it also meant that efforts could be focused more narrowly and, we hoped, would have a more impactful effect.

On December 12, 2013, GVDHD staff pulled mapping and event line-listing reports from NC EDSS for Valley County chlamydia cases from January 1, 2010 through December 11, 2013. De-identified data were provided to the Institute for analysis, after which a baseline report was developed and presented to the team at its January meeting.

Reported cases in the baseline report were events in which Valley County residents had a laboratory-confirmed chlamydial infection and could include cases of reinfection. Cases were selected based on the patient's county of residence at diagnosis (an important point to keep in mind as we eventually map these data, which span a period of five years). Descriptive analyses of these data involved cross-tabulating cases by variables collected in the NC EDSS data set, including year, gender, pregnancy status, age group, race, and reporting providers. Report year was based on the date when the case was reported to the Centers for Disease Control and Prevention. If that data point was missing, the laboratory specimen collection date was used.

Geospatial analysis involved mapping confirmed reported cases to U.S. Census block groups ($n = 34$) and blocks ($n = 166$) in Valley County (**FIGURE 4A-1**). All mapping was performed using 2000 U.S. Census data, because this was the geographic information used for NC EDSS reporting. A cluster and hot spot analysis of all reported cases was performed to

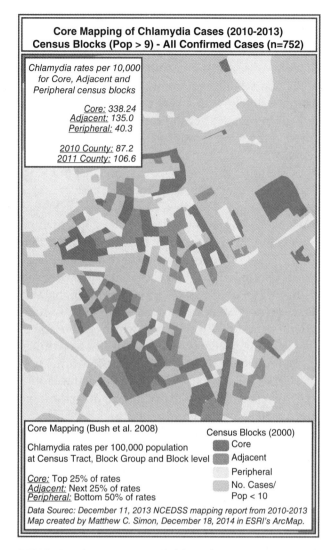

FIGURE 4A-1 Core mapping of chlamydia cases (2010–2013) by U.S. Census blocks (population > 9): all confirmed cases (*n* = 752).

December 11, 2013, NCEDSS mapping report from 2010-2013 Map created by Matthew C. Simon, December 18, 2014 in ESRI's ArcMap.

identify statistically significant spatial clusters of high value (hot spots), cold spots, and spatial outliers. Core mapping was also performed to identify core areas with rates of infection. Finally, census blocks that were identified as core areas, hot spots, or clusters were highlighted as potential intervention neighborhoods.

The methods used are easily replicable but do have some limitations. The final report included only those cases that may have been reported in NC EDSS. Although providers are required to notify the local health department of reportable diseases such as chlamydia, there is the possibility that not all positive cases were reported and entered into NC EDSS. Since chlamydia is often asymptomatic in both males and females, infected persons often do not seek

out health care for this infection and, therefore, their cases would not be reported. In some instances, as the result of missing values or variables, some of the totals in separate cross-tabulations may not agree

In addition, there are several limitations to the geospatial analysis. First, fewer than half of all reported cases in the county had valid address data. Nevertheless, the cases that could be mapped had demographics very similar to those of all reported cases. A second limitation was that only 10 census blocks had more than 10 cases. Blocks with fewer than 10 cases may not be reliable, and sharing the location of these blocks could potentially breach confidentiality. Including all blocks in the analysis ensured valid statistical tests could be performed; however, targeting blocks with fewer than 10 cases was not recommended given the demand on resources. Analysis at the block group level is much more reliable, but the neighborhoods identified are much larger.

▶ Translating Data for Different Audiences: The Ethics of Data Presentation

As focus group discussions continued, Health Department staff noted an opportunity to include health providers throughout the community as a target audience for campaign messages. They decided to focus a large amount of effort on reaching out to these groups before the main kick-off to the campaign. In these efforts, lead staff from the department met with key providers in the town's hospitals and clinics to share our baseline data and campaign materials with them. These messages differed drastically from those that were developed to persuade the at-risk group to get tested.

Additionally, department staff requested the use of a patient survey in its clinic to capture perceptions and potential behavior changes related to exposure to the campaign materials. Because the survey would be administered to every patient age 15–65 years and involved collection of data identified by the UNC institutional review board as being about the person, the survey language had to meet a number of standards.

Finally, the project team spent a great deal of time considering the ethical implications of mapping chlamydia cases and sharing that information with the public. How much information people should see and how the information would be used became guiding questions.

▶ Campaign Development and Implementation

Because persons aged 15–24 years are a key risk group for chlamydia transmission, and because many residents were likely to either know little about the disease or hold stigmatized perceptions about the disease, campaign developers realized this program presented an opportunity to promote free and confidential testing. They also wanted to encourage community-wide norms in favor of testing as a strategy to improve community health. Campaign materials featured bright colors, contemporary formatting (e.g., depicting slogans using text message formatting), and resonance with popular culture current at the time of the campaign. For example, they used the slogan "Keep Calm and Get Tested," which references the resurgence of a World War II slogan from the United Kingdom that was popular in the United States in 2013.

▶ Outcome Evaluation

The North Carolina Institute for Public Health employed a time-based assessment of administrative records to investigate a key proximal outcome of the campaign—namely, chlamydia testing. County chlamydia testing records are kept in the county and have been collected for years. In fact, county officials collect the date and outcome of each test. By conceptualizing a unit of time as a unit of analysis, evaluation researchers were able to assess the testing behavior of the county as a whole over time. Instead of assessing the individual resident as the unit of analysis, the evaluation team assessed an average day in the life of the county as the unit of analysis. They were able to compute the likelihood of testing on a particular day as a function of time period. As a result, they could compare the likelihood of testing immediately prior to the launch of the campaign, and immediately after the campaign was completed. Recognizing that seasonality could lead to month-to-month changes as a function of seasonal constraints such as the start-up of the new school year or holiday schedules, the evaluation team chose to assess the likelihood of testing in a given month after the campaign launched compared to the same month a year earlier (to control for seasonality).

Given that this program was intended to be replicable and sustainable, data had to be easy to capture and easy to get. We experienced some unexpected challenges that reflected state policy, for example, especially with regard to male and female testing. Only female swab testing is done by the state lab in North Carolina (other local health departments, such as that in Boston, Massachusetts, cover both male and female swab testing at no cost). If a North Carolina county wants to use a urine test, which is more acceptable to many residents, then the Health Department is responsible for finding a lab to process urine tests. The Greater-Valley District Health Department opted to do that only during a teen clinic night, in the hopes that it would draw in more people to that event.

Another barrier was that a substantial proportion of the at-risk population—namely, men—is not currently being tested by the county because the Health Department cannot afford to do so and the state lab does not process these specimens. The county was able to secure an additional grant to test male urine samples, but the initial evaluation analysis had to concentrate only on women.

By developing a consistent protocol as to what counted as a measure of testing in the county over time, we were able to ensure a consistent outcome measure for assessment. Nonetheless, this did not eliminate the measurement constraint that policy decisions had imposed, which is an important practical consideration for local social marketing work.

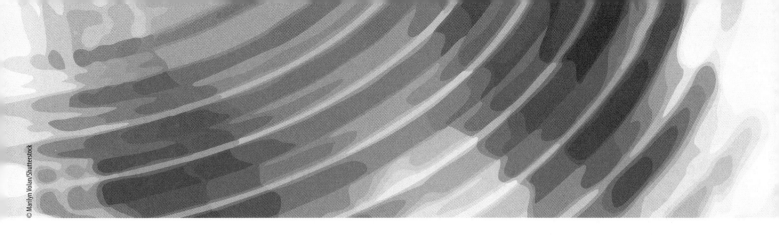

CHAPTER 5

Understanding and Reporting the Science

David E. Nelson

LEARNING OBJECTIVES

By the end of this chapter, the reader will be able to:

- Understand the quality of scientific evidence and the level of consensus among scientists on public health issues.
- Identify credible sources of scientific information.
- Understand factors influencing how lay audiences process and understand scientific information.
- Recognize four questions that the general public usually asks concerning a scientific study or report:
  - What did you find? (Description)
  - Why did it happen? (Explanation)
  - What does it mean? (Interpretation)
  - What needs to be done about it? (Action)
- Use the single overriding communication objective (SOCO) planning approach to shape communication messages from a scientific study and from a major scientific report for different audiences.

▶ Introduction

Public health is based on science and research. The collection, analysis, and interpretation of data using scientific and statistical principles—particularly epidemiologic methods—provide the evidence for recommendations and actions. But for science to lead to improvements in public health, research must be synthesized and communicated to a range of audiences, the majority of whom have little exposure or understanding of advanced science and math. Public health practitioners have two critical but often underappreciated roles[1-3]:

- Assess what is known about a specific topic or issue
- Communicate scientific findings to lay persons, with an eye toward what those findings mean to various audiences

This chapter provides guidance for communicating key scientific findings and conclusions to lay audiences such as policy makers, news media members, organizational representatives, and the public at large.

Evaluating the Quality of Public Health Science

Science is a body of knowledge learned through systemic study using methodologies accepted by others in the same field, which attempts to discover generalized truths about phenomena using hypotheses and deductions. Scientific knowledge is gained through the systematic analysis of quantitative and qualitative data using mathematical and logical principles. Many scientific disciplines, ranging from anthropology to laboratory-based basic science, contribute to public health.[1]

Assessing the quality of scientific knowledge means being able to determine the characteristics of "better science," which can be difficult at times. Occasionally even experts are fooled (e.g., when published studies in prominent journals are retracted because of data falsification or failure to report potential conflicts of interest). Nevertheless, three broad categories of factor must be examined when considering the quality of scientific information: Research design and conduct, scientific consensus, and credibility of the authors and publications in which research is reported. These factors are described further in **TABLE 5-1**.

Research Factors

Study Design

There is strong consensus among scientists that some types of research study designs are stronger than

TABLE 5-1 Factors Influencing the Quality of Science in Public Health

- Research factors
  - Study design
  - Representativeness and causality
- Level of scientific consensus
  - Research syntheses
  - Contextual information
- Source information
  - Authors and their institutions
  - Publications and publishers of scientific work

Adapted from Hill AB. The environment and disease: association or causation? *Proc R Acad Med.* 1965;58(5):295–300; Turnock BJ. *Essentials of Public Health.* 2nd ed. Sudbury, MA: Jones and Bartlett; 2012.

others because they minimize bias.[4,5] Without going into detail, the following types of studies are listed here from strongest to weakest design:

- Experimental studies
- Cohort studies
- Case-control studies
- Time-series studies
- Cross-sectional studies (e.g., surveys)
- Ecologic studies
- Case studies

Experimental studies involve "exposing" group of subjects (e.g., people or animals) to an intervention, such as a new drug, and comparing the results with an unexposed group. With a quasi-experimental design, groups are studied in a natural setting uncontrolled by the researcher, such as comparing a state with a mandatory immunization law to a state without such a law. Cohort studies involve collecting data from individuals prospectively (going forward) or for whom historical data already exist (retrospective or looking backward). In case-control studies, data are collected about past exposures from people with a specific health issue (i.e., a disease or condition) and then compared with data collected from individuals similar to the cases but who do not have the same specific health issue. Time-series studies involve comparing data from the same population at different times, rather than using a comparison group. Typically, results are compared before and after an intervention, such as adoption of a new health policy.

Cross-sectional studies are based on collecting outcome and exposure data from people at one time. Unfortunately, this design can make it difficult to determine if the exposures preceded the outcomes of interest. Ecologic studies typically involve correlating or comparing two types of population-level data. While studies of association can be valuable for generating hypotheses (e.g., "smoking prevalence tends to be higher in geographic areas where residents have low income levels"), they can produce misleading results because association does not mean causation. Case studies involve analyses of data from a small number of people or animals with the same disease or other health condition, which makes it difficult to draw firm (if any) conclusions.

Representativeness and Causality

Another important factor in assessing research is whether the data are applicable or representative on a population basis. For example, animal studies have contributed much to the base of scientific knowledge, even though animal research findings may not be directly applicable to humans. In addition, many scientific studies are conducted using small numbers of people who are often not representative of larger populations, Such research produces results that are suggestive but not broadly generalizable until repeated many times or confirmed by larger studies.

A longstanding issue in interpreting findings from scientific studies is assessing causality. For example, if a study demonstrates that risk factor X is strongly associated with health outcome Y, can we conclude that X caused Y? This is not a simple matter in science, and there are several factors to consider when it comes to causality.[4-6] Since 1965, the nine criteria of causality proposed by Hill have been widely used and adapted in epidemiological research.[6] Chief among them for our purposes are the following four criteria:

- Temporal precedence—risk factor before health outcome. (Causality is unidirectional.)
- Strength of association—for example, a relative risk (RR) estimate much greater than 1.
- Biological gradient—increasing exposure results in increased risk.
- Plausibility—the causal explanation fits the modern understanding of pathological processes.

Level of Scientific Consensus

It is fairly easy to find studies in scientific journals suggesting that "X causes (or prevents) Y," which means it is essential to understand the level of scientific consensus about a particular topic or issue when assessing the quality of research. The past three decades have seen the development of methods to do so, along with an explosion in syntheses and summaries of research findings in an effort to reach evidence-based scientific consensus about specific topics.

Research Syntheses

Given the large number of scientific journals and the sheer volume of research, there is a great need for synthesis of research so that scientists, practitioners, and lay audiences can have information about "the state of the science" and its implications for public health. Research syntheses are invaluable sources of scientifically credible public health information that can be communicated to lay audiences. There are three major types of research syntheses:

- Meta-analyses
- Systematic reviews of the literature
- Comprehensive reports

Meta-analysis refers to a type of study in which researchers analyze data obtained in prior studies.[7] Using a set of rules for selecting studies and data sources on a specific topic, researchers pool data and calculate a summary measure to estimate the level of association (e.g., relative risk) between exposure X and outcome Y (e.g., a person's blood alcohol level and the risk of impaired driving). The benefits of meta-analyses are that they are based on a broader body of evidence, and larger sample sizes, than can be obtained through any one study, and they produce more precise summary (relative risk) estimates.[8] Most meta-analyses are conducted independently and published in scientific journals, but sometimes they are performed under the auspices of sponsoring organizations that are seeking to publish comprehensive reports on a topic.

Unlike traditional literature reviews, which are subject to several types of biases, systematic reviews of the literature involve a detailed plan and strategy, spelled out in advance, to comprehensively identify published or unpublished research studies from scientific literature databases (e.g., PubMed) and other sources about a topic.[9-11] Exclusion criteria and decision-making rules are used to help ensure that only high-quality research studies are included in the analysis.

The third type of research synthesis is a comprehensive report on a health topic. Such reports are developed by a variety of organizations or groups, performed for many different purposes, and use different ways to synthesize and interpret the scientific literature. Such research syntheses are sometimes conducted by expert panels or working groups, and may lead to clinical, policy, or other guidelines or recommendations for individuals, organizations, or policy makers. Not surprisingly given the many different factors that influence them, the quality and credibility of comprehensive reports are highly variable. Perhaps the best-known international example of an organization that focuses on this type of research synthesis is the Cochrane Collaboration. Based in the United Kingdom, this organization publishes reports developed through a highly rigorous process involving systematic literature reviews and meta-analyses.[12,13]

Other research institutions, government agencies, and other organizations also develop or support the development of comprehensive health reports based on evidence-based research reviews. Examples include reports from the National Academy of Medicine (previously known as the Institute of Medicine),[14] the U.S. Surgeon General,[15] the Community Preventive Services Task Force[16] (**BOX 5-1**), and the U.S. Preventive

---

BOX 5-1 The Guide to Community Preventive Services

The Guide to Community Preventive Services (the Community Guide) is a resource sponsored by the Task Force on Community Preventive Services and hosted on a website managed by the Centers for Disease Control and Prevention (CDC). It is designed to help users select programs and policies to improve health and prevent disease in communities. Rigorous, systematic reviews of scientific research studies, with a particular emphasis on the quality of the study designs, are used to determine the effectiveness of programs and policies. The Community Guide includes cost-effectiveness analyses, and other types of economic-related considerations, whenever possible. It is designed to help users answer the following questions:

- Which interventions have and have not worked?
- In which populations and settings has the intervention worked or not worked?
- What might the intervention cost? What should users expect for their investment?
- Does the intervention lead to any other benefits or harms?
- Which interventions need more research before we know if they work or not?

The Task Force hopes that users of the Community Guide will have the following outcomes:

- Use more interventions that have been shown to work
- Use fewer interventions that have been shown not to work
- Understand there are interventions for which there is not enough evidence to say whether they work

Nearly 300 reviews and reports have been completed during the 20-year history of the Community Guide. Recommendations have been issued for the following areas:

Adolescent health	Mental health
Alcohol consumption	Motor vehicle injury prevention
Asthma	Nutrition
Birth defects	Obesity
Cancer prevention and control	Oral health
Cardiovascular disease prevention and control	Physical activity
Diabetes prevention and control	Social environment
Emergency preparedness and response	Tobacco
Health communication and social marketing	Vaccination
Health equity	Violence
HIV/AIDS, sexually transmitted infections, and pregnancy	Worksite health promotion

Community Preventive Services Task Force Web site. http://www.thecommunityguide.org/index.html. Accessed January 23, 2015.

Services Task Force[17] (**BOX 5-2**). Such reports can be invaluable resources for health information communication because they are performed by organizations seen as credible, and the conclusions can often be used to develop messages that are directly relevant for public health practice. Keep in mind, however, that some comprehensive reports have much lower scientific credibility. These include reports from organizations, institutions, or professional societies whose conclusions or recommendations are based primarily or solely on "expert panel" members' opinions, or that fail to describe in sufficient detail the process used to review the literature or reach conclusions.

Contextual Information

Another important question to consider related to the level of scientific consensus is the context in which scientific findings are presented.[3] Today, there is unprecedented, widespread, and rapid availability of scientific information through the Internet, social media, and other sources. Unfortunately, over-generalization and over-interpretation of scientific findings are widespread problems.[18] Probably every reader of this chapter has encountered information trumpeting a fascinating new health finding or breakthrough that was quickly discovered to fall short of those claims.

BOX 5-2 U.S. Preventive Services Task Force Recommendations

Created in 1984, the U.S. Preventive Services Task Force (USPSTF) is an independent, volunteer panel of national experts in prevention and evidence-based medicine. The USPSTF works to improve the health of all Americans by making evidence-based recommendations about clinical preventive services such as screenings, counseling services, and preventive medications. Members of the task force come from the fields of preventive medicine and primary care, including internal medicine, family medicine, pediatrics, behavioral health, obstetrics and gynecology, and nursing. Their recommendations are based on a rigorous review of existing peer-reviewed evidence and are intended to help primary care clinicians and patients decide together whether a preventive service is right for a patient's needs.

The USPSTF assigns a letter grade (an A, B, C, or D grade or an I statement) to each recommendation based on the strength of the evidence and the balance of benefits and harms of a preventive service.[a] The recommendations apply only to people who have no signs or symptoms of the specific disease or condition under evaluation, and the recommendations address only services offered in the primary care setting or referred by a primary care clinician.

Here are some examples of recent recommendations from the USPSTF:

- *Recommends* clinicians screen all pregnant women for HIV, including those who present in labor who are untested and whose HIV status is unknown. *Grade: A recommendation.*
- *Recommends* clinicians screen women of childbearing age for intimate partner violence, such as domestic violence, and provide or refer women who have a positive screen to intervention services. This recommendation applies to women who do not have signs or symptoms of abuse. *Grade: B recommendation.*
- *Does not recommend* automatically performing an in-depth multifactorial risk assessment in conjunction with comprehensive management of identified risks to prevent falls in community-dwelling adults aged 65 years or older because the likelihood of benefit is small. In determining whether this service is appropriate in individual cases, patients and clinicians should consider the balance of benefits and harms on the basis of the circumstances of prior falls, comorbid medical conditions, and patient values. *Grade: C recommendation.*
- *Recommends against* prostate-specific antigen (PSA)–based screening for prostate cancer. *Grade: D recommendation.*
- Current evidence is *insufficient* to assess the balance of the benefits and the harms of combined vitamin D and calcium supplementation for the primary prevention of fractures in men. *Grade: I statement*

a. For a Grade A recommendation, the USPSTF recommends the service because there is high certainty that the net benefit is substantial. For a Grade B recommendation, the USPSTF recommends the service because there is high certainty that the net benefit is moderate, or there is moderate certainty that the net benefit is moderate to substantial. For a Grade C recommendation, the USPSTF recommends selectively offering or providing this service to individual patients based on professional judgment and patient preferences. There is at least moderate certainty that the net benefit is small. For a Grade D recommendation, the USPSTF recommends against the service because there is moderate or high certainty that the service has no net benefit or that the harms outweigh the benefits. For a Grade I statement, the USPSTF concludes that the current evidence is insufficient to assess the balance of benefits and harms of the service because evidence is lacking, of poor quality, or conflicting, and the balance of benefits and harms cannot be determined.

U.S. Preventive Services Task Force Web site. http://www.uspreventiveservicestaskforce.org/. Accessed January 15, 2015.org/index.html. Accessed January 23, 2015.

Given the level of hyperbole and interest that may surround certain scientific findings, it is more important than ever to ascertain from a journal article, oral presentation, news story, or other source whether the contextual considerations for a scientific finding are addressed. **TABLE 5-2** highlights some questions to consider when evaluating new scientific information.[19,20]

Information Sources

A common mental shortcut that people use when considering the quality of information they receive is to take into account the perceived credibility (trustworthiness and expertise) of the information sources.[3] For example, advice from a computer scientist about a software problem is easier to accept than advice from someone with limited or no computer experience. Persons or organizations with potential conflicts of interests are not likely to be credible sources of information. For example, alcohol beverage companies are likely to be viewed as less credible sources of information about the health risks or alleged benefits associated with alcohol use. The same principle holds true when assessing scientific information, because some information sources are far more credible than others.

Source credibility for scientific information can be considered along two dimensions: (1) the scientists and their respective institutions reporting the findings

TABLE 5-2 Contextual Questions to Consider When Evaluating New Scientific Information[19, 20]

- Have findings been included in a scientifically credible publication?
- Are these findings preliminary?
- Are these new findings, or have they been previously reported?
- How do the findings compare with previous research? (If the findings are different, why should these results be considered more believable than prior research?)
- How certain is it that the results are not due to chance?
- What are potential alternative explanations?
- Can these results be generalized to other populations?
- Are supplementary data tables available, and if so, where can they be accessed?
- Are the original data available, and are the researchers willing to share them with others?
- What are the limitations of these findings?
- What is potentially missing?
- Should judgment be withheld until more evidence is available (e.g., completion of other studies, replication of this study)?
- What do other scientific experts in the same field say about these findings?
- Who is promoting these findings?
- Do the promoters have a conflict of interest?

and (2) the publication or publisher of the reports. The credibility of individual scientists is based on their prior research and reputation within their fields. With the widespread availability of searchable databases and Internet search engines, it is fairly easy to gather information about individual scientists.

The prominence of the organization where a scientist works is also important. Persons employed at more renowned scientific research organizations (e.g., Northwestern University, National Institutes of Health) are likely to have higher credibility—although this is certainly not always the case—because obtaining and retaining positions in these organizations is a highly competitive process. Furthermore, scientific documents produced by some governmental agencies go through an extensive review process prior to publication.

Just as credibility can be based on "whether" scientists' research findings are published, so credibility can also depend on "where," or in which publications, the findings are published. Obviously, scientists who publish extensively in more prominent scientific

journals (e.g., *Science, Nature, New England Journal of Medicine, The Lancet*) have more proven track records and are likely to be seen as more credible. As mentioned earlier, comprehensive reports of major research syntheses also have high credibility because of the rigorous process used by these organizations when developing the reports.

A number of organizations, such as advocacy groups, ideologically oriented "think tanks," and industry-supported organizations, seek to produce or contribute to publications, news releases, or other public relations efforts that will garner substantial attention from the news media and others. The major goal for these organizations is typically to gain support for their own preferred outcome(s) or conclusion(s). To achieve this aim, they may "cherry pick" studies (take findings out of context) to promote particular points of view or recommendations.

In sum, many factors influence the quality of science and scientific information. You do not have to be a practicing scientist, however, to assess quality. Careful consideration of the factors described here, and a healthy dose of skepticism, will go a long way toward ensuring you select only high-quality scientific information to communicate to others.

▶ How Lay Audiences Assess Science-Based Public Health Information

Several factors influence how lay audiences process and understand scientific information. A key point to remember, though, is that people are not empty vessels when it comes to providing them with information; rather, they have different health-related experiences, preexisting beliefs about health, and worldviews that affect their reaction to health messages.[3,21]

Level of Interest in Health and Extent of Scientific Knowledge

Readers of this chapter are interested in health issues, but health is of only low to moderate interest to the population at large.[3] Studies show that in the general population, the persons who are most interested in health topics tend to be older, be female, and generally have better personal health. Those who have experienced specific health problems or who have close family members with such problems (a factor called involvement) also tend to pay more attention to health issues.[22]

The level of scientific knowledge among the general population in the United States and elsewhere is fairly limited.[23] For example, approximately half of U.S. adults incorrectly believe antibiotics kill viruses, and one-fourth believe the sun orbits the earth. Remember that most people are not thinking about health on a daily basis, which means that it will take some effort to gain their attention and let them know why they should care about a particular public health issue.

Culture and Worldview

Many of us in public health are unaware of how commonly people form their own theories about health. When coupled with broader societal beliefs, this tendency can complicate communication about scientific findings. Some people have grown up with a completely different tradition of medicine, such as European homeopathy and botanical cures, or southeastern and southern Asian systems that seek equilibrium in bodily humors or energy flow (chi).

Many Americans also have health beliefs that are outside the evidence-based scientific views: Exposure to cold temperatures causes the common cold, stress causes high blood pressure, and large doses of vitamins and "natural foods" are beneficial to health. These and other deeply held beliefs, some of which stem from personal worldviews, can influence individual receptivity to communications about scientific health information. "Worldview" refers to how people perceive their level of control over their own lives and how they think about power and wealth distribution. Examples include fatalism, individualism, egalitarianism, or respect and trust for authority. People with a strong individualistic worldview, for instance, may be opposed to mandatory immunization laws, believing that they are an unacceptable infringement on individual choice. People with a strong fatalistic worldview often do not believe in screening tests, thinking that if they are meant to die of cancer, for example, this represents "God's will" for them. Those who do not "trust the government" might apply their view to all governmental branches and divisions, including health departments. People with these types of worldviews are likely not to attend to, nor believe, rationales or arguments based on scientific evidence.

Trust and Belief

Given the many factors that play into assessing scientific evidence and credible scientific sources, certain individuals may not be inclined to believe or accept the current accepted state of scientific knowledge about a topic. Instead, they may trust their friends, family members, work colleagues, clergy, the mass media, the Internet, community organization leaders, and others before they trust anything a "nerdy scientist" has to say. Personal experience or anecdotes that support existing viewpoints or behaviors (e.g., "My uncle smoked cigarettes and he lived until he was 92") are often believed much more readily than conflicting information based on scientific consensus.

The acceptance or disbelief of health information is strongly influenced by two psychological principles: confirmation bias and selective exposure.[24-26] Confirmation bias means that we tend to interpret messages as confirming what we already believe. A corollary to this tendency is that we may pay no attention to, or even "tune out," messages with which we do not agree. Selective exposure means we like to obtain information from sources with which we agree. Thus, we generally have friends, and choose media and other sources of information, whose beliefs and opinions are similar to our own and who tend to agree with us. Selective exposure is especially challenging to overcome for health communicators because people have many communication sources available, and they can (and often do) choose to be exposed only to those with which they agree. Such preferences make it difficult and expensive to produce a distinctive, scientifically sound public health message that can attract the attention of a non-empathetic or distracted audience.

Information Processing and Interpretation

People's ability to process large amounts of information is limited.[3] When exposed to a lot of information, particularly if the information is complex or unfamiliar, they may "tune it out" or just remember the first item (primacy effect) or the last item (recency effect). As health communication professionals, we need to be careful how much scientific information we include in our messages, and strive to highlight key points without overwhelming people. Except among persons who are highly involved in a particular health issue, providing more information will rarely help audiences better comprehend key messages.

When people seek information, they usually want to get right to the bottom line: What is the key point or gist? This preference is related to satisficing,[24] a term coined to describe what happens when people search for information quickly ("satisfy + suffice"). Because most people do not want to expend much time or energy searching, when they find what they need, they typically end their search. From a communication practice standpoint, it is important to provide information materials that convey the gist of the main message(s) and to ensure that these main messages can be found easily and quickly.

People have a strong desire for certainty.[3] When they hear advice from experts, regardless of their field, they want the advice to be definitive, which can be a challenge in health communication. In acute public health outbreaks, the cause or solution to the problem might take time to discover. In other situations, it can take time to recognize that no action is needed because there is neither a causative agent or nor a solution. When scientists cannot provide definitive answers, or when they provide an answer that suggests "no action is needed," people can become fearful and angry.

A further complication is that many people have difficulty accepting that scientists' explanations or recommendations can change because of more recent research. For example, in the past several years, recommendations for cervical cancer screening have changed; most women no longer need an annual Pap test. Acceptance of these new recommendations has been difficult for some women and their healthcare providers.[27]

As should be clear by now, communicating scientific information in public health is both complex and challenging. Much more is involved than simply explaining findings and making recommendations, and then expecting people will believe what we say and do what we want them to do. Even when a public health intervention is supported by strong scientific evidence and consensus, communicating the science will not necessarily lead to a change in behavior.

▶ Science Communication Fundamentals

Content

An important lesson from the fields of communication research and practice is to carefully consider what audiences want from experts in public health and other areas.[3,28] From a communication perspective, most people want to know answers to the following questions:

- What did you find? (Description)
- Why did it happen? (Explanation)
- What does it mean? (Interpretation)
- What needs to be done about it? (Action)

Description is the journalist's basic "Who, what, where, when, and how?" query. In a hypothetical example, the health communicator might provide a message such as "*More than 50 people experienced a severe bout of gastrointestinal illness within a few days in x state between October 15 and 21, 2015. Further research demonstrated that the affected individuals had* Cryptosporidium *infection*."

Explanation and interpretation are closely related because they attempt to answer the questions "how" and "why." For example, the (hypothetical) explanation for a foodborne outbreak might be "*Research indicates that persons who drank Brand X of apple cider were more much more likely to develop symptoms. Laboratory studies indicated Brand X apple cider was contaminated with* Cryptosporidium *bacteria*." Interpretation typically involves trying to determine why those findings occurred, by presenting hypotheses or theories to explain causal relationships or associations: "*Brand X apple cider was unpasteurized and contained no preservatives. Further investigation found that apples that had dropped to the ground were used in cider presses. All these factors likely contributed to* Cryptosporidium *being found in the apple cider*."

Many scientists focus heavily on description, explanation, and interpretation of scientific information. For the health information professional, however, it is important to remember that messages that raise awareness about a public health problem often create fear, anxiety, or anger. When this happens, people may deny the importance of the problem; become too anxious or, conversely, overly optimistic that they are not at risk; or search for someone or something to blame.

The public, policy makers, the media, and others want public health experts to provide advice or recommendations about what to do to address a problem—that is, which actions are needed. Simply put, people want to know how to use the information they receive to make decisions.[3] At an individual level, this might mean taking steps to avoid certain adverse health effects (e.g., engage in higher levels of physical activity). For policy makers, it might mean enacting (or continuing) a recommendation or policy, such as closing a manufacturing plant that produced contaminated food products, or passing legislation requiring health insurers to cover payment for disease screening or treatment. Providing up-to-date resources and explaining where to find them (e.g., a government agency website, an emergency telephone number) are ways to make additional information available to those most involved or interested in the issue.

Context

Another key aspect of communicating scientific findings is to place them in their proper context. Scientific findings always need to be considered in the context of prior research and recommendations (see the discussion of scientific context earlier in this chapter). In another sense, context can refer to the communication of scientific results in a meaningful context for local communities. For instance, if a major scientific study demonstrated the value of a preventive medication or screening test, health communicators could let local healthcare providers and news media outlets know where people in a given community could go to obtain the medication or test. If news reports describe a disease outbreak occurring in another state, it would be a good idea to share information on specific steps people in the local area could take to reduce their disease risk.

Overload

Interpreting scientific information can be mentally taxing, especially when too much is presented and the information is as complex.[3] To avoid the problem of information overload, it is important to present only the essential information. Carefully consider, for example, whether numbers should be used in messages at all, let alone which numbers are appropriate. Providing short executive summaries, or including key points or conclusions up front in longer written documents, can be especially helpful in circumventing overload.

▶ Putting It All Together

Single Overriding Communication Objective

A wealth of communication tools are available to help you learn to be succinct in writing or speaking about health and science information. The CDC's Media Relations office developed a template called the single overriding communication objective (SOCO) form, which is included in **BOX 5-3**.[29] The choice of the SOCO acronym, which conveys the idea of selecting a message or messages that "socks you in the mouth" (or wherever), was intentional.

Although other communication tools exist, the SOCO form is particularly designed and useful for communicating scientific information to lay audiences. For lay audiences, communicators need to "boil down" the essence of a study or report into a key message and a few main facts. SOCO also emphasizes the

---

BOX 5-3 CDC's Single Overriding Communication Objective (SOCO) Planning Document

In one paragraph, please state the key point or objective of your article or report. This statement should reflect what you, the writer, would like to see as the lead paragraph in a newspaper story or in a broadcast news report:

List three facts or statistics you would like the audience to remember as a result of reading or hearing about your article:

What is the main audience or population segment you would like this article to reach?

■ Primary audience:
■ Secondary audience:

What is the one main message the audience needs to take from your article or report?

Who in your office will serve as the point of contact for media questions?

Name: Degree(s):
Title:
Email:
Phone:
Date(s) and time(s) available:

Sample single overriding communications objective (SOCO) worksheet. Centers for Disease Control and Prevention Web site. www.cdc.gov/.../dwa-comm-toolbox/before/tools/Single-Overriding-Comm-Objective-Worksheet.docx. Accessed January 19, 2015.

importance of identifying the intended audience(s), which helps when developing messages tailored to specific types of individual.

Case Study: Communicating Science from a Research Study Article

A good way to learn how to prepare messages and materials so as to communicate scientific findings to lay audiences based on the information covered in this chapter is to deconstruct actual scientific publications. The first example presented here comes from an article reporting a research study on melanoma (an aggressive form of skin cancer) and indoor tanning, which was published in 2010 in the journal *Cancer Epidemiology, Biomarkers & Prevention*.[30] See http://cebp.aacrjournals.org/content/19/6/1557. This study was conducted by researchers in Minnesota and involved surveys of adults regarding their exposure to indoor tanning among both persons recently diagnosed with melanoma (cases) and people without melanoma who were similar in age and gender (controls).

Assessing the science for health communication purposes involves considering the research factors, the level of scientific consensus, and the information sources. In terms of the research factors for the melanoma study, a case-control study is a moderately strong study design, ranking third behind only experimental and cohort designs. A case-control study is often the best research design when investigating diseases such as melanoma that are relatively uncommon in the general population.[4,5] Representativeness was addressed by identifying individuals with melanoma from the Minnesota statewide cancer registry, and members of the control group from a database of individuals with a driver's license or state identification card. Nevertheless, residents of Minnesota (or any other state, for that matter) are not necessarily representative of the United States as a whole.

Causality is an especially important issue to assess for this study. There is biological plausibility for its cause-and-effect hypothesis because exposure to solar ultraviolet (UV) rays is believed to account for the increase in melanoma incidence that has occurred in recent decades. The overall strength of association between indoor tanning and melanoma risk (assessed using the odds ratio to estimate relative risk) was less than 2 after controlling for other factors, but there was a strong biological gradient because persons exposed for more years, hours, or number of sessions of indoor tanning were at greater risk of developing melanoma.

As for level of scientific consensus, this article describes one study and is not a research synthesis. Even so, it does contain contextual information

to help readers understand where the findings "fit" based on prior research: The International Agency for Research on Cancer (IARC) classifies tanning devices as carcinogenic to humans.[31] This study overcomes major limitations of previous studies (e.g., exposure measurement, dose-response relationship, age of initiation), which had found only weak associations between indoor tanning and melanoma risk.

Assessing the quality of scientific information also involves determining the credibility of the source, which includes the authors and their institutions, along with the publication. Source credibility for this study is quite high. The lead author, Dr. Lazovich, is an associate professor, and director of graduate studies, in the Division of Epidemiology and Community Health at the University of Minnesota School of Public Health.[32] This Division is well known nationally and internationally for conducting high-quality research. *Cancer Epidemiology, Biomarkers & Prevention* is a prominent scientific journal published by the American Association for Cancer Research.[33] Research study manuscripts submitted to this journal undergo peer review by other scientists, who make recommendations about whether they should be published.

After assessing the quality of the science, the process of communication message development begins. Before getting into specifics about indoor tanning and melanoma, the first consideration is to determine the SOCO. There is no simple formula or one "right way" to decide on the SOCO, but here is one suggestion:

> *Indoor tanning causes melanoma, a dangerous form of skin cancer. The risk of developing this skin cancer is much greater among persons who use indoor tanning devices more frequently and over longer periods of time.*

Prior to developing main messages based on this scientific article, it is important to consider whether lay audiences know what melanoma is, and whether they understand the health consequences of developing this disease (Why is it important?). Providing some basic background information about melanoma familiarizes audiences with this type of cancer. Audiences can learn that the number of people with melanoma has increased substantially over the past 20 years, what melanoma looks like, how it is diagnosed and treated by healthcare providers, that it can spread (metastasize) beyond the skin, and that it causes nearly 10,000 deaths per year in the United States.[34]

Use the four key message elements (description, explanation, interpretation, and recommended actions) when communicating information from scientific publications to lay audiences. Here are some examples of descriptive messages from this study (note that they are similar to the SOCO):

- People who had ever tanned indoors had a 75% greater risk of developing melanoma.
- Skin cancer risks were substantially higher among people who used indoor tanning devices over many years, who had more tanning sessions, or who had more total hours of indoor tanning.

Here are some examples of explanatory and interpretive messages:

- Even when accounting for other factors related to skin cancer risk, there is strong evidence that indoor tanning causes melanoma.
- Findings from this study strongly support the International Agency for Research on Cancer's conclusion that indoor tanning causes skin cancer.

As mentioned earlier, people are most interested in the gist, or major results, from a study and the action that needs to be taken as a result of the findings. Although the authors of this particular article did not address individual or policy actions, a public health communicator must always be prepared to address the potential implications of scientific research studies. Here are examples of action messages for individuals and policy makers based on this study:

- People should avoid indoor tanning because it increases their risk of getting skin cancer.
- If you currently engage in indoor tanning user, stop doing so immediately.
- Laws or regulations should be enacted that forbid or limit indoor tanning.

Case Study: Communicating Science from a Comprehensive Report

The 2012 Surgeon General's Report (SGR) titled *Preventing Tobacco Use Among Youth and Young Adults*[35] is an example of a comprehensive scientific report (**FIGURE 5-1**). This 900-page document, which took several years to complete, contains a comprehensive review and synthesis of the scientific research literature about tobacco use prevention for these population groups. **BOX 5-4** highlights the SGR's major conclusions.

BOX 5-4 Major Conclusions of the 2012 Surgeon General's Report on Preventing Tobacco Use Among Youth and Young Adults

1. Cigarette smoking by youth and young adults has immediate adverse health consequences, including addiction, and accelerates the development of chronic diseases across the full life-course.
2. Prevention efforts must focus on both adolescents and young adults because among adults who become daily smokers, nearly all first use of cigarettes occurs by 18 years of age (88%), with 99% of first use occurring by 26 years of age.
3. Advertising and promotional activities by tobacco companies have been shown to cause the onset and continuation of smoking among adolescents and young adults.
4. After years of steady progress, declines in the use of tobacco by youth and young adults have slowed for cigarette smoking and stalled for smokeless tobacco use.
5. Coordinated, multicomponent interventions that combine mass-media campaigns, price increases including those that result from tax increases, school-based policies and programs, and statewide or community-wide changes in smoke-free policies and norms are effective in reducing the initiation, prevalence, and intensity of smoking among youth and young adults.

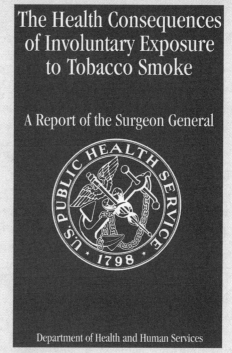

FIGURE 5-1 Cover of the 2012 Surgeon General's Report.

Reproduced from: https://nccd.cdc.gov/OSH_Pub_Catalog/SelectionDetails.aspx?p=XNvEK7UkxLj0Xr%2FPZxFUXS7Y57qW26JlcuLoDM5lexk%3D

U.S. Department of Health and Human Services. Preventing Tobacco Use among Youth and Young Adults: A Report of the Surgeon General. Atlanta, GA: U.S. Department of Health and Human Services, Centers for Disease Control and Prevention, National Center for Chronic Disease Prevention and Health Promotion, Office on Smoking and Health; 2012.

While we still need to assess the science and deconstruct this publication for communication purposes, the process is somewhat different than for the previously described scientific article. In particular, much of the assessment of the science has already been done: The SGR authors reviewed hundreds of studies and carefully assessed the quality of the science and evidence to reach their conclusion and come to consensus. Also, SGRs contain executive summaries highlighting key scientific findings and conclusions, which makes developing communication messages much easier. (Note that SGRs do not make policy or other types of recommendations.)

Assessing the science begins with evaluating the study design and representativeness. These particular factors are not especially problematic for the SGR, because they were carefully evaluated by the report's authors. (If you were interested in a particular topic, such as the tobacco industry's influence on youth tobacco use, then you should carefully examine the scientific quality of the studies reviewed in that section of the report.) Determining causality is a major goal for certain topics within the report (e.g., health effects, tobacco industry influence, prevention approaches), with the strength of the causality evidence being classified as strong evidence, suggestive evidence, inconclusive evidence, or no evidence.

The level of scientific consensus was not an issue, because the report itself represents a consensus. Prior research and other contextual information were taken into account before assigning a rating for causality. As for source information, the lengthy list of authors, editors, and other contributors contains well-known scientific experts in the field of tobacco control from highly credible institutions or organizations. The U.S. Surgeon General and the SGRs on tobacco are considered credible sources of health information. The process for obtaining and reviewing scientific information, as well as the extensive review process for report drafts conducted by federal health agencies representatives and outside scientists not affiliated with the SGR's writing, contribute to the integrity of the findings. It is noteworthy that no conclusion in any Surgeon General Report on Tobacco (the first was published in 1964) has ever been retracted.

Communication planning begins with considering the SOCO. Because of the comprehensiveness of the SGR, there are many potential SOCOs depending on the target audience (the public, healthcare providers, policy makers, news media) and communication objectives, but an excellent starting point would be the five major conclusions from the report (Box 5-5). Here is one simple SOCO:

Previous declines in tobacco use by youth and young adults have stalled, with tobacco marketing being one of the main reasons. But tobacco use among young people can be prevented using proven, broad-scale interventions to reverse these trends.

One of the great values of relying on comprehensive reports such as the SGR is that some communication materials may have already been developed and made available, which saves a lot of time. For this report, a wealth of supplementary written and visual materials is available on the websites of the U.S. Surgeon General (http://www.surgeongeneral.gov) and the CDC's Office on Smoking and Health (http://www.cdc.gov/tobacco). These materials were specifically created to communicate different aspects of the report to different audiences, and they are readily adaptable for use by others.

Unlike the article on indoor tanning and melanoma, which required some background information, there is less need for background information about tobacco use issues among youth and young adults, because most lay audiences will already have a good understanding of this topic. The exceptions would be if the communication effort focused on health effects, or if it emphasized multicomponent prevention interventions (e.g., mass-media campaigns, price increases, school or community smoke-free policies).

Messages based on this report should describe, explain, and interpret the findings and then provide recommendations for action. Here are some descriptive message examples:

■ Nearly 90% of adult smokers begin smoking by age 18, and 99% by age 26. This makes it imperative to prevent tobacco use among young people so they can avoid the many adverse health effects caused by tobacco.
■ Almost one in four high school students and one in three young adults are cigarette smokers.
■ Cigarette smoking causes asthma in children and adolescents.
■ Tobacco company advertising and promotion is associated with the initiation and progression of tobacco use in young people.

Here are some examples of explanatory and interpretive messages from the SGR:

■ Adolescents and young adults are especially susceptible to peer and other influences in their environment, and peer pressure can lead them to begin or continue to smoke.

- Poor school performance is a strong risk factor for adolescents becoming regular smokers.
- Tobacco companies spend more than $10 billion a year on marketing, most of which is used to reduce prices (e.g., discounts).

Given the implications from the findings in this report, here are examples of action messages:

- Because of their proven effectiveness in reducing tobacco use by young people, more funding is needed [or current funding should be maintained] for antitobacco mass-media campaigns, and for comprehensive community and statewide tobacco control programs in the state of X.
- The cigarette tax should be increased by [Y amount] because this will reduce smoking among adolescents and young adults.

Case Study: Interpreting Science for Communication to the Public

The appendix to this chapter presents an example of a government agency going to great lengths to synthesize the scientific knowledge on a subject and develop a set of consensus messages appropriate for public communication. In this case study, Barret, Sprague, and Reimers describe the systematic review and process by which an expert panel was convened by the National Institutes of Environmental Health Sciences and the National

Cancer Institute (both institutes within the National Institutes of Health [NIH]) as part of the Breast Cancer and the Environment Research Project. The science in this case was extremely complex, involving multiple research centers examining the relationships between environmental exposures, particularly in childhood and adolescence, and the potential for genetic mutations leading to breast cancer. The expert panel that was convened to develop the messages included physicians, communication scientists, and representatives of advocacy organizations. Hence the group had to work out the tensions related to sharing information (the scientists considered sharing premature but the advocates felt it would be life-saving) by finding a balance between informing the public and not scaring them to death.

▶ Conclusion

Credible scientific evidence is based on several important characteristics, including how studies were conducted and where and by whom their findings were published. Many factors influence whether and how audiences receive and interpret scientific information. Several approaches may be used to communicate scientific findings to lay audiences, depending on the audience and type of messages, but good planning is always essential. Practicing the recommendations in this chapter can increase the chance that high-quality science, when communicated well, will result in better public health.

Wrap-Up

Chapter Questions

1. Why is it important to consider the quality of science first?
2. What are the three broad categories of factors to consider when assessing scientific quality?
3. Why is it important to present findings from a scientific study or report in context?
4. What is source credibility, and why does it matter so much?
5. What are at least five broad factors that influence how people process and evaluate scientific information?
6. What are the four basic questions about scientific studies or reports that lay audiences want public health scientists, practitioners, or their representatives to answer?
7. Why do you need to develop a SOCO?

References

1. Turnock BJ. *Essentials of Public Health*. 2nd ed. Sudbury, MA: Jones and Bartlett; 2012.
2. Friis RH, Sellers TA. *Epidemiology for Public Health Practice*. 5th ed. Sudbury, MA: Jones and Bartlett; 2013.
3. Nelson DE, Hesse BW, Croyle RT. *Making Data Talk*. New York, NY: Oxford University Press; 2009.
4. Rothman KJ. *Epidemiology: An Introduction*. New York, NY: Oxford University Press; 2012.
5. Gordis L. *Epidemiology*. St. Louis, MO: Saunders; 2013.

6. Hill AB. The environment and disease: association or causation? *Proc R Acad Med.* 1965;58(5):295–300.

7. Schmidt FL, Hunter JE. *Methods of Meta-Analysis: Correcting Error and Bias in Research Findings.* 3rd ed. Washington, DC: Sage; 2014.

8. Murad MH, Montori VM, Ionnidis JPA, et al. How to read a systematic review and meta-analysis and apply results to patient care: users' guides to the medical literature. *JAMA.* 2014;312(2):171–179.

9. Gough D, Oliver S, Thomas, J. *An Introduction to Systematic Reviews.* Washington, DC: Sage; 2012.

10. Uman LS. Systematic reviews and meta-analyses. *J Can Acad Child Adolesc Psychiatry.* 2011;20(1):57–59.

11. Strauss SE, Richardson WS, Glasziou P, Haynes RB. *Evidence-Based Medicine: How to Teach and Practice EBM.* 4th ed. Philadelphia, PA: Churchill Livingstone Elsevier; 2010.

12. Higgins JPT, Green S, eds. *Cochrane Handbook of Systematic Reviews of Interventions.* Chichester, UK: John Wiley & Sons; 2008.

13. Cochrane Collaboration. http://www.cochrane.org/. Accessed January 19, 2015.

14. National Academies of Science, Engineering, and Medicine. http://www.nationalacademies.org/. Accessed January 19, 2015.

15. U.S. Surgeon General. Reports of the Surgeon General, U.S. Public Health Service. http://www.surgeongeneral.gov/library/reports/. Accessed January 19, 2015.

16. Community Preventive Services Task Force. http://www.thecommunityguide.org/index.html. Accessed January 23, 2015.

17. U.S. Preventive Services Task Force. http://www.uspreventiveservicestaskforce.org/. Accessed January 15, 2015.

18. Yavchitz A, Boutron I, Bafeta A, et al. Misrepresentation of randomized controlled trials in press releases and news coverage: a cohort study. *PLoS Med.* 2012;9(9):e1001308. doi:10.1371/journal.pmed.1001308.

19. Nelson DE, Brownson RC, Remington PL, Parvanta C, eds. *Communicating Public Health Information Effectively.* Washington, DC: American Public Health Association; 2002.

20. Health News Review. http://www.healthnewsreview.org/. Accessed January 19, 2015.

21. Guidotti TL. Communication is an essential skill for the scientist. *Arch Environ Occup Health.* 2014;69(4):252–253.

22. Slater MD. Persuasion processes across receiver goals and message genres. *Commun Theory.* 1997;7(2):125–148.

23. National Science Board. Chapter 7. Science and technology: public attitudes and understanding. *Science and Engineering Indicators 2014.* http://www.nsf.gov/statistics/seind14/index.cfm/chapter-7. Accessed January 22, 2015.

24. Plous S. *The Psychology of Judgment and Decision-Making.* New York, NY: McGraw-Hill; 1993.

25. Heath C, Heath D. *Decisive: How to Make Better Choices in Life and Work.* New York, NY: Crown Business Random House; 2013.

26. Sparks GG. *Media Effects Research: A Basic Overview.* 5th ed. Independence, KY: Cengage Learning; 2015.

27. Meissner HI, Tiro, JA, Yabroff KR, Haggstrom DA, Coughlin S. Too much of a good thing? Physician practices and patient willingness for less frequent Pap test screening intervals. *Med Care.* 2010;48:249–259.

28. Remington PL, Nelson D. Communicating epidemiologic information. In: Brownson RC, Petitti D, eds. *Applied Epidemiology.* 2nd ed. New York, NY: Oxford University Press; 2006:327–351.

29. Centers for Disease Control and Prevention. Sample single overriding communications objective (SOCO) worksheet. http://www.cdc.gov/healthywater/emergency/dwa-comm-toolbox/tools-templates-main.html. Accessed January 19, 2015.

30. Lazovich D, Vogel RI, Berwick M, Weinstock MA, Anderson KE, Warshaw EM. Indoor tanning and risk of melanoma: a case-control study in a highly exposed population. *Cancer Epidemiol Biomarkers Prev.* 2010;19:1557–1568.

31. Ghissassi F, Baan R, Straif K, et al. A review of human carcinogens—Part D: radiation. *Lancet Oncol.* 2009;10:751–752.

32. University of Minnesota School of Public Health. Our faculty: DeAnn Lazovitch. http://sph.umn.edu/faculty1/name/deann-lazovich/. Accessed January 23, 2015.

33. American Association for Cancer Research. *Cancer Epidemiology, Biomarkers & Prevention.* http://cebp.aacrjournals.org/. Accessed January 23, 2015.

34. National Cancer Institute. SEER stat fact sheets: melanoma of the skin. http://seer.cancer.gov/statfacts/html/melan.html. Accessed January 23, 2015.

35. U.S. Department of Health and Human Services. *Preventing Tobacco Use Among Youth and Young Adults: A Report of the Surgeon General.* Atlanta, GA: U.S. Department of Health and Human Services, Centers for Disease Control and Prevention, National Center for Chronic Disease Prevention and Health Promotion, Office on Smoking and Health; 2012.

Appendix 5

From Research to Patient Education: Distilling the Science for the Health of the Public

Theresa J. Barrett, PhD, **Robert Sprague**, and **Frances Reimers**

▶ Introduction

Researchers have made great strides in understanding a woman's genetic susceptibility to breast cancer. However, the potential relationships among environmental elements, personal choices, and the risk of developing breast cancer are still unknown. Researchers have recognized that breast cancer likely originates early in life, during times of rapid breast development such as puberty and pregnancy. To further understand these findings, the Breast Cancer and the Environment Research Program (BCERP) was created through the combined efforts of the National Institutes of Environmental Health Sciences (NIEHS) and the National Cancer Institute (NCI) to further the study of how environmental factors may influence breast cancer risk.[1]

BCERP is a multidisciplinary program supporting teams of scientists, clinicians, and community partners who are involved in examining the effects of exposure to environmental factors that may increase a woman's risk of developing breast cancer at some point in her life. BCERP encompasses both laboratory and population-based research to study the environmental effects on puberty and other "windows of susceptibility"[2]—that is, those times when the developing breast may be more susceptible to the effects of environmental exposure.

BCERP is considered unique in part because it embraces both multidisciplinary and transdisciplinary approaches to research. In a multidisciplinary approach to research, scientists from different disciplines (e.g., molecular biology, genetics, epidemiology, bioinformatics) work together at some point during the project, but maintain separate questions and conclusions.[3] Transdisciplinary research allows for the sharing of a common framework and methodology. This encourages scientists from different disciplines to work together to create new "conceptual, theoretical, methodological, and translational innovations that integrate and move beyond discipline-specific approaches to address a common problem."[4,5]

▶ Project Overview

The NIEHS sought to take the findings from BCERP and make them accessible to the general public without inciting undue health concerns. In 2010, NIEHS, with input from NCI, collaborated with a team of experts from PCI and the New Jersey Academy of Family Physicians (NJAFP) to create a communications plan for the dissemination of key messages from BCERP research findings that had already been published in the peer-reviewed scientific literature. The overall objective of the project was to identify key concepts from the BCERP literature, outline a high-level approach for the development of these concepts into key messages, and determine the best methods for dissemination of these messages to the lay target audiences.

▶ First Steps

The first step in the development of the key messages was for NJAFP and PCI (henceforth known as the Communications Team) to begin a review of the published BCERP literature to gain an understanding of the work that had been accomplished by the BCERP scientists. The Communications Team reviewed more than 90 abstracts and articles, published between 2004 and 2010, and categorized them into three main groups: Animal Models, Tissue Culture Systems, and Epidemiological Studies.

The Communications Team then began to search for potential members of an expert panel using NIEHS-approved criteria and protocol. The panel would assist in distilling the vast amount of information available to the Communications Team. The search resulted in the creation of a panel of six individuals with experience and expertise in one or more of the following areas: environmental health, health decision making, breast cancer, and risk communication (**BOX 5A-1**). The charge to the expert panel was to review the BCERP research findings to determine if they included concepts that could be further developed into key messages for the lay public that would have a positive impact on reduction of breast cancer, either by increasing the awareness of risk or by promoting a change in behavior.

BOX 5A-1 Expert Panel Identified by the Communications Team

Angela Fagerlin, PhD
Associate Professor, Department of Internal Medicine, University of Michigan

Jeanne Ferrante, MD, MPH
Associate Professor, Department of Family Medicine, University of Medicine and Dentistry of New Jersey–Robert Wood Johnson Medical School

Lisa Newman, MD, MPH, FACS
Director, Breast Care Center
Professor of Surgery, University of Michigan Comprehensive Cancer Center

Cheryl Osimo
Director of Events and Communication, Massachusetts Breast Cancer Coalition
Founder and Outreach Coordinator, Silent Spring Institute

Claudia Parvanta, PhD
Professor and Chair, Department of Behavioral and Social Sciences
University of the Sciences in Philadelphia

Peter Ubel, MD
Professor of Business, Fuqua School of Business, Duke University

Major stakeholders in the development of the key messages were the Community-Based Outreach and Translation Core (COTC) Teams that were a part of BCERP.[6] These teams were tasked with ensuring that the views and concerns of the breast cancer advocates community were heard and that the research findings were disseminated to the public. To capture input from all stakeholders, and to ensure transparency of the process for developing the key messages, the Communications Team set up a blog site. Emails were sent to the stakeholder community inviting members to log on, review the messages, and provide feedback to the Communications Team on which messages would likely work with their audiences and which messages would not.

The expert panel assembled in March 2011 for a working session. The session began with a list of 56 key messages from the 90 BCERP research and/or review papers; this list had been distilled by the Communications Team, by individual panel members, and through input from the blog participants. The purpose of the working session was to combine, refine, and/or discard any of the 56 ideas into several simple, straightforward sentences that captured the essence of what was to be communicated, with each message being distinct from the others. The work was accomplished through a facilitated discussion and a nominal group technique process (NGT). NGT is a weighted ranking process that allows a group to prioritize a large number of issues within a framework that gives each participant an equal voice. The tool is called *nominal* because there is limited interaction among the members of the group during the NGT process.

After the NGT process, the panel engaged in an impact analysis (**FIGURE 5A-1**) to identify which messages should be developed further so as to assess their impact on behavior and the probability that the message would be acted upon. As the project had both limited time and resources, it was important that the team concentrated on those messages with both high probability and high impact.

	Impact Analysis ← Probability →	
	High	*Low*
High → *Impact*	• High Impact • High Probability of Action	• High Impact • Low Probability of Action
← *Low*	• High Probability of Action • Low Impact	• Low Probability of Action • Low Impact

FIGURE 5A-1 Impact analysis model.

After the Working Session

At the end of the working session, the expert panel had developed nine proposed key concepts (**TABLE 5A-1**). The Communications Team took these nine messages and distilled them into five proposed key messages (**TABLE 5A-2**), which they presented in report form to NIEHS.

Along with presenting the key messages to stakeholders (**TABLE 5A-3**), the report included supporting points (items to provide context for the target audience, which might be developed into body copy), references (supporting the science behind the key messages, which were included only as information

TABLE 5A-1 Summary of the Nine Key Concepts Developed by the Expert Panel

Concept	Meaning
1. Early puberty and breast cancer	Earlier puberty is linked to increased risk of breast cancer; a higher body mass index (BMI) can cause early puberty.
2. BCERC program	Research into environmental exposure can lead to a better understanding of disease; understanding disease can guide further research and improve diagnosis and prevention measures.
3. Early puberty/ chemical exposure	Certain chemicals are associated with early puberty; these are the steps that you can take to reduce exposure.
4. Exposure to radiation	Exposure to radiation has been shown to increase the risk of cancer; exposure to radiation cannot be avoided, but being more informed about radiation levels can help in making more informed choices about exposure. (*Does not link; lower priority.*)
5. Chemical exposure message to moms	Your exposure is your baby's exposure; studies done in animals show a link between chemical exposure and the development of breast cancer.

TABLE 5A-2 Five Key Messages Developed by the Communications Team

1. Your daughter may reduce her risk of breast cancer if she maintains a healthy weight before puberty.
2. You may reduce your daughter's risk of breast cancer if you limit your exposure to certain chemicals while you are pregnant.
3. You may reduce your daughter's risk of breast cancer if you limit your exposure to certain chemicals while you are breastfeeding.
4. You may reduce your daughter's risk of breast cancer if you limit her exposure to certain chemicals before puberty.
5. You may reduce your risk of breast cancer by maintaining a healthy weight throughout life.

and not to be presented to the lay public), a standard statement (one brief line for each deliverable from the key messages that informs the reader about the origin and nature of the information to provide context and assurance that the information is from trusted sources).

▶ Message Development Strategies

Volkman and Silk stated that messages about breast cancer should "incorporate self-efficacy and family appeals to increase message effectiveness."[7] Keeping this premise in mind, the Communications Team presented the following recommendations:

1. *Stress positive action.* Key messages should stress the positive actions one can take to lower the risk of breast cancer.
2. *Messages should be for mothers.* The primary target audience for these messages should be mothers and women of childbearing age.
3. *Use accessible messages.* The language for all resulting materials should be simple and at a grade school level that allows the messages to be assessable to all audiences (eighth-grade reading level recommended as the absolute maximum).

Positive Action

While the idea of lifestyle changes—such as eating wholesome food and engaging in physical

TABLE 5A-3 Example of Key Message Presentation to Stakeholders

Proposed Key Message

Your daughter may reduce her risk of breast cancer if she maintains a healthy weight before puberty.

Supporting Points	References with Initial Message
This is bectause …	Biro FM, Khoury P, Morrison J. Influence of obesity on timing of puberty. *Int J Androl.* 2006;29:272-277.
■ Young girls who are overweight have been shown to enter puberty earlier.	■ Studies have shown that obesity is a contributing factor to early menarche in girls.
■ Studies have shown a link between the earlier onset of puberty and an increased risk of getting breast cancer.	■ A higher BMI combined with environmental factors has been related to an earlier onset of menarche.
Keep in mind …	■ The combination of early menarche and obesity could contribute to the development of breast cancer later in life.
■ Young girls who consume more whole grains and soy are less likely to enter puberty earlier.	Claudio L. Centered on breast cancer. *Environ Health Perspect.* 2007;115(3):A132-133.
Standard Statement	■ Environmental factors, such as diet or exposure to chemicals, could affect when puberty begins and how quickly a girl matures.
■ This cancer-prevention message has been brought to you by the National Institute of Environmental Health Sciences (NIEHS) and the National Cancer Institute (NCI), along with concerned community partners.	

activity—was not new, it was novel in the context of breast cancer prevention. Using lifestyle modification as a message met the objective of avoiding inciting undue health concerns. Stressing positive action also carried the potential of instilling a sense of empowerment in the audience for the message: "I have the ability to reduce my risk."

Messages for Moms

The Communications Team regarded a parental approach as a huge opportunity for message development, as a mother who might not have the drive to make changes in her own life might do so for the sake of her child. This theme aligned with the views of Volkman and Silk, who stated, "Prevention messages should attempt to appeal to the priority of familial safety as it is a potential motivator for action among primary family caretakers."[7]

The importance of making specific recommendations to reach women in areas of lower socioeconomic status was also emphasized by the Communications Team. For example, 27% of African American families live in poverty versus 11% of Caucasian families.[8] Reaching African American mothers was also considered important because black women often have higher risk factors, such as earlier onset of menarche and earlier start for breast development.[9]

Accessible Messages

The Communications Team recommended that materials be developed to correspond to approximately the eighth-grade and fifth-grade reading levels. This recommendation was based on studies that have shown that "most adults read at an eighth-grade level" and "20% of the population reads at or below a fifth-grade level."[10]

▶ Communications Plan

Originally, the government's requirements specified the development of a toolkit for each of the five key messages identified by the expert panel. These toolkits would be designed to be used as outreach materials targeted to lay audiences. However, as the project unfolded, the Communications Team determined that a toolkit for each of the key messages would be redundant and perhaps even cause confusion among the target audience owing to their overlapping calls to action. The Communications Team believed that the five key messages worked best when presented as a unit, so they recommended that the messages be disseminated as a set, with one toolkit developed for each target audience (**BOX 5A-2**). This would allow the messages to be delivered in a way that would ensure each audience "heard" them. For example, the expert panel noted that important cultural variations exist

- Parents of young female children
- Latino parents of young female children
- Educators
- Advocacy groups
- Healthcare providers

among different ethnic populations (e.g., attitudes, language, community values, educational levels), which would make it difficult to reach each audience in exactly the same way.

The Communications Team planned a series of toolkits that would feature materials derived from the same set of key messages, with the items in each toolkit then varying by target audience. Each toolkit was to be deployed on a branded web portal or microsite, with no hard copies of materials actually produced. This would allow community and grassroots organizations to download, customize, and distribute the materials. **TABLE 5A-4** shows the recommended content for the microsite by audience.

The Communications Team decided the first item to be developed would be the brochures aimed at mothers of young girls. The brochure was to be a simple trifold informational piece that would present the key BCERP findings and their implications for mothers with young daughters.

▶ Focus Groups

Working under contract, the Communications Team developed a set of four concepts containing the key messages. It was recommended that these four concepts be part of toolkits specifically developed for each target audience group: (General) mothers of young daughters, Latina mothers of young daughters, black mothers

TABLE 5A-4 Suggested Toolkit Contents by Audience Type

	Suggested Media	General	African American	Healthcare	Advocacy
Print	Engagement guide		X	X	X
	Brochure	X	X	X	X
	Flyer	X	X		
	Direct mail				
	Print PSA	X	X		
	Illustrated novella				
	Coloring book				
	Education/training materials			X	
Outreach/Press	Talking points				X
	Fact sheets			X	X
	Press kits				X
Online	Microsite	X	X (Tab)	X (Tab)	X (Tab)
	Banners				
	Buttons				

(continues)

TABLE 5A-4 Suggested Toolkit Contents by Audience Type		General	African American	Healthcare	Advocacy *(continued)*
	Suggested Media	**General**	**African American**	**Healthcare**	**Advocacy**
Social Media	Social media message scripts				X
	Smartphone app	TBD			
	Online game				
Broadcast Video and Audio	Video vignettes		X		X
	Radio	X	X		X

of young daughters, Asian mothers of young daughters, healthcare providers, policy makers, and educators. NIEHS and NIH reviewed, commented, and provided feedback during the development and implementation of the toolkits. In addition, the decision was made to conduct focus groups to evaluate the toolkits to make sure they met the needs their intended audiences.

Mothers of Young Children was the first focus group conducted to gauge reaction to the toolkit materials as well as to gather suggestions for content or format changes.[11] The following key messages were tested with this focus group:

- Girls who get their periods earlier than average may have a higher risk of breast cancer later in life.
- Certain exposures early in life (foods, chemicals) may affect when a girl gets her first period, which may influence her breast cancer risk later in life. Exposures early in life includes the time when a mother is pregnant or breastfeeding her daughter.
- Parents can take several steps that may help reduce a girl's risk of breast cancer later in life, such as encouraging her to:
  - Eat healthy food (limit high-fat foods; eat whole grains and soy).
  - Maintain a healthy weight.
  - Reduce the use of everyday products concerning certain chemicals (e.g., phthalates, BPA).

One 90-minute focus group discussion was conducted in January 2012, led by a professional, independent moderator. As the key messages focused on the time before a girl gets her first period, all of the participants were mothers with at least one daughter between the ages of 1½ and 11 years. The goal of the focus group was to gauge the mothers' responses

to and comprehension of the toolkits that had been developed. Specifically, the focus group sought to assess the participants' knowledge and assumptions related to the following issues:

- The causes of breast cancer and whether it was preventable
- Their knowledge and assumptions about the factors that may influence when a girl has her first period
- General impressions of the brochure (whether it was meant for them)
- Understanding of the key messages
  - Use of the precautionary principle ("in the absence of definitive information, err on the side of caution")
  - Having daughters avoid certain chemicals and high-fat foods
  - Starting prevention steps for daughters during the mother's pregnancy and breastfeeding
- Thoughts on the source(s) of the information
- Opinions about three alternative visual presentations

Three research questions were used during the focus group: (1) How understandable are the messages presented in the toolkit?; (2) Do the primary users understand and relate to the artifacts as intended?; and (3) Are the correct elements included in the toolkit and in the correct format?

Focus Group Results

The results of the focus group[11] showed that the core messages aligned with the mothers' general belief that there could be a relationship between diet and chemicals and early menstruation and cancer risk. This belief allowed the mothers to agree with the rationale for making changes at home. The results also showed that the idea of a linkage between early menstruation and future breast cancer risk was new to the mothers, and they wanted to know how and why—or at least scientists' current best guesses as to why—this was the case. The mothers' responses to the key content and related recommendations are shown in **TABLE 5A-5**.

TABLE 5A-5 Selected Responses to Key Information/Concepts

Participants' Responses to Key Information/Concepts	Recommendations Related to the Brochure	Recommendations Related to Online or More Detailed Communication Tools
Encourage your daughter to eat healthy foods. ▪ Many mothers felt they were already doing so, and most acknowledged that doing so is generally challenging. ▪ The presence of soy on the list caused several questions among those mothers who had heard that young girls should not have soy and that older women use soy to help with menopause symptoms. ▪ Some mothers wondered whether girls should avoid all high-fat foods (both "good fats" as in avocados and "bad fats" as in fried foods). ▪ Seeing healthy eating mentioned raised questions about why exercise was not mentioned. These were not pressing questions.	▪ If soy remains on the healthy eating list, some mothers will question why.	▪ Consider links to sources such as the U.S. Department of Agriculture (USDA) designed to help parents understand healthy eating principles and find ways to reduce the healthy eating barriers. ▪ If soy remains on the healthy eating list, some mothers will question why. Therefore, it is also a topic to address when more detailed communications are prepared. ▪ Explain whether both "good" and "bad" fats should be avoided. ▪ Support exercise as part of healthy living and briefly note why exercise is not specifically linked to breast cancer risk reduction in this context.
Use products free of phthalates and BPA. ▪ Most mothers seemed to miss the idea that reducing exposure is still good, even if the chemicals cannot be eliminated in day-to-day life. ▪ Many wanted to learn more about how phthalates and BPA are thought to act in the body and cause changes—why were they singled out? ▪ All mothers assumed phthalate- and BPA-free products are more expensive and/or require trips to special stores (e.g., Whole Foods), which are potential barriers to change. ▪ Many mothers felt better able to identify chemicals in personal and household products (with ingredient lists) than in toys. ▪ Some mothers wanted help knowing which alternatives are available.	▪ Emphasize that reducing exposure is still helpful and worthwhile. This topic may be tied to (or help alleviate) concerns about costs and special trips to buy chemical-free products. ▪ Consider whether any additional advice about identifying phthalate- and BPA-free toys is warranted and can fit on the brochure.	▪ Provide explanations for those readers who would like such details about how phthalates and BPA in particular are thought to cause changes in girls' development. ▪ Address concerns about cost and special trips honestly. Again, consider tying the message to reduction if scientifically appropriate, encouraging action within one's budget, and accommodating changes within an already busy schedule. ▪ Give advice about identifying phthalate- and BPA-free toys. In other words, tell readers what to do if there is no ingredient list. ▪ Provide suggested alternatives. Participants wanted product names, but even generic suggestions such as housecleaning with vinegar/water solution may be welcomed. ▪ Tell parents exactly which terms to look for on ingredient lists to identify these unwanted chemicals.

The concept brochures (**FIGURES 5A-2 through 5A-7**) met some key goals, but also raised a shared set of questions. The mothers understood the precautionary principle and were comfortable with the specific changes suggested in the brochures—helping daughters to avoid chemicals and eating a healthier diet. The material that was presented also inspired information-seeking behavior (some mothers indicated they would do further research online) and behavior change (many mothers said they would check at home for phthalates and BPA). The mothers saw the brochure as a tool to build awareness and provide basic action steps. They expected to find answers to their detailed question elsewhere.

Based on the visual cues (i.e., photos of girls and mothers, language mentioning daughters, and visuals of healthy foods and toys), the mothers felt that all three brochures were meant for them. Brochure B was the most favored for the way the rationales/explanations were laid out. Additional feedback from the mothers indicated that a chemical ingredient list would be a valuable tool to help mothers to know what to look for. The focus group participants suggested that the list should include specific terms mothers should look for, such as "phthalate." Based on the results of the focus groups, modifications were made to the content before final production of the materials.

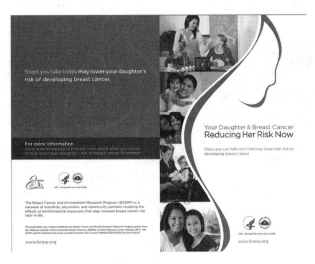

FIGURE 5A-2 Concept brochure 1A.
Courtesy of the Breast Cancer and the Environment Research Program.

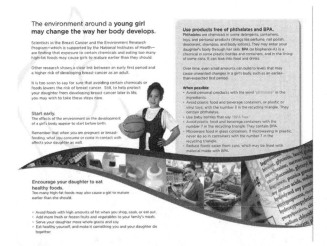

FIGURE 5A-3 Concept brochure 1B.
Courtesy of the Breast Cancer and the Environment Research Program.

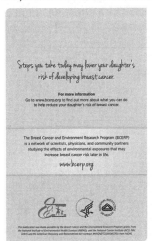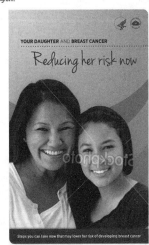

FIGURE 5A-4 Concept brochure 2A.
Courtesy of the Breast Cancer and the Environment Research Program.

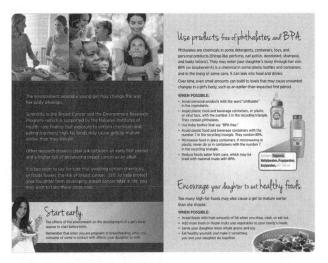

FIGURE 5A-5 Concept brochure 2B.
Courtesy of the Breast Cancer and the Environment Research Program.

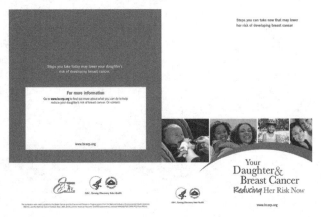

FIGURE 5A-6 Concept brochure 3A.
Courtesy of the Breast Cancer and the Environment Research Program.

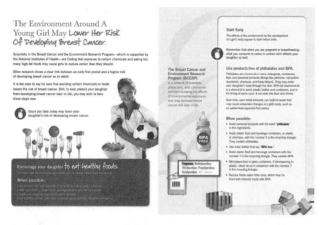

FIGURE 5A-7 Concept brochure 3B.
Courtesy of the Breast Cancer and the Environment Research Program.

▶ Dissemination of Materials

A microsite (http://www.info.bcerp.org/) was developed to house the four toolkits that were developed for the project. The toolkits were aimed at (1) a general audience of parents and caregivers, (2) an African American audience of parents and caregivers, (3) health professionals, and (4) outreach organizations. Each toolkit contains a brochure with language appropriate to the intended audience (**FIGURES 5A-8 through 5A-11**).

The materials were also designed for adaptability depending on the audience. For example, the African American toolkit (**FIGURE 5A-9**) has the same content as the general toolkit (**FIGURE 5A-8**), but has been adapted with photos and images that are relevant to African American parents. Each toolkit contains a PDF version of the full brochure as well as a text-only version. The toolkits also contain flyers and advertisements, as well as more in-depth resources for healthcare professionals and advocacy groups.

Guidance on how to customize the individual documents is provided, and organizations are encouraged to use the BCERP logo to identify the source of the information. If organizations are planning to adapt the material, they are instructed to add the following statement: "This material is adapted from information/materials developed by the Breast Cancer and the Environment Research Program. Additional information on the program can be found at www.bcerp.org." It is also recommended that a BCERP investigator review the material if changes are made to the text to ensure scientific accuracy is maintained.

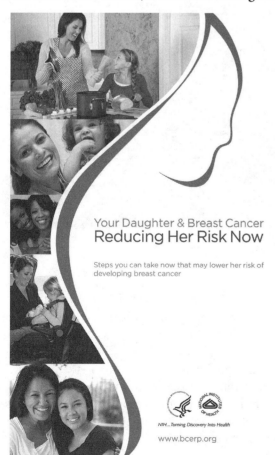

FIGURE 5A-8 General audience brochure.
Courtesy of the Breast Cancer and the Environment Research Program.

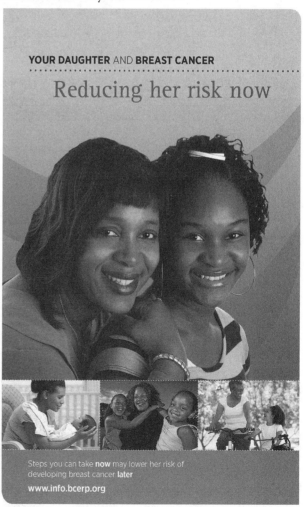

FIGURE 5A-9 African American brochure.
Courtesy of the Breast Cancer and the Environment Research Program.

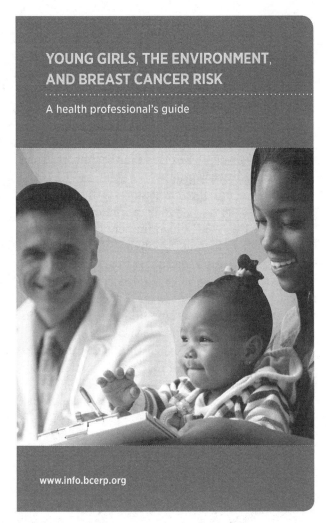

FIGURE 5A-10 Health professional brochure.
Courtesy of the Breast Cancer and the Environment Research Program.

The materials were designed to allow for flexibility to meet the needs of the stakeholders. For example, it was suggested that images could be replaced with locally, culturally appropriate images (organizations are encouraged to make sure the images are not copyrighted, or if copyrighted, permission for use is obtained). Fonts and colors can also be changed. In addition, local contact information, organizational logos, and organizational names can be added.

▶ Conclusion

The literature from the Breast Cancer and the Environment Research Project revealed that most cases of breast cancer develop through a combination of genetic and environmental factors, as opposed to genetics alone. This project aimed to inform individuals that they have the power, through the choices that they make, to influence the chance of whether

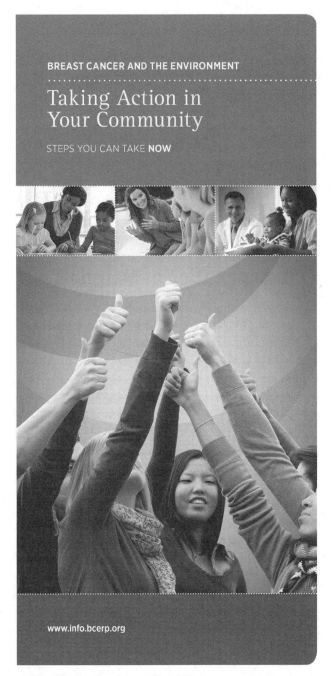

FIGURE 5A-11 Advocacy brochure.
Courtesy of the Breast Cancer and the Environment Research Program.

they or their daughter might develop breast cancer. The creation of the communication toolkits, which were made available to breast cancer advocacy communities throughout the United States as well as to the general public, allowed for the dissemination of important information about environmental factors related to breast cancer to empower women to make the best lifestyle choices for themselves and for their young daughters.

This case study demonstrates one process for taking scientific information and distilling it for use by the general public. Two key components contributed to the success of this project. The first component involved taking the time to clearly articulate the different skill sets that the expert panel would need to review the published literature and make recommendations. The Communications Team determined that the expert panel would need to include individuals who were specialists in environmental health/environmental risk, risk communications, human-centered breast cancer research/risk assessment (e.g., epidemiology), and public health and/or health literacy and cultural competency. The search was then initiated for the right mix of educators and scientists who possessed these skills. The second component that contributed to the success of the project was the implementation of the focus groups. The focus groups ensured that the messages being considered were the right messages, with the right images, for the right audience.

Through careful planning and message testing, the Communications Team was able to create materials that met the needs of NIEHS, NCI, the project stakeholders, and the intended audiences. These materials remain available on the BCERP website. Development of the materials was made possible through Breast Cancer and the Environment Research Program (BCERP) grants from the National Institute of Environmental Health Sciences (NIEHS) and the National Cancer Institute (NCI), which are part of the National Institutes of Health (NIH) and the U.S. Department of Health and Human Services (HHS) and the American Recovery and Reinvestment Act (contract #HHSN273201000070U).

References

1. Breast Cancer and the Environment Research Program. http://www.bcerc.org/index.htm. Accessed March 15, 2015.
2. Breast Cancer and the Environment Research Program. Windows of susceptibility studies. http://www.bcerc.org/granteesWOS.htm. Accessed March 15, 2015.
3. Washington University School of Medicine in St. Louis, TREC Center. What is transdisciplinary research? http://www.obesity-cancer.wustl.edu/en/About/What-Is-Transdisciplinary-Research. Accessed March 15, 2015.
4. Harvard T. H. Chan School of Public Health, Harvard Transdisciplinary Research in Energetics and Cancer Center. Transdisciplinary research. http://www.hsph.harvard.edu/trec/about-us/definitions. Accessed March 15, 2015.
5. Rebbeck TR, Paskett E, Sellers TA. Fostering transdisciplinary science. *Cancer Epidemiol Biomarkers Prevent*. 2010;19:1149–1150.
6. Breast Cancer and the Environment Research Program. Community outreach and translation core. http://www.bcerc.org/cotc.htm. Accessed March 15, 2015.
7. Volkman J, Silk K. Adolescent females and their mothers: examining perceptions of the environment and breast cancer. *J Health Psychol*. 2008;13:1180–1189.
8. Isaacs SL, Schroeder SA. Class: the ignored determinant of the nation's health. *New Engl J Med*. 2004;351:1137–1142.
9. Biro FM, Wolff MS, Kushi LH. Impact of yesterday's genes and today's diet. *J Pediatr Adolesc Gynecol*. 2009;22:3–6.
10. Safeer RS, Keenan J. Health literacy: the gap between physicians and patients. *Am Fam Physician*. 2005;72:463–468.
11. National Cancer Institute. *Final Report on Breast Cancer and the Environment Research Program (BCERP) Focus Group Research: Print Material for Mothers on Reducing Daughters' Breast Cancer Risk*. Rockville, MD: National Cancer Institute, Office of Market Research and Evaluation (OMRE); 2012.

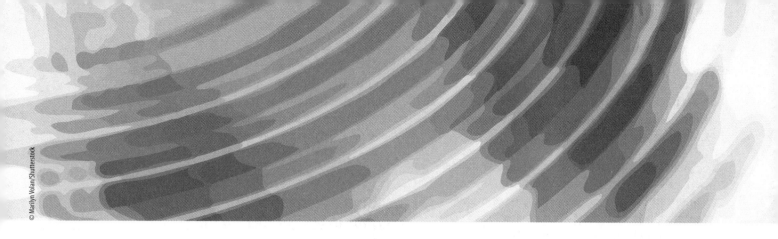

CHAPTER 6

Communicating for Policy and Advocacy[a]

Claudia Parvanta

LEARNING OBJECTIVES

By the end of this chapter, the reader will be able to:

- Understand the importance of policy in influencing health and well-being.
- Describe the role of political action committees (PACs), lobbying, and advocacy in influencing policy decisions.
- Understand the barriers and challenges when communicating with policy makers.
- Describe the policy communication and advocacy strategies used by two leading organizations.
- Identify the role of the message, the messenger, and the modes of delivery in policy communication.
- Conduct an environmental scan.
- Develop selected types of policy and advocacy material.

▶ Introduction

"Never doubt that a small group of thoughtful committed citizens can change the world. Indeed, it is the only thing that ever has."

—Attributed to Margaret Mead, PhD, anthropologist, 1901-1978[1]

In the ecological model, federal and state laws and regulations, as well as local ordinances and policies, shape many of the upstream determinants that affect our health. Health policies can be broad in scope (e.g., the Patient Protection and Affordable Care Act, state laws for indoor air quality), or they may have a narrower focus, involving organizational practices (e.g., workplace paid vacations, school district physical activity policies). Many policies that *affect* health do not come from the health sector at all. Indeed, in recent years, public health has moved away from

---

a. This chapter incorporates material previously published as Brownson R, Jones E, Parvanta C. Communicating for policy and advocacy. In: Parvanta C, Nelson DE, Parvanta SA, Harner RN, eds. *Essentials of Public Health Communication*. Sudbury, MA: Jones and Bartlett; 2011:91-117.

a strictly sectoral policy to a "health in all policies" approach, which requires more collaboration with stakeholders and decision-making entities beyond the health sector. As Rudolf et al. state,

> At any given moment, most governments are discussing or implementing literally hundreds of issues, processes, or initiatives in all kinds of policy areas, many of which offer opportunities to promote health. These create windows of opportunity—or "policy windows"—that may only be open for a short time. You rarely have control over the timing or content of policy windows, but if you look for them, they can provide you with opportunities to engage in intersectoral collaboration for health.[2]

To quote Louis Pasteur from a lecture in 1854, "Chance favors only the prepared mind." This chapter is meant to help you prepare for communicating during those times when policy windows open up for the issues that you care about. While this area is complex, many excellent and free tools are available online that can facilitate communication in this milieu. This chapter makes extensive use of the *Legislative Advocacy Handbook* developed by the American Public Health Association (APHA).[3] Other valuable resources include the *Health Advocacy Toolkit* created by the Connecticut Health Foundation;[b] the *Health in All Policies* guide created by the American Schools of Public Health (ASPH) and partner agencies;[c] and *Tools for Policy Impact: A Handbook for Researchers from the Overseas Development Institute* (United Kingdom).[d]

We have assumed that the reader of this chapter is someone who provides content to inform health policy. This individual may work in a public agency, a nonprofit organization, a research institution, or a for-profit setting. Regardless of the specific work setting, this individual's goal is to share information with policy makers who have the power and responsibility to make decisions. We describe this as the **policy communication** process. We reserve the term **advocacy** for the process of sharing information with stakeholders—aligned organizations, selected members (segments) of the public, or anyone engaged in an issue without law-making ability. Before describing specific approaches and methods, however, we will explore the "big picture"—that is, how policies come

into being. Note that although this chapter describes communication for policy and advocacy in the United States, many of the principles and recommendations will apply in other countries.

How Citizens Shape Public Policy

Indirect Route: Elections, Political Action Committees, and Super PACs

In the U.S. democratic society, "We the People" shape policy indirectly or directly. Indirectly, U.S. citizens elect government representatives, who then enact policy on their behalf at several political levels (e.g., federal, state, county, congressional district, city, territory, and/or tribal unit). U.S. citizens have the right and responsibility to elect into public office those candidates whom they feel best represent their positions. Each registered voter is allowed one vote in each election. As a private citizen, you are free to spend all your time supporting your favorite candidate and can contribute a relatively modest amount of money directly to the candidate's campaign. By comparison, political action committees (PACs) and super PACs have a more profound influence on campaign-related spending and provide an indirect mechanism for individuals to make much larger campaign contributions.

The Federal Election Commission (FEC) recognizes two forms of PACs: separate segregated funds (SSFs) and non-connected committees. SSFs are political committees established and administered by corporations, labor unions, membership organizations, or trade associations that may solicit contributions only from individuals associated with the sponsoring organization. Nonconnected committees, in contrast, are free to solicit contributions from the general public. Fairly strict guidelines govern how much money traditional PACs may raise and for which purposes, but they chiefly support candidates' campaigns.

In July 2010, the U.S. Supreme Court ruling in *SpeechNow.org v. Federal Election Commission* allowed for the creation of so-called super PACs. Because the Supreme Court's decision defined money as "free speech," and corporations as "individuals," super PACs may raise unlimited sums of money from anyone for the purpose of communicating about "issues." Super PACs are prohibited from donating money directly to political candidates. Both PACs and super PACs

b. http://www.cthealth.org/

c. https://www.apha.org/~/media/files/pdf/factsheets/health_inall_policies_guide_169pages.ashx

d. https://www.odi.org/sites/odi.org.uk/files/odi-assets/publications-opinion-files/194.pdf

must report their donors to the FEC on a monthly or quarterly basis. Briffault and others have noted that super PACS have sometimes outspent the candidates whom they support during elections, and they may even allow a few very wealthy individuals to exceed the impact of political parties on the electoral process.[e]

Direct Routes: Lobbying, Advocacy, and Activism

FIGURE 6-1 lays out the legal options that citizens may take to influence policy in the United States.

Once officials are elected and in office, they may enact legislation. (If you do not remember "how a bill becomes a law" from your grade school or middle school civics class, check out the legislative handbook[f] from American Public Health Association.) Now imagine that your organization cannot afford to put millions of dollars into a super PAC for "'issues communication" to influence voting on a particular legislation. The next potential line of influence is through lobbying.

Lobbying, loosely defined, usually refers to the practice in which a sponsoring organization pays someone (ideally a person with government experience and influential contacts) to persuade elected officials to vote according to the sponsor's wishes. As APHA explains,

To be considered lobbying, a communication must refer to and express a view on a specific legislative proposal that has been introduced before a legislative body (federal, state, or local). This means working to influence the outcome of specific legislation—trying to get a bill passed or defeated—by communicating your organization's views or position to those who participate in the formulation of the specific legislation—your Members of Congress, your state legislators, your local elected officials,... staff of policy-makers,... or appointed officers of a regulatory agency.[2]

Restrictions are placed on lobbying by certain types of organizations, especially nonprofits. In particular, the tax code specifies that a charitable organization, defined as one that is tax-exempt under section 501(c)(3) of the Internal Revenue Code, "may not attempt to influence legislation as a substantial part of its activities and... may not participate in any campaign activity for or against political candidates."[g]

The Internal Revenue Service (IRS) offers a way of calculating what is considered "substantial." For example, an organization that spends $1 million on exempt-purpose expenditures may spend up to $175,000 on lobbying activities. However, no

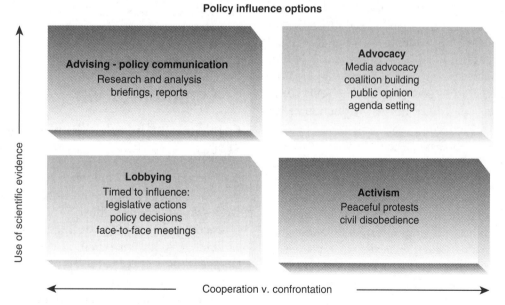

Policy influence options

FIGURE 6-1 Policy Influence Options Matrix

Modified from: Start D, Hovland I. Tools for Policy Impact: A Handbook for Researchers. http://www.odi.org/publications/156-tools-policy-impact-handbook-researchers. The Overseas Development Institute; Research and Policy in Development Programme. ISBN 1850037417. Published September 2004. Accessed August 29, 2015.

e. Briffault R. *Super PACs*. Columbia Public Law Research Paper No. WP 12-298. April 16, 2012. Available at http://ssrn.com /abstract=2040941

f. http://www.iowapha.org/resources/Documents/APHA%20Legislative%20Advocacy%20Handbook1.pdf

g. http://www.irs.gov/Charities-&-Non-Profits/Charitable-Organizations/Exemption-Requirements-Section-501(c)(3)-Organizations

organization (no matter how large) may spend more than $1 million per year on lobbying and maintain its tax-exempt status. In addition, organizations that receive federal funds as grants must adhere to the provisions of the Anti-Lobbying Act (18 U.S.C. § 1913). The National Institutes of Health (NIH) has posted this advice regarding compliance with this act:

> The Anti-Lobbying Act prohibits the direct or indirect use of appropriated funds to pay for any personal service, advertisement, telegram, telephone, letter, printed or written matter or other device, intended or designed to influence in any manner a Member of Congress, a jurisdiction, or an official of any government to favor, adopt, or oppose, by vote or otherwise, any legislation, law, ratification, policy, or appropriation, whether before or after the introduction of any bill, measure, or resolution proposing such legislation, law ratification, policy or appropriation.[h]

The lines between lobbying, advocacy, and policy communications can be thin and sometimes blurry. When an organization of which you are a member sends an email asking you to contact your congressional representatives to urge them to vote a particular way on a bill actively under consideration, this message is considered lobbying by that organization. If, as a private citizen, you take the step of sending the email, calling, or visiting an elected official, that action is considered advocacy because you are representing only yourself, not your organization. Keep in mind you must always use your personal (not organization) address in advocacy messages and send these messages to representatives in the jurisdiction (e.g., county, district) where you live.

If an organization's message does not indicate a preference for which way a policy vote should go—for example, if it simply informs recipients about the issue and says that a vote is pending—this would be considered policy communication. If no vote is pending, and the organization provides information about the pros and cons of a particular issue and what it believes the outcome should be, the message would be considered advocacy. If you go with a group of people and raise your arm in protest, or lie down on Wall Street, or build a house in a tree and refuse to come down, or spam individual webpages, your action would be considered activism. As you can see, the distinctions between lobbying, advocacy, policy communications, and activism are chiefly a matter of timing and intent.

If you work in a government agency, you are required to communicate in a way that informs the public and policy makers without bias. Nongovernmental organizations may take more of a stand, as long as their communications are not designed to influence voting on federal, state, or local legislation.

The bottom line: Make no assumptions about what you may or may not do in advocacy or lobbying without researching your explicit organizational rights in your jurisdiction. You may be able to do more—or less—than you think. As far as activism is concerned, the First Amendment of the U.S. Constitution protects your rights to nonviolent assembly and free speech, as long as that activity takes place on your own time and with your "dime". Later in this chapter, we describe a community-based approach to coalition formation and policy selection originated by the Florida Prevention Research Center that uses social marketing as its framework. Because this is a more grassroots mechanism, it is not subject to the same regulations as nonprofit organizations or government-funded entities.

Organizations That Do Extensive Advocacy

Public health is a field dominated by advocacy efforts. **BOX 6-1** lists some of the major organizations committed to advocating for public health. If you are interested in addressing a public health issue, it is a smart move to start by aligning your own work with the advocacy efforts of one of these, or similar, organizations.

▶ Strategic Policy Communication

Communicating with (Public) Policy Makers

This section presents guidance for those persons in positions barred from doing lobbying or advocacy work—in other words, those persons working in government agencies or government-funded positions. Individuals in less restricted positions may use everything else, as well as the tools covered in the next section, for lobbying and advocacy purposes.

Because politicians are elected and voters may replace them every two years (U.S. representatives, many state legislators), four years (president, state governors), or six years (U.S. senators), it often seems politicians are in a rush to accomplish their goals. In marked contrast, most scientific discoveries are

---

h. https://ethics.od.nih.gov/topics/Lobby-Publicity-Guide.htm

BOX 6-1 Leading Organizations for Public Health Advocacy

This box provides information about some of the leading organizations committed to public health advocacy on a national level, and across a wide range of issues. Neither topic-specific agencies, such as the American Cancer Society and Tobacco Free Kids, nor foundations are included in this brief list. The information here comes from each organization's website.

American Public Health Association (APHA)

https://www.apha.org/

APHA champions the health of all people and all communities. We strengthen the public health profession. We speak out for public health issues and policies backed by science. We are the only organization that influences federal policy, has a 140-plus year perspective, and brings together members from all fields of public health.

Association of State and Territorial Health Officers (ASTHO)

http://www.astho.org/

ASTHO's Federal Government Relations team advocates on behalf of state public health before the U.S. Congress and the administration to inform federal policy to achieve better health outcomes. We provide congressional leaders with key information regarding public health activities in their state/district, support members' advocacy efforts, provide federal testimony and participation in congressional briefings, and educate members and state health agency staff on key budget and public health policy.

National Association of County and City Health Officials (NACCHO)

http://www.naccho.org/

NACCHO informs policy makers of the critical role local health departments play in keeping our communities healthy and safe. As the national voice for local health departments, NACCHO educates policy makers about critical local public health issues, provides members with the latest updates on key public health issues and opportunities to take action, and helps local health departments communicate the value of local public health with their own policy makers.

American College Health Association (ACHA)

http://www.acha.org/

ACHA provides continuous and timely advocacy for policies and programs that support the health and well-being of college students and their campus communities. ACHA's committees, coalitions, and task forces continually identify advocacy issues that are important to those in the college health field. The association provides members with up-to-date information concerning relevant national public policy issues affecting the health of college students. Where necessary and appropriate, ACHA weighs in to influence public policy making (legislative and regulatory) with the continual aim of protecting and advancing students' health. Members of ACHA enjoy the benefits of having a nationally recognized association take on the issues that are important to them.

Association of Schools and Programs of Public Health (ASPPH)

http://www.aspph.org/

As the principal voice of academic public health education, ASPPH has a long-standing partnership with the federal government. ASPPH works with Congress and the Executive Branch in support of sound public health policies directed at the prevention of disease and the enhancement of wellness, domestically and globally. ASPPH's role includes educating policy makers about the science-based evidence available regarding public health policy issues, as well as advocating for specific policies and legislation. Such efforts include advocacy for appropriate levels of federal investment in a wide range of public health programs. Advocacy positions are set by the Association based on recommendations of its Legislative Committee, which is comprised of deans and program directors from almost two dozen schools and programs of public health.

Society for Public Health Education (SOPHE)

http://www.sophe.org/default.cfm

Advocating for public policies conducive to health is part of SOPHE's mission as a health education organization. SOPHE has a responsibility to educate decision makers on national and state legislative issues related to the health of society. Each year SOPHE identifies priority issues on which it will focus its education efforts through sustained communication channels with members and chapters, and by developing and maintaining collaborative partnerships

(continues)

with public and private national organizations. SOPHE also encourages chapters in their own implementation of national, state, and local health education public policy activities. SOPHE has an active Advocacy Committee, with chapter representation, and interested SOPHE members.

Research! America

http://www.researchamerica.org/

Research! America is the nation's largest not-for-profit public education and advocacy alliance committed to making research to improve health a higher national priority. Together with our member organizations that represent a vast array of medical, health, and scientific fields, our goals are: (1) achieve funding for medical and health research from the public and private sectors at a level warranted by scientific opportunity and supported by public opinion; (2) better inform the public of the benefits of medical and health research and the institutions that perform research; (3) motivate the public to actively support medical and health research and the complementary sciences that make advances possible; and (4) promote and empower a more active public and political life by individual members of the research community on behalf of medical and health research, public health, and science overall.

Trust for America's Health (TFAH)

http://healthyamericans.org/

Trust for America's Health (TFAH) is a nonprofit, nonpartisan organization dedicated to saving lives by protecting the health of every community and working to make disease prevention a national priority. From anthrax to asthma, from chemical terrorism to cancer, America is facing a crisis of epidemics. As a nation, we are stuck in a "disease du jour" mentality, which means we lose sight of the bigger picture: building a public health defense that is strong enough to cover us from all points of attack—whether the threats are from a bioterrorist or Mother Nature. By focusing on prevention, protection, and communities, TFAH is leading the fight to make disease prevention a national priority, from Capitol Hill to Main Street. We know what works. Now we need to build the resolve to get it done.

Public Health Institute (PHI)

http://www.phi.org/

As a trusted voice in public health, PHI is committed to developing strategic public policy solutions at the federal, state, and local levels that leverage cutting-edge research and evidence-based analysis. With experience across a range of policy areas and issues, combined with our strong record working side-by-side with business, government, and community-based organizations, PHI and its programs are effective, influential advocates for public health in local, state, and federal policy. Building on this success, PHI is now working to strengthen its role in U.S.-based policy that has implications for health domestically and worldwide. With strategic policy platforms, PHI addresses policy in areas such as obesity prevention, climate change, and health reform. In addition, PHI tracks federal and state legislation, regulations, and budgeting processes across a wide range of issues that impact the public's health, and advances policy solutions that address the social determinants of health.

achieved through incremental advances in knowledge over years or decades. Data from long-term research studies and surveillance systems provide the best picture of what is happening in public health. Unfortunately, press releases about small changes in disease prevalence or behavior from one year to the next may not be punchy enough to generate significant interest in a topic or draw the attention of policy makers.

A further challenge is that policy makers often want quick, absolute answers to complex questions. Two decades ago, the Institute of Medicine determined that decision making in public health is often excessively driven by "crises, hot issues, and concerns of organized interest groups."[4] Indeed, existing public health data from long-term reliable research are often underutilized and sometimes ignored because policy

makers regularly make decisions based on short-term demands—crisis situations—and policies and programs are frequently developed around anecdotal evidence.[5] Changing these patterns should be a concern and priority among public health communicators.

The "Cookbook"

Assuming an organization has a position on a policy and plans to communicate this stance to decision makers, it should use a process similar to that employed with any other type of strategic communication, although the details vary:

1. Determine exactly what you want to accomplish.
2. Decide who you are trying to reach.

3. Research and craft the message.
4. Choose the spokesperson(s).
5. Deliver the message.
6. Evaluate your progress.

We now explore these steps, along with some examples of their use.

1. State What You Want to Accomplish

What do you want the policy makers to do as a result of receiving your communication? In direct policy communication, for example, you might want the recipients to take one or more of the following actions:

- Create new laws or regulations
- Prevent current laws or regulations from being weakened or discontinued

- Enforce existing laws and regulations, including stronger penalties for violations
- Direct more funding to programs
- Raise taxes on products (e.g., cigarettes, sugary soda) to decrease demand for those products
- Change practices that are regulated by government agencies (e.g., in health care, agriculture, or pharmaceutical pricing).

As noted earlier, individuals in government or government-funded positions may not seek to influence the outcome of voting by policy makers directly, so this cannot be one of your explicit goals for policy communication. **BOX 6-2** presents a table from *Health in All Policies* [i] showing a set of legal government processes and indicating how these can be used to create policy windows and partnerships.

BOX 6-2 Government Mechanisms as Opportunities for Change

GOVERNMENT MECHANISMS AS OPPORTUNITIES FOR CHANGE

GOVERNMENT MECHANISM	OPPORTUNITY	POSSIBLE ACTION
DATA	Government agencies collect, standardize, and disseminate information and data. Sharing data or standardizing data elements across agencies can ensure more effective collaboration.	• Improve data sharing and collaborate on data collection between schools and social service agencies to improve access to nutrition assistance programs. • Include indicators related to the social determinants of health (e.g., income and employment, housing, and transportation) in health department reports.
DIRECT SERVICE PROVISION	States, counties, and cities provide direct services to communities and individuals. Departments can expand or create new services, better customize services, link services, and reduce barriers to access.	• Include healthy homes assessments in weatherization programs. • Incorporate health screening into intake processes at youth detention facilities.
EDUCATION AND INFORMATION	Agencies educate and inform the population on topics relevant to individuals, organizations, communities, and businesses.	• Incorporate messages around the importance of physical activity in promotional materials for a park. • Require that nutrition information be either posted or appear on the food labels of all food sold on school grounds or at school-sponsored events.
EMPLOYER	Governments employ staff in offices, parks, schools, and throughout cities, counties, and states. Employee policies can encourage healthy behaviors and also set a positive example for private businesses.	• Provide transit subsidies to encourage employees to use public transportation. • Provide lactation accommodations, including specially designated rooms and refrigerators, to support breastfeeding.

(continues)

---

i. Rudolph L, Caplan J, Ben-Moshe K, Dillon L. *Health in All Policies: A Guide for State and Local Governments.* Washington, DC/Oakland, CA: American Public Health Association and Public Health Institute; 2013.

BOX 6-2 Government Mechanisms as Opportunities for Change *(continued)*

FUNDING	Grants provide funds to support specific projects or activities. Subsidies are assistance (monetary or otherwise) that reduces the need for monetary expenditures. Grants and subsidies can be used to encourage health-promoting actions. This includes payment for health-promoting services (e.g., Medicaid or Medicare).	• Offer childcare subsidies to support workers with children. • Incorporate health and health equity criteria into requests for proposals from agencies outside the public health field.
GUIDANCE AND BEST PRACTICES	Guidelines can be used to encourage communities to implement best practices or proven methodologies.	• Incorporate strategies that promote community health into comprehensive land use and transportation plans or community climate action plans. • Share evidence to inform the adoption of evidence-based and evidence-informed strategies to address crime prevention.
PERMITTING AND LICENSING	Permits and licenses provided by government bodies authorize particular types of activities or development. [90] Zoning, for example, is used to divide land into areas for allowable uses.	• Streamline permitting processes for farmers' markets to provide healthy food in underserved residential neighborhoods. • In the housing element of a comprehensive plan, outline a method for encouraging housing development near public transit hubs.
PURCHASING: PROCUREMENT AND CONTRACTS	Agencies spend significant money purchasing goods like food, supplies, and equipment, and contracting for services like construction and janitorial services. Procurement and contracting policies can promote other desired outcomes such as economic resiliency, and are a way to model behavior for other agencies or private businesses.	• Establish procurement policies that require vending machines on agency property to provide a minimum number of healthy options. • Establish policies supporting contracting with veteran-, minority-, or women-owned businesses.
REGULATION	Agencies can add, abolish, or change regulations, close or open loopholes, improve enforcement, or change complaint mechanisms for the public. Regulation is often useful in situations where consumers lack essential information.	• Improve enforcement of smoking bans in multi-unit housing structures. • Develop a regulation to apply a health analysis to budgetary and legislative decisions.
RESEARCH AND EVALUATION	Agencies may initiate research, or partner on projects with universities, research institutions, and communities. Evaluation can promote best practices and support model programs.	• Conduct economic research on the expected return on investment in terms of health outcomes from specific policies or types of policies. • Research new fuel technologies to identify strategies to improve air quality.
LEGISLATION AND ORDINANCES	State legislation and local ordinances provide funding or authorize new programs, regulations, or restrictions. Government agencies vary in their legal ability to support the passage of legislation and ordinances.	• Amend a local ordinance to allow mobile produce vending in a residential area. • Pass legislation to support access to safe, clean, and affordable water.
TAXES AND FEES	Governments can add new taxes, change or abolish existing taxes, or change the tax base to finance needed services.	• Increase vehicle licensing fees to raise revenue for supporting transit projects. • Raise cigarette taxes and use the revenue to pay for health care services and discourage tobacco use.
TRAINING AND TECHNICAL ASSISTANCE	Agencies provide training and technical assistance to support local programs in working toward ongoing goals, and as programs and policies change. Both interagency and intra-agency training are essential to support collaboration.	• Educate non-health staff on how their work relates to health outcomes. • Provide technical assistance to regional transportation agencies on how to incorporate health considerations and outcomes into transportation modeling.

Courtesy of Health in All Policies: A Guide for State and Local Governments. Washington, DC and Oakland, CA: American Public Health Association and Public Health Institute; 2015:97-99

2. Define the Audience

As in all communication, understanding the recipients of the information and the context in which their decisions are made are keys to getting the message right. By doing some online legwork, you can accumulate quite a bit of information about the party affiliation, length of service, voting record, birthplace, age, and other factors to help you understand the person you hope to persuade.

Your first interactions with elected officials will most likely occur through their staff members. Their job is to keep policy makers and administrators informed about the issues and the potential pitfalls of proposed legislation.[7] Some of these staff members may have in-depth knowledge of health issues or an interest in specific health issues, but most will not. When interacting and working with these staff, the communicator's role is to present a compelling argument that leads to a desired action. Also, you should look at *your* job as being devoted to making *their* job as easy as possible in terms of presenting your thoughts to their boss. When possible, your message should be concise and tied to a policy action. Using sound bites that a policy maker or staffer can repeat later is often helpful in distilling the essence of your message. Many public health messages are complicated, so policy-making staff members will want to be able to explain their position in simple terms and then call upon experts, such as you or others, to add the details.

3. Research and Craft the Message

The message needs to be direct, definitive, and defensible (backed up by the science).[8] It should be framed in a context that is both easily understood by policy makers and actionable—that is, capable of being implemented in the real world. Public health practitioners often work in a context of prevention and treatment in which results are achieved only in 10 or more years, whereas elected officials work in an environment driven by election cycles and legislative calendars.

To narrow the message and make it compelling for policy makers, it is often useful to consider three questions that are usually most relevant to policy audiences:

- Is there a problem?
- Do we know what to do about the problem?
- How much will it cost to solve the problem?

While it might not be explicitly stated, the policy maker will be balancing the answers to these questions against his or her own perceptions of the electorate. Thus, you should anticipate the policy maker's unspoken questions:

- How does this help my constituency?
- Will this make me look good (to the media, to my electorate, and to the powerful interests that shape my region)? (You will need to be subtle about this point.)

BOX 6-3 offers some new analyses on what matters in policy communication to state legislators and lobbyists.

Framing   One of the most studied topics in communication science, particularly as it pertains to policy, is message framing—that is, emphasizing some aspects of a subject over others based on the same set of facts. The simplest form of message framing focuses on the gains from performing a behavior versus the losses associated with nonperformance of that behavior. Maibach and colleagues at George Mason University's Center for Climate Change have spent years studying the value of message frames in communicating about science. They state, "when climate change is introduced as a human health issue, a broad cross-section of audiences—even segments otherwise skeptical of climate science—find the information to be compelling and useful."[9] Framing research can identify not only which frames are likely to be effective, and with whom, but also which are likely to "boomerang." For example, several studies have confirmed that messages emphasizing catastrophic, dire consequences or threats that are geographically remote can reduce the audience's level of concern and increase its sense of hopelessness.[10]

BOX 6-4 features some alternative frames for communicating about science.[j]

Telling Stories   In the context of advocacy to increase physical activity, but applicable to other public health issues, Stamatakis et al.[6] suggest that a "well-executed, evidence-based story may improve the translation of research evidence into policy by:

- … Enhancing the understanding of quantitative evidence that describes the extent of the problem [of physical inactivity] and the impact of policy interventions on promoting health in the population, with an emphasis on involuntary aspects of

---

j. Nisbet MC. Communicating climate change: why frames matter for public engagement. *Environment: Science and Policy for Sustainable Development*. 2009;51:2, 12-23.

BOX 6-3 What Do State Legislators Value in Policy Communication?

TABLE 6-1 shows factors considered to be important in advocacy communications by state legislators who participated in a study of evidence-based policy making. In this particular study, female respondents and those 55 years of age or older were most likely to be moved by the needs of their constituents as well as the scientific evidence.

TABLE 6-1 What Matters to State Legislators in Evidence-Based Policy Making?

1 = unimportant and 5 = very important

Total	N	Scientific Evidence	Constituent Needs	Health Impact	Personal Interest	Local Leader	Advocacy Groups
Total	75	4.5	4.5	4.2	3.9	3.7	3.6
Men	57	4.4	4.5	4.4	3.9	3.7	3.6
Women	18	4.7*	4.8*	4.2	4.0	3.6	3.7
55+	47	4.7**	4.7*	4.3	4.0	3.7	3.7

*$p < 0.10$, ** $p < 0.05$

Data from Dodson EA, Stamatakis KA, Chalifour S, Haire-Joshu D, McBride T, Brownson RC. State legislators' work on public health-related issues: what influences priorities? *J Public Health Man.* 2013 Jan-Feb;19(1):25-9. Table 1.

Another set of authors conducted in-depth interviews with three Democrats, three Republicans, and three health organization lobbyists about what influenced their decisions about tobacco control funding in North Carolina after 2011. The following themes emerged from their qualitative analysis: "(1) High awareness of tobacco-related health concerns but limited awareness of program impacts and funding, (2) the primacy of economic concerns in making policy decisions, (3) ideological differences in views of the state's role in tobacco control, (4) the impact of lobbyist and constituent in-person appeals, and (5) the utility of concise, contextualized data."[1] The authors concluded that it makes sense to "build relationships with policymakers to communicate ongoing program outcomes, emphasize economic data, and develop a constituent advocacy group."

Reference

1. Schmidt AM, Ranney LM, Goldstein AO. Communicating program outcomes to encourage policymaker support for evidence-based state tobacco control. *Int J Environ Res Public Health.* 2014;11(12):12562-12574.

physical activity behaviors (e.g., structural barriers, environmental determinants);

■ Humanizing or anchoring the problem in real-life examples from the constituency, thereby promoting commitment to solving the problem;

■ Packaging the evidence in a mode of communication that is familiar to policy makers, so they may in turn easily communicate to constituents and other stakeholders; and

■ Bolstering advocates and policy champions by improving content of messages and materials used for communicating with policy makers."[6]

These authors have characterized such stories in terms of their use to support a specific stage of policy making. **Upstream stories** focus on a project that is proposed or just beginning. In such a story, the supporting data come from an early pilot program or from estimates based on available science. At this early stage, policy makers want to know about support for the program, funds leveraged, and the potential for success. **Midstream stories** explain the progress of a program already in place. At this point, policy makers want to hear about utilization of funds, beneficiaries of the program, public support, and positive impact on their public image. If funds are needed to continue or expand the program, midstream stories can help to make the case. After a program has had a long period in service, **downstream stories** describe the impact that the program has had on the population served. At this stage, policy makers are interested in health impact, economic

BOX 6-4 Communicating Climate Change: Why Frames Matter for Public Engagement

Typology of frames applicable to climate change	
Frame	Defines science-related issue as...
Social progress	A means of improving quality of life or solving problems; alternative interpretation as a way to be in harmony with nature instead of mastering it.
Economic development and competitiveness	An economic investment; market benefit or risk; or a point of local, national, of global competitiveness.
Morality and ethics	A matter of right or wrong; or of respect or disrespect for limits, thresholds, or boundaries.
Scientific and technical uncertainty	A matter of expert understanding or consensus; a debate over what is known versus unknown; of peer-reviewed, confirmed knowledge versus hype or alarmism.
Pandora's box/Frankenstein's monster/runaway science	A need for precaution of action in face of possible catastrophe and out-of-control consequences; or alternatively as fatalism, where there is no way to avoid the consequences of chosen path.
Public accountability and governance	Research or policy either in the public interest or serving special interests, emphasizing issues of control, transparency, participation, responsiveness, or ownership; or debate over proper use of science and expertise in decisionmaking ("politicization").
Middle way/alternative path	A third way between conflicting or polarized views or options.
Conflict and strategy	A game among elites, such as who is winning of losing the debate; or a battle of personalities or groups (usually a journalist-driven interpretation).

W.A. Gamson and A. Modigliani, "Media Discourse and Public Opinion on Nuclear Power: A Constructionist Approach," *American Journal of Sociology* 95, no. 1 (1989): 1–37; U. Dahinden, "Biotechnology in Switzerland: Frames in a Heated Debate," *Science Communication* 24, no. 2 (2002): 184–97; J. Durant, M.W. Bauer, and G.Gaskell, *Biotechnology in the Public Sphere: A European Sourcebook* (Lansing, MI: Michigan State University Press, 1998);M.C. Nisbet and B.V. Lewenstein, "Biotechnology and the American Media: The Policy Process and the Elite Press, 1970 to 1999," *Science Communication* 23, no. 4 (2002): 359–91; and M.C. Nisbet, "Framing Science: A New Paradigm in Public Engagement," in L. Kahlor and P. Stout, eds., *Understanding Science: New Agendas in Science Communication* (New York: Taylor & Francis, 2009).

Reproduced from Nisbet MC. Communicating Climate Change: Why Frames Matter for Public Engagement. Environment. March-April 2009. http://www.environmentmagazine.org/Archives/Back%20Issues/March-April%202009/Nisbet-full.html.

impact, sustainability, public support, and added value of the program. Downstream stories that address these issues may make the case for continued funding or expansion of the program to new populations.

4. Choose the Spokesperson

The credibility of the messenger is as important as the strength of the message. It helps if this person is a "voter" as well as a spokesperson for the issue, although this factor is of less importance when the messenger is representing a government agency and speaking to a policy maker in a national position. Whatever the information, it should be presented in a forthright, nonconfrontational manner, regardless of the prior stated positions of either the official or the spokesperson. Messengers are most effective when they have earned the respect of legislators and have a reputation for providing information that is accurate and timely, and presented in a manner that is free of rancor.

Government agency representatives are frequently asked to provide testimony to congressional subcommittees (e.g., testimony about tobacco control and prevention). If the message is intended to persuade decision makers to engage in a thoughtful review of health policy options, the outcome is less about awareness and more about action. The pressing question then becomes, "To whom will they listen?" Knowing the preferences of policy makers and their staff can facilitate the selection of trusted communicators. In a testimony scenario, the most compelling and effective messenger might not be a public health official, but rather might be a respected scientist, a trusted community leader, a constituent, a business leader, an adolescent, or even a celebrity, depending on the topic or issue. A comprehensive communication strategy might involve several layers of messengers, including health leaders, political insiders, and constituents. Sometimes you will want to bring someone who has been affected by a program or law to speak on its behalf. **BOX 6-5** highlights the use of individual spokespersons and their true-life stories by one of the most successful advocacy programs of its kind—the truth campaign.

BOX 6-5 The Power of the Personal: Storytelling in Strategic Communications

Patricia McLaughlin, MA
Former AVP, Communications
Legacy Foundation

Introduction

In our social media–driven age, the desire to share information and tell stories has been given new wings. Whether through 140-character anecdotes on Twitter, video-sharing on YouTube, texting or picture-sharing on our mobile phones, we are a "share and share some more" society. The popularity of reality television also reinforces the simple truth that people want to talk about themselves—and will seek out ways to do so.

Personal stories can be a colorful way to shape communications and further your message or cause. With more communication channels than ever, marketers are losing control of their message, and members of the public are becoming more empowered to make their own decisions—whether that occurs through the brands they select, the causes they support, or the media outlets they choose to consume. Sharing personal stories that are relevant and credible to specific audiences is a way to drive engagement, foster loyalty, and potentially turn consumers into advocates for your issue or cause.

Integrated campaigns centered on storytelling can be conducted through advertising, public relations, and personal appearances, or via social networking and social media channels. Ideally, your communications campaign can incorporate all of the various public relations and marketing elements, allowing you to utilize many virtual and in-person touchpoints to best reach your intended audience.

Story Time for a Cause

At the Legacy Foundation, the largest U.S. public health foundation devoted to keeping young people from starting to smoke and helping smokers quit, personal stories are an integral part of the communications outreach. Throughout the organization's 15-year history, storytellers have conducted media interviews, fronted its advertising campaigns, led its grassroots outreach on the ground, and helped with fundraising efforts to reduce smoking. Two of the early quit-smoking campaigns—"Bob Quits" and "Mary Quits"—followed Bob from New York City and Mary from the Washington, D.C., area as they shared their personal struggles to quit smoking (**FIGURE 6-2**). Through TV, print and radio ads, videos and website content, personal appearances and media interviews, Bob's and Mary's stories helped the Legacy Foundation share best practices on how to quit smoking and served as catalysts for other smokers to quit.

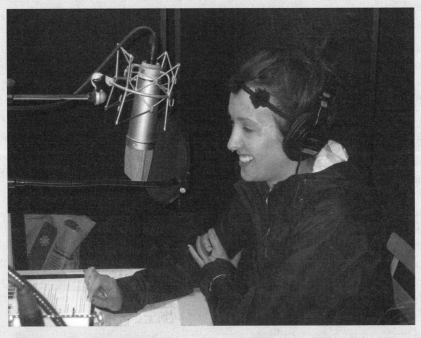

FIGURE 6-2 Chelsee at the Mike
Truth tour rider Chelsee Warneke participates in a radio media tour, sharing her personal story around tobacco use in her family.

Courtesy of Patricia McLaughlin, MA, Legacy® Foundation.

The long-running truth youth smoking-prevention campaign taps storytellers every summer to represent the campaign with the youth target audience as they tour the country with popular music and sporting events like the Vans Warped Tour, skateboarding, and surfing events (**FIGURE 6-3**). In the field, the truth "crew" shares their personal stories with young people around the issue of tobacco use, as well as during media interviews and at personal appearances—from meetings with Capitol Hill staff to branded entertainment shows for media properties like MTV, Fuse, and Fuel.

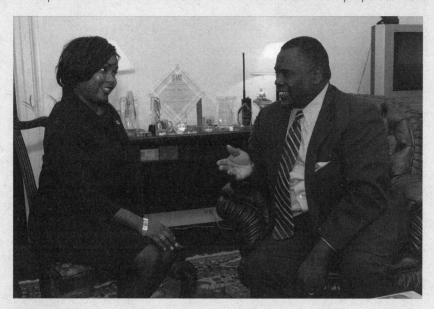

FIGURE 6-3 "Mary Quits": Tonya with Congressman

Courtesy of Patricia McLaughlin, MA, Legacy® Foundation.

How to Do This?

Storytelling starts with having a compelling storyteller. In the digital age, it is somewhat easy to find appropriate personalities:

- *Tap personal networks.* Let family, friends, and coworkers know that you are looking for a certain type of storyline or storyteller. Be specific about the criteria, but welcome all suggestions. Sending a group email or distributing the request and your criteria via social networks such as Facebook, LinkedIn, or Twitter makes the process a few simple clicks away.
- *Use your local resources.* Community groups and service organizations that have a vested interest in your issue can be helpful sources in identifying relevant speakers.
- *Speak with strangers.* You may find yourself in a "target-rich" environment where people connected to your issue already gather. For instance, if you are trying to line up an advocate on green issues for an environmental organization's storytelling campaign, look to your community for events such as clean-ups or green-living education sessions where potential storytellers may naturally gather.
- *Monitor social media channels.* Oftentimes, potential speakers are already in your organization's "universe," having reached out on their own. They may be posting comments on your organization's Facebook page, sending emails in which they organically share a story, or sharing stories as part of a donation to your organization. Have your social media monitoring team or fundraising teams be on the lookout for potential storytellers who may be right under your nose.
- *Create a storytellers database.* Keeping an active and comprehensive database of potential speakers is a way to grow your network and have speakers at the ready as a request or need comes up. Be mindful of putting as much relevant information as possible into your database, including full contact details for the storyteller, background and personal history, and relevant actions or outcomes.

Showtime!

Once you have identified spokespeople with authentic, relatable stories who are willing to share them, it is important to prepare storytellers for sharing their stories:

- Provide basic media training, educating them on tips and techniques that will help them to work best with journalists and online media.
- Pair your storyteller with an organizational spokesperson for both appearances and media interviews, when appropriate. Having an organizational representative along often gives the new or beginning storyteller an increased

(continues)

BOX 6-5 The Power of the Personal: Storytelling in Strategic Communications   *(continued)*

comfort level. It also ensures relevant organizational messages or statistics are conveyed properly, freeing the personal storyteller to focus strictly on his or her own tale.

- For both media interviews and personal appearances, provide a briefing sheet to the storyteller in advance. On the sheet, outline talking points and key messages, and provide detailed information about event venues, reporter background, the audience whom the storyteller will be addressing, and any and all logistical details (e.g., when and where to arrive, parking information, on-site contact, dress code).

Story Extensions

- Media interviews: With the large number of media outlets—both traditional and digital—out there today, there are ample opportunities to engage media with your storyteller. But think of where that story would be most relevant: hometown newspapers, local community talk shows, college or university publications, ethnic media? Online Q&A opportunities, affinity groups looking for guest bloggers, and video testimonials are also ways to spread your message.
- Personal appearances: Beyond conducting media interviews, look at other forums where your storyteller can speak—for example, the local Lions Club or youth club meeting, schools, or community events. Affinity groups are often looking for experts in a certain subject area to come and speak at meetings; search for like-minded groups relevant to your issue and offer up your storyteller as a guest speaker.
- Social media: Use digital platforms to spread your storyteller's story even further. Highlight testimonial videos on your website, have your speakers do guest blog posts, and have them share the content through their own social networking sites as well.

Proceed with Caution

Before entering into any relationship with a storyteller, it is important that organizations and companies do some homework upfront. First and foremost, both the storyteller and the story should reflect your organization's values. Make sure your storytellers share your company's or organization's mission and philosophy, and truly want to share their stories as a way to help further that mission or cause. Be very clear from the beginning about whether this is a paid or unpaid opportunity. Many storytellers truly want to speak just to be of help, or to honor a loved one or highlight a cause close to their hearts. Unfortunately, that dynamic can change when money is involved or is not discussed fully before the relationship takes shape. Be clear about your organization's expectations, time commitment, and financial compensation, if any, and clarify what you can provide to the storyteller in the form of support or opportunities to share his or her story.

It is always helpful to have a basic release form that outlines the nature of the relationship and what the storytellers are agreeing to do. Clearly outline the parameters around rights to use their image, their story, photos or videos from their appearances, and the venues where that content will be shared or distributed (e.g., company website, annual report, social media sites).

While you always want your storytellers to speak from the heart and be authentic, it is important that the organization be authentic from the beginning in managing expectations with storytellers and making clear their role moving forward with the organization. Together, you will then craft your own unique story!

Courtesy of Patricia McLaughlin, MA, Legacy® Foundation.

5. Deliver the Message

Every profession has its own language, and public health is no different. When delivering your message, it is important to avoid jargon because it may confuse an audience and project an attitude of elitism. Not everyone will understand technical terms; you cannot afford to lose one individual who might be a potential ally and advocate for your position. Do not use words that are in vogue (e.g., "infrastructure," "modality"). Such words are overused and may project the disagreeable impression of an overly academic or bureaucratic style. You should seek to express, not impress.

Giving formal testimony at a congressional or state legislative hearing is not likely something that you would be asked to do early in your career. Nevertheless, you may be the most qualified person to speak about an issue that is important to your organization.

You can use many different modes to communicate your message to public health administrators and policy makers. Such communications may occur in highly structured or less structured settings. The techniques and amount of preparation needed may differ depending on the setting. An example of a highly structured and formal setting is a legislative hearing. In such a hearing, a group of elected officials gather in a committee meeting room to hear testimony from experts (witnesses) in the public health field. The witness is usually given just a few minutes to present his or her position. **BOX 6-6** provides some suggestions of what to keep in mind when speaking with elected officials.[7]

BOX 6-6 Tips for Face-to-Face Meetings with Policy Makers

When preparing for an interaction with an elected official, try to develop a positive working relationship with his or her legislative staffer(s). These individuals often have a great deal of influence in shaping the activities and priorities of an elected official. When meeting with an elected official, specifically remember to take these steps:

- Make an appointment.
- Select a primary spokesperson if a group is meeting the official.
- Go with a specific purpose and be prepared.
- Be brief and cover only one or two topics.
- Have a few pieces of key data at your fingertips that support your position.
- Provide an illustration of the program or policy impact—a human interest story often works best.
- Know precisely what you want your elected official to do.
- Anticipate questions so that your answers are thoughtful and thorough.
- Provide written data or a fact sheet.
- Be cordial and always thank the official for his or her time.
- Follow up later with a brief thank-you note.

In addition to the content and language you use, your tone of voice and body language are powerful communication tools. Here are a few techniques to remember:

- *Shake hands and make eye contact*. When meeting an official, shake hands and greet him or her with eye contact. In a formal presentation, you should attempt to maintain eye contact with your audience. When you have a large audience, you should address the committee chairperson or other person in charge of the meeting. Avoid darting your eyes across the room or to your notes.
- *Sit upright in the chair*. Appear interested and involved. Be relaxed and confident and at ease with your subject and your audience.
- *Dress professionally*. Your appearance and the manner in which you present your message are clear reinforcements to your message. It is generally good practice to dress conservatively; wear simple, not ornate jewelry; select solid colors over flashy patterns; never wear a hat; avoid shaded or dark glasses unless medically required; and use makeup sparingly. Most importantly, it is essential that you look professional and that your physical appearance does not detract from the message.
- *Start with your message*. Give your conclusion early, and follow with supporting data and information.
- *Involve the audience*. Make your message relevant to the audience at hand. When presenting an abstract concept, such as the value of disease prevention, choose concrete examples that bring the concept home to the audience. For example, when testifying about the impact of premature mortality from chronic disease in a given city, you might frame the issue in the following way: "Last year, more people died from chronic diseases in [this state] than live in [a local city of a smaller size]."

Tips on Letter Writing

In addition to the preceding approaches to presenting information in written and oral form, there are several points to keep in mind when writing a letter to an elected official. It is also important to select the signatory for the letter who will have the most sway with the recipient. Letters are likely to be more effective if they are tailored to the policy maker and come from the policy maker's known constituents.

Tips on Electronic Communication

The explosion in information technologies over the past few decades has greatly enhanced the ability to communicate nearly instantaneously with persons who can influence public health programs. **Electronic communication** (usually email) is more likely to be effective at the national level than at the state level, more likely to be used by staff than by elected officials, and more likely to be used by younger persons than by older individuals. In addition, state legislators are more likely to use email with constituents and political insiders than with intermediary groups, including advocacy organizations, lobbyists, and the media.[18] Email messages from constituents, advocacy organizations, and political insiders are viewed differently by policy makers. Many advocacy groups have developed networks that they can use to alert their members of key issues needing attention.

Barriers and Challenges in Communicating with Policy Makers

Several barriers and challenges are important to consider when communicating directly with policy makers:

- Trends in the legislative arena (e.g., term limits) and other leadership changes (e.g., the rapid turnover in state health officers) will influence the timing and intensity of efforts to effectively communicate public health data.

(continues)

- Social determinants of health are individual characteristics (e.g., income, education, race/ethnicity) that often have a powerful effect on one's health status or health outcomes, yet the policy solutions to address these determinants are not straightforward.[19]
- Public health leaders and policy makers need to take a "long view" of health. Such a vision is needed because many of the "modern epidemics" such as cancer and HIV/AIDS are manifested over the course of years or decades. Also, working with many populations requires a substantial commitment of time and energy to build the necessary trust between public health practitioners and community members.
- Effective methods of communication may also be affected by the organizational "climate"—that is, the dynamics and structure of the organization. For example, a highly formal organization with a strong chain of command would imply that communication with higher-level administrators would be highly structured and channeled through one or more intermediate supervisors.
- Within an organization, practitioners may be affected by previous failures or present restrictions on efforts to make an important policy change. For example, employees at the middle or lower levels within an organization may have official or unofficial restrictions on policy or advocacy efforts related to their programmatic area.
- Reliable data for small-area analyses (e.g., a rural county or a legislative district) often do not exist, which may lead to frustration for both administrators and policy makers. Increasingly, public health agencies are aware of the need for more extensive and timely small-area data.[20]

Nelson DE, Brownson RC, Remington PL, Parvanta C, Eds. Communicating Public Health Information Effectively: A Guide for Practitioners. Washington, DC: American Public Health Association; 2002.

6. Evaluate Your Progress

There are many ways to keep track of the policy, legislation, or action for which you have advocated. Some advocacy organizations keep a close watch on specific policies as they move through congressional or state-level channels. **BOX 6-7** lists a few commonly used metrics.

When taking a "health in all policies" approach, process and impact measures will accommodate the critical formation of coalitions across sectors and health outcomes will be incorporated into policy decisions in other areas. **BOX 6-8** lists some of the process and outcome measures when taking this approach.

Preparing and Delivering a Policy Presentation

Research indicates that the vast majority of policy makers at the national and state levels prefer face-to-face communication. For example, in their systematic review of health policy makers, Innvaer and colleagues reported personal contact, timeliness, and summaries with policy recommendations facilitated use of information.[11] One-fourth of the policy makers surveyed mentioned the poor quality of health policy information as an important communication barrier. Sorian and Bough found that among state-level policy makers, the preferred ways of receiving information were summaries or brief reports,

The following list can be used for tracking the success of policy communications along the process over time:

- Number of knowledge-sharing/dissemination events
- Number of people reached
- Number of high-level policy makers engaged
- Number of news media stories
- Number of citations or other web metrics data
- Number of stakeholders and policy makers present at the launch/dissemination workshop
- Number of actionable policy recommendations
- Number of articles and policy brief downloads
- Number of policy maker invitations to present the findings
- Number of citations in government/donor agency strategy documents
- Documented instances of policy changes consistent with the organization's recommendations
- Level of interest from the implementing partner to conduct an impact evaluation

BOX 6-8 Evaluation for Health in All Policies

Process Evaluation

Process evaluation can provide important information about the collaborative aspects of a "health in all policies" effort, the extent to which partners and stakeholders feel that the process meets their individual and organizational needs, and opportunities for improving the functioning of a group or process, including mid-course adjustments. The following questions might be asked in a process evaluation:

- Did the meetings meet the needs of participants?
- Did partners and stakeholders feel they had sufficient opportunities to participate? Did they feel their input was heard and incorporated?
- Did agency partners perceive that their agency's priorities and needs were taken into consideration?
- What value did agency partners see from participation?
- Which components of the process were most or least useful?
- Which external processes or events helped or hindered "health in all policies" efforts?
- What opportunities lie ahead?
- How can this effort be made more effective?
- Were deliverables produced on time?

Process evaluation can also be used to explore the success of applying a health or equity lens, in which case it will be useful to ask questions such as how the analysis worked, whether the health or equity analysis met the needs of all partners involved, and whether the analysis supported the development of a collaborative climate.

Impact Evaluation

"Health in all policies" initiatives ideally have multiple outcomes, ranging from creating a more collaborative and health-oriented organizational culture, to promoting healthy public policy and decision-making processes, to ultimately improving population health and equity. An impact evaluation will look at those policy and organizational outcomes that may have occurred as a result of the "health in all policies" approach or a specific policy. Such an evaluation can measure the changes that are likely to lead to health improvements and determine the effectiveness of health or equity analysis. It might also look for evidence that health and equity considerations have been incorporated into policies or programs as a result of the analysis. The following questions might be used to assess outcomes related to *organizational and cultural change*:

- Has participation led to increased trust among partner organizations and agencies?
- Has participation led to a perceived or measurable increase in collaboration across sectors?
- How do partner agencies see the relationships among health, equity, sustainability, and their own objectives?
- How have health experts been consulted on decisions made by nonhealth partners?
- Which steps have partner agencies taken to impart health, equity, and sustainability knowledge to their staff?

The following questions can help to assess *policy outcomes, including structural changes to decision-making processes*:

- How have other agencies used a health or equity lens in their assessment of a particular project, program, or policy? Which elements of this work have been collaborative across agencies?
- What progress has been made toward incorporating a health or equity lens into the decision-making process of sectors or partners outside the public health field, including agency partners, city councils, or legislatures?
- How have health, equity, and sustainability criteria been incorporated into the funding or program evaluation criteria of partners outside public health?
- How have health, equity, and sustainability explicitly been incorporated into government guidance or policy documents?
- Have there been legislative actions to support use of a health and equity lens in decision making?
- Have other organizations or groups developed new initiatives that build upon your "health in all policies" work?

Health Outcome Evaluation

Because "health in all policies" is a strategy for improving population health, it is important to use outcome evaluations to measure changes in health status that relate to policy changes and improve your initiatives accordingly. Unfortunately, changes in population health status are difficult to measure, as they are influenced by many factors that may be difficult to disentangle, and they can take a long time to unfold. To compensate for these difficulties, it is important to identify intermediate health outcomes that can help demonstrate progress. Measuring changes in

(continues)

the social determinants of health, for example, can support collaborative work by showing improvements that are relevant to partners both inside and outside the public health field. Health outcome evaluations can also use proxy measures to identify medium- to long-term changes, such as whether partner agencies' policy priorities have shifted to consider health.

For example, suppose you have evidence that violence and perceptions of violence contribute to rates of diabetes and other diseases by negatively impacting people's likelihood of engaging in physical activity. It would be difficult to measure the direct causal impact of a specific change in criminal justice policy on those disease rates. Instead, you might focus your evaluation efforts on intermediate outcomes such as changes in rates of violence or perceptions of violence. You could even go one step further and look at the correlation between those changes and rates of physical activity, even if those changes are too new to be reflected in rates of chronic disease.

From *Health in All Policies: A Guide for State and Local Governments*. Washington, DC and Oakland, CA: American Public Health Association and Public Health Institute; 2015:97-99.

reports from similar states, and reports on states in the region.[12] In this study, state policy makers were found to have read in detail only 27% of the health policy material they received; they "never got to" 35% of the material they were given. These findings suggest a role for relationship-building between public health communicators and policy makers to increase readership of desired materials.[13]

Doing Your Research: The First Step in Tailoring a Presentation to the Policy Maker

Media Scanning In the "good old days," **media scanning** was done by manually clipping print news articles (and collecting data on broadcast media) about an issue of interest. Today, the amount of information available online about any issue has made media scanning both easier and more complicated. It is easier because most media resources can be accessed online in a matter of minutes and there are free tools to help. It is more complicated because separating actual news and expressions of opinion from multiple repetitions of the same item across a range of media platforms is difficult. Twenty-four-hour news channels may repeat the same story, or add barely noticeable differences to freshen it up. Blogs and Twitter feeds are tracked, taking care to separate the real from the hype and the authentic from the fabricated.

Because the amplification of a story by the media (through repetition) can be so extreme, you might need to conduct an independent survey to see what the public is truly thinking about an issue. Almost all news agencies subscribe to **polling surveys** such

as the Gallup Poll[k] or Harris Interactive[l] for weekly national polling on critical issues. The Centers for Disease Control and Prevention (CDC) has worked closely with Harvard University's Robert Blendon to conduct time- and region-specific surveys around critical health emergencies and preparedness.[m] There is often a mismatch between how the media portray public opinion—which can be shaped by a few people standing in front of a camera waving signs, with the same images being shown over and over again—versus an entirely different majority opinion that is not making headlines.

Online Tools The power of **Google trends** seems to be fading, but is still useful to get a macroscopic look at issues. A trend analysis between October 2014 and August 2015 using the following search terms: Supreme Court and marriage, the Patient Protection and Affordable Care Act (ACA), health insurance, and Unemployment yields an interesting discovery. Without actually performing this trend analysis, it might have seemed that 'everyone' was concerned about the marriage equality act or "Obamacare." However, using search activity on Google as a proxy reveals that many more people were concerned about unemployment than either of these two other issues except for right after the June 26 Supreme Court decision requiring states to license marriages, and recognize out of state marriages, for two persons of the same sex. Very quickly all searches returned to pre-announcement levels, with numbers increasing for unemployment into August 2015.

Twitter is a highly popular media channel for messaging, and a number of tools are available to

k. http://www.gallup.com/home.aspx
l. http://www.harrispollonline.com/
m. http://www.hsph.harvard.edu/research/horp/project-on-the-public-and-biosecurity/

measure who is following whom or what. In addition, more specific measures can analyze the content being tweeted.[n] Nevertheless, it is difficult to know what these statistics actually mean in terms of real impact, because a clear relationship between tweeting messages and taking action has not been demonstrated.

Despite these measurement-related challenges, you can gain some idea of how an elected official might interpret the same information by comparing the volume of positive and negative postings on an issue, using online tools. When this analysis is taken together with the official's record, you may be able to decide whether an elected official might want to support your issue.

Of course, there is no law against calling and speaking to staff to help you prepare more effectively for a meeting. When asked a question during your presentation, you want to be able to say, "I thought you might ask about that, and I have prepared this analysis." As much as possible, you want to avoid having to say, "I will have to get back to you on that."

Writing the Policy Brief

Stamatakis and colleagues provide excellent guidance on the elements of a policy brief.[6] **BOX 6-9** summarizes what they consider to be the essential elements in such a brief.

▶ Advocacy

We have just described the most effective ways to communicate about public health directly with policy makers. Many times, however, that option might not be available to you. The issue about which you are concerned might not seem that important to an elected official. In such a case, how do you get your issue on the official's radar? The primary method is through grassroots advocacy, which is done by working with a group of concerned citizens. This kind of group attempts to work through the media to amplify their voices so that they are heard.

A number of "cookbooks" for this process, which once seemed highly mysterious, are now available. For example, the American Public Health Association (APHA) has published a useful advocacy guide for its membership,[o] and state and other national organizations have developed many other types of materials, including websites[l] and advocacy toolkits.[p]

The actual advocacy process is somewhat similar to the process for presenting information to policy makers and to the persuasive communication process (to be described in the next section). They differ in the amounts the of effort devoted to (1) forming an effective coalition, (2) conducting an in-depth study of the issue, (3) identifying potential solutions, (4) creating events, (5) working with local news media representatives and (6) framing the discussion based on your objectives. Government agencies do not lead advocacy initiatives, although they may play key roles in providing data and information to organizations or groups, such as those striving to increase funding for programs within their jurisdiction.

Explicit objectives can also be set for the process of advocacy itself. Some examples follow:

- Getting an issue onto the radar—that is, getting it onto an agenda for discussion
- Reframing an issue to support the public health position
- Discrediting the opponents of public health objectives
- Bringing important, different voices into debates
- Introducing new key facts and perspectives calculated to change the focus of a debate

---

BOX 6-9 Essential Elements of a Policy Brief

1. Title: The hook, a demand for attention
2. Story: Making it real, appealing, and emotional
3. Problem: Risk, scope, and epidemiology
4. Benefits: Public health prevention and impact
5. Options: Summaries of the literature, reviews, and authoritative sources
6. Recommendations: A specific policy solution or a range of options
7. Sources: Scientific sources, websites, and model legislation

Based on Stamatakis K, McBride T, Brownson R. Communicating prevention messages to policy makers: The role of stories in promoting physical activity. *J Phys Act Health.* 2010 Mar;7 Suppl 1:S99-10

Community-Based Prevention Marketing for Policy Development: A New Planning Framework

The Florida Prevention Research Center (PRC), which is supported by the CDC, and working in concert with its community partners, developed an

---

BOX 6-10 Community-Based Prevention Marketing Policy Development Framework

1. Build a strong foundation for success.
2. Review evidence-based policy options.
3. Select a policy to promote.
4. Identify priority audiences among beneficiaries, stakeholders, and policy makers.
5. Conduct formative research with priority audiences.
6. Develop a marketing plan for promoting the policy.
7. Develop a plan for monitoring implementation and evaluating impact.
8. Advocate for policy change.

A web-based training program that walks through each of these steps in a manner suitable for community engagement is available at http://health.usf.edu/publichealth/prc/policy/policy-development.htm.

Community-Based Prevention Marketing. University of South Florida, Florida Prevention Research Center website. Available at http://health.usf.edu/publichealth/prc/policy/policy-development. Accessed October 8, 2015

---

eight-step process for community coalitions to identify, select, tailor, and promote evidence-based policies (**BOX 6-10**).[14] The focus of the community-based prevention marketing (CBPM) approach for policy development is to allow community members to assess the "return on investment" of their energies and time in selecting their advocacy focus. The CBPM relies on community development and social marketing principles. It also teaches coalitions to use public health advocacy tools to promote policy change at the organizational, local community, and state levels. The Florida PRC has applied CBPM to tobacco and alcohol prevention, childhood obesity prevention, "tween" nutrition and fitness, and citrus workers' health while working with different counties and communities across the state.

In California, Change Lab Solutions (changelabsolutions.org), develops innovative approaches and useful tools to engage communities in policy action. **BOX 6-11** shows two pages from its Healthy Planning Guide. For a negative health outcome, such as poor or inadequate nutrition, the guide identifies long-term health impacts, relationships to the built environment, policy recommendations, action steps for public health, and suggested partners.

Use of New and Traditional Media

New Media Advocacy

In recent years, social media have become the primary way of engaging others in advocacy topics. Guo and Saxton analyzed how 188 nonprofit organizations were using social media in 2014.[15] Apart from the relatively rare video or tweet that "goes viral," the organizations

they studied all embraced social media as a daily experience. The authors created a three-stage typology to describe nonprofits' work of "reaching out to people, keeping the flame alive, and stepping up to action" predominantly through use of Facebook, LinkedIn, Twitter, and YouTube. In their analysis of one month of Twitter feeds (which they used as a proxy for overall social media use), Guo and Saxton found that organizations used this channel to increase the number of "followers" or "friends" (average of 2465; range from 0 to more than 83,000). The organizations sent an average of 103 tweets during the 4-week period studied, or about 3.5 tweets per day. Somewhat less than half of the tweets were categorized by the researchers as containing public education information.[14]

Despite social media's popularity, there is a cautionary tale in the actual numbers and return on investment realized from these channels in terms of time. Even the largest organizations reach far fewer individuals via social media than any mass-media channel can access. Social media can be part of the health communication mix, but should not be the sole channel used to disseminate messages.

The Community Toolbox offers guidance in this area.[q] The advice for using social media for advocacy does not differ from the advice for other uses of these channels. Social media are about two-way conversations and engagement—that is, both listening to information and sharing it outward. A few specific tips for advocacy are provided here:

- *Set your objectives.* Is your goal narrow (publicizing an event) or broad (building and engaging with a community or coalition)?

---

q. http://www.aahperd.org/naspe/advocacy/governmentRelations/toolkit.cfm

■ *Identify the audiences.* Are you primarily communicating with people who are already familiar with your group or cause, such as your members and volunteers? Or are you reaching out to people in other locations whom you have identified as potential members and supporters?

■ *Select a mix of social media platforms.* This decision should be guided by your objectives and intended audience. Facebook provides a stable base and archive that can be refreshed periodically. Twitter, Instagram, and similar platforms require updating and are most effective for promoting events.

■ *Appoint a team to manage your social media presence.* Social media require constant updating with new content and messages. This is a big job that may need to be done by more than one person to prevent early burnout.

Traditional Media Advocacy

Traditional media advocacy focuses on local TV, radio stations, and newspapers. As when engaging with policy makers, it is important to know the people responsible for researching, reporting, and presenting the news and feature stories in your area. Call ahead and try to make an appointment for an **informational interview** with them. You want to know what each reporter's "beat" is (e.g., health, food, beauty and fashion, science, the environment, violence prevention, local interest, and even entertainment might all be relevant) so that you can frame stories for their audience.

BOX 6-11 Healthy Planning Guide Example

lack of physical activity

Negative Health Outcomes	Relation to build Environment	Policy recommendations	Action steps for public health	Partners
·· Attention deficit disorder ·· Cancer ·· Depression ·· Diabetes ·· Heart disease ·· Obesity ·· Stress ·· Stroke	**Community access** ·· Limited or no open space or parks ·· Limited access to parks or open space due to distance to or from transit ·· School land unavailable for recreation after school hour **Safety concerens** ·· Poorly maintained parks ·· Physical activity discouraged by neighborhood safety issues ·· Outdoor activity limited by air pollution **Auto dependency** ·· Separation of jobs, housing, schools and essential services means time spent commuting diminishes time for other activity ·· Public transit is inefficient or expensive	**General & Area plans** ·· Create convenient, safe physical activity opportunites for residents of all ages, abilities, and income ·· Promote transit-oriented and compact, mixed-use development **Zoning** ·· Adopt mixed-use residential, commercial, and office zoning where appropriate ·· Adopt complete streets design guidelines Require walking, biking, and wheelchair facilities in new developments **Redevelopment** ·· Develop parks and open spaces accessible to all users **Economic development** ·· Incentivize mixed-use, compact developemnt **Transportation** ·· Plan for and invest in pedestrian and bicycling infrastructure and transit-oriented development ·· Adopt design guidelines that enhance street connectivity ·· Reduce parking requirment for transit-oriented developments ·· Establish parking maximum (vs. minimum) requirements ·· Expand safe routes to school programs **Parks & Recreation** ·· Ensure access to safe, well-maintained parks and recreation facilities ·· Pursue join use agreements to share facilities with schools ·· Establish and fund a high "level-of-service" maintenance standard for parks **Schools** ·· Develop joint use agreements to provide access to school land after hours	**Assessment** ·· Map walkable routes and transportation options ·· Compile evidence base linking public transit use to health outcomes **Outreach & Education** ·· Provide testimony and data to decision-makers on link between built environment and physical activity **Participation in planning process** ·· Establish an official advisory role for public health in palnning processes ·· Work with school boards and administrators to promote small schools and joint use agreements ·· Collaborate with local agencies to implement safe routes to schools ·· Work with local jurisdictions to adopt bike and pedestrian master plans ·· Partner with law enforcement and neighborhood watch groups to reduce crime	**Public agencies** ·· Planning department ·· Economic/community development department ·· Redevelopment agency ·· Local/regional transportaion agency ·· School boards ·· Parks and recreation **Community partners** ·· Neighborhood watch groups ·· Community-based organizations ·· Nonprofit groups ·· Community benefit organizations

www..changelabsolutions.org | www.barhii.org

Pages from the Healthy Planning Guide used with permission from ChangeLab Solutions (changelabsolutions.org).

(continues)

BOX 6-11 Healthy Planning Guide Example *(continued)*

alcohol and tobacco use

Negative Health Outcomes	Relation to build Environment	Policy recommendations	Action steps for public health	Partners
·· Alcoholism ·· Cancer ·· Communicable diseases ·· Heart disease ·· Liver disease ·· Mental health problems ·· Teen pregnancy ·· Violance	**Community access** ·· Concentration of liquor stores, convenience stores, and bars **Marketing** ·· Proliferation of alcohol and tobacco advertising	**General & Area plans** ·· Reduce concentrated exposure to alcohol and tobacco **Zoning** ·· Restrict approvals of new retailers selling alcohol for off-sites consumption near high-crime areas, schools, and parks ·· Enforce compliance with community standards through conditional use permits and "deemed approved" ordinance ·· Create smokefree workplaces, multiunit housing, and outdoor spaces to eliminate secondhand exposure **Redevelopment** ·· Incentivize the development of health retail outlets in all neighborhoods as an alternative to alcohol and tobacco vendors **Economic development** ·· Provide incentives to small stores who limit alcohol and tobacco and offer more healthy choices **Parks & Recreation** ·· Adopt smokefree ordinances for parks and recreation areas **Schools** ·· Mandate universal smokefree campuses **Licensing** ·· Ensure that California's Alcoholic beverage Control (ABC) and local planning commissions limit the number of off-sale liquor stores in overconcentrated areas ·· Mandate use of public health criteria in ABC licensing process ·· Enact local licensing ordinance to control location and operations of tobacco retailers **Law enforcement** ·· Enforce laws regulating storefront and window signage	**Assessment** ·· Work with community groups to identify stores that sell alcohol and tobacco products in neighborhoods **Outreach & Education** ·· Educate community members and policy makers on relationship of built environment to alcohol and tobacco use **Participation in planning process** ·· Coordinate work with timelines of local plan updates, redevelopment, and community meetings ·· Work with small corner stores to shift to healthier business models ·· Integrate public health injury prevention with tobacco and alcohol prevention programs	**Public agencies** ·· Planning department ·· Economic/community development department ·· Redevelopment agency ·· California Department of Alcoholic beverage Control (ABC) **Community partners** ·· Local business organizations (e.g., Chambers of Commerce) ·· Community-based organizations ·· Local schools and universities ·· Neighborhood and community clinics

www..changelabsolutions.org | www.barhii.org

Pages from the Healthy Planning Guide used with permission from ChangeLab Solutions (changelabsolutions.org).

You need to also know their deadlines and news cycles. All reporters have one thing in common: They want to bring important information to their audience. If you are working to support a national public health campaign activity, it is essential to tell news media representatives why the campaign is important *in your area*. This can be done by using local data, spokespersons, and visual images.

As with **earned media** (publicity gained through promotional efforts rather than paid advertising), you usually need to initiate an event to attract media coverage. If you want television reporters to attend the event, make sure they have good visual and on-air interview opportunities. Similarly, when seeking to engage with radio reporters, be sure that you have an interesting soundscape and that the event is not so noisy that you cannot hold a quiet interview nearby. Print media (newspapers or magazines) are somewhat different, in that you can send a report or announcement to the editor or reporter, who might just need to call you to check a few facts. Contact the reporters well in advance to build relationships and give them time to arrange for someone to cover the event.

Media that reach out to specific populations, such as Spanish- or Asian-language print media or African American radio stations, might take a particular interest in an issue that disproportionately affects their audience. Reporters or editors at these outlets might be willing to become champions for your issue, volunteer to be speakers or presenters, or add some pizzazz (attention) to a community event in other ways. This kind of give-and-take is also good because a larger crowd may attend because of the local celebrity's appeal and the media networks will be more likely to cover the event.

Media Relations Tools[r]

Media relations relies on a key set of tools, including the following written pieces:

- A **press release** is generally issued for "hard news," which means a new finding, report, or release of data on your issue. (See **BOX 6-12** for an example.)
- A **media alert** is a kind of invitation to promote a special event. It highlights what you would put in a party invitation: the "who, what, when, where, and why" of your event. Assignment and calendar section editors can use this news alert to plan coverage and fill out "community happenings" listings. (See **BOX 6-13** for an example.)
- A **backgrounder** usually has more detailed information about your issue, event, or campaign from

which the media can pull out relevant facts. (See **BOX 6-14** for an example.)
- Optional items:
  - Fact sheets on different topics
  - "Frequently asked questions" (FAQs) and answers
  - Biographies of organizational leaders and spokespersons
  - "Real-life stories" of individuals affected by the issue (these individuals, if they are willing, can serve as spokespersons)

Data Collections and Report Cards

Advocacy groups will often conduct an assessment, or collect data, to point out the deficiencies in a program. Many efforts use a "report card" to highlight the problems and compare the targeted entity being evaluated to others in its class.

Anticipating Audience Questions

Regardless of how much information seems to be available, preparing a strategy related to an issue requires grasping what members of the relevant public are saying about it. In addition, elected officials' questions to you are likely to be driven by their reading of the media, as well as what the polls are indicting. Clearly, then, you need to be prepared with this information as part of your strategy and to have data and other types of information handy. **FIGURE 6-4** shows a strategy for analyzing issues that can be applied to media coverage, blogs, or polling data.

▶ Example of a Successful Policy Change Communication Campaign

Box 6-14 is an example of a policy change communication campaign implemented by the Maternity Care Coalition. This organization works to make Philadelphia a safe and supportive place for working breastfeeding mothers. Its campaign materials include a photo of the city's mayor signing the bill that the organization had sought to pass (**FIGURE 6-5**). The examples of the media alert, press release, and backgrounder come from this program.

BOX 6-12 Sample Press Release

Courtesy of Maternity Care Coalition

---

r. http://ctb.ku.edu/en/table-of-contents/advocacy/direct-action/electronic-advocacy/main

BOX 6-13 Sample Media Alert

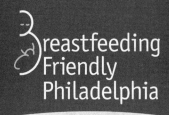

reastfeeding
Friendly
Philadelphia

Please Join Maternity Care Coalition
For the Breastfeeding-Friendly Business Awards

Presented by
Dr. Donald F. Schwarz
Deputy Mayor, Health & Opportunity
Health Commissioner, City of Philadelphia

Wednesday, September 29, 2010
3:00 PM to 5:00 PM
The College of Physicians of Philadelphia
19 South 22nd Street, Philadelphia, PA 19103

Featuring 2010 Awardees

Health Federation of Philadelphia, Early Head Start Program
The Children's Hospital of Philadelphia
Trolley Car Diner

Representing the U.S. Department of Labor
Sara Manzano-Diaz
Director of the Women's Bureau

On Behalf of Human Resource Professionals
Kelley Cornish, MA, CCPD
President of Philly SHRM

Hors d'oeuvres and beverages will be served.

Please RSVP by September 22nd to 215.989.3564 or kpigur@momobile.org.

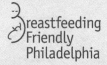

reastfeeding
Friendly
Philadelphia

As part of the Philadelphia Department of Public Health's
Get Healthy Philly initiative, Maternity Care Coalition is
promoting the health and economic benefits of breastfeeding to
help create and strengthen breastfeeding support in the workplace.

2010 Nominees
Defense Supply Center at Naval Support Activity Philadelphia
Drexel University
Health Partners, Inc.
Nationalities Services Center
Pennsylvania Hospital
Penn Sleep Center
Philadelphia Youth Network
University of Pennsylvania School of Nursing

Campaign Partners

Maternity Care Coalition | COMMUNITIES PUTTING PREVENTION TO WORK

Event Sponsors

The Pennsylvania
Breastfeeding Coalition

This project is made possible by funding from the Department of Health and Human Services
and *Get Healthy Philly*, an initiative of the Philadelphia Department of Public Health.

Courtesy of Maternity Care Coalition

BOX 6-14 Breastfeeding Friendly Philadelphia; Subtitle: Supporting Breastfeeding Moms Makes Good Business Sense

Breastfeeding Works A Minimal Investment for a Healthy Return

Majority Interests
In 2008, 56.4% of mothers with children under age one participated
in the labor force. For many working mothers, returning to work is
a major barrier to breastfeeding.

Added Value
Mothers need minimal support to continue breastfeeding when they return to work.
Employers that offer supportive work environments for breastfeeding employees have
discovered that the return in cost savings and productivity is worth the investment.

The Bottom Line
Do the math. Breastfeeding employees + supportive employers = healthier moms,
babies, families, workplaces and communities.
It's a win-win situation!

Legal Matters
Section 4207 of the Patient Protection and Affordable Care Act, signed into law on
March 23, 2010, includes a provision that employers shall provide reasonable, unpaid
break time and a private, non-bathroom place for an employee to express breast milk for
her nursing child for one year after the child's birth. Employers with less than 50 employees are not subject to the requirement if it would cause undue hardship related to the
size, financial resources, nature, or structure of the employer's business.

Join Other Employers in creating a Breastfeeding-Friendly Philadelphia!
email: breastfeeding-friendly@momobile.org or call 215-989-3564.

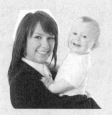

Courtesy of Maternity Care Coalition

reastfeeding
Friendly
Philadelphia

Wednesday, September 29, 2010
3:00 PM to 5:00 PM
The College of Physicians of Philadelphia

Featuring 2010 Awardees
Health Federation of Philadelphia, Early Head Start Program
The Children's Hospital of Philadelphia
Trolley Car Diner

Presented by
Dr. Donald F. Schwarz
Deputy Mayor, Health & Opportunity
Health Commissioner, City of Philadelphia

Hosted by
Linda Munich
Vice President of Public Affairs for GABC

Representing the U.S. Department of Labor
Sara Manzano-Diaz
Director of the Women's Bureau

On Behalf of Human Resource Professionals
Kelley Cornish, MA, CCPD
President of Philly SHRM

Rosemarie O'Malley Halt, RPH, MPH

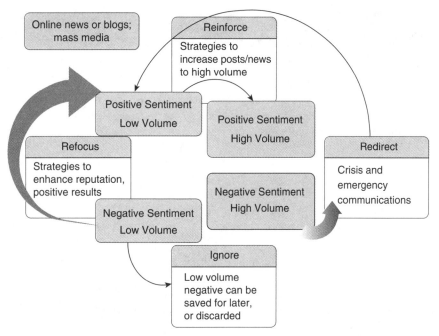

FIGURE 6-4 Media Scanning Strategies

BOX 6-15 Breastfeeding Friendly Philadelphia Campaign

Rosemarie O'Malley Halt, RPh, MPH

Maternity Care Coalition Background

Founded in 1980, Maternity Care Coalition (MCC) is a nonprofit organization with the mission to improve maternal and child health and well-being through the collaborative efforts of individuals, families, providers, and communities. Our comprehensive approach includes research, public policy initiatives, and services for families. MCC has assisted more than 95,000 families throughout southeastern Pennsylvania since its founding, focusing particularly on neighborhoods with high rates of poverty, infant mortality, health disparities, and changing immigration patterns.

Breastfeeding Friendly Philadelphia Campaign

Breastfeeding is the healthiest first food for babies, critical for the development of healthy individuals and communities. The World Health Organization and the American Academy of Pediatrics have identified breastfeeding as the optimal method of infant feeding, ideal for fostering nutritional, immunological, and emotional health. Both organizations recommend exclusive breastfeeding for six months, followed by continued breastfeeding as complementary foods are introduced, with continuation of breastfeeding for one year or longer as mutually desired by mother and infant.

Philadelphia's breastfeeding rates continued to decrease while its early child health outcomes worsened. MCC responded to this need by identifying a lack of workplace policies to support breastfeeding mothers when they returned to work. We launched a breastfeeding-friendly businesses and hospitals initiative by establishing a multifaceted advocacy campaign. The cumulative effort of MCC and key stakeholders resulted in the signing of Philadelphia City Council Bill 130922 on September 3, 2014, by Philadelphia Mayor Michael Nutter. Key provisions of the bill included that breastfeeding accommodations be made for all nursing employees (hourly paid and salaried) regardless of size of business, and that businesses must include a private, clean space (not a bathroom) and provide appropriate break time for women to express milk. A major breakthrough was that violations are now subject to penalties, making this bill stronger than the current federal nursing break law. According to Katja Pigur, Director of Clinical and Breastfeeding Services, MCC, "The key to success in the Breastfeeding Friendly Philadelphia Campaign was inspiring change through relationship building. That meant bringing critical partners together—the health department, businesses, hospitals, maternal child health advocates, politicians, funders, and mothers, all working together for a common goal."

(continues)

BOX 6-15 Breastfeeding Friendly Philadelphia Campaign *(continued)*

Inspiring Change

While MCC had a successful history of advocacy around the issue of breastfeeding, it was not until the passage of the federal Affordable Care Act (ACA) that the political and social environment seemed right to advance the issue in Philadelphia. ACA integrated supporting nursing mothers in the workplace for businesses with 50 or more employees. The accommodation applies until the child is one year of age.

Funding Change

MCC as a nonprofit lacked the financial resources to conduct a citywide breastfeeding campaign. We formed partnerships to finance the activity. In March 2010, MCC partnered with the Philadelphia Department of Public Health and launched the Breastfeeding Friendly Philadelphia campaign as a part of the Get Healthy Philly initiative, funded through the CDC's "Communities Putting Prevention to Work" Grant, to improve city-wide breastfeeding rates through a twofold approach:

1. Encouraging hospitals to implement evidence-based policies and practices to support and promote breastfeeding
2. Promoting the health and economic benefits of breastfeeding within the business community and helping employers create and strengthen lactation support policies and programs for their worksites

Developing Change

MCC faced the tremendous challenge of developing a campaign with two different target audiences. However, common threads existed to coordinate the campaign:

1. Analyze the target audiences' perceptions and policies around breastfeeding.
2. Utilize diverse networking to form strategic partnerships.
3. Identify "champions" within organizations, businesses, and hospitals.
4. Form advisory groups and task forces to develop target audience messages, share ideas, and identify concerns, problems, and solutions in implementing breastfeeding programs.
5. Assist in developing breastfeeding policy documents and strategies for employers and hospitals and the process to implement them.

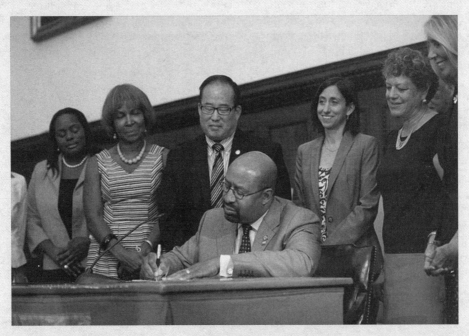

FIGURE 6-5 Mayor Michael A. Nutter enacts Bill No. 130922, ensuring breastfeeding accommodation in Philadelphia workplaces, witnessed by (left to right) Saniah M. Johnson, Councilwoman Blondell Reynolds Brown, Councilman David Oh, Rue Landau, JoAnne Fischer, and Letizia Amadini Lane, vice president and global head, Employee Value Proposition, Office of CEO and Corporate Strategy, GlaxoSmithKline.

6. Tailor technical assistance to the individual organizational needs and internal processes.
7. Seek policy makers' support and sponsorship of legislation for breastfeeding in Philadelphia.
8. Implement a multifaceted media campaign (radio, TV, social media photo campaign, and videos), to build momentum with stakeholders and the broader community.
9. Recognize achievements and model implementation of breastfeeding initiatives on a regular basis.
10. Analyze results and identify methods to improve, continue, and expand programs over the long term.

Challenges with Change

Advocacy campaigns can be challenging, particularly on what is perceived to be a private issue. Change in the public arena does not happen overnight; indeed, it can take years to move the bar forward on issues. MCC was extremely successful utilizing limited resources to effect citywide change on the issue of breastfeeding.

Challenges during the process were many, including lack of buy-in from some hospitals, employers, and business organizations. The ongoing difficult economic environment placed added strain on limited resources. Compounding the inherent problems was the controversial nature of the ACA, including the provision of breastfeeding accommodations in the workplace and the perceived increase in costs to employers. Hospitals offered unique challenges with developing acceptance of breastfeeding-friendly environments for patients. The requests for support from administrators and extra education directed to doctors and nurses on best practices for breastfeeding were not always met enthusiastically. Fortunately, by using evidence-based processes for breastfeeding support and maintaining and nurturing relationships, MCC was able to steer problems to equitable solutions that continue to impact thousands of mothers and babies in the Philadelphia region. This collaborative approach successfully built a foundation for normalizing breastfeeding and increasing breastfeeding rates so that the health and societal benefits of breastfeeding can be experienced across a large, urban environment.

▶ Conclusion

Effective communication of public health information to key policy makers is a challenging task. To produce change in public health policy we need to communicate with policy makers in a manner that is clear, articulate, and inspiring. Strategic use of scientific information and narratives in these types of communication can greatly enhance their impact. Although there is no single "recipe" that is appropriate for every audience and setting, the principles and approaches outlined in this chapter provide a basis for more effective communication with decision makers.

Wrap-Up

Chapter Questions

1. What are two (or more) factors that elected officials have to juggle when developing or voting on policy that affects their constituency?
2. Why is it important to get to know a policy makers and their staff before presenting information to them?
3. Describe some ways that you can anticipate the questions or concerns of a policy maker about your issue.
4. What are three essential elements of an effective policy presentation?
5. What is meant by "framing" an issue? Do you consider framing to be ethical?
6. Besides serving food, how else can you attract the news media to an event?
7. What is meant by "search engine optimization," and why is it such an important tool for advocacy?

s. Much of the information in this section is based on the CDC's guide for partners to work with the media on folic acid campaigns: *Media Campaign Implementation Kit: A Guide to Media Outreach and Placement for Your Health.*

References

1. Lutkehaus NC. *Margaret Mead: The Making of an American Icon*. Princeton, NJ: Princeton University Press; 2008:261.

2. Rudolph L, Caplan J, Ben-Moshe K, and L. *Health in All Policies: A Guide for State and Local Governments*. Washington, DC/Oakland, CA: American Public Health Association and Public Health Institute; 2013:2.

3. American Public Health Association Government Affairs Department. *APHA Legislative Advocacy Handbook: A Guide for Effective Public Health Advocacy*. Washington, DC: American Public Health Association; 2005.

4. National Conference of State Legislatures. Full- and part-time legislatures. Updated June 2009. http://www.ncsl.org/default.aspx?tabid= 16701

5. O'Neill T, Novak J. *Man of the House*. New York: Random House; 1987; 387pp.

6. Stamatakis K, McBride T, Brownson R. Communicating prevention messages to policy makers: the role of stories in promoting physical activity. *J Phys Act Health*. 2010;7 (suppl 1):S99-S107.

7. Nelson DE, Brownson RC, Remington PL, Parvanta C, eds. *Communicating Public Health Information Effectively: A Guide for Practitioners*. Washington, DC: American Public Health Association; 2002.

8. Woolf SH. Social policy as health policy. *JAMA*. 2009; 301(11):1166-1169.

9. Maibach E, Leiserowitz A, Roser-Renouf C, Mertz CK. Identifying like-minded audiences for climate change public engagement campaigns: an audience segmentation analysis and tool development. *PLoS One*. 2011;6(3):e17571. doi: 10.1371/journal.pone.0017571.

10. Myers TA, Nisbet MC, Maibach EW, Leiserowitz AA. A public health frame arouses hopeful emotions about climate change. *Climatic Change*. 2012;113(3-4):1105-1112.

11. Innvaer S, Vist G, Trommald M, Oxman A. Health policy-makers' perceptions of their use of evidence: a systematic review. *J Health Serv Res Policy*. 2002;7(4):239-244.

12. Richardson L, Cooper C. E-mail communication and the policy process in the state legislature. *Policy Stud J*. 2006;34(1):113-129.

13. Sorian R, Baugh T. Power of information: closing the gap between research and policy. When it comes to conveying complex information to busy policy-makers, a picture is truly worth a thousand words. *Health Aff (Millwood)*. 2002;21(2):264-273.

14. Center for Health Improvement. Health policy guide: bringing policy change to your community. 2009. Available at http://www.healthpolicyguide.org/advocacy.asp?id=23

15. Guo C, Saxton GD. Tweeting social change: how social media are changing nonprofit advocacy. *Nonprofit Vol Sector Qtly*. 2014;43:57-79.

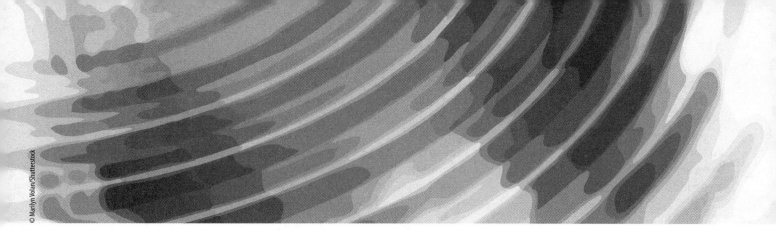

CHAPTER 7

Health Literacy and Clear Health Communication

Erika M. Hedden

Erika M. Hedden

LEARNING OBJECTIVES

By the end of this chapter, the reader will be able to:

- Define basic literacy, health literacy, and numeracy.
- Describe the factors that affect health literacy.
- Define the current state of health literacy in the United States.
- Discuss health literacy policy initiatives in the United States.
- Describe tools for assessing health literacy in research and practice.
- Apply readability tools.
- Use the CDC's Clear Communication Index to rate and revise materials.

▶ Introduction

Literacy refers to an individual's ability to make sense of information in any form in which it is presented. While the ability to sign your name once sufficed to be considered literate, in modern times the definition has acquired a larger meaning of social competence. As we will see later in this chapter, too few high school graduates in the United States—let alone those persons with only an elementary education—possess adequate levels of literacy to make sound financial, legal, medical, or other complex decisions. This social disparity must be addressed outside of the health sector, although much of its impact is felt there.

In recent years, a paradigm shift has occurred regarding the importance of health literacy. We now think of health literacy as a "right," defining it as "the degree to which individuals can obtain, process, understand, and communicate about health-related information needed to make informed health decisions."[1]

A great deal of research demonstrates the negative effects of low health literacy. For example, lower literacy is associated with increased emergency department and hospital use as well as decreased screening rates for cervical and breast cancer, influenza immunization, and access to insurance. Among older adults, a strong association exists between lower health literacy and a higher risk of mortality. In addition, a moderate level of evidence supports a relationship between low health literacy in the elderly and the inability to take medications properly or interpret labels and health messages.[2] The costs of low health literacy are estimated to range from $106 billion to $238 billion annually, representing 7% to 17% of all personal healthcare expenditures.[3]

A further challenge is that persons with limited health literacy may feel ashamed about their lack of skills and are unlikely to voluntarily report when they do not understand information presented to them. Moreover, there is a human cost at the individual level that cannot be fully portrayed with findings from research studies.

The implications are clear: Communicators need to be aware of the problem of low health literacy and shape health messages to meet the needs of audiences with low health literacy levels. In a clinical practice or pharmacy setting, noticing "red flags" of low health literacy may provide an indication as to whether a person requires further assistance with understanding materials and instructions. It may also suggest that your organization's materials need to be revised.

Modeling Health Literacy

There are several frameworks that lay out the determinants, applications and outcomes for health literacy. **FIGURE 7-1** shows the model developed by Sørensen and others.[4] This model emphasizes the elements of the definition above in their application to health care, disease prevention and health promotion domains at the individual and population level. Health literacy goes beyond basic skills and really refers to a knowledge base, as well as to our ability to add information to that to make health-related decisions. So, it is important to first understand how we create that knowledge base in the first place.

Human Learning and Development

Infants learn to interpret the world through sensory perception and motor development. Children subsequently become aware of the ability to manipulate objects and learn to think logically and in terms of organized systems. Primary education uses an information-building approach known as "scaffolding" to assist children in retaining and adding to their knowledge in specific areas.[6]

Humans are limited in how much information they can actually process in a given period of time. Millions of bits of new information pass by our sensory apparatus daily—all the sights, sounds, smells, tastes, and textures that we either recognize as "information" or ignore. On a higher level, thousands of words, numbers, and other organized packets of information pass by us, only some of which we process. But on top of our learned or inherent predilection to ignore most of the communication we receive on a daily basis, *individual* limitations affect our ability to use complex information. The key to

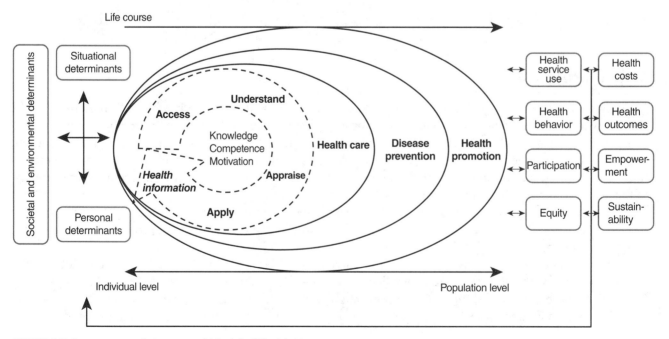

FIGURE 7-1 Sørensen et al.'s Integrated Model of Health Literacy

Sørensen K, Van den Broucke S, Fullam J, Doyle G, Pelikan J, Slonska Z, Brand H. Health literacy and public health: A systematic review and integration of definitions and models. BMC Public Health 2012, 12:80.

using such information is simplifying it, and linking new information to what we already possess in our brains. Once we have managed to "learn" something, our brain uses shortcuts to pull that knowledge into active use. An extensive literature focuses on the heuristics (shortcuts, logical rules) of decision making, including the well-known book by Kahneman, Slovick, and Tversky.[7] The basic idea is that we interpret anything new in terms of what we already know, and we make inferences based on the way in which information has been presented to us.

Attention

In addition to our basic cognitive structures and capacity to learn from an early age, our ability to pay attention to information is affected by how much we care about that information,[8] as well as the conditions in which we are reviewing the information. Information that we are perfectly capable of processing while in the quiet of our home can become unintelligible if we are tired, in a noisy or distracting environment, or under stress or duress, such as in a medical office. Since individual cognitive abilities are difficult to modify, health communicators should focus on relieving the cognitive burden by simplifying the materials presented to consumers.[9] Ways to do this are discussed in detail below.

▶ Basic Literacy and Its Components

The Educational Testing Service (ETS) has developed a framework for defining and assessing different forms of literacy in the United States. Its most basic definition of *literacy* is task based: using printed and written information to function in society, to achieve one's goals, and to develop one's knowledge and potential. Performing these tasks requires successful use of word-level reading skills and higher-level literacy skills.[10]

Types of Literacy

ETS distinguishes three types of literacy, or proficiency scales:

- **Prose literacy** is the ability to read sentences and paragraphs.
- **Document literacy** is the ability to interpret tables, forms, graphs, or other structured formats.
- **Quantitative literacy (QL)** is the ability to understand information that requires a mathematical operation for its interpretation.[11]

Quantitative literacy is a subset of **numeracy**. Numeracy applies mathematical reasoning and knowledge within varied contexts and purposes. Math may include numbers, operations, patterns, functions, algebra, measurement, geometry, statistics, and probability. The cognitive and affective processes necessary to use math proficiently include conceptual understanding; reasoning about the relationships across, within, or between ideas; strategic competence or problem-solving skills; procedural fluency for the necessary calculations; and a productive disposition, or perseverance to solve a problem. Numeracy examples range from taking measurements for building construction, to interpreting the sensitivity and specificity of a new diagnostic test for cancer, to preparing and maintaining a household budget, to examining the costs and benefits of a variety of health insurance options and making a decision based on the individual context.[11]

How Literate Is the U.S. Public?

The U.S. Department of Education conducted the first National Adult Literacy Survey[12] in 1993 and the second such survey, known as the National Assessment of Adult Literacy (NAAL),[13,14] in 2003. NAAL surveyed a representative sample of U.S. adults age 16 and older to assess their functional literacy abilities, scoring literacy tasks and skills across three types of literacy (prose, document, and quantitative). In 2003 (the most recent year for NAAL results are available), approximately 93 million Americans—43% of the total population—were estimated to read at or below the *basic* level of literacy, 34% had comparable document literacy and 55% had quantitative literacy at or below basic level.[13,14] Few changes in these rates were reported in the decade between the 1993 study and the 2003 NAAL. With an 8% increase in the average score, quantitative literacy was the only measure reporting a significant change from 1993 to 2003.[14]

More recently, the National Center for Education Statistics released results from a 2012 international survey conducted by the Program for the International Assessment of Adult Competencies (PIAAC). PIAAC examined four domains: literacy, reading components, numeracy, and problem solving in technology-rich environments. The report compiled information for the United States from a nationally representative sample of 5000 adults aged 16 to 65 years. These data were compared to samples from other partner countries from the Organization for Economic Cooperation and Development (OECD). PIAAC used a scale from 0 to 500, with six levels identified from "below level 1" to "level 5." **TABLE 7-1** shows the levels and literacy tasks assessed in this study.

The U.S. average literacy score was 270, with 12 countries having higher averages and five countries having lower averages.[15] Overall U.S. percentages by level can be viewed in **FIGURE 7-2A**. As can be seen in **FIGURES 7-2B** through **7-2D**, persons not born in the United States, those with less than a high school education, and minorities had disproportionately lower literacy, numeracy, and problem-solving scores, as measured by level 1 (reading sentences and paragraphs) or below level 1 (reading brief texts, basic vocabulary) performance.

▶ Determinants of Health Literacy

Factors from many domains affect health literacy, including functional literacy, communication skills, knowledge or beliefs about health topics, cultural and linguistic factors, socioeconomic status, public health and healthcare system demands, and contextual factors. These domains interact at all levels of the ecological model, ranging from individual factors, to the surrounding community, to the policies that shape our national healthcare climate.

TABLE 7-1 PIAAC Proficiency Levels on the Literacy Scale	
Proficiency Levels and Cut Scores for Literacy	**Literacy Task Descriptions**
Level 5 (score of 376–500)	At this level, tasks may require the respondent to search for and integrate information across multiple, dense texts; construct syntheses of similar and contrasting ideas or points of view; or evaluate evidence-based arguments. Application and evaluation of logical and conceptual models of ideas may be required to accomplish tasks. Evaluating reliability of evidentiary sources and selecting key information is frequently a key requirement. Tasks often require respondents to be aware of subtle rhetorical cues and to make high-level inferences or use specialized background knowledge.
Level 4 (score of 326–375)	Tasks at this level often require respondents to perform multiple-step operations to integrate, interpret, or synthesize information from complex or lengthy continuous, noncontinuous, mixed, or multiple-type texts. Complex inferences and application of background knowledge may be needed to perform successfully. Many tasks require identifying and understanding one or more specific, noncentral ideas in the text to interpret or evaluate subtle evidence-based claims or persuasive discourse relationships. Conditional information is frequently present in tasks at this level and must be taken into consideration by the respondent. Competing information is present and sometimes seemingly as prominent as correct information.
Level 3 (score of 276–325)	Texts at this level are often dense or lengthy, including continuous, noncontiguous, mixed, or multiple pages. Understanding text and rhetorical structures becomes more central to successfully completing tasks, especially in navigation of complex digital texts. Tasks require the respondent to identify, interpret, or evaluate one or more pieces of information, and often require varying levels of inference. Many tasks require the respondent to construct meaning across larger chunks of text or perform multistep operations to identify and formulate responses. Often tasks demand that the respondent disregard irrelevant or inappropriate text content to answer accurately. Competing information is often present, but it is not more prominent than the correct information.
Level 2 (score of 226–275)	At this level, the complexity of text increases. The texts may be digital or printed, and may consist of continuous, noncontiguous, or mixed types. Tasks at this level require respondents to make matches between the text and information, and may require paraphrasing or low-level inferences. Some competing pieces of information may be present. Some tasks require the respondent to cycle through or integrate two or more pieces of information based on criteria, compare and contrast or reason about information requested in the question, or navigate within digital texts to access and identify information from various parts of a document.

Proficiency Levels and Cut Scores for Literacy	Literacy Task Descriptions
Level 1 (score of 176–225)	Most of the tasks at this level require the respondent to read relatively short digital or print continuous, noncontiguous, or mixed texts to locate a single piece of information that is identical to or synonymous with the information given in the question or directive. Some tasks may require the respondent to enter personal information onto a document, in the case of some noncontiguous texts. Little, if any, competing information is present. Some tasks may require simple cycling through more than one piece of information. Knowledge and skill in recognizing basic vocabulary, evaluating the meaning of sentences, and reading of paragraph text is expected.
Below level 1 (score of 0–175)	The tasks at this level require the respondent to read brief texts on familiar topics to locate a single piece of specific information. Only basic vocabulary knowledge is required, and the reader is not required to understand the structure of sentences or paragraphs or make use of other text features. There is seldom any competing information in the text, and the requested information is identical in form to information in the question or directive. While the texts can be continuous, the information can be located as if the text were noncontiguous. In addition, tasks below level 1 do not make use of any features specific to digital texts.

Data from Goodman, M., Finnegan, R., Mohadjer, L., Krenzke, T., and Hogan, J. (2013). Literacy, Numeracy, and Problem Solving in Technology-Rich Environments Among U.S. Adults: Results from the Program for the International Assessment of Adult Competencies 2012: First Look (NCES 2014-008). U.S. Department of Education. Washington, DC: National Center for Education Statistics. Retrieved December 21, 2014. Available from: http://nces.ed.gov/pubs2014/2014008.pdf.

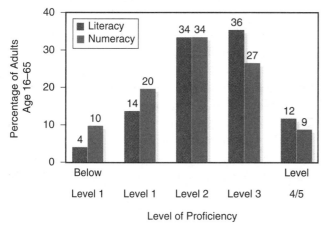

FIGURE 7-2A Overall U.S. PIAAC Literacy and Numeracy Scale Survey Results

Data from Goodman, M., Finnegan, R., Mohadjer, L., Krenzke, T., and Hogan, J. (2013). Literacy, Numeracy, and Problem Solving in Technology-Rich Environments Among U.S. Adults: Results from the Program for the International Assessment of Adult Competencies 2012: First Look (NCES 2014-008). U.S. Department of Education. Washington, DC: National Center for Education Statistics. Retrieved December 21, 2014. Available from: http://nces.ed.gov/pubs2014/2014008.pdf.

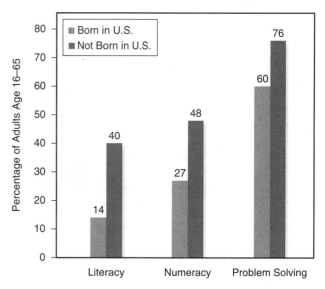

FIGURE 7-2B U.S. PIAAC: Percentage at Level 1 or Below by Native U.S. Status

Data from Goodman, M., Finnegan, R., Mohadjer, L., Krenzke, T., and Hogan, J. (2013). Literacy, Numeracy, and Problem Solving in Technology-Rich Environments Among U.S. Adults: Results from the Program for the International Assessment of Adult Competencies 2012: First Look (NCES 2014-008). U.S. Department of Education. Washington, DC: National Center for Education Statistics. Retrieved December 21, 2014. Available from: http://nces.ed.gov/pubs2014/2014008.pdf.

Communication Skills

In the context of health literacy, communication skills are those needed to use language (spoken, written, signed, or otherwise communicated) for interaction with others, including basic reading, writing, listening, speaking, and comprehension skills. With the proliferation of online health information, the ability to navigate search engines and websites has become an increasingly important communication skill. Persons with limited reading ability will be less able to use written information on websites or printed health materials or to navigate a typical healthcare setting with its numerous signs. If they have trouble writing, they will be less able to fill in forms in medical settings. Reduced verbal ability will make it difficult for them to explain a health concern or raise questions

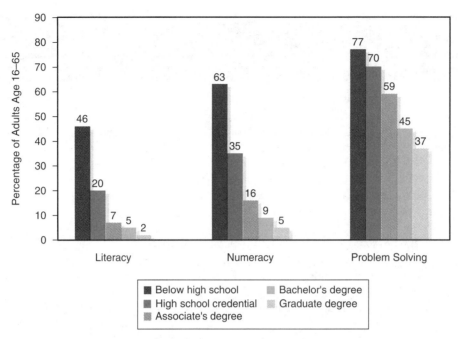

FIGURE 7-2C U.S. PIAAC: Percentage at Level 1 or Below by Education Level

Data from Goodman, M., Finnegan, R., Mohadjer, L., Krenzke, T., and Hogan, J. (2013). Literacy, Numeracy, and Problem Solving in Technology-Rich Environments Among U.S. Adults: Results from the Program for the International Assessment of Adult Competencies 2012: First Look (NCES 2014-008). U.S. Department of Education. Washington, DC: National Center for Education Statistics. Retrieved December 21, 2014. Available from: http://nces.ed.gov/pubs2014/2014008.pdf.

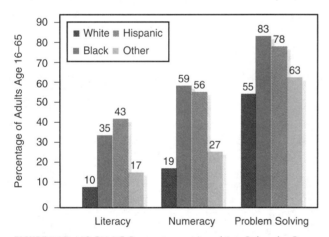

FIGURE 7-2D U.S. PIAAC: Percentage at Level 1 or Below by Race

Data from Goodman, M., Finnegan, R., Mohadjer, L., Krenzke, T., and Hogan, J. (2013). Literacy, Numeracy, and Problem Solving in Technology-Rich Environments Among U.S. Adults: Results from the Program for the International Assessment of Adult Competencies 2012: First Look (NCES 2014-008). U.S. Department of Education. Washington, DC: National Center for Education Statistics. Retrieved December 21, 2014. Available from: http://nces.ed.gov/pubs2014/2014008.pdf.

with healthcare providers. Health information is often conveyed orally, especially at the point of care, and communication skills are needed to speak, listen, and negotiate effectively.[3]

Knowledge

In health literacy, knowledge runs the spectrum from learning about a specific topic (e.g., the warning signs of a heart attack, the sign of the skull and crossbones on a bottle meaning "poison") to a general

understanding of cause-and-effect or the scientific method. The greater challenge in working with persons with low health literacy is not their inability to read, but rather their lack of an explanatory framework, or schema, to use as a starting place for explanation of a complex health topic. Health literacy experts suggest the use of "living room language," referring to language that uses commonplace words and analogies to explain phenomena that are outside common personal experience. Use of ordinary language is closely related to, but does not completely overlap with, the use of cultural explanations and experience.

Culture

Health is a culturally constructed phenomenon. Language and culture, in turn, provide a context for understanding health information. People learn how to define health and illness, who to seek out for care, what constitutes a symptom, what causes illness and what supposedly cures it, and how to describe physical symptoms from their families and larger social groups. Furthermore, willingness to use health technology, medicines, or therapies may be determined by religious or cultural rules, just as the practice of certain risk behaviors or adherence to medical advice will have cultural dimensions.[16] Contrast the health-protecting behaviors of Seventh Day Adventists, who are asked not to smoke, drink, or engage in extramarital sex, with the high-risk behaviors of certain street gangs, which require use of hard drugs, unprotected sex, or other tests of belonging. In terms of health literacy, knowledge describes what a person knows, while culture reveals what a person believes or values. Someone might have learned in school about genetics and the value of screening for birth defects (knowledge), yet absolutely oppose screening if it would mean terminating a pregnancy (culture). How people evaluate health information for themselves or their family, which forms of health information they prefer, and who they trust to convey health information are all filtered through the lens of culture.

Local Language Proficiency

The 2010 census of the U.S. population revealed that 60.6 million people, or 21% of the U.S. population 5 years or older, spoke a language other than English at home. This rate represents a 3% increase from the rate found in the 2000 census. Overall, 58% of those respondents said they also spoke English "very well," though this rate varied by language spoken at home. Spanish (including Spanish Creole) is by far the foreign language most frequently spoken in the United States, with 37.6 million speakers in 2010. Of these Spanish speakers, 56.3% also said they spoke English "very well."[17]

Some patients might be perfectly literate in their native language, and even have a high degree of health literacy, but have limited ability to communicate in English. To respond to the needs of those persons with **limited English proficiency (LEP)**, the U.S. Office of Minority Health developed a standard set of language access services that all healthcare providers are encouraged to employ, and that medical facilities receiving federal funding must provide per Title VI of the Civil Rights Act of 1964.[18]

Numerous resources serve as guides for public health facilities and personnel regarding how to implement **culturally and linguistically appropriate services (CLAS)**. **BOX 7-1** describes the recommended standards for CLAS in health care in the United States.

Providing CLAS is important for routine health communication, but particularly important in the case of emergencies. **BOX 7-2** presents an example in which the Massachusetts Department of Public Health incorporated a CLAS approach for people with LEP as part of its "Show Me: A Communication Tool for Emergency Shelters" initiative.

Context

A specific setting or situation can make someone feel fearful or stressed. Perhaps the person is in an unfamiliar or intimidating environment, or perhaps the individual possesses a mental or physical impairment. These factors are especially critical when people find themselves unexpectedly facing a serious illness or injury and have to interact with people and systems that can be difficult and often impersonal. Even persons with a high degree of literacy and education may become less able to process health information when given bad medical news or when in a stressful setting, such as placing a loved one in a skilled nursing facility.

Most elderly patients must contend with multiple comorbidities, chronic conditions, and normal changes in cognition that accompany aging. Normal changes in cognition include reduced information processing speed, a greater tendency to be distracted, and a reduced capacity to process and remember new information at the same time (i.e., working memory). Cognitive abilities include fluid (processing speed, working memory, inductive reasoning, long-term

---

BOX 7-1 Recommended National Standards for Culturally and Linguistically Appropriate Services in Health Care

Competent Care

1. Healthcare organizations should ensure that patients/consumers receive from all staff members effective, understandable, and respectful care that is provided in a manner compatible with their cultural health beliefs and practices and preferred language.
2. Healthcare organizations should implement strategies to recruit, retain, and promote at all levels of the organization a diverse staff and leadership that are representative of the demographic characteristics of the service area.
3. Healthcare organizations should ensure that staff at all levels and across all disciplines receive ongoing education and training in CLAS delivery.

Language-Access Services

4. Healthcare organizations must offer and provide language-assistance services, including bilingual staff and interpreter services, at no cost to each patient/consumer with LEP at all points of contact and in a timely manner during all hours of operation.

(continues)

BOX 7-1 Recommended National Standards for Culturally and Linguistically Appropriate Services in   *(continued)*
Health Care

5. Healthcare organizations must provide to patients/consumers in their preferred language both verbal offers and written notices informing them of their right to receive language-assistance services.

6. Healthcare organizations must ensure the competence of language assistance provided to limited-English-proficient patients/consumers by interpreters and bilingual staff. Family and friends should not be used to provide interpretation services (except on request by the patient/consumer).

7. Healthcare organizations must make available easily understood patient-related materials and post signage in the languages of the commonly encountered groups and/or groups represented in the service area.

Organizational Supports

8. Healthcare organizations should develop, implement, and promote a written strategic plan that outlines clear goals, policies, operational plans, and management accountability/oversight mechanisms to provide CLAS.

9. Healthcare organizations should conduct initial and ongoing organizational self-assessments of CLAS-related activities and are encouraged to integrate cultural and linguistic competence-related measures into their internal audits, performance improvement programs, patient satisfaction assessments, and outcomes-based evaluations.

10. Healthcare organizations should ensure that data on the individual patient's/consumer's race, ethnicity, and spoken and written language are collected in health records, integrated into the organization's management information systems, and periodically updated.

11. Healthcare organizations should maintain a current demographic, cultural, and epidemiological profile of the community as well as a needs assessment to accurately plan for and implement services that respond to the cultural and linguistic characteristics of the service area.

12. Healthcare organizations should develop participatory, collaborative partnerships with communities and utilize a variety of formal and informal mechanisms to facilitate community and patient/consumer involvement in designing and implementing CLAS-related activities.

13. Healthcare organizations should ensure that conflict and grievance resolution processes are culturally and linguistically sensitive and capable of identifying, preventing, and resolving cross-cultural conflicts or complaints by patients/consumers.

14. Healthcare organizations are encouraged to make available regularly to the public information about their progress and successful innovations in implementing the CLAS standards and to provide public notice in their communities about the availability of this information.

Reproduced from U.S. Department of Health and Human Services. Office of Minority Health. Healthcare Language Services Implementation Guide. Available from: https://hclsig.thinkculturalhealth.org/page/view.rails?name=Section+2:+Page+2,3.

memory, prospective memory) and crystallized (verbal) ability. Fluid abilities comprise cognitive traits that facilitate information processing where prior general knowledge is not useful. Crystallized abilities reflect general background knowledge stored in long-term memory. Diminished levels of both forms of cognition have been associated with low health literacy.[19,20]

Evidence also suggests that a 1-standard-deviation decrease in episodic memory results in an education-level decrease of nearly 4 years. An executive function decline of 1 standard deviation reduces the total literacy score by nearly 2 years of education.[21] Declining executive function makes it more difficult to develop, carry out, and make necessary changes to goal-related plans.

As elderly patients attempt to navigate the complex Medicare system, they must understand differences among coverage options; decide whether to buy prescription coverage; identify doctors and hospitals that can provide services for their specific needs; navigate within a plan; choose the most appropriate treatment options; and understand their rights and responsibilities. Low health literacy is a major complicating factor when addressing these tasks. Recognizing the challenges faced by older adults in trying to navigate the healthcare system, the U.S. Department of Health and Human Services (DHHS) has made several recommendations to improve health literacy communication specific to the elderly population (**BOX 7-3**).

Complexity of Health Care

The challenges inherent in accessing healthcare services and benefits and navigating healthcare settings are demanding at multiple levels. The U.S. healthcare system is highly fragmented, with intrinsically complex relationships existing between organizations and individuals.

BOX 7-2 Creating Picture-Based Communications

Clear communication is the lifeline of emergency response. In Massachusetts, state public health officials needed a tool to facilitate communication between first responders and people who have hearing impairments, limited English proficiency, or cognitive delays during an emergency. In these circumstances, using plain language does not go far enough.

The Massachusetts team took a **user-centered design** approach to develop the tool. In other words, they involved users as co-creators. The team began the design process by conducting in-depth interviews and focus groups to determine what needed to be communicated in an emergency situation. Then they worked through multiple iterations of icons to find those that would be most widely understood. Next the team designed and tested several prototypes (drafts), observing first responders and individuals with communication challenges using the tool to complete tasks. Finally, they created a mobile app version of the tool that could be used in multiple emergency settings, including evacuations and emergency shelters.

Involving end users in the design process ensures the communication will be understood—and can facilitate health literacy among vulnerable populations.

Watch this demo to see how the app works: https://www.youtube.com/watch?v=gS5vMJjvvI4&feature=youtu.be.

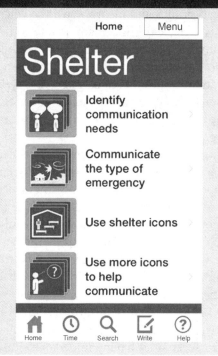

Individuals may not know all of the services available to them or recognize whether they are eligible for different forms of care or insurance. For example, a low-income woman who is pregnant may not understand her eligibility for benefits under the Women, Infants, and Children (WIC) program, a federal supplementary food program. To take advantage of those benefits, first she must be aware of the service and who provides it, and then she must have the self-efficacy to contact the provider. One strategy to encourage self-efficacy and uptake of a health behavior is to use a conversational tone, incorporating real members of the audience into the health communication message. An example of how this strategy can be implemented is demonstrated by the Growing Healthy Website that the American Academy of Pediatrics (AAP) developed for parents.

The American Academy of Pediatrics Institute for Healthy Childhood Weight (Institute) developed key messages for parents related to obesity prevention for children ages 0 to 5 years. The Institute wanted to make sure their messages were accepted and

BOX 7-3 Quick Guide to Health Literacy and Older Adults: Cognitive Challenges

- *Repeat essential "true" information.* Repetition and subsequent familiarity with false information can create the sense of it being true, so concentrate on what is true and what should be done.
- *Focus on important details*, such as timing and order and making sure they are understood.
- *Emphasize desired actions* to be taken rather than things to avoid.
- *Use plain language.* Consider the effects of stress and fatigue. For instance, stress comes with illness, and self-care can make anyone tired. Understand that mistakes in judgment, errors, and depressed mood may result more from sickness than cognitive changes.
- *Be aware of the effects of illness and recovery.* For example, cancer chemotherapy can temporarily reduce cognitive function, reducing the ability to self-manage treatment. Other conditions can permanently affect executive function. Be sensitive to individual needs. Not every older adult is the same, so it is important to individualize your communication, just as you would your care plan.
- *Be sensitive to individual needs.* All older patients are not the same. Clarify the areas in which they need.
- *Provide adequate time for instruction.* You may need more time to explain instructions—for example, at a slower pace and with reinforcement.

Quick Guide to Health Literacy and Older Adults. US Department of Health and Human Services Website. http://health.gov/communication/literacy/olderadults/cognitive.htm Accessed Dec 28, 2015.

understood by all parents, including those with limited health literacy skills. To do this, the team conducted focus groups and incorporated the voices of real parents to make the information more authentic. To communicate messages clearly, increase understanding of specific concepts and to provide personalized information the team created interactive web content and a myth-busting quiz for parents. To learn more, visit the Growing Healthy Website at www.healthychildren.org/growinghealthy.

Sometimes patients are overwhelmed by the complexity of negotiating what might seem like simple appointments. If they are seeking a new provider, a specialist, or some type of diagnostic test, they may not know where to start. Patients frequently find it difficult to understand and complete written health forms. In fact, rates of comprehension of written or verbal information at "first pass" in low-health-literacy populations are low, ranging from 17% to 45%.[22]

Informed consent forms are notoriously difficult to understand, even by college graduates. To illustrate, even after having undergone simplification, the National Cancer Institute's informed consent template is 29 pages long![23] The mean grade level of informed consent materials is estimated to be 10.6. While many institutions have grade-level standards for consent form development, one study found that only 8% used the standard to develop their informed consent materials. Some exceeded their own standard by 2.8 grade levels.[24]

This problem is so well known that informed consent was the subject of a 2014 Institute of Medicine (IOM) Consent Workshop. During this workshop, stakeholders discussed the latest best practices and processes for research and treatment, as well as the disproportionate impact on already disenfranchised populations.[25] Technology may allow for improved understanding, with multimedia programs now becoming available for smaller computer devices (e.g., *Enroll* by Mytrus) that take a patient through the informed consent process using pictures, words, and frequent assessment of understanding. Nevertheless, a meta-analysis using random effects modeling of 22 studies found mixed results depending on the approach used. Multimedia approaches increased understanding scores, but not significantly (standardized mean difference [SMD] = 0.30). Use of an enhanced consent form did significantly improve understanding, as did use of extended discussion (SMD = 0.53).[26]

After giving consent, being admitted to the hospital, and undergoing a medical procedure, patients are discharged with a set of instructions that they may or may not understand. Not being able to follow the instructions can lead to readmissions or worse. At a 2014 IOM After Visit Summary and Discharge Instructions Workshop, experts discussed the challenges of low patient self-efficacy (whether procedure-related, age-related, or due to the overwhelming amount of documentation); lack of physician understanding of patient limitations; mechanistic pathways; lack of access to patient portals; lack of centralized records maintained by a primary care provider (especially for vulnerable populations in a clinic setting); LEP and cultural differences; the fluid nature of post-discharge changes; and lack of health literacy as a priority in development of electronic health record (EHR) programs.[27] Recommendations for improved communications include physician involvement in patient discharge; structured content, presented verbally, with written and visual cues to enhance recall; customization of approaches based on patient need (including language and reading level); and confirmation of understanding before the patient leaves.[28-31]

Researchers at Boston University and the Agency for Healthcare Research and Quality (AHRQ) have developed a toolkit for hospitals to enable them to replicate their re-engineered discharge (RED) process, which has been proven to reduce readmissions and emergency department visits. This toolkit includes process planning, implementations and simplified templates for patient discharge materials.[32]

▶ Improving Health Literacy Through National Policy

Healthcare and public health professionals have an ethical responsibility toward the patients whom they serve, including vulnerable populations affected by low health literacy. This responsibility as related to health communication has been succinctly summarized by the American Medical Association (**BOX 7-4**).

As access to healthcare services expands and the environment changes, more responsibility is being transferred to individual patients for their own well-being. Managing this responsibility successfully requires not only that the individual be able to find relevant and trustworthy information, but also that the information presented be "written in a clear, concise, well-organized manner" to aid in decision making.[33] A substantial disparity between the readability level of health information materials and the health literacy level of individuals persists, however.[33] Recent policy initiatives reflect the need to address

"Patients have the right to understand healthcare information that is necessary for them to safely care for themselves, and to choose among available alternatives. Healthcare providers have a duty to provide information in simple, clear, and plain language and to check that patients have understood the information before ending the conversation."

American Medical Association. 2005 White House Conference on Aging: Part 2, Pre-conference Events, Executive Summary. Washington, DC: Mini-Conference on Long-Term Care. April 2005:73. Available from: http://permanent.access.gpo.gov/lps74930/05_Report_3.pdf.

health literacy as a systems issue, rather than see it as an "individual patient deficit"—that is, to view health literacy as a complex interaction that involves navigating a fractured healthcare system and understanding complicated health information.[33]

Plain Writing Act of 2010

This law requires all U.S. government agencies to write and present information using clear communication that the public can understand and use. It applies to all federal agencies including the Department of Health and Human Services, which encompasses the CDC, Administration for Children and Families (ACF), and Centers for Medicare and Medicaid (CMS), to name a few subsidiaries.

The CDC developed the **Clear Communication Index (CCI)** to comply with the Plain Writing Act of 2010 and achieve the goals set forth in its own Action Plan to Improve Health Literacy. CCI provides a set of research-based criteria to develop and assess public communication products.[34] The CCI is discussed in more detail, in the section on developing materials to enhance health literacy.

Patient Protection and Affordable Care Act

The Patient Protection and Affordable Care Act (ACA) contains both direct and indirect references to health literacy. The direct references can be found in four sections:

- Section 3501 requires AHRQ research to be made "available to the public… [and] to reflect varying needs of… providers and consumers and diverse levels of health literacy."
- Section 3506 amends the Public Health Services Act and authorizes a program, administered by

the CDC and National Institutes of Health (NIH), to update patient decision aids to "reflect varying needs of consumers and diverse levels of health literacy."

- Section 3507 directs the Secretary of Health and Human Services to examine prescription drug labeling and print advertising and consult with various stakeholders and "experts in health literacy" to improve the presentation of benefit and risk information.
- Section 5301 permits the Secretary of Health and Human Services to make training grants to qualified medical applications, with preference being given to those related to improving cultural competence and health literacy.[35,36]

Additional indirect references to concepts involving health literacy were found and organized into six domains within the ACA: (1) Insurance Reform, Outreach, and Enrollment; (2) Individual Protections, Equity in Special Populations; (3) Workforce Development; (4) Health Information; (5) Public Health, Health Promotion, and Prevention and Wellness; and (6) Innovations in Quality and Delivery and Costs of Care. For example, one ACA Insurance Reform provision requires the development of consistent coverage descriptions and definitions. This type of materials development benefits greatly from incorporating health literacy concepts to improve access, understanding, and, ultimately, decision making for the consumer or patient.[35]

Healthy People 2020

Healthy People is the culmination of a multiyear process that incorporates stakeholder feedback from public health and prevention experts; federal, state, and local government officials; a consortium of more than 2000 organizations; and members of the public. Most of the Health Communication and Health Information Technology (HC/HIT) objectives in *Healthy People 2020* include aspects of health literacy, with the overarching goals to improve health outcomes and quality and to attain health equity.[37] Details of the health literacy-specific objectives can be seen in **BOX 7-5**.

National Action Plan to Improve Health Literacy

In 2010, the U.S. Department of Health and Human Services' Office of Disease Prevention and Health Promotion proposed a National Action Plan to

BOX 7-5 *Healthy People 2020*: First Health Communication and Health Information Technology Objective

HC/HIT-1 (Developmental) Improve the health literacy of the population.

- HC/HIT-1.1 (Developmental) Increase the proportion of persons who report their healthcare provider always gave them easy-to-understand instructions about what to do to take care of their illness or health condition.
- HC/HIT-1.2 (Developmental) Increase the proportion of persons who report their healthcare provider always asked them to describe how they will follow the instructions.
- HC/HIT-1.3 (Developmental) Increase the proportion of persons who report their healthcare providers' office always offered help in filling out a form.

Healthy People 2020 [Internet]. Washington, DC: U.S. Department of Health and Human Services, Office of Disease Prevention and Health Promotion [cited March 15, 2015]. Available from: https://www.healthypeople.gov/2020/topics-objectives/topic/health-communication-and-health-information-technology/objectives.

BOX 7-6 Goals of the National Action Plan to Improve Health Literacy

1. Develop and disseminate health and safety information that is accurate, accessible, and actionable
2. Promote changes in the healthcare system that improve health information, communication, informed decision making, and access to health services
3. Incorporate accurate, standards-based, and developmentally appropriate health and science information and curricula in child care and education through the university level
4. Support and expand local efforts to provide adult education, English language instruction, and culturally and linguistically appropriate health information services in the community
5. Build partnerships, develop guidance, and change policies
6. Increase basic research and the development, implementation, and evaluation of practices and interventions to improve health literacy
7. Increase the dissemination and use of evidence-based health literacy practices and interventions

U.S. Department of Health and Human Services, Office of Disease Prevention and Health Promotion. (2010). National Action Plan to Improve Health Literacy. Washington, DC. Available from http://www.health.gov/communication/hlactionplan/. Accessed March 15, 2015.

Improve Health Literacy (NAP). NAP provides goals and strategies that organizations and healthcare professions can use to transform jargon-filled, dense, and complex health information into clearer, more easily understood messages. The two key principles underpinning the plan are (1) everyone has the basic right to health information to help them make informed decisions and (2) understandable health services delivery is beneficial to health, longevity, and quality of life. NAP includes seven goals, which are summarized in **BOX 7-6**.

The strategies included in NAP are extensive and detailed for each profession, including, but not limited to, health professionals, payers, pharmacies, as well as agencies that prepare their materials, educators, and librarians. NAP recommends adopting user-centered design, involving members of the target audience in development, using a universal precautions approach (i.e., assuming most patients have low health literacy), targeting and tailoring information, and making changes at the organizational level.[38,39] The CDC has proposed several steps that can move organizations toward making those changes, including identification of the goals and strategies that are most relevant for the organization, briefing colleagues, drafting and proposing action steps, planning and implementing the approved actions, evaluating their effectiveness, and sharing any findings widely.[40]

Assessing Health Literacy

There are practical limits to assessment of health literacy in a healthcare context compared to a research setting. Participants in research or surveys have consented to complete these tests, which might take a considerable amount of time, and they have been assured of anonymity. In contrast, in a clinical practice setting, such assessments may be more difficult to perform. The Weiss health literacy toolkit created for the American Medical Association Foundation includes several videos in which patients describe their discomfort or shame at not being able to read well or write[41]—a factor that may make them reluctant to submit to such assessments in a healthcare setting. Nevertheless, there are non-shaming ways to incorporate health literacy screening into clinical assessment and patient records,[42] and several tools for doing so are discussed after we profile those instruments used more commonly in research.

Instruments to Measure Health Literacy

Three "standard" instruments are used to measure health literacy across a range of research contexts:

the Rapid Estimate of Adult Literacy in Medicine (REALM), the Test of Functional Health Literacy in Adults (TOFHLA), and the Newest Vital Sign (NVS). Newer instruments used for this purpose include the eHealth Literacy Scale (eHEALS), the Numeracy Understanding in Medicine Instrument (NUMi), and the Health Literacy Skills Instrument (HLSI).

REALM

The Rapid Estimate of Adult Literacy in Medicine is a word-recognition test of 66 medical words and is one of the oldest and most widely used health literacy assessment tools.[43] It starts with easy words (e.g., fat, flu, pill) and then moves on to difficult words (e.g., osteoporosis, impetigo, potassium). Patients are asked to pronounce each word out loud. The test makes no attempt to determine if patients actually *understand* the meaning of the word. REALM can be administered in approximately 3 minutes, and it is available only in English. The number of correctly pronounced words is used to assign a grade-equivalent reading level.

REALM-R[44] is a shorter version of the REALM consisting of these words:

Fat	Osteoporosis	Anemia	Colitis
Flu	Allergic	Fatigue	Constipation
Pill	Jaundice	Directed	

Fat, flu, and *pill* are not scored and are positioned at the beginning of the REALM-R to decrease test anxiety and enhance confidence. Unlike the REALM instrument, which must be purchased, all materials related to the REALM-R may be downloaded for free from the American Society on Aging and American Society of Consultant Pharmacists Foundation website.

TOFHLA

The Test of Functional Health Literacy in Adults has traditionally been the instrument of choice when a detailed evaluation of health literacy is needed for research purposes.[45] It is available in both English and Spanish. The full-length form requires 20 minutes to complete; the short version takes approximately 12 minutes. The full-length TOFHLA includes two parts: multiple-choice questions to test document and numeracy and fill-in-the-blank questions (the "Cloze" procedure) to test reading closure. A testing kit may be ordered from the distributor, Peppercorn Books.

NVS

The Newest Vital Sign instrument is available in English and Spanish, and can typically be completed by patients in approximately 3 minutes.[46] Many patients find the "ice cream label challenge" acceptable as part of standard medical care, with more than 98% of patients agreeing to undergo the assessment during a routine office visit. The NVS can be obtained online at no cost from the Partnership for Clear Health Communication.

eHEALS

The eHealth Literacy Scale (eHEALS) is an 8-item measure of e-health literacy that assesses combined knowledge, comfort, and perceived skills at finding, evaluating, and applying electronic health information to health problems.[47] It has been used in several studies to evaluate e-health literacy and communications programs, and has been adapted to the Japanese and Dutch languages.[48-52]

NUMi

The Numeracy Understanding in Medicine Instrument was developed by Shapira and colleagues at the University of Pennsylvania. This 20-item pencil-and-paper test measures most of the quantitative challenges a patient may face in health care. Items include reading the numbers on a digital thermometer, interpreting an icon array and a simple bar chart and line graph, and answering multiple-choice questions pertaining to reading labels and estimating probability. The NUMi has been validated with 1000 patients. An 8-item version is available at no charge with access through the validation publication.

HLSI

The Health Literacy Skills Instrument was developed by McCormack and a team of other national health literacy experts. The HLSI measures print literacy as well as oral and Internet-based information seeking skills that U.S.-based adults are likely to face routinely in the context of health care. The 25-item HLSI can be self-administered via a computer in approximately 12 minutes. A 10-item version is also available.

Health Literacy Tool Shed

The Health Literacy Tool Shed was constructed by Boston University with funding from the National Library of Medicine.[53] It contains more than 100 tools for specific applications and allows users to access specific instruments by health literacy domain, health context, administration time, modality of administration, language (many are available), and more. Users are invited to submit validated tools to the site for use by fellow researchers and practitioners.

Health Literacy in Clinical Practice

It is important to assess a patient's health literacy so as to comply with quality of care standards within a profession or facility, select appropriate educational materials (e.g., video, foreign language), and rule out other complications, such as cognitive impairment or hearing or visual loss. The assessment instruments just described were developed for research but some may be used cautiously in practice. One- or two-question tests may have good predictability in the healthcare setting,[54] although studies have found that multiple-question tests are more effective than those consisting of a single question. Here are three questions that have performed well together:

1. How often do you have problems learning about your medical condition because of difficulty understanding written information? (always, often, sometimes, occasionally, or never)
2. How often do you have someone help you read hospital materials? (always, often, sometimes, occasionally, or never)
3. How confident are you filling out medical forms by yourself? (extremely, quite a bit, somewhat, a little bit, or not at all)

Health Literacy Universal Precautions Toolkit[55]

Experts agree that demonstrating sensitivity to patients' feelings about being judged as "uneducated" is more important than obtaining results from a finely tuned measure of health literacy. Several factors were determined to be critical for successful implementation of a prototype toolkit in clinical practice, including forming a team and generating awareness of the toolkit, practice assessment and strengthening areas of weakness, and prior knowledge of the implementation model.[56] The consensus is that three "universal precautions" for health literacy should be applied in healthcare settings:

- Strive to communicate clearly with everyone.
- Avoid reliance on visual estimates of a person's ability to understand health information in the practice setting.
- Confirm understanding with everyone.

It is recommended that all healthcare providers use plain language (e.g., "high blood pressure" instead

of "hypertension") and focus on the two or three most important concepts during an interaction. Afterward, the provider should confirm patient understanding using a "teach-back" or "ask–educate–ask" method. The teach-back step seeks to verify that the provider has been clear without seeming to be "testing" the patient.[57-60]

▶ Developing and Assessing Materials

As in all health communication, understanding the intended audience is essential when creating materials that are easier to understand. End-user inputs will determine how you create your materials and which channels you choose for dissemination of information. It will also be important to test your materials with the intended users and revise them as needed based on this feedback.

Key Principles

- Limit the number of objectives, which will help you to keep the message simple.
- Make sure the document is not text dense, by using lots of white space.
- Choose fonts that are easier to read, such as serif fonts (e.g., Times New Roman) that are 12 points or larger in size.
- Use bold and underline to highlight important text, but remember that text written in all capital letters, script fonts, and italics is more difficult to read.
- Use present-tense and active verbs, cutting unnecessary words where ever you can.
- Write the way you speak; do not worry about grammatical perfection.
- Use examples, pictures, or stories that are appropriate to the audience instead of difficult words.

Most of these elements will carry over into any social media communications that you plan. Selection of social media communication channels depends on the overall communications strategy, your audience, and available resources. For example, the National Cancer Institute developed a smoking cessation program (https://smokefree.gov) that spans many digital communication channels and targets specific hard-to-reach audiences (see **APPENDIX 7C**).

At this point, you should understand the literacy level of your audience or have taken the universal precautions approach (i.e., assume everyone has a low health literacy level). You have developed the materials to be used for communicating, whether in print, electronic, or verbal form. The next step is to assess those materials or interactions. The following subsections briefly describes the most commonly used measures for evaluating communication materials.

Clear Communication Index

The CDC's Clear Communication Index is a key tool for evaluating a draft material and determining whether it is working on several levels. **BOX 7-7** describes the origins and development of the CCI, and **APPENDIX 7A** and **APPENDIX 7B** provide before and after examples of how to use the CCI.

The **Flesch-Kincaid Grade Level Readability Test** was originally formulated for the U.S. Navy.[61,62] It uses words per sentence and syllables per word as part of a formula to determine the reading grade level of the text. The formula is calculated as (0.39 × Average sentence length) + (11.8 × Average number of syllables per word) − 15.59, where a score of 8.3 would indicate an eighth-grade reading level. Electronic calculators for this test are available through the Internet. The formula is also built into the Microsoft Word software, although the Word version is not able to determine any grade above 12.

The **Suitability Assessment of Materials** is an instrument that has been validated across several cultures and is used to measure the suitability of a set of healthcare instructions for a particular population.[63] Completing the SAM instrument takes an estimated 30 to 45 minutes. There are several steps, the first of which is to review the SAM factors and criteria. Next, examining the material to identify its purpose and key

---

BOX 7-7 CDC Clear Communication Index

The CDC Clear Communication Index is a research-based tool to help people develop and assess public communication materials. It was originally designed for CDC staff who write, edit, design, and review communication products, but anyone can use it to assess and revise materials or to help guide the development of new materials. The CCI can be used for materials that are intended for use by consumers, patients, or professional audiences such as clinicians, health department staff, or policy makers.

An extensive process was used to develop the CCI that included the following steps:

- Reviewing health literacy guidelines
- Obtaining input from experts in the field
- Searching and reviewing research findings about items
- Cognitive testing
- Review by the CDC's Associate Directors of Communication
- User testing including inter-rater reliability
- Consumer testing of materials developed with and without the index

The end result of this process is a 20-item index. All items are supported by research, expert review, and testing. In addition, they represent the most important characteristics that can enhance and aid people's understanding of information. The index assesses materials in six areas:

1. MBK Main message and call to action language (7 items)
2. Information design (3 items)
3. State of the science (1 item)
4. Behavioral recommendations (3 items)
5. Numbers (3 items)
6. Risk (3 items)

A unique component of the CCI is the initial cover sheet, which contains four open-ended questions to be answered before you begin scoring. These questions help identify your **primary audience** and their health literacy skills, motivation, beliefs, and current behaviors. Knowing your audience and the challenges they face in accessing health information is critical to developing materials they can understand and use in health decision making. Formative research can provide insights into the knowledge, attitudes, beliefs, and behaviors of the audience. If you are unable to conduct formative research, proceed as if your audience has limited skills.

The CCI worksheet also asks you to write out your **primary communication objective**. A communication objective is what you want the audience members to think, feel, or do after they receive the message or material. The primary communication objective will guide development of the material's **main message**. The main message is the one thing you would like audience members to remember after reading, viewing, or using the material.

(continues)

BOX 7-7 CDC Clear Communication Index   *(continued)*

Using the CCI to Guide Materials Development

The CCI can also be used to guide the development of a communication product from its inception. The CDC has provided an online user guide that defines the 20 items making up the CCI and explains how to score them: http://www.cdc.gov/ccindex/pdf/clear-communication-user-guide.pdf.

Modified Version of the CCI

A shorter version of the CCI is available that has only 13 items. It was created for use with shorter materials, such as social media messages, podcast and call center scripts, and infographics. It can be obtained at the following website: http://www.cdc.gov/ccindex/pdf/modified-index-scoresheet.pdf.

Data from the CDC.

---

points allows the evaluator to decide if the material is short enough to review the entire piece, or if samples from the material should be used in the evaluation. The SAM evaluation scores 22 factors in 6 areas (content, literacy demand, graphics, layout and type, learning stimulation and motivation, and cultural appropriateness), with the scores in the 6 areas being tallied to create the final score. The final step is to determine the effect of the deficiencies and any changes to be made to improve the communication.

The **SMOG** (Simple Measure of Gobbledygook) instrument provides an estimate of the number of years of education needed to understand a prose text, including website copy.[64,65] This rigorous assessment focuses on word length and sentences. If analyzing 30 sentences or more, the following formula is used: Grade = 1.043 $\sqrt{30 \times (\text{Number of polysyllables} / \text{Number of sentences})}$ + 3.1291. The formula may be modified for fewer than 30 sentences as well. The SMOG tool is available at http://prevention.sph.sc.edu/tools/smog.pdf.

As discussed earlier, the **healthcare environment** itself can present overwhelming barriers for those consumers with low health literacy.[66,67] Several tools are available to assist in assessing hospitals, healthcare centers, and pharmacies for challenges to these consumers. Assessment categories include navigation, such as the telephone system and directional signage; print communication, including writing style, font size, and use of graphics; oral exchange, or how the staff interacts with the patient, so that the patient can understand; and technology, such as different uses of videos or computers to help orient or educate patients.

Conclusion

An understanding of health literacy and numeracy is a component of audience analysis and is essential for planning effective communication interventions. This chapter presented a framework of guiding concepts and practical tools to assist you in communicating more clearly with everyone.

Wrap-Up

Chapter Questions

1. Define literacy, health literacy, and numeracy.
2. Why is low health literacy a critical communication consideration?
3. With which adverse health outcomes has low health literacy been associated?

4. What are the implications of low numeracy levels for communication?
5. What are the best available ways to assess health literacy in a healthcare setting?
6. How are verbal and written communications measured to determine their health literacy level?

References

1. Berkman ND, Davis TC, McCormack L. Health literacy: what is it? *J Health Comm*. 2010;15(suppl2): 9-19.

2. Berkman ND, Sheridan SL, Donahue KE, et al. Health literacy interventions and outcomes: an updated systematic review. *Evid Rep Technol Assess*. 2011;199:1-941.

3. National Library of Medicine. Economic impact of low health literacy. 2014. http://nnlm.gov/outreach/consumer /hlthlit.html#A5. Accessed December 14, 2014.

4. Sørensen K, Van den Broucke S, Fullam J, Doyle G, Pelikan J, Slonska Z, Brand H. Health literacy and public health: a systematic review and integration of definitions and models. *BMC Public Health*. 2012;12:80.

5. Squiers L, Peinado S, Berkman N, Boudewyns V, McCormack L. The health literacy skills framework. *J Health Comm*. 2012;17(suppl 3):30-54.

6. Borzekowski DL. Considering children and health literacy: a theoretical approach. *Pediatrics*. 2009;124 (suppl 3):S282-S288.

7. Kahneman D, Slovick P, Tversky A. *Judgment Under Uncertainty: Heuristics and Biases*. Cambridge, UK: Cambridge University Press; 1982.

8. Petty RE, Brinol P. The elaboration likelihood model. In: Van Lange PAM, Kruglanski AW, Higgins ET, eds. *Handbook of Theories of Social Psychology: Collection*. Thousand Oaks, CA: Sage; 2011:224-245.

9. Wolf MS, Curtis LM, Wilson EA, et al. Literacy, cognitive function, and health: results of the LitCog study. *J Gen Intern Med*. 2012;27(10):1300-1307.

10. Educational Testing Service. Types of literacy. 2015. https://www.ets.org/literacy/research/literacy_types/. Accessed March 14, 2015.

11. Institute of Medicine. *Health Literacy and Numeracy: Workshop Summary*. Washington, DC: National Academies Press; 2014.

12. Kirsch IS, Jungeblut A, Jenkins L, Kolstad A. *Adult Literacy in America: A First Look at the Findings of the National Adult Literacy Survey*. Washington, DC: U.S.Department of Education, Office of Educational Research and Improvement; April 2002.

13. Kutner M, Greenberg E, Baer J. *A First Look at the Literacy of America's Adults in the 21st Century*. Washington, DC: National Center for Education Statistics, Institute of Education Sciences, U.S. Department of Education; 2006.

14. U.S. Department of Education, Institute of Education Sciences, National Center for Education Statistics. National Assessment of Adult Literacy: demographics, overall, average scores. 2007. http://nces.ed.gov/naal/kf _demographics.asp. Accessed May 10, 2015.

15. National Center for Education Statistics, U.S. Department of Education. *Literacy, Numeracy, and Problem Solving in Technology-Rich Environments Among U.S. Adults: Results from the Program for the International Assessment of Adult Competencies*. Washington, DC: NCES 2014-008. 2012.

16. Singleton K, Krause E. Understanding cultural and linguistic barriers to health literacy. *Online J Issues Nurs*. 2009;14(3):11.

17. U.S. Census Bureau. 2010 census data. 2013. http:// www.census.gov/2010census/data/. Accessed March 15, 2015.

18. U.S. Department of Health and Human Services, Office of Minority Health. Healthcare language services implementation guide. 2013. https://hclsig.thinkcultural health.hhs.gov/. Accessed May 21, 2015.

19. Smith SG, O'Conor R, Curtis LM, et al. Low health literacy predicts decline in physical function among older adults: findings from the LitCog cohort study. *J Epidemiol Community Health*. 2015:jech-2014-204915.

20. Serper M, Patzer RE, Curtis LM, et al. Health literacy, cognitive ability, and functional health status among older adults. *Health Serv Res*. 2014;49(4):1249-1267.

21. Boyle PA, Yu L, Wilson RS, Segawa E, Buchman AS, Bennett DA. Cognitive decline impairs financial and health literacy among community-based older persons without dementia. *Psychol Aging*. 2013;28(3):614.

22. Tamariz L, Palacio A, Robert M, Marcus EN. Improving the informed consent process for research subjects with low literacy: a systematic review. *J Gen Intern Med*. 2013;28(1):121-126.

23. National Cancer Institute. NCI consent form template for adult cancer trials. 2013. http://cdp.cancer.gov/resources /elsi/docs/NCI_Consent_Form_Adult_Cancer_Trials.pdf. Accessed May 10, 2015.

24. Paasche-Orlow MK, Taylor HA, Brancati FL. Readability standards for informed-consent forms as compared with actual readability. *N Engl J Med*. 2003;348(8):721-726.

25. Institute of Medicine. Informed consent and health literacy: a workshop. 2014. https://www.nap.edu/catalog /19019/informed-consent-and-health-literacy-workshop -summary. Accessed December 14, 2014.

26. Nishimura A, Carey J, Erwin PJ, Tilburt JC, Murad MH, McCormick JB. Improving understanding in the research informed consent process: a systematic review of 54 interventions tested in randomized control trials. *BMC Med Ethics*. 2013;14(1):28.

27. Institute of Medicine. *Facilitating Patient Understanding of Discharge Instructions: Workshop Summary*. Washington, DC: National Academies Press; 2014.

28. Buckley BA, McCarthy DM, Forth VE, et al. Patient input into the development and enhancement of ED discharge instructions: a focus group study. *J Emerg Nurs*. 2013;39(6):553-561.

29. Coleman EA, Chugh A, Williams MV, et al. Understanding and execution of discharge instructions. *Am J Med Quality*. 2013;1062860612472931.

30. Lindquist LA, Yamahiro A, Garrett A, Zei C, Feinglass JM. Primary care physician communication at hospital discharge reduces medication discrepancies. *J Hosp Med*. 2013;8(12):672-677.

31. Samuels-Kalow ME, Stack AM, Porter SC. Effective discharge communication in the emergency department. *Ann Emerg Med*. 2012;60(2):152-159.

32. Re-engineered discharge (RED) Toolkit. 2014. http:// www.ahrq.gov/professionals/systems/hospital/red/toolkit /index.html. Accessed May 27, 2015.

33. Martin LT, Parker RM. Insurance expansion and health literacy. *JAMA*. 2011;306(8):874-875.

34. Centers for Disease Control and Prevention. Clear Communication Index user guide. 2014. http://www.cdc.gov /ccindex/tool/index.html. Accessed December 22, 2014.

35. Somers SA, Mahadevan R. *Health Literacy Implications of the Affordable Care Act*. Hamilton, NJ: Center for Health Care Strategies; 2010.

36. Food and Drug Administration. Office of Prescription Drug Promotion (OPDP) Research. 2014. http://www.fda.gov/AboutFDA/CentersOffices/OfficeofMedicalProductsandTobacco/CDER/ucm090276.htm. Accessed December 13, 2014.

37. U.S. Department of Health and Human Services. About Healthy People. 2014. https://www.healthypeople.gov/2020/About-Healthy-People. Accessed December 13, 2014.

38. U.S. Department of Health and Human Services. HHS releases national plan to improve health literacy. 2010. http://wayback.archive-it.org/3926/20131126162912/http://www.hhs.gov/ash/news/20100527.html. Accessed December 13, 2014.

39. U.S. Department of Health and Human Services, Office of Disease Prevention and Health Promotion. *National Action Plan to Improve Health Literacy*. Washington, DC: U.S. Department of Health and Human Services, Office of Disease Prevention and Health Promotion; May 2010.

40. Baur C. *National Action Plan to Improve Health Literacy*. Washington, DC: U.S. Department of Health and Human Services, Office of Disease Prevention and Health Promotion; 2010.

41. Weiss BD. *Help Patients Understand*. Chicago, IL: American Medical Association; 2007.

42. Cawthon C, Mion LC, Willens DE, Roumie CL, Kripalani S. Implementing routine health literacy assessment in hospital and primary care patients. *Jt Commission J Quality Patient Saf*. 2014;40(2):68-68.

43. Davis TC, Long SW, Jackson RH, et al. Rapid estimate of adult literacy in medicine: a shortened screening instrument. *Fam Med*. 1993;25(6):391-395.

44. Bass PF, Wilson JF, Griffith CH. A shortened instrument for literacy screening. *J Gen Intern Med*. 2003;18(12):1036-1038.

45. Baker D, Williams M, Nurss J. The Test of Functional Health Literacy in Adults: a new instrument for measuring patients' literacy skills. *J Gen Intern Med*. 1995;10:537-541.

46. Weiss BD, Mays MZ, Martz W, et al. Quick assessment of literacy in primary care: the Newest Vital Sign. *Ann Fam Med*. 2005;3(6):514-522.

47. Norman CD, Skinner HA. eHEALS: The eHealth Literacy Scale. *J Med Internet Res*. 2006;8(4):e27.

48. Choi NG, Dinitto DM. The digital divide among low-income homebound older adults: Internet use patterns, eHealth literacy, and attitudes toward computer/Internet use. *J Med Internet Res*. 2013;15(5):e93.

49. Ghaddar SF, Valerio MA, Garcia CM, Hansen L. Adolescent health literacy: the importance of credible sources for online health information. *J School Health*. 2012;82(1):28-36.

50. Mitsutake S, Shibata A, Ishii K, Oka K. Association of eHealth literacy with colorectal cancer knowledge and screening practice among Internet users in Japan. *J Med Internet Res*. 2012;14(6):e153.

51. Noblin AM, Wan TT, Fottler M. The impact of health literacy on a patient's decision to adopt a personal health record. *Persp Health Info Manage*. 2012;9:1-13.

52. van der Vaart R, van Deursen AJ, Drossaert CH, Taal E, van Dijk JA, van de Laar MA. Does the eHealth Literacy Scale (eHEALS) measure what it intends to measure? Validation of a Dutch version of the eHEALS in two adult populations. *J Med Internet Res*. 2011;13(4):e86.

53. Health Literacy Tool Shed. http:\\healthliteracy.bu.edu. Accessed December 29, 2015.

54. Wallace LS, Rogers ES, Roskos SE, Holiday DB, Weiss BD. Brief report: screening items to identify patients with limited health literacy skills. *J Gen Intern Med*. 2006;21(8):874-877.

55. Brega AG, Barnard J, Mabachi NM, et al. *Health Literacy Universal Precautions Toolkit*. 2nd ed. (Contract No. HHSA290200710008, TO#10. AHRQ Publication No. 15-0023-EF). Rockville, MD: Agency for Healthcare Research and Quality; 2015.

56. DeWalt DA, Broucksou KA, Hawk V, et al. Developing and testing the health literacy universal precautions toolkit. *Nurs Outlook*. 2011;59(2):85-94.

57. Abrams MA, Earles B. Developing an informed consent process with patient understanding in mind. *North Carolina Med J*. 2007;68(5):352-355.

58. National Quality Forum. *Safe Practices for Better Healthcare—2010 Update: A Consensus Report*. Washington, DC: National Quality Forum; 2010.

59. Shekelle PG, Wachter RM, Pronovost PJ, et al. Making health care safer II: an updated critical analysis of the evidence for patient safety practices. *Evid Rep Technol Assess*. 2013(211):1-945.

60. Shojania KG, Duncan BW, McDonald KM, Wachter RM, Markowitz AJ. Making health care safer: a critical analysis of patient safety practices. *Evid Rep Technol Assess (Summary)*. 2001;43:i-x, 1-668.

61. Kincaid JP, Fishburne Jr RP, Rogers RL, Chissom BS. *Derivation of New Readability Formulas (Automated Readability Index, FOG Count and Flesch Reading Ease Formula) for Navy Enlisted Personnel*. Millington, TN: DTIC Document; 1975.

62. ReadabilityFormulas.com. The Flesch Grade Level Readability Formula. 2014. http://www.readabilityformulas.com/flesch-grade-level-readability-formula.php. Accessed December 22, 2014.

63. Doak CC, Doak LG, Root JH. *Teaching Patients with Low Literacy Skills*. Philadelphia, PA: J. B. Lippincott; 1996.

64. McLaughlin GH. SMOG grading: a new readability formula. *J Reading*. 1969;12(8):639-646.

65. Harvard School of Public Health, Health Literacy Studies. SMOG overview. 2010. http://cdn1.sph.harvard.edu/wp-content/uploads/sites/135/2012/09/smogoverview.pdf. Accessed December 22, 2014.

66. Jacobson KL, Gazmararian J, Kripalani S, McMorris K, Blake S, Brach C. *Is Our Pharmacy Meeting Patients' Needs? A Pharmacy Health Literacy Assessment Tool: User's Guide*. (Prepared under contract No. 290-00-0011 T07.) AHRQ Publication No. 07-0051. Rockville, MD: U.S. Department of Health and Human Services, Public Health Service, Agency for Healthcare Research and Quality; 2007.

67. Rudd RE, Anderson JE. *The Health Literacy Environment of Hospitals and Health Centers. Partners for Action: Making Your Healthcare Facility Literacy-Friendly*. Cambridge, MA: National Center for the Study of Adult Learning and Literacy; 2007. http://cdn1.sph.harvard.edu/wp-content/uploads/sites/135/2012/09/healthliteracyenvironment.pdf.

Appendix 7A

CDC Clear Communication Index Before and After Example: NVDRS

National Violent Death Reporting System (NVDRS)
FY 2014 Background Document

NVDRS Data Saves Lives

Violence is not inevitable and can be prevented. The National Violent Death Reporting System (NVDRS) is a state-based surveillance system developed by the Centers for Disease Control and Prevention, National Center for Injury Prevention and Control (CDC Injury Center). NVDRS collects facts from different sources about the same violent death to provide a more complete picture of the circumstances of the event. State and local violence prevention practitioners use these data to guide their prevention programs, policies, and practices including:

- Identifying common circumstances associated with violent deaths of a specific type (e.g., gang violence) or a specific area (e.g., a cluster of suicides);
- Assisting groups in selecting and targeting violence prevention efforts;
- Supporting evaluations of violence prevention activities; and
- Improving the public's access to in-depth information on violent deaths.

Public Health Problem

Preventing violence is a critical public health goal because violence inflicts a substantial toll on individuals, families, and communities throughout the United States. No one is immune to violence. It affects people across the lifespan-from infants to the elderly. CDC Injury Center data indicates:

- In 2010, violence claimed more than 55,000 American lives, translating into more than six people dying each hour from a homicide or suicide.
- In 2010, 38,364 people died by suicide.
- In 2010, homicide claimed more than 16,000 people in the United States.
- Violence-related deaths, assaults, and acts of self-harm cost the United States an estimated $84.3 billion in medical care and lost productivity every year.

Strategies that Work

NVDRS aids in violence prevention through the creation of a reliable violence surveillance system synthesizing multiple data sources into one uniform system, which can be used to inform decision makers and program planners about the magnitude, trends, and characteristics of violent deaths so appropriate prevention efforts can be put into place. It also facilitates the evaluation of state-based prevention programs and strategies. Capturing data from various sources allows us to: link records on violent deaths occurring in the same incident to help identify risk factors for multiple homicides or homicides-suicides, provide timely preliminary information on violent deaths (currently data is not available until 2 years after death), describe in detail the circumstances, which may contribute to a violent death such as job loss, physical and mental health problems, family and other stressors.

1

FIGURE 7A-1 NVDRS Original

Changes made to the original material to increase the index score:

- Emphasized the main message in large, purple font.
- Added an image with a caption to support the main message.
- Placed the call to action in a blue box to highlight how public health department staff can use NVDRS data.

- Used only words that public health department staff are familiar with.
- Summarized the most important information in the first section of the material.
- Explained the statistics on the first page.

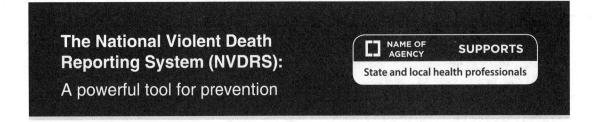

The National Violent Death Reporting System (NVDRS):

A powerful tool for prevention

NAME OF AGENCY   **SUPPORTS**

State and local health professionals

The National Violent Death Reporting System (NVDRS) provides data that can help state and local health departments develop evidence-based strategies for reducing violent deaths.

Violence is a public health problem that affects individuals, families, and communities throughout the United States. Too often, violence results in death by homicide or suicide. According to data from the Centers for Disease Control and Prevention, National Center for Injury Prevention and Control (CDC Injury Center):

- **More than 55,000 Americans died because of homicide or suicide in 2010 — that's an average of more than 6 people dying a violent death every hour.**

- **Violence-related deaths, assaults, and acts of self-harm are expensive. They cost the United States an estimated $107 billion in medical care and lost productivity every year.**

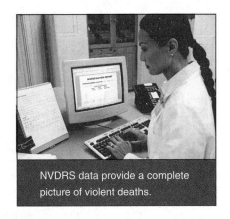

NVDRS data provide a complete picture of violent deaths.

The good news is that violence can be prevented—and accurate information about violence is the key to directing, designing, implementing, and evaluating prevention efforts. NVDRS provides this information to state and local health departments.

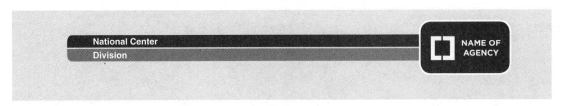

National Center

Division

NAME OF AGENCY

FIGURE 7A-2 NVDRS Updated

Appendix 7B

CDC Clear Communication Index Before and After Example: Thimerosal

Changes made to the original material to increase the index score:

- Developed a main message and presented it at top of page.
- Reduced jargon and added language familiar to the primary audience (detailed explanation of ethylmercury removed).

- Consolidated and reorganized information to present the most important information first.
- Inserted a stronger call to action.
- Added an image related to the main message.
- Reduced passive voice.
- Added a numbered list.
- Added a statement on the state of the science.
- Added information on the meaning of "risk."

A-Z Index A B C D E F G H I J K L M N O P Q R S T U V W X Y Z #

Vaccine Safety

Vaccine Safety
Vaccines Safety Basics
Addressing Common Concerns
  Adjuvants
  Autism
  CDC Statement on Pandemrix
  Fainting (Syncope)
  Febrile Seizures
  GBS
  IOM Assessment of Studies on Childhood Immunization Schedule
  IOM Report on Adverse Effects of Vaccines
  Pregnancy and Influenza Vaccine Safety
  Sudden Infant Death Syndrome (SIDS)
  Thimerosal
    Vaccines & Immunoglobins & Risk of Autism
    Infant & Environmental Exposures to Thimerosal
    ▶FAQs about Thimerosal
    Timeline: Thimerosal in Vaccines (1999-2010)
    Publications
  FAQs about Multiple Vaccines and the Immune System
  FAQs about Vaccine Recalls
  FAQs about Vaccine Safety
Vaccine Monitoring
Activities
Special Populations
Resource Library

Vaccine Safety > Addressing Common Concerns > Thimerosal

Recommend 88   Tweet 16   Share

Frequently Asked Questions About Thimerosal (Ethylmercury)

There are two, very different, types of mercury which people should know about: **methylmercury** and **ethylmercury**.

Mercury is a naturally occurring element found in the earth's crust, air, soil, and water. Since the earth's formation, volcanic eruptions, weathering of rocks and burning coal have caused mercury to be released into the environment. Once released, certain types of bacteria in the environment can change mercury into **methylmercury**. Methylmercury makes its way through the food chain in fish, animals, and humans. At high levels, it can be toxic to people. For more information about methylmercury: please read "What You Need to Know about Mercury in Fish and Shellfish ⌧" from the Environmental Protection Agency (EPA).

Thimerosal contains a different form of mercury called **ethylmercury**. Studies comparing ethylmercury and methylmercury suggest that they are processed differently in the human body. Ethylmercury is broken down and excreted much more rapidly than methylmercury. Therefore, ethylmercury (the type of mercury found in the influenza vaccine) is much less likely than methylmercury (the type of mercury in the environment) to accumulate in the body and cause harm.

On this Page
- What is thimerosal?
- Why is thimerosal used as a preservative in vaccines?
- How does thimerosal work in the body?
- Is thimerosal safe?
- What are the possible side-effects of thimerosal?
- Does thimerosal cause autism?
- Do MMR vaccines contain thimerosal?
- Do all flu vaccines contain thimerosal?
- How can I find out if thimerosal is in a vaccine?

What is thimerosal?
Thimerosal is a mercury-based preservative that has been used for decades in the United States in multi-dose vials (vials containing more than one dose) of medicines and vaccines.

Top of page

Why is thimerosal used as a preservative in vaccines?
Thimerosal is added to vials of vaccine that contain more than one dose to prevent the growth of could cause severe local reactions, serious illness or death. In some vaccines, preservatives are added during the manufacturing process to prevent microbial growth.

Top of page

How does thimerosal work in the body?
Thimerosal does not stay in the body a long time so it does not build up and reach harmful levels. When thimerosal enters the body, it breaks down, to ethylmercury and thiosalicylate, which are easily eliminated.

Top of page

Is thimerosal safe?
Thimerosal has a proven track record of being very safe. Data from many studies show no convincing evidence of harm caused by the low doses of thimerosal in vaccines.

Top of page

What are the possible side-effects of thimerosal?
The most common side-effects are minor reactions like redness and swelling at the injection site. Although rare, some people may be allergic to thimerosal. Research shows that most people who are allergic to thimerosal will not have a reaction when thimerosal is injected under the skin (Wattanakrai, 2007; Heidary, 2005).

Top of page

Does thimerosal cause autism?
Research *does not* show any link between thimerosal in vaccines and autism, a neurodevelopmental disorder. Although thimerosal was taken out of childhood vaccines in 2001, autism rates have gone up, which is the opposite of what would be expected if thimerosal caused autism.

Top of page

Do MMR vaccines contain thimerosal?
No, measles, mumps, and rubella (MMR) vaccines do not and never did contain thimerosal. Varicella (chickenpox), inactivated polio (IPV), and pneumococcal conjugate vaccines have also never contained thimerosal.

Top of page

Do all flu vaccines contain thimerosal?
No. Influenza (flu) vaccines are currently available in both thimerosal-containing and thimerosal-free versions. The total amount of flu vaccine without thimerosal as a preservative at times has been limited, but availability will increase as vaccine manufacturing capabilities are expanded. In the meantime, it is important to keep in mind that the benefits of influenza vaccination outweigh the theoretical risk, if any, of exposure to thimerosal.

Top of page

How can I find out if thimerosal is in a vaccine?
For a complete list of vaccines and their thimerosal content level, you may visit the U.S. Food and Drug Administration. Additionally, you may ask your health care provider or pharmacist for a copy of the vaccine package insert. It lists ingredients in the vaccine and discusses any known adverse reactions.

Top of page

References
Please see References for a list of published articles on thimerosal.

Email   Print   Updates

Page last reviewed: March 1, 2010
Page last updated: October 14, 2011
Content source: **Centers for Disease Control and Prevention**
National Center for Emerging and Zoonotic Infectious Diseases (NCEZID)
Division of Healthcare Quality Promotion (DHQP)

Home   A-Z Index   Site Map   Policies   Using this Site   Link to Us   All Languages   CDC Mobile   Contact CDC

Centers for Disease Control and Prevention   1600 Clifton Rd. Atlanta, GA 30333, USA
800-CDC-INFO (800-232-4636) TTY: (888) 232-6348 - Contact CDC-INFO

FIGURE 7B-1 Thimerosal Original

Reproduced from The CDC Clear Communication Index: Example Materials. August 11, 2014. Available from: http://www.cdc.gov/ccindex/examplematerial/index.html. Accessed May 2015.

Anatomy of a Material

The following example illustrates how multiple Index items work together to make a material easier to understand and use.

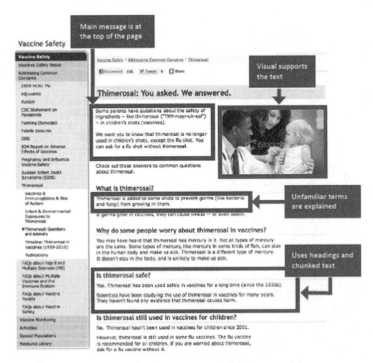

FIGURE 7B-2 Thimerosal Updated: Anatomy of a Material

Reproduced from The CDC Clear Communication Index: Example Materials. August 11, 2014. Available from: http://www.cdc.gov/ccindex/examplematerial/index.html. Accessed May 2015.

Appendix 7C

Case Study – Smokefree.gov

Linda Squiers (RTI), Erik Augustson (NCI), and **Amy Sanders (ICF International)**

FIGURE 7C-1 SmokefreeTXT
Courtesy of Smokefree.gov.

The capacity of digital platforms and the prevalence of cell phones expands each year. This expansion has led to 87% of Americans using the Internet and 90% owning a mobile device.[1] Mobile devices offer unprecedented capacity to reach large populations and populations that were previously deemed "hard to reach." Apps and text messaging programs promoting and supporting healthy behaviors are widespread and can provide immediate feedback and data in real time.

The National Cancer Institute (NCI) has developed a smoking cessation program, smokefree.gov, that spans the digital world by using the web, social media, apps, and text messaging. The goal of this program is to increase the proportion of smokers who quit smoking by providing engaging and accessible support services. Specific programs under the smokefree.gov umbrella incorporate many principles of health communication such as targeting and message framing:

- The Smokefree.gov website offers a variety of tools designed to help people quit smoking. Site features include an online step-by-step cessation guide, phone numbers for telephone support, a link to instant messaging with NCI counselors, facts about quitting and smoking, and self-help materials with links for downloading or ordering.

FIGURE 7C-2 Smokefree Banner Ad
Courtesy of Smokefree.gov.

Smokefree.gov was developed by NCI and received assistance from CDC. The site is free to the public.

- Smokefree Women is an extension of smokefree.gov. It is intended to help you or someone you care about quit smoking. The site offers a special focus on topics important to women. The information and professional assistance available on the website can help to support both your immediate and long-term needs as you become, and remain, a nonsmoker. The website also contains an interactive feature with Facebook to cultivate an online support community for women trying to quit. The Facebook group, Smokefree Women, contains a number of social encouragement applications and allow "fans" to share the quit resources with other women.

- Smokefree Teen is a teen-oriented smoking cessation program and provides teens who smoke with evidence-informed resources. The initiative consists of four core components: teen.Smokefree.gov; SmokefreeTXT, a text message–based intervention; QuitSTART, an interactive quit tracking application that features games to play during cravings; and Smokefree Teen-branded social media pages on Twitter, Facebook, and Tumblr. Many of these components use mobile technology given teens' unique usage patterns of emerging mobile technologies, social media, and text messaging. The use of text messaging to deliver cessation treatment is seen as a core feature of the teen site.

- Espanol.smokefree.gov is a website featuring evidence-based smoking cessation information and interactive tools designed for Spanish speakers in the United States. SmokefreeTXT en Español is one of the major features of the new website, which provides smoking cessation tips, information, and support in Spanish. Users can enroll in the free text

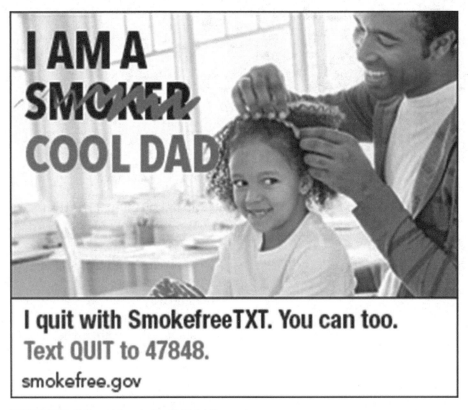

FIGURE 7C-3 Tailored SmokefreeTXT Ad Example
Courtesy of Smokefree.gov.

messaging service by signing up online or by texting the word LIBRE to 47848. SmokefreeTXT en Español provides 24/7 encouragement, advice, and tips to help Spanish-speaking smokers quit.

■ SmokefreeTXT is a mobile text messaging service designed for adults and young adults across the United States who are trying to quit smoking. The program was created to provide encouragement, advice, and tips to help smokers quit smoking and stay quit. The program, available 24 hours a day, 7 days a week, focuses on providing actionable strategies and fact-based information, serving as an engagement tool delivering two-way communication. The SmokefreeTXT program helps smokers select a quit date (i.e., a day they commit to stop smoking). Then, 2 weeks prior to a smoker's selected quit date, the text messaging program begins to send messages. Smokers receive messages to help prepare them for their quit date. Smokers receive multiple supportive messages on their quit date and continue to receive text messages for 6 weeks after their quit date.

Throughout the program, smokers receive texts that cover a variety of content areas including tips, informational content, motivational messaging, and keyword responses. Examples of these messages can be found in **TABLE 7C-1**.

TABLE 7C-1 Examples of Text Messages Sent for SmokefreeTXT

Message Type	Message
Quit day reminders	QuitTXT: The countdown begins! 2 weeks until you quit smoking. We are here to help you prepare & follow through.
Cravings assessments	QuitTXT: Cravings are real. They will not go away immediately, but giving in will only make them stronger. What's your craving level? Reply: Hi, Med, or Low
Unprompted keyword reminder	QuitTXT: Many smokers say quitting is the hardest thing they have ever done. When it gets hard, you can text CRAVE, MOOD, or SLIP for support.

Message Type	Message
Quit day reminders; motivational messaging	QuitTXT: Today is your quit day. The big day is here—you can do this! You are stronger than you think, so stay positive.
Smokefree tips; motivational messaging	QuitTXT: Stress can make you want to smoke. Knowing your smoking triggers will help you stay smokefree. Write down your top 3 & make a plan to avoid them.
Smokefree tips; motivational messaging	QuitTXT: Calculate how much money you spend on cigs every week, every month, & every year. Soon you can use that money for something else.
Smokefree tips	QuitTXT: There are people, places, and things that make you want to smoke. Identify your triggers and make a plan to deal with them on quit day.
Smokefree tips	QuitTXT: Take anything that reminds you of smoking out of your home, car, office, etc. Lighters, matches, and ashtrays too. Everything.

Since 2011, SmokefreeTXT has had more than 109,000 subscribers and sent more than 8 million messages. A recent evaluation of different versions of the text messaging program found that the full program, which is currently being implemented by NCI, was most effective in helping study participants quit smoking, compared two other versions of the program that sent fewer text messages over time.

References

1. Fox S, Rainie L. *The Web at 25 in the U.S. The overall verdict: the Internet has been a plus for society and an especially good thing for individual users.* Pew Research Center; 2014. http://www.pewinternet.org/2014/02/27/the-web-at-25-in-the-u-s/. Accessed May 28, 2015.

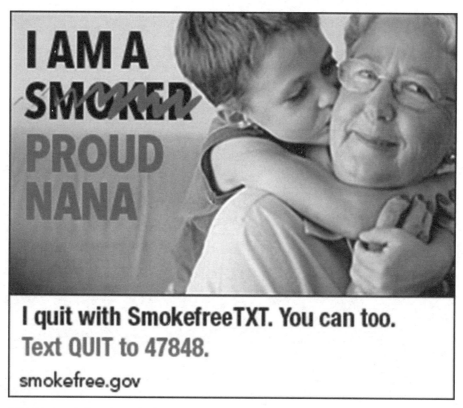

FIGURE 7C-4 Tailored Smokefree TXT Ad Example
Courtesy of Smokefree.gov.

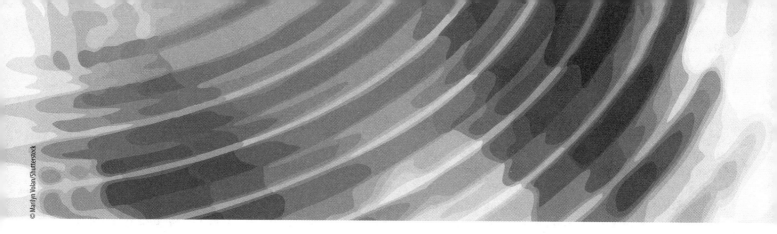

CHAPTER 8

Behavior Change Communication: Theories, Models, and Practice Strategies

Claudia Parvanta

LEARNING OBJECTIVES

By the end of this chapter, the reader will be able to:

- Describe the disciplinary sources of leading theories in health communication.
- Explain why theory is used in health communication planning.
- Create alternative message frames.
- Describe the key theories of behavior change used most commonly in public health communication.
- Use intervention mapping to identify theory-based methods and practice strategies.
- Grasp the fundamentals of social marketing.
- Find cutting-edge research at the National Institutes of Health on behavior change.

▶ Introduction: The Power (?) of Persuasion

Public health practitioners put a lot of effort into trying to convince others to modify their behaviors. Some writers have questioned the ethics of this approach,[1] with scores of articles being written on the "paternalism" of the "nudge."[2] The nudge—that is, "giving a little push" to people to get them to do the right thing—brings behavioral economics into the field of social psychology, and applies both disciplines to public health.[3] Since public health embraces the utilitarian philosophy of the greatest good for the greatest number,[4] health communicators have embraced the moral obligation of "informing and empowering people to make healthy choices." If only we humans were so rational that all we needed was information and a few resources to do the right thing for ourselves!

Health communicators do not have to choose between the views espoused by Daniel Kahneman, the Nobel laureate in behavioral economics, and Albert Bandura, the social psychologist who, among other things, created the construct we call "self-efficacy." Over time, such communicators have incorporated evidence from economics, psychology, and other fields into their own work to develop persuasive behavior change communication strategies.

For some voluntary behaviors, such as those involving road traffic or infant safety, the state applies laws and fines to motivate adoption of the socially sanctioned behavior. Some behaviors are easy to do, cost little, and make such a huge difference—such as purchasing and using only iodized salt[a]—that most people are persuaded to adopt this simple behavior when they are provided with appropriate information. Milk consumption is another food example, but it involves two levels of intervention. First, the U.S. government provides a choice of milk-fat levels and tries to educate people to choose the lower-fat versions. At the same time, the U.S. Department of Agriculture (USDA) requires fortification of milk with vitamins A and D because "public health" advocates gave up trying to explain how to get those critical fat-soluble nutrients into our diets nearly a century ago.

If you look for a totally rational plan as to when public health uses laws and fines, when practitioners use education, when they merely "nudge," and when they utilize a more persuasive approach, you will be frustrated. Our advice: Accept that persuasion in public health communication is a necessary strategy, and do it well and in an ethical manner.

The rationale for this approach can best be appreciated by considering the following data: According to researchers at the University of Southern California (USC), Americans are *exposed* to all forms of media for a staggering 15.5 hours per person per day, *not counting* workplace time. The amount of media data delivered exceeds 8.75 zettabytes (74 gigabytes) annually, which is equal to approximately nine DVDs being sent to the average consumer on a typical day.[4] How many of these media messages do we actually attend to? How many convince us to run out and buy or do anything? To answer this question, think about your own behavior. For public health communicators to cut through the clutter and make any impact with their own messages, they must use the best strategies and tools available, beginning with the body of theory.

▶ Theory in Health Communication for Behavior Change

The Value of Theory in Health Communication

In the early days of health education, program directors would tell their staff, "We need a poster" or "We need a brochure" to get (fill in the blank *audience*) to (fill in the blank *behavior*). In contrast, today's program directors might ask for the latest social media app for an intervention without any basis for thinking that channel or medium would be appropriate for the audience, the context, and the change intended. As an antidote to such automatic responses, more savvy health communicators may call upon "theory"—that is, the vast canvas of behavior change approaches that are continually tested in public health. Those theories, or systematic ways of understanding what causes an individual or group to behave in certain ways in specific situations, are made up of "propositions that explain or predict events by illustrating the relationships among variables."[6(p4)]

According to Glanz and Rimer,[6] the most successful health-promotion interventions incorporate theories of both problem and change. Health communicators use tools from epidemiology and community-based assessment (such as the PRECEDE–PROCEED model) to diagnose a problem's locus in an ecosystem, including the predisposing, enabling, and reinforcing factors that create or maintain it within a population. They search for explanatory models of why problems exist and which interventions might bring about change. As in any other scientific enterprise, these hypotheses of causality and change must be tested systematically in multiple populations and contexts to generate theory. Once something has been observed to work in a number of applications, it may be elevated to the level of a working model or "grand theory." Grand theories are the basis of the methods and practice strategies that health communicators choose for their interventions. They allow us to plan in a systematic way and evaluate whether a program is working the way we intend or falling short of the desired goal. Moreover, if a strong logic model is available that shows how our theory-based methods lead to results, we should be able to identify what needs to be altered to make the program more effective.

Sources of Theory in Health Communication

Theories relevant to health communications spring from several different lines of research.

■ Psychologists research **mediators** and **moderators** of human behavior in an experimental or clinical setting, with their results informing the majority of the individual behavior change theories. (**BOX 8-1** explains these terms.) Much of this

---

a. Iodine in salt helps prevent iodine deficiency, which is associated with thyroid cancer, IQ deficits, goiter, and the health of the multiple physiological systems.

work is adapted into interpersonal counseling therapies. Public health applications include individual change theories, such as social cognitive theory and the Stages of Change Model, as well as applications of those theories to entertainment education, online coaching, and targeting and tailoring efforts.

- Academic communications research is increasing, with international scholars (with different perspectives) claiming more space in the field's journals over the past five years. Communication theories used in public health tend to focus on message wording (framing), the "richness" of communications content and the means in which it is used, and spokesperson and media channel credibility.

- Marketing research conducted over the past century has provided understanding of demand creation, including most recently the transformation of what was once perceived as a unidirectional "marketing funnel" into today's concept of the peripatetic "customer journey." Marketing research is to economics what engineering is to physics—namely, the application of science to solve problems. Thus, while behavioral economics has contributed to marketing for a long time, it is also having a decade of being in the spotlight by itself.

- Practitioners, often working in international settings, have created a theory of praxis[7,b] focused on participatory and practical approaches to accomplish behavior change goals in communities. This work often occurs within a social marketing framework.

Collectively, the fields of psychology, communication, and marketing—together with a healthy dose of social praxis—form the basis of our theory toolkit in health communication.

BOX 8-1 Moderators and Mediators of Behavior[1]

Alesha G. Hruska, MPH, MS, MCHES

In cause-and-effect research, investigators often detect the actions of other variables, sometimes referred to as "third variables,"[1,2] which may either confound or help to explain the relationship between the independent and dependent variables. Researchers may actively investigate these potential mediators or moderators depending on which questions they seek to answer.

Helping to answer the questions "how," "why," or "through which process," *mediators* allow for understanding of the mechanisms through which the independent variable affects the dependent variable.[3] Mediators are most commonly psychological or biological characteristics. However, within some research areas such as patient-centered communication, mediating variables can also include contextual factors such as access to care and high-quality medical decisions.[4]

Moderators, or interaction variables, affect the magnitude and direction of change between the predictor variable (or independent variable in experimental research) and the outcome variable (or dependent variable) and can answer such questions as "when" or "for whom" does this intervention work.[2] In general, trait characteristics such as age or sex, or relatively stable variables such as socioeconomic status, may moderate the effect on the outcome variable, depending on the level of interaction between the moderator and the predictor variable.[2]

Although "third variables" are applicable in various types of research, including clinical and experimental studies, mediators and moderators are particularly salient in intervention research designed with theory in mind. Both can be integrated into the planning stage of an intervention study to test and refine the theory used as the basis for the study design and are critical for testing the external validity and applicability of theory.[1,2]

References

1. Kazdin AE. *Research Design in Clinical Psychology*. 4th ed. Boston, MA: Allyn & Bacon; 2003.

2. MacKinnon DP. Integrating mediators and moderators in research design. *Res Soc Work Prac*. 2011;21(6):675–681.

3. Karazsia BT, Berlin KS, Armstrong B, Janicke DM. Integrating mediation and moderation to advance theory development and testing. *J Pediatr Psychol*. 2014;39(2):163–173.

4. Epstein RM, Street RL Jr. *Patient-Centered Communication in Cancer Care: Promoting Healing and Reducing Suffering*. NIH Publication No. 07-6225. Bethesda, MD: National Cancer Institute; 2007.

---

b. Starting with the likes of Paolo Freire and others, "praxis-oriented research involves the community or group under study in the research process… [an] explicit goal is to empower marginalized peoples and help them challenge their oppression… By engaging in collaborative research, researchers may help participants acquire the critical tools to transform their own lives."[7]

Behavior Change Theory

The models and theories described in this section are presented in the approximate chronological order of their uptake into public health.

Health Belief Model

The **Health Belief Model (HBM)** was one of the first models in the field of public health to explain individual health behaviors, particularly individual decisions to participate in public health services such as free tuberculosis screening programs.[8,9] In the HBM, several sets of beliefs either motivate or discourage people from demonstrating certain health behaviors:

- Perceived susceptibility: The individual's sense of personal risk for a health condition.
- Perceived severity: The individual's belief about how serious this condition is.
- Perceived benefits of interventions: The individual's perception of the effectiveness of taking action.
- Perceived barriers or costs of interventions: The individual's perception of the monetary, physical, or psychosocial costs to perform a behavior.
- Cues to activate behavior change: Specific messages or indicators that might prompt the individual to take action.
- Self-efficacy to perform the behavior: The individual's confidence about performing this specific action.

The HBM fell out of favor for a few decades, particularly among practitioners who were developing interventions for adolescents and young adults. Now, however, the HBM appears to be coming into wide use again, particularly in developing interventions for smoking cessation for adults and for "baby boomers" who are entering into the years when chronic disease onset is most likely and who have a heightened sense of "susceptibility."

The CDC created a Screen for Life campaign for colorectal cancer prevention. The key message for this intervention is that if you are 50 years of age or older, you are more susceptible to colorectal cancer. Everyone believes that cancer is serious. A colonoscopy is positioned as a 'cure waiting to happen,' by removal of polyps that can lead to cancers of the colon. Colorectal cancer screening is the poster child for application of the HBM.

Despite celebrity endorsements, specific programs have found the need to use multiple theory-based initiatives (including those discussed later in this chapter) to persuade reluctant adults to perform one of the American Cancer Society's recommended screening tests.

Transtheoretical Model

The awkwardly named **Transtheoretical Model (TTM)**,[10] also known as the **Stages of Change (SOC) Model**, indicates that individuals move through a specific process when deciding to change their behavior and then actually changing their behavior. There are five stages in this process:

1. Precontemplation
2. Contemplation
3. Preparation
4. Action
5. Maintenance

Different individuals may be at different stages along this process and, therefore, must receive differently tailored interventions or communications according to their attitudes. For example, smokers who are in the precontemplation stage have no intention of quitting smoking in the next six months, so information about cessation aids such as nicotine patches will not facilitate their cessation behavior. In contrast, smokers in the contemplation stage do plan to quit smoking in the next six months, so positively reinforcing this goal with enabling information should be more effective at this point. Descriptions of the other stages and appropriate health communication, education, and intervention strategies appear in **TABLE 8-1**.[6] Many interventions combine TTM with social cognitive theory constructs, or other models, to deliver messages to prompt audiences to take a next step.

Subsequent work that combined the TTM with social cognitive theory eliminated the supposition that the TTM represents a smooth transition from one stage to the next, with different stages being influenced through quantity, not quality of message.[11]

Social Cognitive Theory

Social cognitive theory (SCT) hypothesizes that individual behavior is the result of constant interaction between the external environment and internal psychosocial characteristics and perceptions.[12] Albert Bandura originally named this social learning theory in 1962, then later published it as SCT in 1986. "The theory takes into account a person's past experiences, which factor into whether behavioral action will occur. These past experiences influence reinforcements, expectations, and expectancies, all of which shape whether a person will engage in a specific behavior and the reasons why a person engages in that behavior."[12] Many constructs included in SCT are included in **TABLE 8-2**. Self-efficacy ("I can do it"), for example, is an SCT construct that has become an end in itself for many behavior change interventions (e.g., teens

TABLE 8-1 Transtheoretical (Stages of Change) Model Stages

Stage	Definition	Potential Change Strategies
Precontemplation	Has no intention of taking action within the next six months	Increase awareness of need for change; personalize information about risks and benefits
Contemplation	Intends to take action in the next six months	Motivate; encourage making specific plans
Preparation	Intends to take action within the next 30 days and has taken some behavioral steps in this direction	Assist with developing and implementing concrete action plans; help set gradual goals
Action	Has changed behavior for less than six months	Assist with feedback, problem solving, social support, and reinforcement
Maintenance	Has changed behavior for more than six months	Assist with coping, reminders, finding alternatives, avoiding slips/relapses (as applicable)

Reproduced from National Cancer Institute. Theory at a Glance, A Guide for Health Promotion Practice, 2nd ed. NIH Publication No. 05-3896; 2005, p. 15. http://www.cancer.gov/PDF/481f5d53-63df-41bc-bfaf-5aa48ee1da4d/TAAG3.pdf.

TABLE 8-2 Social Cognitive Theory

Concept	Definition	Potential Change Strategies
Reciprocal determinism	The dynamic interaction of the person, the behavior, and the environment in which the behavior is performed	Consider multiple ways to promote behavior change, including making adjustments to the environment or influencing personal attitudes
Behavioral capability	Knowledge and skill to perform a given behavior	Promote mastery learning through skills training
Expectations	Anticipated outcomes of a behavior	Model positive outcomes of healthful behavior
Self-efficacy	Confidence in one's ability to take action and overcome barriers	Approach the behavior change in small steps to ensure success; be specific about the desired change
Observational learning (modeling)	Behavioral acquisition that occurs by watching the actions and outcomes of others' behavior	Offer credible role models who perform the targeted behavior
Reinforcements	Responses to a person's behavior that increase or decrease the likelihood of reoccurrence	Promote self-initiated rewards and incentives

Reproduced from National Cancer Institute. Theory at a Glance, A Guide for Health Promotion Practice, 2nd ed. NIH Publication No. 05-3896; 2005, p. 20. http://www.cancer.gov/PDF/481f5d53-63df-41bc-bfaf-5aa48ee1da4d/TAAG3.pdf.

avoiding high-risk behaviors or women negotiating condom use with their partners). Vicarious (observational) learning is another well-recognized construct in the SCT model, often used to teach people incremental behavior skills through role modeling. It is hard to overestimate how often SCT has been used explicitly or implicitly in behavior change communication programs. As health communicators, we all owe a huge debt of gratitude to Albert Bandura.

The Precaution Adoption Process Model

The **Precaution Adoption Process Model (PAPM)** looks quite similar to the TTM in that it consists of distinct stages between a lack of awareness and completed preventive action.[13] According to its originators, the PAPM includes seven stages:

1. Unaware of the issue
2. Aware of the issue but not personally engaged
3. Engaged and deciding what to do
4. Planning to act but not yet having acted
5. Deciding not to act
6. Acting
7. Maintenance

The PAPM asserts that these stages represent qualitatively distinct patterns of behavior, beliefs, and experience and that the factors that produce transitions between stages vary depending on the specific transition being considered. The "deciding not to act" stage is unique to the PAPM, which was developed in reference to environmental hazards—hence the inclusion of the term "precaution adoption" in the model's name. The PAPM has been extensively applied to communicating about testing for radon in homes, installing smoke detectors, and the like. In addition, the PAPM is being increasingly used in cancer screening communication.

Integrative Model (Theory of Reasoned Action and Theory of Planned Behavior)

The **Integrative model (IM)**[14] represents an evolved version of Fishbein and Ajzen's *theory of reasoned action (TRA)*.[15] Ajzen developed the *theory of planned behavior (TPB)*[16] as an extension of the TRA. Fishbein and Ajzen worked together to develop the IM, which they also referred to as the *reasoned action approach*.[17] **FIGURE 8-1** depicts the concepts of the IM.

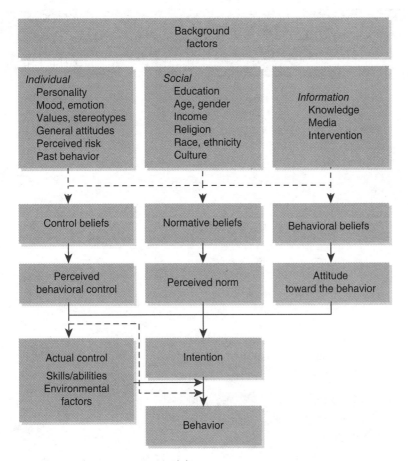

FIGURE 8-1 The Integrative Model

The most important assumption of the IM is that the best predictor of behavior is the intention to perform the behavior. This model focuses on the antecedents (predictors) of an individual's intention to perform (or not perform) a behavior. The IM focuses on the following beliefs:

- **Behavioral beliefs** are expectancies about positive or negative outcomes related to performing the behavior. They lead to the formation of **attitudes**.
- **Normative beliefs** are perceptions about what relevant others think about performing the behavior, or beliefs about what others are doing. Together, these beliefs determine a concept of *perceived normative pressure* related to the behavior.
- **Control beliefs** relate to whether there are barriers or facilitators to performing the behavior. They are directly associated with an individual's *perceived behavioral control*, or *self-efficacy*, when performing the behavior.

The IM also takes into account various background factors, which influence the constructs in the model differently. These background factors include race, gender, personality, education, income, and past behavior, among others. Factors such as media exposure can also be included—which is where health communication messages fit in.

These components of the intervention work together within the IM. When performing research subject screening interviews or initial surveys of the intended audience, the health communicator seeking to utilize the IM should take the following steps:

- Determine which of the direct antecedents of intention (attitude, perceived norms, self-efficacy) best predict the audience members' intention.
- Elicit the audience members' beliefs underlying the attitudes, norms, and self-efficacy.
- Design the health communication message or messages to influence these antecedent beliefs.

Of course, if the subject screening and surveys reveal that the audience already intends to perform the behavior, then the health communicator need not go through all the steps of the IM. In this case, it is not likely that their beliefs, attitudes, or self-efficacy are preventing them from adopting healthy behaviors. Instead, environmental factors, skills, or knowledge—that is, factors that take *actual* control over the behavior—are likely precluding their behavior change. If environmental barriers exist, for example, rather than designing the communication campaign to change intentions in a population, you might need to focus the campaign on changing policies that affect the population's opportunities to perform the behavior.[c]

Elaboration Likelihood Model

Petty and Cacioppo's Elaboration Likelihood Model of Persuasion (ELM)[18] may be used to design content to inform a user. The ELM predicts that individuals will "elaborate," or think about new information more, if they are already concerned about or interested in the subject. If not, then other symbolic references valued by the intended user, such as spokespersons, images, settings, colors, or language, may be used to capture the individual's attention. These other references are called **peripheral cues**, because they do not deal directly with the subject matter (cancer screening or prevention of sexually transmitted disease, for example), but more call out to the intended user —"Hey, look at me. I'm speaking to YOU." **TABLE 8-3** shows the differences postulated between central-route and peripheral-route processing of a piece of content. The theory behind the ELM suggests that if you can get someone's attention with peripheral cues, that person will then move into a more central processing route as he or she starts to pay attention and think about the material.

Diffusion of Innovations

All the preceding theories and models focus on individual behavior; the **diffusion of innovations (DI)** theory addresses change in a group.[19] Developed by E. M. Rogers in 1962, DI is one of the oldest social science theories used in public health. Rogers constructed the theory after studying how new agricultural techniques spread among farmers. DI describes how new ideas, or innovations, are spread within and among people, organizations, or communities. According to this theory, innovations spread via different communication channels within social systems over a specific period of time. For their purposes, health communicators should focus on specific aspects of an innovation, such as the *relative advantage, compatibility, complexity, trialability*, and *observability* of the innovation. The innovation should seem better than "the leading brand," be compatible with its specified audience, and be easy to adopt. People should also be able to "try it out" before committing to it, and the changes should be obvious enough to permit their measurement.

Successful diffusion often relies on media communication as well as interpersonal communication

---

c. This summary of the IM is based on the last book by Fishbein and Ajzen, published in 2010.

TABLE 8-3 Elaboration Likelihood Model of Persuasion: Two Routes

	Central-Route Processing	Peripheral-Route Processing
Route	Central	Peripheral
Elaboration	High	Low
Information processing	Contents of message are closely examined by the receiver	Receiver is influenced by factors other than the contents of the message
Attitude	Will change or be reinforced based on message characteristics such as strength of argument and relevancy	Might change or be reinforced based on the effectiveness of factors other than the message
Strength of attitude formed/reinforced	More enduring and less subject to counterarguments	Less enduring and subject to change through future persuasive messages

Reproduced from Victor Yocco, A List A part. http://alistapart.com/article/persuasion-applying-the-elaboration-likelihood-model-to-design#section2.

and social networking. Messages should be targeted to specific segments of the overall audience, because some members are likely to adopt the innovation early, whereas others will do so late. Still other audience members will be the innovators who diffuse the behavior change and will be receptive to very different kinds of messages.

Malcolm Gladwell's popular book *The Tipping Point* extends diffusion theory by suggesting that the "innovators" in Rogers's terminology are indeed trendsetters who can create so much buzz around a new idea that it spreads very rapidly throughout a population.[20] This pattern is similar to the actions of the more traditional group that Rogers called "early adopters," who lead the majority into adopting a behavior.

▶ Theory Derived from Communication Studies

We have already presented a few important theories that dealt directly with "informing" audiences. In our discussion of health literacy, we introduced information processing theory as what we have learned about how people take in information, organize it mentally, and make sense of it. Here we focus on communication theories that pertain to persuasion.

Message Framing

Framing a message is giving it a context or even suggesting a point of view or an interpretation through which it is to be understood. Whether consciously or unconsciously, even as we speak, we "frame" information to make it more interesting, more palatable, or more frightening for our audience. The frame itself has been demonstrated to have a direct impact on how someone hears, processes, and acts on information. As such, framing is an important technique for persuasive health communication, in addition to advocacy and politics.

"Framing bias" is sometimes seen in a negative light, as something that can be done to manipulate an audience's interpretation of numerical data. For example, if we say that 1 in 20 people "die," many people will think the death rate is worse than if we said 19 out of 20 people "survive." **Gain-framed** appeals state the advantages of taking an action (chance of survival), whereas **loss-framed** appeals state the disadvantages of not taking an action (chance of death).

Using the human papillomavirus (HPV) vaccine as an example, Gainforth and colleagues found that framing the HPV message in terms of the benefits of engaging in the behavior (gain frame) was more important to mothers of boys than the costs of failing to engage in the behavior (loss frame).[21] In contrast, an earlier study of college-age women found they were more motivated by loss-framed messages if they identified themselves as sexually active. The CDC Features website's September 2015 headline read, "Put 'HPV Cancer Prevention' on Your Back-to-School Checklist,"[22] thereby framing the HPV vaccine (1) as a routine immunization for school and (2) as cancer prevention. Opponents of the HPV vaccine frame its use as a "controversy" or an "ethical decision" based on the fact that individuals who are not sexually active have little risk of acquiring HPV.

Message framing can be much more nuanced. **BOX 8-2** shows an example from the Get Yourself Tested program, which frames sexually transmitted diseases (STDs) as an issue for the target audience.

Inoculation Theory

Nietzsche's statement, "What does not kill us makes us stronger," is the concept behind vaccines: A weak dose of a virus causes our bodies to create an immune

---

BOX 8-2 Communicating to Vulnerable Populations: Results from a National Message Framing Study Involving Sexually Active African Americans

Allison Friedman, Jennifer Uhrig, Booker Daniels, Carla M. Bann, and **Jon Poehlman**

Background

African Americans bear a heavier burden of reported STDs than any other racial/ethnic group in the United States. Although behavioral factors play a role, STD rates are also driven by underlying social and structural determinants—for example, poverty, education, health literacy, stigma, gender imbalances, and incarceration rates, among other factors. These factors may not only hinder access to appropriate and quality STD/HIV testing, treatment, and care, but can also influence an individual's sexual network (exposing low-risk individuals to high-risk partners) and limit behavioral choices or ability to negotiate safer sex. Experts have advocated for raising awareness of health disparities as "a necessary first step" to mobilize at-risk communities and prompt behavior change. Others have cautioned against the dissemination of racially comparative STD data, arguing that it may increase public blame for those groups most affected by these disease and foster hopelessness, powerlessness, and distress among vulnerable populations.

Little is known about the effects of racially comparative STD data on African American audiences' affect and behavioral intent, or whether these outcomes are influenced by differential message framing. The CDC's exploratory research with African American adults found that racially comparative STD information may prompt defensive reactions and contribute to stigmatization both between and within groups. Despite these potentially negative outcomes, most study participants believed it would be important to inform their communities about racial disparities in STDs as a "wake-up call" to action.

Objective

The CDC sought to assess the relative effectiveness of STD rates framed in absolute, progress (positive), and disparities (negative) frames; and to measure the impact on audiences' affect, STD-related knowledge, motivations, and behavioral intent.

Methods

African American adults, ages 18 to 30 years, were recruited through a survey research firm using a nonprobability-based quota sample. An online survey ($N = 551$) was used to test respondents' reactions to a mock news article about gonorrhea, framed one of three ways:

- Impact—described the impact and consequences of gonorrhea in the African American community in absolute terms
- Progress—emphasized improvements in gonorrhea rates among African Americans over time
- Disparity—highlighted the disproportionate impact of gonorrhea among African Americans compared to whites

Participants were randomly assigned to view one of the article formats and asked to respond to questions assessing knowledge, trust, emotions, behavioral intent, and offensiveness of the article. All but the latter question were closed-ended, using a five-point Likert scale to assess level of agreement with 10 statements (1 = strongly disagree; 5 = strongly agree). Mean scores were calculated and compared across frame types for each statement.

Results

A total of 170 respondents read the progress version; 184 respondents read the impact version; and 197 read the disparity version. Statistically significant differences ($p < 0.05$) were found for all but three of the constructs (motivated condom use, knowledge that gonorrhea can be life threatening, and perceived offensiveness). Trust in the article's information was rated higher by those who read the impact version (3.99) compared with the disparity version (3.79). The impact version was more likely to make someone want to learn more (4.03), compared to the progress version (3.82). The progress version was both less upsetting (2.64) and more encouraging (3.96) than either the impact version (3.36 and 3.57, respectively) or the disparity version (3.36 and 3.38, respectively). Respondents who read the

(continues)

BOX 8-2 Communicating to Vulnerable Populations: Results from a National Message Framing Study Involving Sexually Active African Americans   *(continued)*

impact version were more likely than those who read the progress or disparity versions to report wanting to get tested (3.93 versus 3.70 and 3.66, respectively) and planning to talk to friends about the article (3.71 versus 3.37 and 3.47, respectively). Level of agreement scores for the statement about gonorrhea rates being higher among African Americans was highest among those who read the impact version (3.80) compared to the disparity (3.71) and progress (3.26) versions. A small minority of participants found the information to be offensive, regardless of which frame was used.

Conclusions

The findings suggest using either an impact or progress frame to communicate about the STD burden with vulnerable populations. The impact version was most likely to motivate readers to learn more, get tested for STDs, and talk to friends about the article. When communicating about STD rates to vulnerable populations, statistics should be supported by explanations of the underlying social determinants that may constrain sexual networks, individual choices, and access to care to help audiences understand that racial differences in STD rates are not simply a function of individual behavior; and by concrete solutions for addressing STD disparities to empower individuals and communities for change.

Progress Message Frame	Impact Message Frame	Disparity Message Frame
Gonorrhea among African Americans declines over the past decade.	**Gonorrhea affects African Americans at a high rate.**	**African Americans are affected by gonorrhea at higher rates than whites.**
Over the past decade, rates of gonorrhea among African Americans have declined. This may be due in part to growing numbers of African Americans using condoms and getting regular STD testing.	Gonorrhea is a common STD, affecting 170,000 African Americans each year in the United States. The heavy burden of STDs on African Americans is believed to result from individual behavior, as well as broader social problems.	Gonorrhea is a problem in the African American community. It impacts African Americans at 17 times the rate of whites. In fact, African Americans account for 70% of all reported gonorrhea cases in the United States. These differences are believed to result from individual behavior, as well as broader social problems.
Although many people with gonorrhea have no symptoms at all, it can lead to serious and permanent problems if left untreated—such as painful or swollen testicles in men, and infertility (problems having babies) in women. Gonorrhea can also spread to the blood or joints, which can be life threatening.	Although many people with gonorrhea have no symptoms at all, it can lead to serious and permanent problems if left untreated—such as painful or swollen testicles in men, and infertility (problems having babies) in women. Gonorrhea can also spread to the blood or joints, which can be life threatening.	Although many people with gonorrhea have no symptoms at all, it can lead to serious and permanent problems if left untreated—such as painful or swollen testicles in men, and infertility (problems having babies) in women. Gonorrhea can also spread to the blood or joints, which can be life threatening.
Gonorrhea remains a common STD. But, according to one expert, "The African American community is taking steps to make our communities healthier and stronger. As each of us takes responsibility for our sexual health—by using condoms, reducing our number of partners, and getting tested regularly— fewer African Americans will suffer from diseases like gonorrhea."	According to one expert, "STDs like gonorrhea are a big problem in African American communities. We need to work together to find ways to get more of us using condoms, reducing our number of partners, and testing regularly for STDs—to reduce their impact in our communities."	According to one expert, "We, as African Americans, need to take action to change this inequity. We can take control of our sexual health—by using condoms, reducing our number of partners, and getting regular STD testing— to reduce the impact of gonorrhea in our communities."

Limitations

This study had several limitations. The progress frame did not include data on gonorrhea burden. Information presented did not include a clear explanation of underlying social/structural causes of STDs. This study measured behavioral intent, not actual behavior change. Finally, the research focused on reactions of at-risk African American adults to STD information and may not be generalizable to other populations or health topics.

References

1. Aubrun A, Grady J. *Thinking About Race: Findings from Cognitive Elicitations.* Washington DC: Frameworks Institute; August 2004. http://www.frameworksinstitute.org/assets/files/PDF_race/cognitive_elicitations.pdf

2. Friedman AL, Uhrig J, Poehlman J, Scales M, Hogben M. Promoting sexual health equity in the United States: implications from exploratory research with African-American adults. *Health Educ Res.* 2014;29(6):993-1004.

3. Jones CP. Invited commentary: "race," racism, and the practice of epidemiology. *Am J Epidemiol.* 2001;154(4):299-304.

4. Nicholson RA, Kreuter MW, Lapka C, et al. Unintended effects of emphasizing disparities in cancer communication to African Americans. *Cancer Epidemiol Bio Prev.* 2008;17(11):2946-2953.

Courtesy of Allison Friedman, Jennifer Uhrig, Booker Daniels, Carla M. Bann, and Jon Poehlman.

response. McGuire applied the same concept to what we learned about the "brain washing" of Korean War American prisoners.[23,24] That is, psychological warfare came of age when conceptual inoculation was developed as a way to defend against it.

Inoculation theory has since been used extensively in communication, with hundreds of applications to not only health, but also politics and advocacy. A meta-analysis done in 2010 found "across a sample of 41 published and unpublished research reports involving over 10,000 participants… [a] weighted mean effect size comparing inoculation treatments to no-treatment… of Cohen's d =.43, or a small magnitude effect."[25(p302)] This small effect has been increased by manipulating various components of the messaging used in inoculation.

Inoculation theory fits well with social cognitive theory in providing individuals with chances to think through and rehearse their arguments to those attempting to get them to do something against their wishes, such as engage in teen smoking or unprotected sex. **BOX 8-3** provides an example of an inoculation

---

BOX 8-3 Translating Theories into Practice: The Secret of Seven Stones

Ross Shegog

The Secret of Seven Stones is a game that is designed to provide sexual health skills training to youth (11 to 14 years) and to encourage parent and youth engagement in a more meaningful dialogue around sexual health topics. In focus group discussions with parents and their children, a number of important themes emerged.[1] Primarily, parents were found to regard sexual health issues (puberty, relationships, reproduction, and sex) as very important topics. This opinion is certainly validated by data indicating that youth in the United States account for nearly half of all new STD diagnoses, 5% of new HIV diagnoses, and approximately 7% of pregnancies (to teenage girls younger than age 20).[2,3] Parents indicated they want to be central in their children's sexual education.

While school-based sexual health education can reduce sexual risk behaviors, it may not come into play at critical precoital timing or may lack sufficient power or breadth to be effective.[4-6] An additional emergent theme found by researchers was that while sexual health programs have been initiated in school and clinic settings, there are relatively few interventions designed for use in the home, or interventions that facilitate parent and child communication. While parents want to be central to their children's sexual education, they also want to be credible, confident, and knowledgeable about sexual health topics and know how to conduct a dialogue on these subjects. Both parents and children have acknowledged that they feel considerable discomfort in discussing sexual health issues. Moreover, both parents and youth agree that a common technological approach that provides "common ground" for discussion might offer advantages.

Improved parent–child communication can improve adolescent sexual health outcomes, including later age of sexual debut and increased condom and contraceptive use.[7-12] Unfortunately, parents often fail to initiate timely

(continues)

BOX 8-3 Translating Theories into Practice: The Secret of Seven Stones *(continued)*

communication regarding risk reduction (delayed sexual debut, condom and contraceptive use). More than 40% of youth have engaged in sexual activity prior to any discussion of sexual education topics with their parents.[13] For parents to effectively engage in successful communication, they must feel confident in their skills to communicate, believe that communicating will affect their children's behavior, and recognize that communicating about sexual issues is approved by other people considered as important.[14] Interventions that target communication skills training and involve parents have been shown to increase sexual risk communication and youth knowledge, confidence, and comfort regarding communication.[15–18] However, delivery through face-to-face and multi-session group-based channels limits program reach and fidelity.[19–22] *The Secret of Seven Stones* (SSS) was developed as a way to provide sexual health education in the home setting by harnessing parents' and youth motivation to use technology to obtain sexual health information.[23]

Intergenerational Video Game to Promote Parent–Youth Communication at Home

SSS is a National Institutes of Health (NIH)–funded intergenerational game (IGG) that aims to provide sexual health skills training for youth and resources for parents, and that promotes parent–youth sexual health communication. Video games can facilitate interactions between parents and children, promote positive communication,[17,24–26] influence sexual behavior (i.e., delayed initiation of sex or risk-reduction behaviors in sexually active youth), and impact determinants of these behaviors (i.e., knowledge, attitudes, and intentions).[27–34]

Game-based interventions have traditionally targeted youth. SSS takes an intergenerational approach by providing an inclusive and shared experience for parents and youth to provide a common "meeting ground" for sexual health discussion.[35–38] In an IGG, both parents and youth can play an active role in winning the game. In the health field, and particularly in the realm of sexual health education, IGG-based interventions are rare.

SSS was designed to take advantage of the positive aspects of IGGs, including the intergenerational interactions they invoke,[39,40] the flexibility of the available player roles (e.g., youth can adopt leadership roles and be mentored by older players),[35,40] and collaborative engagement in which intergenerational player dyads act more cooperatively than same-aged dyads.[41]

In developing SSS, the researchers collaborated with a parent–youth advisory group who provided feedback and ideas on game play. Critical advice was that SSS accommodate the busy lifestyle of parents, many of whom are juggling numerous family and professional obligations.[1]

SSS is played on Internet-accessible devices through the Adobe Air framework. Youth adopt an avatar to negotiate the town of Seven Stones, liberating the town's inhabitants from an evil nemesis. The town's inhabitants suffer from deficiencies in their ability to select and protect their personal rules for their life, including keeping healthy friendships, understanding puberty and reproduction, having healthy dating relationships, refusing sex, and negotiating safe sexual practices. The player liberates the inhabitants of Seven Stones in "battles" in which the player uses his or her wisdom, skills, and social support (**FIGURE 8-2**). To be successful, players must "power up" their wisdom, skill, and support (represented in the game as battle cards) in a dojo, under the tutelage of Alfred the Dojo Master, where they master life skills related to sexual health through a series of mini-games, role modeling, and talking-head videos.

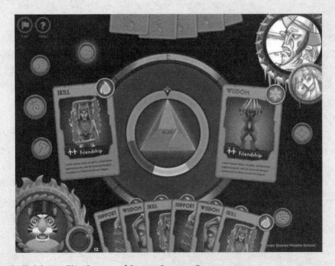

FIGURE 8-2 Battle Table in *The Secret of Seven Stones* Game

Courtesy of Ross Shegog. Acknowledgements: This research was funded by NIH/CICHD grant # 1R42HD074324 and with appreciation to the parents and youth you contributed SSS development.

At seven critical milestones in the game, players are cued to have PEP (prepare–engage–plan) talks with their collaborating parent. These talks focus on the content covered by the player in SSS and introduce seven consecutive character traits that are important in succeeding in choosing and adhering to life decisions (e.g., persistence, responsibility, courage, caring, and vision). Parents are notified through text prompts on their phones as to their children's progress through the game. In addition, parents receive cues to receive resources to guide communication with their children and are alerted when it is time to have a PEP talk. In this context, the parent becomes a gatekeeper in the program. The parent website provide parents with progress updates as well as support-oriented videos and resources dealing with how to successfully engage in PEP talks.

SSS comprises 18 game levels with 50 interactive skills training clusters, 54 "battle" sequences, and 7 game-mediated parent–youth PEP talks. The game provides behavioral skills training in 15 domains (drawn from 135 performance behaviors and more than 1300 learning objectives), encompassing responsible decision making about friendships, dating relationships, and sex. It is founded on social cognitive theory,[42] the theory of triadic influence,[43] normative theories,[44,45] and motivational theory.[46] SSS was developed using the intervention mapping framework.[47] It employs a variety of theoretical methods and practical applications needed to achieve the desired parent and youth outcomes, including computer tailoring, consciousness raising, role modeling, guided practice, goal setting, and ways to stimulate communication to mobilize social support.[48]

Usability and feasibility testing with 10 parent–youth dyads of two "proof-of-concept" game levels of SSS over a three-week period yielded positive usability results from both parents and youth for credibility (accuracy of information and trustworthiness), perceived impact to make healthy choices, and motivational appeal. Most parents and youth indicated they would play the game again and tell others about SSS. Youth compared the two-level SSS "proof-of-concept" as more fun than other school computer programs, but less fun than their favorite computer games. They rated the SSS prototype as easy to play and understandable, as did their parents. This testing informed modifications of SSS to streamline navigation and layout, provide a more obvious causal association between the dojo training and the degree of "power up" of battle cards, and troubleshoot program bugs to improve the gaming experience.

SSS is intended to help parents and their children go beyond "the sex talk" to engage in an ongoing, developmentally appropriate HIV, STD, and pregnancy prevention education experience. It represents a unique home-based resource for meeting a challenge faced by every family with sexually maturing youth. In addition to providing developmentally appropriate sexual health education for middle school youth, SSS is positioned to mitigate the discomfort and uncertainty of parents who lack the confidence or skills to adequately provide effective information and skills training to help their children make healthy and responsible decisions about healthy friendships, dating relationships, and sex.

The efficacy of SSS in altering parent–child communication and behavioral intentions to delay initiation of sex is currently being assessed in a randomized controlled field trial with 80 parent–youth (11 to 14 years) dyads. This project addresses a significant public health problem by focusing on the gap between the needs of families in preparing their sexually maturing youth and the developmentally appropriate intervention resources currently available to support them. This work contributes to the dearth of research on the application of intergenerational games to address home-based life skills training to impact pregnancy prevention for middle school youth mediated by parental involvement.

Acknowledgments

This research was funded by NIH/CICHD grant #1R42HD074324. We extend our appreciation to the parents and youth who contributed to the development of SSS.

References

1. D'Cruz J, Santa Maria D, Dube S, et al. Promoting parent–child sexual health dialogue with an intergenerational game: parent and youth perspectives. *Games Health J.* 2015;4(2):113–122. doi: 10.1089/g4h.2014.0080.

2. Kost K, Henshaw S. US teenage pregnancies, births and abortions, 2010: national and state trends by age, race and ethnicity. Guttmacher Institute; 2014. https://www.guttmacher.org/sites/default/files/report_pdf/ustptrends10.pdf.

3. Kann L, Kinchen S, Shanklin SL, et al. Youth risk behavior surveillance—United States, 2013. *MMWR.* 2014;63 (suppl 4):1–168.

4. Landry DJ, Singh S, Darroch JE. Sexuality education in fifth and sixth grades in US public schools, 1999. *Fam Plan Persp.* 2000;32(5):212–219.

5. Mueller TE, Gavin LE, Kulkarni A. The association between sex education and youth's engagement in sexual intercourse, age at first intercourse, and birth control use at first sex. *J Adolesc Health.* 2008;42(1):89–96.

(continues)

6. Kirby D. The impact of schools and school programs upon adolescent sexual behavior. *J Sex Res*. 2002;39(1):27–33.

7. Kirby D, Lepore G. Sexual risk and protective factors: factors affecting teen sexual behavior pregnancy childbearing and sexually transmitted disease: which are important? which can you change? National Campaign To Prevent Teen and Unplanned Pregnancy; 2005. http://www.thenationalcampaign.org/ea2007/protective_factors_FULL.pdf.

8. Resnick MD, Bearman PS, Blum RW, et al. Protecting adolescents from harm: findings from the National Longitudinal Study on Adolescent Health. *JAMA*. 1997;278(10):823–832.

9. Sieving RE, McNeely CS, Blum RW. Maternal expectations, mother–child connectedness, and adolescent sexual debut. *Arch Pediatr Adolesc Med*. 2000;154(8):809–816.

10. Borawski EA, Ievers-Landis CE, Lovegreen LD, Trapl ES. Parental monitoring, negotiated unsupervised time, and parental trust: the role of perceived parenting practices in adolescent health risk behaviors. *J Adolesc Health*. 2003;33(2):60–70.

11. Cohen DA, Farley TA, Taylor SN, Martin DH, Schuster MA. When and where do youths have sex? The potential role of adult supervision. *Pediatrics*. 2002;110(6):e66.

12. McNeely C, Shew ML, Beuhring T, Sieving R, Miller BC, Blum RW. Mothers' influence on the timing of first sex among 14-and 15-year-olds. *J Adolesc Health*. 2002;31(3):256–265.

13. Beckett MK, Elliott MN, Martino S, et al. Timing of parent and child communication about sexuality relative to children's sexual behaviors. *Pediatrics*. 2010;125(1):34–42.

14. Katherine Hutchinson M, Wood EB. Reconceptualizing adolescent sexual risk in a parent–based expansion of the theory of planned behavior. *J Nurs Scholar*. 2007;39(2):141–146.

15. Villarruel AM, Loveland-Cherry CJ, Ronis DL. Testing the efficacy of a computer-based parent–adolescent sexual communication intervention for Latino parents. *Fam Relations*. 2010;59(5):533–543.

16. Turnbull T, van Schaik P, Van Wersch A. Exploring the role of computers in sex and relationship education within British families. *Cyberpsychol Behav Soc Network*. 2013;16(4):309–314.

17. Lustria MLA, Cortese J, Noar SM, Glueckauf RL. Computer-tailored health interventions delivered over the Web: review and analysis of key components. *Patient Educ Counsel*. 2009;74(2):156–173.

18. Pappa D, Dunwell I, Protopsaltis A, Pannese H, de Freitas S, Rebolledo-Mendez G. Game-based learning for knowledge sharing and transfer: the e-VITA approach for intergenerational learning. In: Felicia P, ed. *Handbook of Research on Improving Learning and Motivation through Educational Games: Multidisciplinary Approaches*. Hershey, PA: Information Science Reference (an imprint of IGI Global), 2011.

19. Akers AY, Holland CL, Bost J. Interventions to improve parental communication about sex: a systematic review. *Pediatrics*. 2011;127(3):494–510.

20. Burrus B, Leeks KD, Sipe TA, et al. Person-to-person interventions targeted to parents and other caregivers to improve adolescent health: a Community Guide systematic review. *Am J Prev Med*. 2012;42(3):316–326.

21. Wight D, Fullerton D. A review of interventions with parents to promote the sexual health of their children. *J Adolesc Health*. 2013;52(1):4–27.

22. Downing J, Jones L, Bates G, Sumnall H, Bellis MA. A systematic review of parent and family-based intervention effectiveness on sexual outcomes in young people. *Health Educ Res*. 2011;26(5):808–833.

23. Guilamo-Ramos V, Lee JJ, Kantor LM, Levine DS, Baum S, Johnsen J. Potential for using online and mobile education with parents and adolescents to impact sexual and reproductive health. *Prevent Sci*. 2014:1–8.

24. Itō M. *Hanging Out, Messing Around, and Geeking Out: Kids Living and Learning with New Media*. Cambridge, MA: MIT Press; 2010.

25. Shegog R, Brown K, Bull S, et al. Serious games for sexual health: roundtable discussion. *Games Health J*. 2015;4(2):69–77. doi: 10.1089/g4h.2014.0139.

26. DeSmet A, Shegog R, Van Ryckeghem D, Crombez G, Baranowski T, De Bourdeaudhuij I. A systematic meta-analytic review of serious digital games for sexual health promotion. *Games Health J*. 2015;4(2):78–90. doi: 10.1089/g4h.2014.0110.

27. Evans AE, Edmundson-Drane EW, Harris KK. Computer-assisted instruction: an effective instructional method for HIV prevention education? *J Adolesc Health*. 2000;26(4):244–251.

28. Kiene SM, Barta WD. A brief individualized computer-delivered sexual risk reduction intervention increases HIV/AIDS preventive behavior. *J Adolesc Health*. 2006;39(3):404–410.

29. Kirby D. *Innovative Approaches to Increase Parent–Child Communication About Sexuality: Their Impact and Examples from the Field*. New York, NY: Sexuality Information and Education Council of the United States; 2002.

30. Paperny DM, Starn JR. Adolescent pregnancy prevention by health education computer games: computer-assisted instruction of knowledge and attitudes. *Pediatrics*. 1989;83(5):742–752.

31. Tortolero SR, Markham CM, Peskin MF, et al. It's Your Game: keep it real: delaying sexual behavior with an effective middle school program. *J Adolesc Health*. 2010;46(2):169–179.

32. Markham CM, Tortolero S, Peskin MF, et al. Sexual risk avoidance and sexual risk reduction interventions for middle school youth: a randomized controlled trial. *J Adolesc Health*. 2012;50;279–288.

33. Shegog R, Peskin MF, Markham C, et al. "It's Your Game-Tech": toward sexual health in the digital age. *Creative Educ*. 2014;5(15):1428–1447. http://dx.doi.org/10.4236/ce.2014.515161.

34. Peskin MF, Shegog R, Markham CM, et al. Efficacy of It's Your Game-Tech: a computer-based sexual health education program for middle school youth. *J Adolesc Health*. 2015;56(5):515–521. doi: 10.1016/j.jadohealth.2015.01.001.

35. Voida A, Greenberg S. Collocated intergenerational console gaming. *Universal Access in the Information Society*. 2009:1–24.

36. Voida A, Greenberg S. Console gaming across generations: exploring intergenerational interactions in collocated console gaming. *Universal Access in the Information Society*. 2012;11(1):45–56.

37. Derboven J, Van Gils M, De Grooff D. Designing for collaboration: a study in intergenerational social game design. *Universal Access in the Information Society*. 2012;11(1):57–65.

38. Chen Y, Wen J, Xie B. "I communicate with my children in the game": mediated intergenerational family relationships through a social networking game. *J Community Informatics [Online]*. 2012;8(1).

39. Chiong C. *Can video games promote intergenerational play and literacy learning*. Paper presented at Joan Ganz Cooney Center at Sesame Workshop; 2009.

40. Othlinghaus J, Gerling KM, Masuch M. Intergenerational play: exploring the needs of children and elderly. Paper presented at Mensch & Computer Workshopband; 2011.

41. Rice M, Tan WP, Ong J, Yau LJ, Wan M, Ng J. The dynamics of younger and older adult's paired behavior when playing an interactive silhouette game. In: *Proceedings of the SIGCHI Conference on Human Factors in Computing Systems*; 2013.

42. Bandura A. *Social Foundations of Thought and Action: A Social Cognitive Theory*. Englewood Cliffs, NJ: Prentice-Hall; 1986.

43. Flay BR, Petratis J. The theory of triadic influence: a new theory of health behavior with implications for preventive interventions. In Albrecht GS, ed. *Advances in Medical Sociology: A Reconsideration of Models of Behavior Change*, Vol. IV. Greenwich, CT: JAI Press; 1994:19–44.

44. Perry CL. *Creating Health Behavior Change: How to Develop Community-Wide Programs for Youth*. Thousand Oaks, CA: Sage; 1999.

45. Komro KA, Perry CL, Williams CL, Stigler MH, Farbakhsh K, Veblen-Mortenson S. How Did Project Northland reduce alcohol use among young adolescents? Analysis of mediating variables. *Health Educ Res*. 2001;16:59–70. http://dx.doi.org/10.1093/her/16.1.59.

46. Lepper MR, Malone TW. Intrinsic motivation and instructional effectiveness in computer-based education. In: Snow RE, Farr MJ, eds. *Aptitude, Learning, and Instruction, III. Conative and Affective Process Analysis*. Hillsdale, NJ: Lawrence Erlbaum; 1987:255–286.

47. Bartholomew LK, Parcel GS, Kok G, Gottlieb N. *Planning Health Promotion Programs: An Intervention Mapping Approach*. 3rd ed. San Francisco, CA: Jossey-Bass; 2011.

48. Ceglio L. *The Secret of Seven Stones: applying intervention mapping for the development of an intergenerational, online game to prevent HIV/STI and pregnancy in middle-school youth*. Thesis for master of public health, University of Texas School of Public Health; 2015.

Courtesy of Ross Shegog. Acknowledgements: This research was funded by NIH/CICHD grant # 1R42HD074324 and with appreciation to the parents and youth you contributed SSS development.

application in a teen gaming intervention, known as *The Secret of Seven Stones* (SSS). While the game was constructed using social cognitive, norming, and other psychological theories, children get to actively test their resilience to suggestions to behave against their wishes while playing the game—theoretically inoculating them against the effects of such influence in their real lives.

Extended Parallel Process Model

Humans are motivated to minimize fear. In turn, communications that attempt to scare people into action can backfire due to the effects that Witte described in the Extended Parallel Process Model (EPPM).[26] When presented with information about a threat, people initiate two parallel lines of thinking: (1) Am I susceptible to this threat and how dangerous is it to me? (based on the Health Belief Model) and (2) Is there an action I know that I can take to avoid this threat?

This second track is based not only on knowledge of a tactic to avoid the threat, but also self-efficacy in performing it. If people do not believe that they can side-step the threat, they might justify inaction in this circumstance by telling themselves that the threat does not pertain to them or is not especially serious, or they may ignore information about the threat all together.

The EPPM is used extensively to develop risk and emergency messages.[27] Describing an unusual use of the model, **BOX 8-4** summarizes an analysis by Emery and colleagues, who evaluated tweets about the CDC's Tips from Former Smokers campaign. They concluded that viewers who tweeted about the campaign did not reject or dismiss the information despite its graphic and emotionally charged content. To some extent, it is possible that the concept of message sensation value (discussed next in this section) might be driving the extensive uptake of this information by young people.

BOX 8-4 "Are You Scared Yet?": Analyzing Tweets About Tips

Emery et al. looked at tweets about the CDC's Tips from Former Smokers campaign using Witte's Extended Parallel Process Model as their theoretical framework. While fear appeals are popular in public health, the EPPM suggests that some level of concern is necessary for people to pay attention to a health message, but if people are too frightened, self-protective "deflector shields" may go up so that the message is ignored. According to Emery et al., "The Tips campaign contained high levels of fear appeals represented by graphic descriptions of health effects such as cancer, facial damage, stoma, amputation and hair loss." The researchers examined tweets to see if the right balance of scaring people just enough to react and not tune out the message was attained.

The researchers obtained their data through Gnip, Inc. (http://www.gnip.com), which was licensed to provide access to the entire corpus of Twitter data, using a data-streaming process referred to as the "Firehose." According to Emergy et al., "Firehose provides real-time access to 100% of all tweets and metadata. Potentially relevant tweets were filtered from the Firehose using a broad set of content-specific keywords, following methods proposed by Stryker and colleagues (Stryker, Wray, Hornik, & Yanovitzky, 2006)." This study design required a team of six researchers to preview the Tips ads prior to the campaign launch and develop a comprehensive keyword list. Trained coders also worked with machine classification to eliminate false-positives and to train a computer-based classifier.

Here are their reported results:

- After considerable filtering and analysis, there were 193,491 relevant tweets for the Tips campaign.
- Approximately 87% (167,867) of the Tips-relevant tweets were classified as message acceptance, 7% (14,281) as message rejection, and 6% (11,521) as message disregard. Thus a majority of Twitter messages related to Tips displayed a high perceived threat (94%) as opposed to a low perceived threat or disregard. Moreover, the results indicate that there was more message acceptance than message rejection among high-perceived threat tweets.
- This study provides strong evidence that the controversial Tips from Former Smokers campaign was neither rejected nor dismissed by viewers, despite its use of graphic and emotionally evocative imagery and themes. A corpus of 193,491 Tips-relevant tweets was collected during the course of the 2012 campaign, and the vast majority of these tweets reflected message acceptance.
- This research provides strong evidence that Twitter reactions to Tips gave the campaign life beyond the ads; each of the nearly 200,000 tweets about the campaign created a ripple effect that extended the ads' reach. Beyond that, Emery et al.'s study showed that the graphic emotional approach employed by Tips had the desired result of jolting the audience into a thought process that might have some impact on future behavior.

Highlights and interpretations of: Emery SL, Szczypka G, Abril EP Kim Y, Vera L. Are you Scared Yet?: Evaluating Fear Appeal Messages in Tweets about the Tips Campaign. *J Commun.* 2014; 64: 278–295.

(Media) Uses and Gratifications Theory

Uses and gratifications theory (UGT), which was first introduced by Lasswell in 1948, is seeing a resurgence of interest in the face of the new media options available today. UGT looks at the full range of social needs and wants for which people use media. For example, in an in-depth study involving 25 self-identified social media consumers, Whiting and Williams identified 10 uses and gratifications: social interaction (88%), information seeking (80%), pass time (76%), entertainment (64%), relaxation (60%), communicatory utility (56%), expression of opinions (56%), convenience utility (52%), information sharing (40%), and surveillance and watching of others (20%).[28] In public health, health communicators tend to view media channels as merely conduits for bringing information to recipients, whereas media users are more purposeful in selecting media to gratify a range of needs and desires—and being informed is only one of those rationales (*Call of Duty*, anyone?).

Message Sensation Value and Sensation Seeking

The theory of message sensation value and sensation seeking is related to UGT; indeed, one of the early proponents of UGT (Palmgreen) played a key role in its development. University of Kentucky researchers are associated closely with the work in this area, and have described the concepts as well as some recent work with this theory to enhance antidrug messages for youth. Here is an excerpt from their longer piece, which appears in **APPENDIX 8A**:

> According to Harrington et al., sensation seeking is defined as "the seeking of varied, novel, complex, and intense sensations and experiences, and the willingness to take physical, social, legal, and financial risks for the sake of such experience"... The activation model of information exposure... guides an approach to designing messages for audiences that seek stimulation... If audience members do not reach and maintain an "optimal level of arousal" from watching a message—if it is too boring or too overwhelming—they probably will stop watching and look for something more suited to their needs. If the message does meet their needs for arousal, though, they probably will stick with it... High sensation seekers will prefer messages that are more arousing, while low sensation

seekers will not. The construct that captures a message's arousal potential is called message sensation value (MSV). MSV is defined as a message's ability to elicit sensory, affective, and arousal responses in audience members... High sensation value (HSV) messages should be novel, creative, intense, ambiguous, and suspenseful; low sensation value (LSV) messages should be more familiar, predictable, and clear.

Media Richness Theory

In 1984, Daft and Lengel introduced an information processing theory that describes the comparability of different communication channels in terms of their ability to convey complex or ambiguous information.[29] An ambiguous message can be interpreted in more than one way. As anyone who has used email or text messages knows, it is challenging to convey what you really mean in such a "lean" medium—hence the introduction of emoticons to signal the intended tone of messages. For a sender and a receiver to truly understand each other, they need to interpret symbols and words in the same way. For this reason, messages that are more complex or ambiguous are best communicated through a medium that allows for inclusion of more clues as to what the sender intends. In contrast, messages that are derived from a cultural consensus can be communicated effectively through a lean medium—for example, a stop sign.

FIGURE 8-3 shows a set of criteria for media richness. Later we will discuss ways to combine media richness with the theory of gratification and uses so as to select appropriate media channels for interventions.

▶ Applying Theory to Practice Strategies

According to Rimer and Glanz, "Because different theoretical frameworks are appropriate and practical for different situations, selecting a theory that 'fits' should be a careful, deliberate process."[6(p6)] You might really love social cognitive theory, for example, but that does not mean this theory is appropriate in every circumstance. Before applying a specific framework, you need to ask if that theory is "logical, consistent with everyday observations, similar to those used in previous successful programs, and supported by research in the same or related areas."[6(p7)] It is also essential to apply theories to the correct level of the

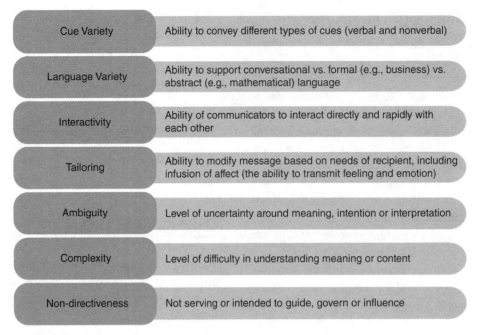

Cue Variety	Ability to convey different types of cues (verbal and nonverbal)
Language Variety	Ability to support conversational vs. formal (e.g., business) vs. abstract (e.g., mathematical) language
Interactivity	Ability of communicators to interact directly and rapidly with each other
Tailoring	Ability to modify message based on needs of recipient, including infusion of affect (the ability to transmit feeling and emotion)
Ambiguity	Level of uncertainty around meaning, intention or interpretation
Complexity	Level of difficulty in understanding meaning or content
Non-directiveness	Not serving or intended to guide, govern or influence

FIGURE 8-3 Media Richness

The Health Communication Capacity Collaborative HC3. (2014) A theory-based framework for media selection in demand generation programs. Baltimore: Johns Hopkins Bloomberg School of Public Health Center for Communication Programs. p:10 (USAID government doc.)

ecological model: individual (intrapersonal) change, interpersonal change (i.e., dyads or group dynamics) or societal change.

Intervention Mapping

According to intervention mapping (IM), **theory-based methods** are derived from empirical research on how changes in the behavior of individuals or groups occur. Individual studies use theory in different ways, creating theory-informed methods. One example of a theory-informed method is using "vicarious learning" (i.e., learning from another's experience) to promote constructs from social cognitive theory.

A **practice strategy** delivers a particular method in an intervention. For example, role-model stories, which are identified as a form of **entertainment education (EE)**, are practice strategies built upon the construct of vicarious learning from social cognitive theory. Practice strategies can also be delivered through activities (or channels)—for example, plays mounted by community theater groups, photo-novels, or radio or television soap operas. Specific media (the play, the picture novel, the radio or TV script and production) will then be created to implement these activities.

TABLE 8-4 provides some examples that highlight the distinctions between theoretical methods, practice strategies, and activities or channels.

From Theory-Based Methods to Practice Strategies

Participatory Approach

Botta et al.'s hand-washing case study provides a good example of how investigators might choose a theory-based method to suit what they learned in their formative research. **BOX 8-5** describes these researchers' choice of the Theory of Planned Behavior (TPB)—in particular, the "norming" of a little practiced behavior. They also selected a highly participatory approach to build sustainability into the program that they developed.

Entertainment Education

Since the mid-1970s, extensive work has been done with entertainment education (EE),[30] beginning with Miguel Sabido's development of *telenovelas* aired in Mexico based on his analysis of the hugely popular Peruvian television soap opera known as *Simplemente María*. Singhal and Rogers have defined entertainment education as "the process of purposely designing and implementing a media message both to entertain and educate, in order to increase audience members' knowledge about an educational issue, create favorable attitudes, and change overt behavior. Entertainment-education seeks to capitalize on the appeal of popular media to show individuals how they can live safer, healthier, and happier lives."[30]

TABLE 8-4 Theoretical Methods, Practice Strategies, and Activities

Theory-Based Method	Practice Strategy	Activity/Channels
Vicarious learning	Education entertainment	Role-model narrated stories, photo-novels, TV or radio serial drama, social media posts
Extended parallel process (fear + ease of solution)	Risk communication raising fear of outcome (e.g., skin cancer) and ease of solution (e.g., sunscreen)	TV, radio, and print public service announcements (PSAs) or native advertising in social media
Elaboration Likelihood Model	Targeting of peripheral cues consisting of images, music, channels, or spokespersons Tailoring to individual criteria	Neighborhood outdoor advertising; targeted print, radio, or TV stations Personalized letters, materials, and interactions; patient navigation, tailoring, and social media channels
Stage-based behavioral adoption	Motivational interviewing; goal setting and rewards	In-person, phone, or online counseling sessions between a trained counselor and a client; group meetings (Alcoholics Anonymous, Weight Watchers); criteria-based texting
Norming (bring attention to actual normative behavior versus perception of minority behavior as norm)—particularly for youth	Education entertainment, buzz (viral) marketing	Channel-specific programming (e.g., MTV, VH1, YouTube, Facebook)
Agenda setting (media such as TV) influences public perception of subject proportional to air-time devoted to subject	Media advocacy, public relations	Radio or TV appearances by leaders, personalities; organization of real or phony (e.g., Astro-Turf) grassroots demonstrations
Self-efficacy for skills	Breaking complex behavior into smaller steps	Do-it-yourself episodes, youth media channels, online communities, rewards programs
Diffusion of innovation; positive deviance	Target to early adopters; train-the-trainer models	Agricultural extension, online media, group "sensitization" through community organization partnerships

BOX 8-5 Theory-Based Methods: Practice Strategies

Renée A. Botta, PhD, Kelly Fenson-Hood, MA, Leah Scandurra, MA, Rina Muasya, MA Candidate

Abstracted from *A Campaign to Sustain Hand Washing Behaviors in an Urban Informal Settlement in Kenya*

Behavior Change Theories Used in the Development of the Campaign

The development of the campaign included the use of the Theory of Planned Behavior (TPB),[1] which seeks to explain how and why behavior change occurs by focusing on a set of key beliefs related to the desired behavior that, as a set, predict intentions to perform the behavior. By increasing positive attitudes, subjective norms, and perceived control about a particular behavior, TPB predicts there will be a subsequent increase in the intention to perform that behavior, which will lead to the adoption of the behavior.[1,2] Attitudes about the behavior follow from beliefs about the behavior's

(continues)

BOX 8-5 Theory-Based Methods: Practice Strategies   *(continued)*

likely consequences. Subjective norms follow from normative expectations from important others about performing the behavior. Perceived behavioral control follows from the presence of factors that control behavioral performance.

How important others see the behavior constitutes a normative belief. For example, do those important to the target audience believe hand washing is a good idea? Do they use proper hand washing techniques? How motivated is the target audience to comply with these important other people's beliefs about proper hand washing?

Control beliefs are the extent to which the target audience believes the issue is in their control and that they have the ability to properly wash their hands. It is necessary to determine their barriers to hand washing. Other theorists and behavior change specialists use a similar concept called self-efficacy, which has been defined as the confidence in one's own ability to carry out a behavior.

Behavioral beliefs are the target audience's attitudes about the behavior and its outcomes. For example, what do they expect to occur as a result of doing the desired behavior? These attitudes can be either positive or negative. For example, audience members could believe proper hand washing reduces diarrhea (positive) or they could believe proper hand washing wastes precious water (negative).

TPB suggests that if control beliefs, behavioral beliefs, and normative beliefs are all positive, the target audience should have a positive intention to perform the behavior—in this case, proper hand washing—and that increased intentions will lead to increased performance of the behavior. Thus, if we can establish positive normative expectations, ensure positive outcome evaluations, and reduce barriers to practicing hand hygiene, then we should be able to increase hand hygiene practices within the community.

…

Practice Strategies

Train-the-trainer sessions were conducted with community health workers and focused on hygiene KAP (knowledge, attitudes, practices) and health behavior change activities. Health messages and communications reinforced this training.

We worked with Kenya's Ministry of Health (MOH) to develop the training. MOH chose 10 of its community health education workers to participate in a week-long workshop in which we developed the training, which was designed to operate in an interactive and small-group format. A key tool involved in completing the training was a set of picture cards created by a local artist utilizing local visual cues about situations and behaviors within the community. Each set contained 50 cards to allow for a variety of responses to the various training cues. Activities were structured using the drawings, creating stories, and group discussions. We also created hygiene manuals for the trainers, which were written in English and in Kiswahili (the local language). Our head trainer was Kenyan and thus fluent in Kiswahili, and was helpful in not just translating the manual but making sure it was culturally appropriate.

According to Tufte and Mefalopulos, "Public participation is based on the belief that those who are affected by a decision have a right to be involved in the decision-making process. Public participation is the process by which an organization consults with interested or affected individuals, organizations, and government entities before making a decision. Public participation is two-way communication and collaborative problem solving with the goal of achieving better and more acceptable decisions."[3] These authors argue that participatory communication strategies are more likely to result in (1) increased feelings of ownership of a problem and a commitment to do something about it; (2) improvement of competencies and capacities required to engage with the defined development problem; and (3) actual influence on institutions that can affect an individual or community. Participatory communication emphasizes involving the stakeholders in the development process and the process of determining outcomes, rather than imposing pre-established (i.e., already decided by external actors) outcomes and processes.[3] "It requires academic members to become part of the community and community members to become part of the research team, thereby creating a unique working and learning environment before, during, and after the research."[3]

An advantage of participatory communication is that it takes into account four (rather than one) quadrants of knowledge in building communication campaigns. The Johari Window, proposed by Joseph Luft and Harry Ingham, and described by Tufte and Mefalopulos,[3] suggests the first quadrant involves dialogue based on the common knowledge shared by all parties, The second quadrant represents knowledge of the local players who have a stake in the campaign, which is not known by the outside experts. The third quadrant is knowledge from the outside experts that is shared with local stakeholders. The final quadrant represents that which is unknown to both groups. At this point, the knowledge, experiences, and skills of key stakeholders and campaign developers come together to develop the most appropriate options and solutions that will lead to the desired change.

When the team of outside academic experts and local MOH experts had completed the development of the hygiene training, a manual was written in both English and Kiswahili to facilitate a simpler process in conducting the trainings. The hygiene training consisted of five steps, each which included two or more group activities.

The first step is problem identification, in which groups talk about diarrhea-related health problems in the community and discuss potential solutions to the health problems. The purpose of the first activity was to enable the community health workers to identify important diarrhea-related issues and problems in their community. The purpose of the second activity was to enable the community health worker participants to identify methods for solving diarrhea-related issues and problems facing their community.

The second step in the training is problem analysis and consists of two hand-hygiene activities. The step also includes a safe water activity and sanitation practices activity, which are part of the larger project rather than the focus of this case study about hand hygiene. These activities are designed to enable the community health worker participants to closely examine common hygiene practices. Through this examination, participants identify normative practices in the community and discuss how practices may be good or bad for health, as well as the advantages and disadvantages of each practice. In the first activity of this step, the community health workers discuss what they believe constitute all kinds of good and bad hygiene behaviors. In the second activity, they discuss hand hygiene more specifically; in the third activity, they discuss safe water use; and in the fourth activity, they discuss community sanitation practices.

The third step is planning for solutions and includes an activity focused on identifying the spread of disease, an activity in which the community health worker participants discuss blocking the spread of disease, an activity focused on barriers to blocking the spread of disease, and an activity in which they discuss ways to overcome those barriers. These activities are focused on their community—how they see disease being spread within their community, potential ways to block the spread of disease within their community, and recognizing and finding solutions for the barriers that people in their community face for stopping the spread of diarrheal disease. Participants analyze the effectiveness of the behaviors that block disease transmission and discuss how easy or difficult the behaviors are to practice in their daily lives in their community.

The final activity in this step is making hygiene messages. It is meant to help participants identify how to introduce, encourage, and reinforce positive hygiene behaviors in the community. Groups develop songs that incorporate hand hygiene guidelines, and they create posters using local artists' renditions to spread the word about hand hygiene, safe water practices, and hygienic sanitation practices…. The community health worker participants create hygiene posters by thinking through what they would say to others to help motivate and remind them to practice good hygiene behaviors. They are given a set of large posters with locally drawn pictures that correspond to hygiene in the community. Groups choose pictures they think will work best for posters and request additional pictures they would like to see drawn. Finally, they write their messages on them. The messages are then placed on the pictures via computer program and returned to the community health workers to serve as hygiene promotion posters displayed in the community for the remainder of the campaign.

Step four is demonstrating hygiene guidelines and practices. There are four main purposes of this step. The first is hand and water hygiene education. The second is to work with participants in making their own portable hand washing station, known as a leaky tin. The third is to work with participants to make their own safe water storage container and demonstrate water purification techniques. The last purpose is to teach participants how to make liquid soap at a cost significantly cheaper than bar soap as a way to reduce the cost barrier for hand washing with soap.

Step five is planning for change. In this step, the community health worker participants develop their own single-day trainings, and discuss and practice peer education, motivational interviewing, and role playing. They are encouraged to use these communication techniques during their own training.

References

1. Ajzen I. The theory of planned behavior. *Org Behav Hum Decision Proc*. 1991;50(2):179–211.

2. Ajzen I. The theory of planned behavior. In: Lange PAM, Kruglanski AW, Higgins ET, eds. *Handbook of Theories of Social Psychology*, Vol. 1. London, UK: Sage; 2012:438–459.

3. Tufte T, Mefalopulos P. *Participatory Communication: A Practical Guide*. Washington, DC: World Bank Publications; 2009.

Abstracted from: A campaign to sustain hand washing behaviors in an urban informal settlement in Kenya. (See full case in Appendix 11A.)

The bulk of EE was done in international settings until nearly 20 years ago, when the CDC initiated its Hollywood, Health, and Society (HH&S) program. This program, which is managed by the Norman Lear Center of the University of Southern California (USC), has flourished and acquired a slate of philanthropic leaders (e.g., the Bill and Melinda Gates Foundation, the Barr Foundation) and organizations (National Cancer Institute, Substance Abuse and Mental Health Services Administration, California Endowment, and others) as funding partners.[31] In the spirit of EE, rather than writing out a full explanation, we suggest that you view Norman Lear Center Director and Chair in Entertainment, Media, and Society (USC) Martin Kaplan's YouTube video[32] "Tell Me a Science." As "Marty" says, "You don't bring a data set to a food fight"—a shorthand way of saying that scientists need to tell their stories more dramatically if they are to capture the hearts and minds of the public.

In public health, EE interventions have ranged from school and community theater productions, to embedded storylines in national prime-time and daytime dramas, to radio dramas, to Internet serial episodes. This broad range is evidenced by the winners of the Sentinel Awards, which HH&S bestows on an annual basis. While narrative lies at the heart of EE, this approach has evolved into an "immersive engagement for behavior change model" (**BOX 8-6**) to support trans-media storytelling.

Note that "immersive engagement" is closely linked to the uses and gratifications theory of media consumption—EE is powerful because people want to be deeply immersed and engaged by a story. All in all, entertainment education is an extremely powerful practice strategy for transforming society—perhaps the most enduring one in human civilization.

Elaboration Likelihood Model Applications

After do-it-yourself (or participatory) approaches and entertainment education, applications of the Elaboration Likelihood Model (ELM) are the most ubiquitous types of messages used in health communication. The ELM is the cornerstone of targeting and tailoring, based on the simple finding that in small media, such as newsletters and brochures, people pay more attention to speakers and situations that resemble themselves when they do not yet identify with the subject matter. In contrast, in big media, such as movies and television, viewers tend to prefer "lifestyles of the rich and famous" to storylines that echo their own lives. The ELM also predicts that people who are not attracted to information along a primary route (i.e., the message) may be attracted along a peripheral route with which they identify. This can be a variation in any other element in the content/message/channel mix.

Demographic Targeting As a media channel strategy, targeting is still widely used in both commercial and social marketing. In the United States, some radio,

---

BOX 8-6   The Immersive Engagement for Change Model

Nedra Weinreich (http://social-marketing.com/immersive-engagement.html) has laid out the elements of Immersive Engagement that need to be present for a story to be optimized for behavior change:

- *Behavior change model.* Start by identifying which action you want the audience to take as a result of being engaged and motivated, and how you intend to get there. By using a proven individual or social change model, you will have a framework for what you need to include in the experience to effectively motivate the adoption of the key actions. In a long-term, story-centered project, you can follow the Sabido method, which has been used successfully for decades to drive development of entertainment education content and brings together behavioral, communication, and learning theories, or you can apply other relevant models.
- *Good storytelling.* Engagement starts with a good story; without that element, the rest of the pieces will fall flat. A good story does not just mean an issue that you feel is important for people to know about. Give a lot of thought to who the key characters are, what the conflict is, how the story arc will play out, and how best to present different parts of the narrative for maximum effect. Otherwise, your audience will lose interest in your project.
- *Ubiquitous media.* By offering your content in the places where the audience members are already spending their time, your story can become seamlessly integrated into their day. In addition, your selected platforms must work together to support the story strategically and synergistically based on their strengths and weaknesses, and how your audience uses them.
- *Participatory experience.* Design opportunities for the audience to go beyond just consuming what you create—that is, enable them to participate by interacting with the content or even submitting their own contributions to the story. Though most will likely prefer to watch from the outside, giving those who are most enthusiastic about the project ways to join in will deepen their immersion. This could include activities such as playing an online game that moves the narrative forward, interacting with characters, connecting with others via a discussion forum to talk about the project, or sharing their own real stories.
- *Real world.* Ideally, the audience should be able to draw the lessons from the story world and apply them to their own lives. This may involve using skills demonstrated in the story, finding local resources such as a medical clinic or community-based organization that provides assistance, or joining a movement to take action on issues portrayed in the story. Your project can connect them to those opportunities.

Weinreich N, 2014, http://social-marketing.com/immersive-engagement.html.

television, Internet, and print media reach out *exclusively* to children (of all ages), whereas others target a spectrum of adults from first-time parents to seniors. Media may also be segmented by gender identity, ethnic identity, and language (there are approximately 50 different in-language media). And, of course, there are media dedicated to special-interest, narrowly focused topics (from *Aikido* to zippers). But how different are the message and creative strategies developed for these different media and channels?

In the early days of advertising, little was done to actually change the "creative" (images, copy, sound) component that went out to different media. The effectiveness of *ethnic target marketing*, however, soon made itself clear to commercial advertisers. Whether advertisers were selling niche products (e.g., cosmetics or hair care products designed to meet the needs and desires of a specific market) or mass-market products, the positive return on investment they enjoyed supported this form of targeting.

Public health was another story, however. Program managers questioned whether audience segments were large enough to warrant using different media and channels, and whether they could be reached effectively by these means. More often than desired, a multi-ethnic campaign was created because the use of differentiated media, from production to dissemination, was too expensive for public health communicators.

Partnership Strategies In response to this dilemma, the National Diabetes Education Program (NDEP) created a partnership stakeholder model that is still in use today.[33] NDEP originally worked with representatives of minority-serving organizations to create media strategies and products that would resonate the most strongly with these distinct audiences. This effort has evolved into an open invitation for collaborators. While multimedia materials for different demographic and ethnic groups can still be accessed from the NDEP website, the organization's "Stories About Managing Diabetes" feature individuals with distinctly different ethnic identities who share their key characteristics, such as their favorite healthy foods and their weaknesses, and narrate a podcast. In addition, NDEP has developed many materials specifically for teens and children with diabetes.[34]

Make It Your Own More recently, the National Institutes of Health (NIH) helped create a wonderful resource to help programs and healthcare providers develop and send cancer prevention–related materials that can be customized based on several demographic and ethnic features. This "Make It Your Own" (MIYO) initiative is based at the Health Communication Research Laboratory at Washington University in St. Louis. MIYO is described further in **BOX 8-7**.

Behavioral Targeting Sometimes demographic distinctions are less important than behavioral intention, or having an illness or condition. For example, women who hope to become pregnant will pay attention to just about anything with a baby in it; women who are not thinking about procreation are likely to skip over the ads for prenatal vitamins, diapers, and the like. This behavior has been a challenge for health promotion programs that focus on "pre-conceptional health," including taking folic acid prior to conceiving to prevent neural tube defects, eating a healthy diet,

---

BOX 8-7 MIYO: A Communication Tool for Reducing Health Disparities

FIGURE 8-4

Health Communication Research Laboratory at the Brown School, Washington University in St. Louis.

Make It Your Own (MIYO; pronounced "mee-yo") is a web platform that allows users to customize evidence-based interventions to the different audiences whom they serve. Users can create a variety of small media and client reminders recommended by the Guide to Community Preventive Services,[1] and adapt them in a step-by-step manner by making choices about images, messages, and designs to be used. Applying concepts and tactics from the world of marketing, MIYO provides health-related organizations with a communication tool for reducing health disparities.

The MIYO Creed

MIYO's approach is guided by three key assumptions: (1) Every community is unique; (2) customizing interventions to match the unique characteristics of communities increases effectiveness; and (3) the individuals and organizations best

(continues)

suited to make customization decisions are those working in or with a local community. The theoretical and conceptual bases for MIYO follow from this philosophy, and reflect ideas from community development, marketing, and digital commerce.

Developed at the Health Communication Research Laboratory (HCRL) in 2007, MIYO has evolved significantly. The initial versions of MIYO were decidedly low-tech, with users selecting options from a printed catalogue. Today, MIYO is an online tool that offers a variety of modifiable design templates for posters, flyers, inserts, question cards, postcards, and web banners. Users select a template and follow a series of steps to customize their own communication products with a photo, a message, a call to action, and their agency's contact information and logo/branding. Using the MIYO tool, they can choose from large, diverse libraries of audience-tested messages and images. MIYO then renders a final, electronic document that users can download and distribute as printed or digital media.

Currently, MIYO supports five health topic areas: colorectal cancer screening, breast cancer screening, cervical cancer screening, human papilloma virus (HPV) vaccination, and tobacco cessation. Typical MIYO users include state and local public health agencies, government agencies, hospitals, community health centers, research centers, American Indian/Alaska Native tribal organizations, nonprofits, and other health organizations. An HCRL professional graphic design team creates the MIYO templates, thereby assuring that organizations and agencies with limited funding and/or technical expertise can still generate professionally designed materials. MIYO builds user capacity to implement high-quality, evidence-based interventions to promote health.

Evidence Base and Underlying Principles

MIYO uses Community Guide–recommended strategies for client- and provider-directed interventions to increase colorectal, breast, and cervical cancer screening through the use of small media and client reminders.[2,3] Small media such as checklists, letters, patient education materials, brochures, and newsletters both inform and motivate people to be screened for cancer, especially when they are targeted to specific populations. Client reminders such as postcards help providers and health agencies remind patients of important health screenings.

MIYO applies principles of community-based participatory research (CBPR) by promoting partnerships between organizations and the communities they serve; providing tools for target populations so that they can take an active role in planning interventions; and placing decision-making power in the hands of the community so members can shape priorities, share resources, and build capacity.[4–8] MIYO users control which products they make and how they shape interventions to meet the needs of the populations they serve. Having driven the decision-making process, users feel confident about using MIYO products in their communities.

MIYO also employs co-creation—a concept borrowed from business and marketing in which consumers become directly involved in constructing a product or service.[9] NikeID, a web-based system in which consumers build their own shoes by choosing everything from style to materials to colors, is a widely recognized example of this approach.[10,11] Because co-creation encourages consumers to become more intimately involved in the decision-making process, they are expected to have a stronger connection to the final product; be more engaged with, dedicated to, and satisfied by the brand; be more likely to share the product with others; and have an increased level of trust in the organization.[9,12–14] MIYO applies co-creation principles both to engage users in design decisions and to obtain feedback about how the system is used.

MIYO in Practice

Co-creation is evident not just in the simple process of creating a product within MIYO, but also in the ongoing partnership between users and the MIYO team. Diana Redwood, PhD, MPH, is the program director for the Alaska Native Tribal Health Consortium's (ANTHC's) Colorectal Cancer (CRC) Control Program and an early adopter of MIYO. ANTHC is a nonprofit organization that provides health services across Alaska in partnership with regional tribal health organizations. ANTHC's CRC Control Program works with seven regional tribal health organizations specifically on the prevention and control of CRC. When Redwood first introduced MIYO to her organizational partners, they were intrigued. The incidence rate for colorectal cancer is two times higher among Alaska Native people than among white Americans; moreover, CRC is the second leading cause of cancer-related deaths in these communities.[15] There was just one problem: The MIYO image library included only photos of American Indians from the lower 48 states—not photos of Alaska Native populations, who are culturally diverse. "The initial pictures of American Indians just didn't have the emotional impact that Alaskan photos would. Even a picture of someone from Southeast Alaska won't necessarily resonate with Alaska Native people from the Arctic coast, which is why it was so important to have pictures available from multiple Alaskan communities," said Redwood. When ANTHC brought this feedback to the Health Communication Research Laboratory, the HCRL quickly partnered with a local photographer to take appropriate photos across Alaska.

As Redwood noted, "We were able to get images that worked better for our context, and we brought it back to our organizations, saying, 'Hey look! Here are these great images, what do you think?'" ANTHC's partner organizations thought the photos were a major improvement and asked ANTHC for MIYO products to use with their communities.

First, the organizations decided that postcards and direct mail would be the most efficient way to reach their widespread patient populations. Then, staff from regional partner tribal health organizations reviewed the new photos on MIYO and selected images they thought would resonate with the communities they served. One photo included a group of women picking berries against an Alaskan landscape (**FIGURE 8-5**). ANTHC also selected reminder messages to prompt patients to schedule an appointment for colorectal cancer screening. Today, patient navigators continue to send the postcard in Figure 8-5 and other MIYO creations to patients. Redwood has found the postcards particularly useful at health fairs, where she asks attendees to write down their name and address on a postcard and offers to send it to them when they are eligible for screening. "We find that strategy is very effective for outreach," says Redwood, "a lot of times they're due for screening right then!"

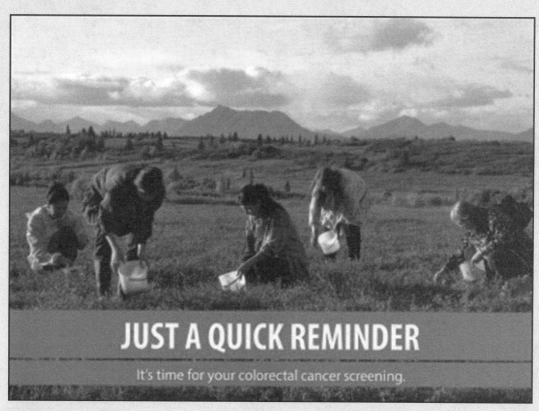

FIGURE 8-5 ANTHC used MIYO to create postcard reminders for Alaska Native clients to get screened for colorectal cancer.

Health Communication Research Laboratory at the Brown School, Washington University in St. Louis.

MIYO users hail from across the United States, representing diverse communities with unique preferences, strengths, and challenges. A MIYO user, for example, may need to create a cervical cancer screening insert for an audience that consists of primarily African-American women. After selecting an insert in MIYO, the user can narrow the system's numerous image options, selecting "African American," "30 to 49" years old, and an "outdoors" setting. MIYO then displays only the photos that fit these criteria. In this example, the user might choose an image of a young mother and her daughter. Next, the user chooses a message that will grab the attention of this target audience and convey the importance of cervical cancer screening. Given the chosen image, the user selects a message that uses a "family" theme. For the "call to action"— a short message highlighting a concrete step toward preventing cervical cancer—the user chooses a message urging the readers to get a Pap test. Finally, the user enters his or her contact information and uploads a logo to incorporate the local agency's brand. **FIGURE 8-6** shows an example of what a MIYO insert could look like for this population.

The same MIYO template—a "talk bubble insert" promoting cervical cancer screening—is used in Figures 8-7, 8-8, and 8-9, albeit customized for different populations. Another user might search for images that are "Hispanic or Latino,"

BOX 8-7 MIYO: A Communication Tool for Reducing Health Disparities *(continued)*

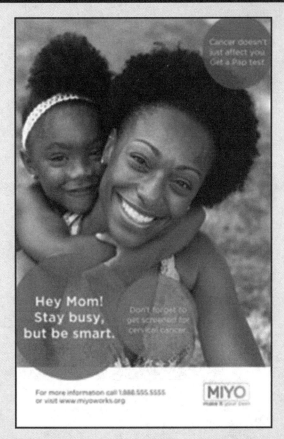

FIGURE 8-6 MIYO users narrow image searches to fit the criteria of their target audiences—in this case, African-American women from 30 to 49 years old.

Health Communication Research Laboratory at the Brown School, Washington University in St. Louis.

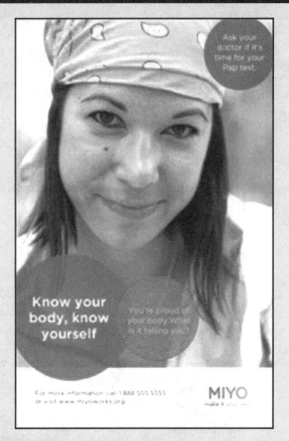

FIGURE 8-7 Using the same template as in Figure 8-6, a different user can create a cervical cancer screening tool for Hispanic and Latina populations.

Health Communication Research Laboratory at the Brown School, Washington University in St. Louis.

and "happy." **FIGURE 8-7** is a product with an image matching these criteria that encourages young Hispanic and Latina women to pay attention to what their bodies are telling them and get screened for cervical cancer.

In **FIGURE 8-8**, a MIYO user creates materials promoting cervical cancer screening that aim to reduce anxiety about cancer. Again, the overall design remains the same, but the content of the insert changes based on the needs of the different target audience.

These examples show just three possibilities for using a single template in MIYO. Given that MIYO offers 15 to 25 templates per health topic in numerous sizes and layouts and scores of images and message choices, the number of potential combinations quickly climb into the thousands.[16]

A Strategy for Addressing Health Disparities: The Long-Tail Effect

The "long tail" concept refers to a distribution of product sales in which a few blockbuster successes have wide appeal and generate substantial sales, followed by a much greater number of niche products, each of which has a narrower appeal and generates only nominal sales (i.e., the long tail of the distribution).[17] In many cases, the collective sales from these niche products in the long tail actually rival those of products with mass appeal. In public health, long-tail thinking can be applied to addressing health disparities, which disproportionately affect a long and diverse "tail" of "niche" populations whose needs may not be adequately met by a handful of approaches designed for the general population.[18]

Researchers from the HCRL applied long-tail analysis to MIYO data on products created from 2011 to 2013.[18] The analysis revealed that MIYO products in the popular, blockbuster "head" of the distribution were more likely to feature images of white subjects.[18] Meanwhile, images of people in minority groups and groups at higher risk for colorectal cancer were more likely to fall in the "long tail" (**FIGURE 8-9**).[18] As predicted, the images, messages, and products in the long tail combined to outnumber the most popular selections. MIYO's long-tail approach helps users address health disparities by making it just as easy to create evidence-based resources for underserved populations as for the masses.[18]

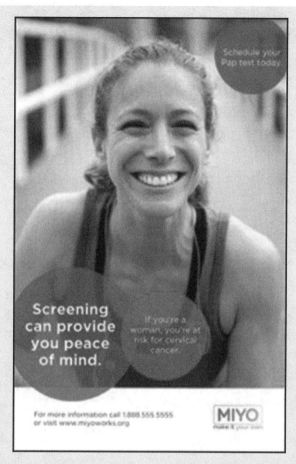

FIGURE 8-8 A third variant of the same MIYO template leads to a product focused on reducing anxiety about cervical cancer.

Health Communication Research Laboratory at the Brown School, Washington University in St. Louis.

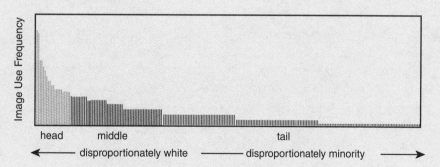

FIGURE 8-9 Race/Ethnicity of Images Used in MIYO Documents by Head, Middle, and Long Tail of the Distribution

Health Communication Research Laboratory at the Brown School, Washington University in St. Louis.

Next Steps

MIYO currently supports communications related to five cancer prevention and health promotion topics. Developers at the Health Communication Research Laboratory are actively expanding MIYO to other Community Guide– recommended interventions in areas such as vaccinations and injury prevention, and topic areas requested by MIYO users, such as clinical trial recruitment. HCRL researchers also aim to evaluate the system's impact on organizational practice and community-level outcomes. By combining technology, marketing principles, and evidence-based approaches, MIYO is building the capacity of organizations across the United States to prevent and control cancer and reduce health disparities.

(continues)

BOX 8-7 MIYO: A Communication Tool for Reducing Health Disparities *(continued)*

References

1. Zaza S, Briss PA, Harris KW. *The guide to community preventive services: What works to promote health?* New York, NY: Oxford University Press; 2005.

2. Task Force on Community Preventive Services. Recommendations for client- and provider-directed interventions to increase breast, cervical, and colorectal cancer screening. *Am J Prev Med*. 2008;35(1s):S21–S25.

3. Baron RC, Rimer BK, Coates RJ, et al. Client-directed interventions to increase community access to breast, cervical, and colorectal cancer screening: a systematic review. *Am J Prev Med*. 2008;35(1):S56–S66.

4. Minkler M, Wallerstein N. Introduction to community based participatory research. In: Minkler M, Wallerstein N, eds. *Community Based Participatory Research for Health*. San Francisco, CA: Jossey Bass; 2003:3–26.

5. Green L, George M. *Review and Recommendations for the Development of Participatory Research in Health Promotion in Canada*. Vancouver, BC: Royal Society of Canada; 1994.

6. Israel B, Schulz A, Parker E, Becker A. A review of community-based research: assessing partnership approaches to improve public health. *Annu Rev Public Health*. 1998;19:173–202.

7. Goodman R, Speers M, McLeroy K, et al. Identifying and defining the dimensions of community capacity to provide a basis for measurement. *Health Educ Behav*. 1998;25(3):258–278.

8. Israel B, Eng E, Schulz A, Parker E. *Methods in Community-Based Participatory Research for Health*. San Francisco, CA: Jossey-Bass; 2005.

9. Jaworski B, Kohli A. Co-creating the voice of the customer. In: Lusch RF, Vargo SL, eds. *The Service-Dominant Logic of Marketing: Dialog, Debate, and Directions*. Armonk, NY: M. E. Sharpe; 2006:109–117.

10. Ramaswamy V. Co-creating value through customers' experiences: the Nike case. *Strategy & Leadership*. 2008;36(5):9–14.

11. Sanders EB-N, Stappers PJ. Co-creation and the new landscapes of design. *CoDesign: International Journal of CoCreation in Design and the Arts*. 2008;4(1):5–18.

12. Prahalad CK, Ramaswamy V. Co-creation experiences: the next practice in value creation. *J Interactive Marketing*. 2004;18(3):5–14.

13. Ramaswamy V, Gouillart F. Building the co-creative enterprise. *Harvard Business Review*. 2010. http://hbr.org/2010/10/building-the-co-creative-enterprise/ar/1. Accesssed September 21, 2016.

14. Ramaswamy V, Gouillart F. *The Power of Co-Creation*. New York, NY: Free Press; 2010.

15. Kelly JJ, Alberts SR, Sacco F, Lanier AP. Colorectal cancer in Alaska Native people, 2005–2009. *Gastrointest Cancer Res*. 2012;5(5):149–164.

16. Kreuter MW, Fernandez ME, Brown M, et al. Increasing information-seeking about HPV vaccination through community partnerships in African American and Hispanic communities. *Fam Community Health*. 2012;35(1):15–30.

17. Anderson C. *The Long Tail: Why the Future of Business Is Selling Less of More*, 2nd ed. New York, NY: Hyperion; 2008.

18. Kreuter MW, Hovmand P, Pfeiffer DJ, et al. The "long tail" and public health: new thinking for addressing health disparities. *Am J Public Health*. 2014;104(12):2271–2278.

Health Communication Research Laboratory at the Brown School, Washington University in St. Louis.

and avoiding alcohol, drugs, or tobacco to give a baby and mother the best start.

In another example of how having an illness or condition affects attendance to health messages, women who have recently learned they have breast cancer usually pay little attention to the ethnicity of the person on the cover of a brochure. Instead, they prefer to see and hear from women of any background who have survived the disease.

Such differences based on behavior can be used to shape the messages delivered to consumers. As an

example, **FIGURE 8-10** shows a new CDC HIV risk-assessment tool that can be customized according to criteria related to HIV risk. With this tool, the information that is displayed is customized to the profile a user develops, including the terminology used to describe various circumstances.

In summary, targeting is a mass-media strategy. When we use targeting, we try to create materials that appeal to particular audience segments that share certain characteristics. The goal is that our intended audience will recognize themselves in these materials and

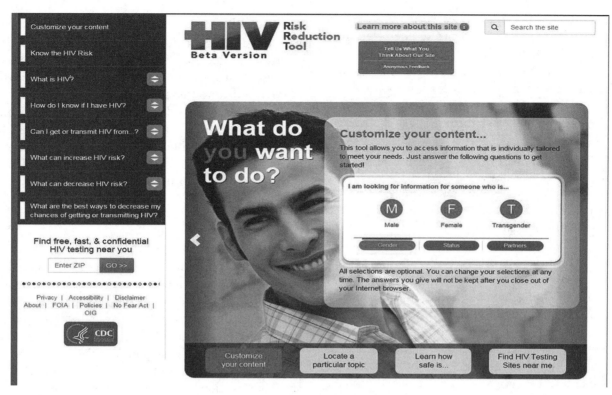

FIGURE 8-10 The CDC's Customizable HIV Risk-Assessment Tool

respond positively, even though we know that we will not reach everyone we planned to reach. At the same time, people whom we did not expect to identify with the messages and materials will also find them useful.

Tailoring

Rimer and Kreuter define tailoring as a process for creating individualized communications by gathering and assessing personal data related to a given health outcome so as to determine the most appropriate information or strategies to meet that person's unique needs.[35] Tailored material is shared with one individual through a direct channel, such as the mail, in-person interaction, the Internet, and, most commonly now, a smartphone. As Jensen et al.[36(p4)] explain:

> Perceived message relevance—the extent to which people view some communicative stimuli being related or applicable to a person and/or situation—has often been proposed as a key mediator of tailoring effects[37]... Tailored communication has been frequently situated... within the elaboration likelihood model (ELM)... which posits that personal involvement with a topic or message dictates processing style.

Tailoring can be an extreme actualization of the ELM if several noncentral elements, such as demography and cultural references, are included in the tailoring factors. In addition to these, most tailored materials rely on theory-based elements such as an adoption readiness stage, self-efficacy and outcome expectations, and message frames. Finally, the central information pertaining to the intervention of most relevance to this individual is included as part of the tailoring. Recent reviews[40] and meta-analyses[41] have reported incremental benefits for tailored versus nontailored interventions in the literature as a whole.[38]

The University of Michigan's Center for Health Communications Research recently brought out its third version of the tailoring system.[42] Its website includes videos to explain what you need to know about tailoring health communication messages and materials.

▶ Social Marketing

We have placed social marketing in its own category because, while it can be considered a "practice strategy" à la IM, it relies on many theories in the delivery of audience-focused interventions. At the heart of social marketing is behavioral economics, including the concept of an exchange. The Community Guide has endorsed health communication campaigns including mass media and health-related product distribution—social marketing in its purest form—as having strong evidence of effectiveness in changing health behavior.[43] Social marketing (and its derivatives, prevention marketing and community-based prevention marketing[44]) creates a basic universe in which we build models of how things work and how we hope to alter them to make the world a better place.

Social marketing adapts the strategies and tactics used to create and sell products commercially so as to promote prosocial ideas and healthy behaviors. Lefebvre and Flora defined it as "[t]he design, implementation, and control of programs aimed at increasing the acceptability of a social idea, [or] practice [or product] in one or more groups of target adopters. The process actively involves the target population who voluntarily exchange their time and attention for help in meeting their needs as they perceive them."[45]

The idea of social marketing is generally attributed to a psychologist, G. D. Wiebe, who was famously quoted as asking, "Can brotherhood be sold like soap?"[46] Wiebe suggested that the public would be likely to adopt a socially beneficial idea to the extent its promoters used commercial marketing practices. Later, Kotler and colleagues,[47] including Rothschild,[48] Bloom and Novelli,[49] and Andreasen,[50] applied marketing principles to a range of social issues and products. They found that as an offering becomes more tangible (i.e., the more it is actually like "soap"), the more applicable is the marketing mix of price, placement, and product positioning in determining success. Communication is transformed into promotion, and is used to make consumers aware of a product and its benefits. By comparison, more abstract offerings, such as "brotherhood" or "safe sex," require more metaphorical use of the marketing mix.

Immutable Laws of Social Marketing

Andreasen,[51] and later French and Blair-Stevens,[52] set out benchmark criteria that can be used to determine if an approach is consistent with best practices in social marketing.[d] These criteria are profiled in this section.

Customer Orientation

The individual who is being asked to make a behavior change "knows best" what will motivate him or her to make this change. The job of the social marketer is to figure out this customer orientation by conducting research.

Behavior

Social marketing focuses on achievement of a behavior—not just its antecedent knowledge, attitudes, or beliefs. Behaviors must be clearly defined and possibly broken into steps that are then addressed by promotional efforts. What the individual does now instead of the desired behavior is considered the "competing product"—for example, smoking instead of not smoking. The marketer then has to use tools, described later in this section, to increase the value of the proposed behavior relative to the current one.

Segmentation

Audience segmentation is a data-based method of identifying groups of people who share characteristics relevant to the proposed offering. Marketers in the private sector often subscribe to marketing databases that divvy up the U.S. public into very narrowly defined segments based on shopping, media choices, census tracts, and other data that are collected (increasingly without our knowledge) every time we use a credit card, place a phone call, go online, or complete a direct survey. Transforming these big data (i.e., the data collected through formative research) into usable targets of opportunity then requires making hard choices, as few programs have ample enough budgets to reach everybody.

Lefebvre, an experienced social marketer, uses three questions to guide the segmentation strategies used in such scenarios: (1) Who are the people at highest risk? (2) Who are the people most open to change? (3) Who are the critical-for-success groups?[53] Such a strategy can also be used in public health, where practical constraints exist regarding the policy makers, intermediary organizations, and others are vested in a program's success. Lefebvre also describes several other critical features that should be taken into account as part of segmentation:

- Demographics are merely a guide and should never be the whole story.
- The segmentation is based on the specifics of the behavior, not generalized to irrelevant behaviors.
- Segmentation provides guidance on how to position the offering for this group, which barriers must be overcome, and which incentives will motivate the target audience.

Partner-based segmentation—that is, working through intermediary groups whose constituencies include the desired audience—is commonly used to

---

d. http://www.thensmc.com/

simplify logistics and reduce marketing costs. For the same reasons, channel segmentation, which is based on personal media preferences, is extremely popular. Since the advent of the Internet, the potential for channel segmentation has increased dramatically. For maximum impact, most programs use behavioral readiness, or other psychosocial indicators, to create segments.

Targeting is a shorthand way of saying that you are deploying a segmentation strategy to reach specific audiences. Personalization uses individually collected information, such as from forms completed on websites and product purchases. Somewhere between these two worlds is the idea of "personas" (the marketing world's spelling of the plural of persona); like *dramatis personae*, marketing-based personas are fleshed-out characters. As an example, **FIGURE 8-11** presents the adolescent "tween" personas developed by the CDC.[54] These kinds of personas should be the foundation of health communicators' creative message and dissemination strategy.

Tweens at-a-Glance

These composites are for illustrative purposes only.

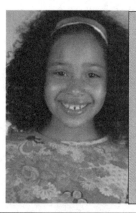

"I'd be lost without my cell phone. That's how I stay in touch with all of my friends. We send text messages and Tweet all the time. I'm on Facebook and never go a day without checking it."

Raven Boxter (The "Talented" Tween)
Raleigh, North Carolina

Fifth Grade, Age: 11

- Multi-tasks with media (texts, Tweets, watches TV).
- Admits she's a "teen wannabee" and does not see herself as a child.
- Her parents still play an important role in her life.
- Goes to a summer camp, where she's learning about acting and photography.
- Pays close attention to her weight. Is on the soccer and swim teams.

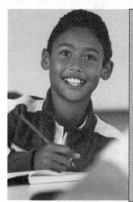

"I really miss my dad. In the meantime, I'll work hard at school to make him proud. I don't sleep well at night, but my mother doesn't know."

Denzel Moss (The "High Achiever" Tween)
Atlanta, Georgia

Sixth Grade, Age: 12

- His father is in the U.S. Army in Afghanistan, and stays in touch with him online via Skype.
- Gets excellent grades in school and has a strong support group of friends and teachers.
- Helps out at home by watching his younger sister after school.
- Wants to go to basketball summer camp, but is concerned his asthma will be a challenge.

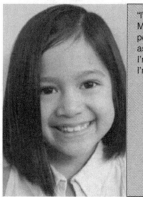

"I've never lived in Mexico, but when people meet me, they assume that's where I'm from. I'm proud I'm an American."

Maria Francisca Davila (The "First-Generation Mexican Amercian" Tween)
San Antonio, Texas

Fourth Grade, Age: 10

- Her parents emigrated from Mexico; she was born five years after they arrived in the U.S.
- Learned to speak English in school, but speaks Spanish with her family at home.
- Enjoys TV and watches Hannah Montana and Disney programs.
- Fits in well with her American friends and introduces them to aspects of her Mexican-American culture.
- Is in good health, but worries about her mother's type 2 diabetes.

FIGURE 8-11 Tween Personas

CDC, ADC, Division of Communication Services. http://www.cdc.gov/healthmarketing/resources.htm#insights

BOX 8-8 provides an example of using a highly targeted segmentation strategy to market tobacco prevention and cessation. Rather than personas, Rescue (a behavior-change marketing agency) created the idea of "peer crowds" as a means to identify market segments for the program.

BOX 8-8   Case Study: Changing Behaviors Through Peer Crowd Norms

Behavior Change Introduction

Teen health behavior change comes in many forms. Policy change and health education are the most commonly used strategies, but they are certainly not the only strategies available to public health practitioners. In fact, some behaviors, such as smoking and binge drinking, persist despite a strong policy environment advocating for their abolition and their widely understood negative health consequences. With these kinds of hard-to-eradicate behaviors, social norms often function as barriers between an individual and change. At the same time, these norms can be harnessed to drive the very changes they inhibit in these populations. This case study reviews how the Virginia Foundation for Healthy Youth (VFHY) is currently using advanced knowledge of teen cultures and norms to deliver highly targeted behavior change messages with its marketing partner, Rescue.

Lessons from the Tobacco Industry

The tobacco industry has used marketing to normalize tobacco use for more than 100 years. A classic example of this approach was an initiative in 1929 to increase smoking among women in the United States called "Torches of Freedom." At that time, it was taboo for women to smoke. To change this perception, the American Tobacco Company hired Edward Bernays, a pioneer in public relations, to associate the women's suffrage movement with tobacco use. As part of his strategy, Bernays informed the press that during that year's New York City Easter Day Parade young women would be protesting for their rights by lighting "torches of freedom." He then hired young women to perform this act, dramatically lighting their cigarettes during the parade. The plan worked brilliantly. Newspaper headlines across the country associated the women's suffrage movement with tobacco use, creating a new norm almost overnight. Suddenly tobacco use became associated with the image of independent women, exerting pressure on women who identified with the suffrage movement to use tobacco. After that stunt, tobacco sales to women began to rise.[1]

Today, the tobacco industry continues to employ marketing strategies to associate individuals' identities with tobacco use. For example, images of manly cowboys, artistic rockers, and hip-hop DJs are regularly associated with smoking by brands such as Marlboro, Camel, and Kool, respectively. New brands are created to appeal specific subcultures of potential new users. In fact, dozens of cigarette brands are available today, appealing to people of all walks of life. In 1929, a single, symbolic act may have been sufficient to motivate thousands of women to smoke; by comparison, today's diverse brand options allow the industry to build deeper and more nuanced relationships with its customers. These brands are so powerful that they continue to motivate individuals to begin smoking despite strong policy-based constraints and widespread knowledge of tobacco's health risks. In turn, the pro–tobacco-use norms created by these brands must change if we are to further reduce teen tobacco use from the current levels.

Identity, Smoking, and Peer Crowds

According to data provided by the CDC's Youth Risk Behavior Survey (YRBS), the rate of high school student smoking reached an all-time low of 15.7% in 2013. While fewer than 1 in 6 teens smokes, teen smokers are not equally distributed across every social group. In fact, some teen social groups likely have almost no smokers, whereas the majority of members of other groups may smoke. These differences are consistent with well-documented research that shows people are powerfully influenced by the behaviors of their social group.[2] Consequently, to further reduce teen tobacco use, we must understand which teen social groups continue to be at risk of smoking and which are no longer at risk.

While there are millions of individual teen social groups in the United States, these groups generally share many similarities. Research conducted by Rescue, a behavior-change marketing agency, shows that teens are organized into roughly five different "peer crowds" throughout the country. Peer crowds are defined as the macro-level connections between peer groups with similar interests, lifestyles, influencers, and habits. While a teen has a local peer group he or she socializes with, the teen and his or her peer group also belong to a larger "peer crowd" that shares significant cultural similarities across geographic areas. Rescue discovered these peer crowds using a photo-based research method that allows youth to visually depict the organization of social groups in their school and/or community. Using this method in studies across 20 different states, Rescue found that nearly all teens identify with one or more of the following five peer crowds: Mainstream, Preppy, Hip Hop, Country, and Alternative.

Unique interests, values, and habits define these peer crowds, and these characteristics should be considered when developing marketing messages directed toward them. When a campaign is designed to reach "all teens," it is not able to reflect the nuances of each specific peer crowd. Consequently, campaigns to reach "all teens" tend to appeal more to those in the center of teen culture, which Rescue has found to be Mainstream or Preppy teens. In contrast, the 1 in 6 teens who are using tobacco tend to be at the fringes of teen culture, which primarily include the Alternative, Country, and Hip Hop peer crowds. Consequently, a campaign that primarily reaches the Mainstream or Preppy peer crowds would not be the most effective means to reach teens who currently smoke.

With a focus on finding a more effective approach to reaching at-risk teens, the VFHY funded a statewide survey in Virginia of high school juniors and seniors that measured tobacco use by peer crowd. The study included 3537 students and found large discrepancies by group, as illustrated in **TABLE 8-5**.

TABLE 8-5 Current Cigarette Smoking by High School Juniors and Seniors*—Virginia, United States, 2011	
Peer Crowd	**Past 30-Day Cigarette Smoking Rate**
Mainstream	9%
Preppy	15%
Hip Hop	25%
Country	28%
Alternative	30%

* Percentage of high school students who smoked cigarettes on 1 or more of the 30 days preceding the survey. Data first collected in 2011.

Courtesy of Rescue Social Change Group

Consistent with Rescue's qualitative findings throughout the United States, this study revealed that Mainstream and Preppy teens were significantly less likely to smoke cigarettes. In fact, the more a teen self-identified with the Mainstream or Preppy peer crowd, as determined by a numerical score obtained during the photo-based research method, the less likely the individual was to smoke. In contrast, the higher a teen's Hip Hop, Country, or Alternative score, the more likely he or she was to smoke. This discovery revealed a challenge for VFHY and Rescue in developing an antitobacco campaign: While a broadly targeted teen campaign would reach the largest number of teens, those teens would largely be Mainstream or Preppy and, therefore, at lower risk of smoking. A different approach was needed to reach high-risk teens.

Peer Crowd Segmentation: Values and Interests

Segmentation is the process of classifying a population into distinct segments that behave in similar ways or have similar needs. Typically in public health, populations are segmented based on age, gender, race/ethnicity, and/or income. However, when it comes to teen tobacco use, these demographic segments may not provide the full story. The Virginia study showed that peer crowds were highly predictive of their member teens' tobacco use. Consequently, the VFHY decided to create three priority segments for intervention: Country, Hip Hop, and Alternative teens. While these three peer crowds represent only 49% of Virginia teens, they include 84.4% of all teen smokers, according to the statewide study.

To reach these three peer crowds, VFHY would have to implement three different campaigns. While this approach would require more work upfront, the potential benefits were seen as largely outweighing the need for additional resources. A key benefit of segmentation by peer crowd is the ability to communicate in a more authentic way with each peer crowd. For example, a campaign that is designed to reach "all teens" must be careful to depict generic situations, images, or environments so that as many teens as possible can relate to them. Messaging in such campaigns must be similarly broad, as it must be understood by almost any teen who encounters it. In contrast, a campaign designed to reach a single peer crowd, such as Alternative teens, can show images of Alternative teens in culturally relevant environments rejecting tobacco use for reasons that reflect the particular interests, values, and habits of that peer crowd. This kind of tailoring can give the impression that the campaign's messages are emanating from within the peer crowd itself rather than from an outside "adult" authority, such as a health department, that may or may not possess sufficient cultural relevancy to be effective.

(continues)

Peer crowd-targeted efforts are particularly authentic because they speak to the unique values of that peer crowd. For example, Rescue's research found that Country teens value independence and freedom, whereas Alternative teens have strong counterculture and anti-big industry values. Based on this information, a message about tobacco industry manipulation would likely fall flat with Country teens because they believe in personal responsibility and the rights of U.S. companies to market their products however they please. In contrast, that same message may be particularly effective with Alternative teens because they typically reject the overtures of big corporations that act unethically. A campaign that treated all teens as a homogenous group would not be able to appeal to these competing values, but instead would be forced to either abandon one segment of its audience or avoid the message all together. This "lowest common denominator" messaging approach prevents generally targeted campaigns from delivering deep and impactful messages to those most in need. Peer crowd–targeted campaigns, in contrast, can develop authentic messages that use the peer crowd's unique values to motivate its members to change. VFHY and Rescue worked together to do just that, developing three separate tobacco prevention campaigns that communicated authentically to each of Virginia's high-risk peer crowds.

"Social Branding" to Reach Three Distinct Peer Crowds in Virginia

To reach the hardest-to-reach teens, Rescue used a strategy it calls Social Branding. Social Branding is a behavior change marketing strategy that relies on peer crowd–targeted brands to associate healthy behaviors with certain desirable lifestyles through interactive and highly stylized marketing tactics. Similar to any commercial brand (including cigarette brands), a "social brand" is designed to appeal specifically to one group. The social brand acts as the organizing element for the campaign, and its personality embodies all the characteristics positively valued by the group. The goal of a Social Branding campaign is to change what it means to be a member of a particular peer crowd by breaking the association between an unhealthy behavior and the peer crowd's identity.

In Virginia, three social brands were developed to target three different peer crowds shown to be at the highest risk of tobacco use: Alternative teens, Country teens, and Hip Hop teens. Each brand was designed to break the association between tobacco use and the peer crowd's values.

Social Brand 1: Syke

The "Syke" campaign was developed to reach the Alternative (Alt) peer crowd and has been implemented in Virginia since 2009 (**FIGURE 8-12**). Syke is implemented in places where Alt teens socialize and engage in tobacco use, such as rock concert venues, as well as traditional and digital media channels where Alt teens are using messages that associate

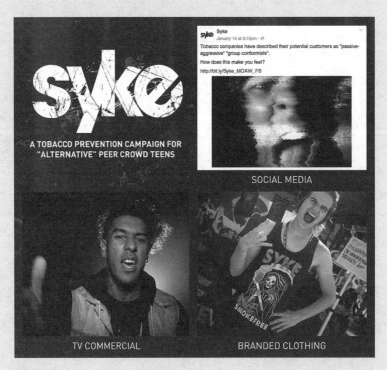

FIGURE 8-12 Social Brand 1: Syke
Courtesy of Rescue Social Change Group.

the peer crowd's values with living a tobacco-free life. The Syke campaign uses a variety of approaches to reach the target audience:

- Experiential marketing, which includes in-person interactive experiences at organized rock concerts where Alt teens can experience a message directly
- Brand ambassadors, who are socially influential youth members of the Alt peer crowd trained to conduct peer-to-peer antitobacco messaging
- Direct mail, which allows messaging to be delivered in an uncluttered and uncompetitive manner, since teens rarely receive their own postal mail
- Web, paid digital media, and facilitated social media, which includes strategic messaging and engagement on Facebook, Instagram, Twitter, and YouTube, with the goal of building relationships with Alt teens, creating interest, reinforcing media/messaging, and generating overall discussions about campaign messages
- Traditional media, which expand Syke's message to a larger, statewide audience while reinforcing the campaign's cultural authority to those who experience it through one of the other strategies

To test this campaign's effectiveness in reducing tobacco use, a baseline survey was conducted at rock music venues in Richmond and Northern Virginia using a time–location sampling method, and four follow-up surveys were conducted from 2011 to 2014 at "all ages" rock concerts. Awareness of and receptivity to Syke, along with the relationship between the Syke campaign and smoking behavior, were examined.

Prior to the campaign's launch, 37.6% of teens at rock concerts were current smokers—nearly twice the state prevalence of 19.7%. From 2011 to 2014, there was a 35.9% reduction in past 30-day smoking rates among all teens at rock concerts. This decline was most prominent for Alternative teens, whose smoking rates declined 49.7%. Non-Alternative teens had only a 26.7% reduction.

Social Brand 2: Down and Dirty

Rural teens are more likely to use tobacco, including chew and cigarettes. Mass media campaigns and policies directed at reduction of tobacco use appear to be less successful at reaching this population, as demonstrated by a slower decline of tobacco use rates among rural teens compared to urban and suburban teens.[3] Among rural teens, the Country peer crowd is at highest risk of tobacco use and is the predominant teen group in rural areas. Formative research found that Country teens identify with a lifestyle embodied by living outdoors, hunting, and engaging in "mudding" events in their trucks. In addition, research showed that past counter-tobacco marketing campaigns have been ignored within this group because they do not see their culture or values reflected in those campaigns.

To address this disparity and gap in tobacco prevention, a campaign called "Down And Dirty" was developed specifically for Country teens in Virginia (**FIGURE 8-13**). Since Facebook was found to still be the preferred social media

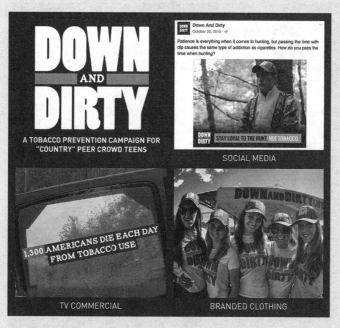

FIGURE 8-13 Social Brand 2: Down and Dirty
Courtesy of Rescue Social Change Group.

(continues)

platform of choice for Country peer crowd teens, the Down and Dirty campaign uses it to reach and engage its audience through paid digital advertising and facilitated online discussions. Using demographic-, geographic-, and interest-based targeting, the campaign can cost-effectively target Country teens and eliminate waste by only reaching those who are at increased risk of tobacco use.

Similar to Syke, Down and Dirty uses a mix of different content online that includes culturally relevant lifestyle posts designed to attract the audience and show these teens that Down and Dirty is part of their culture. Often, this content focuses on Country-related activities such as hunting and driving four-wheel-drive vehicles ("4 × 4-ing") through the mud. Tobacco prevention content focuses on messages that are based on Country teens' values, including how using tobacco influences younger siblings and gets in the way of living a free and independent life. In addition, Down and Dirty uses in-person event sponsorships at Country events to reach teens directly and engage them in the campaign. Lastly, traditional media are used, including TV and radio advertisements, to deliver messages that associate Country values with tobacco-free lifestyles. For this peer crowd in particular, highly targeted mass media are a critical vehicle to spread the message across rural areas.

The Down and Dirty campaign has attracted more than 25,000 Country teens to follow its Facebook page in Virginia, and its videos have been viewed more 500,000 times. Annual online evaluations of Down and Dirty have documented reductions in tobacco use after the campaign's first two years in the market.

Social Brand 3: Fresh Society

The third high-risk peer crowd in Virginia is the Hip Hop peer crowd. Today, the Hip Hop peer crowd supports a multibillion-dollar industry that influences every level of culture in the United States, from politics to fashion to technology innovations. A culture that may have started on the fringes of society has now become so deeply embedded in contemporary teen culture that the majority of American teens' lives have been directly shaped or touched by hip-hop. Whether directly part of the Hip Hop peer crowd or not, teens are getting ideas, products, fashion, imagery, and more from artists at every level of hip-hop culture.[4] As hip-hop invades every layer of teens' lives, its influence is both explicit and implicit—including how tobacco use is portrayed.

Rescue's peer crowd research revealed that Hip Hop teens use tobacco as a way to show strength and toughness in a culture that highly values respect. Armed with insights about the audience, Rescue developed a digital, social, and traditional media campaign called "Fresh Society" (**FIGURE 8-14**). Fresh Society was implemented in Virginia to counteract ongoing efforts of the tobacco industry to associate hip-hop culture with tobacco use by instead linking hip-hop values to living a tobacco-free life.

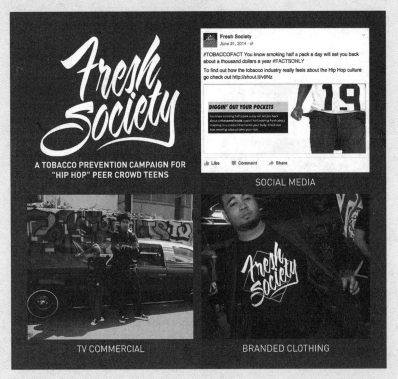

FIGURE 8-14 Social Brand 3: Fresh Society
Courtesy of Rescue Social Change Group.

Fresh Society works toward becoming an embraced, celebrated social leader within the Hip Hop peer crows, creating a platform to deliver hard-hitting anti-tobacco messaging that will reach Hip Hop teens in an authentic way. Online, the campaign uses Twitter, Facebook, Tumblr, and YouTube to deliver its message. Online contests are used to drive engagement, while traditional media reinforced messages throughout the state.

Together, Syke, Down and Dirty, and Fresh Society deliver messages and engaged teens at the fringes of teen culture. By segmenting teens based on their own identities and social groups, the Virginia Foundation for Healthy Youth and Rescue is able to tailor and target messages to include at-risk youth's unique values and, they hope, reduce tobacco use rates to new lows.

References

1. Amos A, Haglund M. From social taboo to "torch of freedom": the marketing of cigarettes to women. *Tob Control*. 2000;9.1. http://tobaccocontrol.bmj.com/content/9/1/3.full.pdf+html. Accessed April 28, 2010.

2. Eaton DK, Kann L, Kinchen S, et al. Youth Behavior Surveillance—United States, 2011. *MMWR Surveill Summ*. 2012;61(SS04):1–162.

3. Lantz PM, Jacobson PD, Warner KE, et al. Investing in youth tobacco control: a review of smoking prevention and control strategies. *Tob Control*. 2000;9:1, 47–63.

4. Klein N. No logo. http://www.naomiklein.org/no-logo. Accessed April 28, 2010.

Courtesy of Rescue Social Change Group.

Exchange: Benefits, Barriers, and Competition

A key contribution from commercial marketing to the health communication field is the emphasis on the central position of the consumer's perspective of a product or service. An old advertising slogan coached salesmen to "Sell the sizzle, not the steak." Rarely do you see a hunk of raw meat used to promote a restaurant. Instead, you see juicy, perfectly browned meat sputtering over a grill. This strategy is used because a product's attributes, which are created by the manufacturer, are not equivalent to the benefits of the product as perceived by the consumer. Thus, toothpaste marketers do not promote the chemical compounds making up their toothpastes' minty flavors, but rather emphasize the benefits of fresh breath directly and sex appeal indirectly. Soap, which made of some combination of oils, surfactants, and perfume, is marketed as a product that makes your skin soft and smooth, makes you smell nice, and, yes, gives you more sex appeal. As these examples illustrate, it is the benefits of a product, service, or idea (not the chemical composition or other dry details) that must outweigh the barriers to the product's use, or compete with something else being used in its place. Advertisers in the private sector have learned to ask consumers what they want or like in a product and then shape their marketing messages based on those desires—and public health communicators need to do the same.

Most barriers, like benefits, are in the mind of the consumer. The economic concept of price elasticity of demand[55] suggests that barriers are not universal, nor are they necessarily stable for an individual. Cost is often seen as the most important barrier to acquisition of a product. Even so, if consumers value a product sufficiently, they will pay just about any price for it. The concept is a little counterintuitive, but high price elasticity suggests that when the price of a good goes up, consumers buy less of it, whereas when the price goes down, consumers buy more. Low price elasticity implies that change in price had little influence on product demand. It is beginning to appear that cigarettes have relatively low price elasticity, whereas green vegetables and fruit have a higher price elasticity. On the one hand, the strategy of increasing tax surcharges on tobacco products did reduce adult smoking, but now seems to have less impact on younger smokers. On the other hand, the principal barriers to consumption of fruits and vegetables seem to be the availability and price of these foods across many population segments. Many public health practitioners blame the obesity epidemic, in part, on the high price elasticity of fast food—people consume much more of it when it is available at cheaper prices.

Cost is far from the only barrier affecting the adoption of a health behavior. In many cases, the major barriers are psychological, including preexisting attitudes and perceived social norms. For young people in particular, the idea of what their friends will think, or what they believe their friends are doing, is essential to a behavior change. Health communicators need to find and promote perceived benefits to offset the many perceived barriers to even an obvious health choice.

Finally, competition refers to what the intended user is doing now, or using now, instead of the behavior or product being promoted to improve their health. Sometimes this is just using brand X instead of brand Y. At other times, competition is a bit further apart from the original behavior or product—using our teeth instead of scissors, or drinking sugary soda instead of low-fat milk. As these examples suggest, what we have learned from marketing is that competing products or services may come from completely different domains. We might not be able to imagine that they compete with the healthy idea we are proposing to a target audience. This substitution of products or services from different domains is particularly important when introducing health concepts in developing countries. The habitual or preferential use of supernatural or ineffective natural products in place of contraceptives, vitamins, immunizations, and other public health interventions has to be considered respectfully in every health communication strategy.

Examples and Resources

Numerous examples of social marketing campaigns can be cited, including the "Friends don't let friends drive drunk" campaign, recycling and other green product ventures, and most of the subsidized health products marketed in developing countries (e.g., oral rehydration salts, contraceptives, insecticide-treated bed nets). For recent examples, see the websites of the Health Communication Capacity Collaborative (HC3)[e] and the Knowledge for Health[f] project. These USAID-funded programs provide technical resources and case studies in social marketing for health in developing countries.

The field of social marketing is large and the literature extensive. The elements described in this section have been selected because they are essential to health communication planning and cannot be overlooked, whether one is taking part in patient–provider communication, health education, or social mobilization.

▶ Conclusion: What Is Next?

Theories in the sense of starting points of inquiry live long and die hard…. When comparing theories we should not only ask what they have explained and how much evidence for [their] truth has been compiled in the past, but also how they can be criticized and which problems are they supposed to solve in the future.[56(p53)]

As R. Schwarzer suggests, we tend to hold onto theories in health communication for a long time, perhaps past the point that they can be used to predict how things might turn out. It is only the most academic health communication researchers who design studies to actually test theory. The vast majority of work that gets published focuses on applications of theory constructs to specific populations and problems. When experiments based on "tried and true" theoretical constructs, such as "creating self-efficacy," do not work out the way we expect, we tend to look for confounding factors or faults in the design; we seldom blame the theory.

Head and Noar have made the following suggestions concerning behavioral theory, using the Reasoned Action Approach as their case study:[57]

- Theoretical domains for theories should be clarified. Is the theory meant to predict behavior or to be used to create an intervention?
- The utility of a theory for a particular application (e.g., works well for persons with cancer but not for those with HIV) should trump its generalizability across many behaviors.
- Clear criteria are needed for adding, amending, or removing variables from a theory—in particular, when using data generated from meta-analyses.
- Organizations that lead health behavior research, such as NIH, should consider managing developments in theory and submitting them to consensus or expert panel evaluation.

Hannawa, Kreps, and others have also suggested that we are underperforming in generating new theory, possibly due to the applied nature of much health communication research[58] (e.g., it is extremely difficult to get government funding to study the communication mechanisms that apply to more than one disease or condition "silo") as well as to the overall lack of long-term funding in this area. To stimulate development in this area, the National Cancer Institute has created a Grid-Enabled Measures Database[59] to facilitate sharing research measures linked to defined theoretical constructs. With this database, if you are trying to apply a specific theoretical construct, such as "attitude," within a problem such as tobacco control, you can access theory-linked measures that are widely used

e. http://healthcommcapacity.org/about/usaidmissions/
f. https://www.k4health.org/about-k4health

and respected. When researchers work with the same measures, their specific studies can also be more easily included in meta-analyses of intervention effects.

The Office of Behavioral and Social Science Research (OBSSR) at NIH has recently adopted an "experimental medicine approach" to testing specific drivers and assays (ways of measuring) of self-regulation, stress reactivity and stress resilience, and interpersonal/social processes—what the OBSSR defines as the three key domains of behavioral control.[60] **BOX 8-9** presents the

---

BOX 8-9 National Institute of Health Common Fund's Science of Behavior Change Domains

Self-Regulation

The nomological network in which the concepts of self-regulation and self-control reside is broad and includes constructs that figure centrally as hypothesized mechanisms, targets, or behavioral phenotypes in research on health behavior and behavior change across a wide range of conditions and developmental phases. Constructs in the target class of self-regulation appear to be indexing multiple mechanisms and processes, some likely distinct, others overlapping, and for which the developmental trajectory is not fully mapped out. This suggests—at a minimum—the need for more *cross-validation* to confirm findings by repeating experimental manipulations in one project using an independent assay technique from other research, as well as *cross-calibration*, to permit comparisons across projects where self-regulation/self-control has been measured differently, and where reassessment is not possible. The goal of such work would be to determine the extent to which various measures of self-control and self-regulation are tapping distinct or overlapping mechanisms, and whether measures are performing similarly across populations, laboratories, and age groups. Work is also needed to determine which measures are appropriate for which contexts, which are redundant, and which truly assess targets that are engaged by interventions in ways that are meaningfully related to behavior change.

Stress and Stress Reactivity

Both chronic and acute stress exposures have been associated with maladaptive health behavior profiles. Heightened sensitivity to threat may constitute a stress-reactive phenotype that predisposes individuals to maladaptive behavioral and psychological responses when confronted with stressors. Although in many situations stress is closely related to processes involved in self-regulation, researchers have noted that the stress response system may have its own set of targets and downstream behavioral and physiological consequences—which suggests additional potential intervention and moderation strategies. Yet current measures of stress exposures and stress reactivity (e.g., inventories of stress exposures, diurnal cortisol rhythms) have been inconvenient or difficult for behavior change researchers to include in actual trials. Future technological advances in stress measurement for observational and clinical studies hold promise for inclusion in behavior change research.

Interpersonal and Social Processes

The influence of social partners and social network members on health behaviors is a topic of substantial research, and numerous mechanisms have been identified that account for social influences on individual behavior. There are powerful social variables that can support or undermine health behaviors (e.g., attachment alliance, social grouping for safety, loneliness/social connectedness). People are sensitive to the social signal in a message and the social value of behavior. In addition to assays of individual consequences of interpersonal mechanisms (e.g., self-reports, physiological or neural responses in individuals), thorough assessment of interpersonal mechanisms requires systematic observational coding of putative causal processes.

Environmental Factors as Moderators

Prominent among the approaches to behavior change that have targeted the environment are those based on *behavioral economics*. Behavioral economics involves the study of the psychological, social, cognitive, and emotional factors that drive choice, including choice related to health-related behaviors (e.g., eating unhealthful foods, engaging in sedentary versus physically active behaviors). Research has demonstrated that individuals' decisions are sensitive to cognitive biases, such as default bias, that may be difficult to intervene on directly (i.e., within the individual) but might be possible to exploit via an intervention targeting the environment (i.e., a manipulation of the "choice architecture" in which a particular decision or behavior is enacted). Discussion [has] explored how environmental manipulations can be leveraged to induce large-scale behavior change and possible approaches to examining the interaction between environmental factors and behavior change targets at the individual (e.g., self-regulation, stress reactivity) and interpersonal levels.

NIH Common Fund, Science of Behavior Change Domains http://commonfund.nih.gov/behaviorchange/meetings/sobc06232014/index.

NIH Common Fund's Science of Behavior Change definitions of these domains.

As this work is just beginning to be funded, we may anticipate an increase in theory testing and refinement as our understanding of the links among neuroscience, cognition, and action grows. In the meantime, practitioners can feel confident about applying behavior change theories and approaches that are regularly associated with positive outcomes in their health communication strategies.

Appendix 8A provides a good example of research on message sensation value.

Wrap-Up

Chapter Questions

1. Explain why theory is used in health communication planning, and cite a specific example from the chapter.

2. How is the Integrative Model different from Social Cognitive Theory or the Transtheoretical Model?

3. How are theories/models of persuasion in health communication different from behavior change theories/models?

4. Why can communications and interventions designed to scare their intended audiences backfire? Which type of messages is this approach useful for?

5. Describe the distinctions between theoretical methods, practice strategies, and activities or channels.

6. What can public health communicators learn from the private sector about the perspective of the consumer?

References

1. Blumenthal-Barby JS, Burroughs H. Seeking better health care outcomes: the ethics of using the "nudge." *Am J Bioethics*. 2012;12(2):1–10.

2. Thaler RH, CR Sunstein. *Nudge. Improving Decisions About Health, Wealth, and Happiness.* New Haven, CT: Yale University Press; 2008.

3. Finighan R. Beyond nudge: the potential of behavioral policy. Melbourne Institute Policy Brief No. 4/15; July 2015. https://www.melbourneinstitute.com/downloads/policy _briefs_series/pb2015n04.pdf. Accessed January 20, 2016.

4. Anderson K. Utilitarianism: the greatest good for the greatest number. May 27, 2004. https://www.probe.org /utilitarianism-the-greatest-good-for-the-greatest -number/. Accessed December 20, 2015.

5. Short JE. How much media? 2013 report on American consumers. October 2013. http://classic.marshall.usc.edu /assets/161/25995.pdf. Accessed December 20, 2015.

6. National Cancer Institute. Theory at a glance: a guide for health promotion practice, 2nd ed. NIH Publication No. 05–3896; 2005. http://cancercontrol.cancer.gov/brp/research /theories_project/theory.pdf. Accessed December 20, 2015.

7. Tierney WG, Sallee MW. Praxis. In: *The Sage Encyclopedia of Qualitative Research Methods.* Thousand Oaks, CA: Sage; 2008. http://www.markfoster.net/struc/praxis.html.

8. Hochbaum BM. *Public Participation in Medical Screening Programs: A Socio-Psychological Study.* Washington, DC: U.S. Department of Health Education, and Welfare; 1958.

9. Rosenstock IM. Historical origins of the Health Belief Model. *Health Educ Monogr.* 1974;2:328–335.

10. Prochaska JO, DiClemente CC. Stages and processes of self-change of smoking: toward an integrative model of change. *J Consult Clin Psychol.* 1983;51(3):390–395.

11. Maibach EW, Cotton D. Moving people to behavior change: a staged social cognitive approach to message design. In: Maibach EW, Parrot EL, eds. *Designing Health Messages: Approaches from Communication Theory and Public Health Practice.* Thousand Oaks, CA: Sage; 1995:41–64.

12. Boston University School of Public Health. Social cognitive theory. January 6, 2016. http://sphweb.bumc.bu.edu/otlt /MPH-Modules/SB/SB721-Models/SB721-Models5.html. Accessed January 20, 2016.

13. Weinstein ND, Sandman PM. A model of the precaution adoption process: evidence from home radon testing. *Health Psychol.* 1992;11(3):170–180.

14. Ajzen I, Albarracin D, Hornik R. *Prediction and Change of Health Behavior: The Reasoned Action Approach.* Mawah, NJ: Lawrence Erlbaum Associates; 2007.

15. Fishbein M, Ajzen I. *Belief, Attitude, Intention, and Behavior: An Introduction to Theory and Research.* Reading, MA: Addison-Wesley; 1975.

16. Ajzen I. The theory of planned behavior. *Org Behav Hum Decision Proc.* 1991;50:179–211.

17. Ajzen I, Albarracin D, Hornik R. *Prediction and Change of Health Behavior: The Reasoned Action Approach.* Mawah, NJ:Lawrence Erlbaum Associates; 2007.

18. Petty RE, Cacioppo JT, The elaboration likelihood model of persuasion. *Adv Exp Soc Psychol.* 1986;19. http://www.psy.ohio-state.edu/petty/documents /1986ADVANCESsPettyCacioppo.pdf. Accessed January 20, 2016.

19. Rogers EM. *Diffusion of Innovations*, 4th ed. New York, NY: Free Press; 1995.

20. Gladwell M. *The Tipping Point. How Little Things Can Make a Big Difference.* New York, NY: Time Warner Book Group; 2002.

21. Gainforth HL, Cao W, Latimer-Cheung AE. Message framing and parents' intentions to have their children vaccinated against HPV. *Public Health Nurs.* 2012;29(6):542–552.

22. Centers for Disease Control and Prevention. Put vaccination on your back-to-school-list. August 5, 2015. http://www.cdc.gov/features/hpvvaccine. Accessed December 28, 2015.

23. McGuire WJ. The effectiveness of supportive and refutational defenses in immunizing and restoring beliefs against persuasion. *Sociometry.* 1961;24:184–197.

24. McGuire WJ. Resistance to persuasion conferred by active and passive prior refutation of the same and alternative counterarguments. *J Abnorm Soc Psychol.* 1961;63:326–332.

25. Banas JA, Miller G. A meta-analysis of research on inoculation theory. *Comm Monogr.* 2010;77(3):281–311.

26. Witte K. Fear as motivation, fear as inhibition: using the extended parallel process model to explain fear appeal successes and failures. In: Anderson PA, Guerrero LK, eds. *Handbook of Communication and Emotion: Research, Theory, Applications, and Contexts.* San Diego, CA: Academic Press; 1998:423–450.

27. World Health Organization, Regional Office for the Eastern Mediterranean. *Health Education: Theoretical Concepts, Effective Strategies and Core Competencies: A Foundation Document to Guide Capacity Development of Health Educators.* Nasr City: Cairo: World Health Organization, Regional Office for the Eastern Mediterranean, 2012.

28. Whiting A, Williams D. Why people use social media: a uses and gratifications approach. *Qual Market Res.* 2013;16(4):369.

29. Daft RL, Lengel RH. Information richness: a new approach to managerial behavior and organization design. *Res Organ Behav.* 1984;6:191–233.

30. Singhal A, Rogers EM. Entertainment-education. In: *A Communication Strategy for Social Change.* Mahwah, NJ: Lawrence Erlbaum Associates; 1999:9.

31. Hollywood Health and Society. https://hollywoodhealthandsociety.org/. Accessed December 28, 2015.

32. Kaplan M. Tell me a science [Video]. *YouTube.* January 22, 2015. https://www.youtube.com/watch?v=B2gRlZgqTgE. Accessed December 28, 2016.

33. National Institute of Diabetes and Digestive and Kidney Diseases. Stakeholder groups. http://www.niddk.nih.gov/health-information/health-communication-programs/ndep/about-ndep/partnership-network/stakeholder-groups/Pages/stakeholdergroups.aspx. Accessed January 10, 2016.

34. National Institute of Diabetes and Digestive and Kidney Diseases. Stories about managing diabetes. http://www.niddk.nih.gov/health-information/health-communication-programs/ndep/living-with-diabetes/stories-managing-diabetes/Pages/volunteers.aspx. Accessed January 10, 2016.

35. Rimer BK, Kreuter MW. Advancing tailored health communication: a persuasion and message effects perspective. *J Comm.* 2006;56:S184–S201.

36. Jensen JD, King AJ, Carcioppolo N, Davis L. Why are tailored messages more effective? A multiple mediation analysis of a breast cancer screening intervention. *J Comm.* 2012;62(5):851–868. doi: 10.1111/j.1460-2466.2012.01668.x.

37. Kreuter MW, Wray RJ. Tailored and Targeted Health Communication: Strategies for Enhancing Information Relevance. *Am J Health Behav.* 2003;27(suppl 3):S227–S232(6).

38. Petty RE, Wegener DT. The elaboration likelihood model: current status and controversies. In: Chaiken S, Trope Y, eds. *Dual-Process Theories in Social Psychology.* New York, NY: Guilford; 1999:41-72.

39. Updegraff JA, Sherman DK, Luyster FS, Mann TL. The effects of message quality and congruency on perceptions of tailored health communications. *J Exp Soc Psychol.* 2007;43:249–257.

40. Noar SM, Benac CN, Harris MS. Does tailoring matter? Meta-analytic review of tailored print health behavior change interventions. *Psychol Bull.* 2007;133(4):673–693.

41. Krebs P, Prochaska JO, Rossi JS. A meta-analysis of computer-tailored interventions for health behavior change. *Prev Med.* 2010; 51 (3–4): 214–221.

42. Center for Health Communications Research. The Michigan Tailoring System. http://chcr.umich.edu/mts/. Accessed January 19, 2016.

43. Robinson MN, Tansil KA, Elder RW et al. Mass media health communication campaigns combined with health-related product distribution: a community guide systematic review. *Am J Prev Med.* 2014;47(3):360–371.

44. Community-Based Prevention Marketing, University of South Florida. Policy development. http://health.usf.edu/publichealth/prc/policy/policy-development. Accessed January 10, 2016.

45. Lefebvre RC, Flora JA. Social marketing and public health intervention. *Health Educ Qtly.* 1988;15:299–315.

46. Weibe GD. Merchandising commodities and citizenship on television. *Pub Opin Qtly.* 1951;15(4):679.

47. Kotler P, Zaltman G. Social marketing: an approach to planned social change. *J Marketing.* 1971;35:3–12.

48. Rothschild ML. Marketing communication in nonbusiness situations or why it's so hard to sell brotherhood like soap. *J Marketing.* 1979;43:1–20.

49. Bloom PN, Novelli WD. Problems and challenges in social marketing. *J Marketing.* 1981;45:79–88.

50. Andreasen AR. *Marketing Social Change: Changing Behavior to Promote Health, Social Development and the Environment.* San Francisco, CA: Jossey-Bass; 1995.

51. Andreasen A. Marketing social marketing in the social change marketplace. *J Public Policy Marketing.* 2002;21(1):3–13.

52. French J, Blair-Stevens C. *Social Marketing National Benchmark Criteria.* UK: National Social Marketing Centre; 2006. http://www.thensmc.com/sites/default/files/benchmark-criteria-090910.pdf.

53. Lefebvre RC. *Social Marketing and Social Change: Strategies and Tools for Health, Well-Being, and the Environment.* San Francisco, CA: John Wiley & Sons; 2013.

54. Centers for Disease Control and Prevention. Gateway to health communication and social marketing practice. http://www.cdc.gov/healthmarketing/resources.htm#insights. Accessed December 28, 2015.

55. Case KE, Fair RC. *Principles of Economics*, 5th ed. Upper Saddle River, NJ: Prentice-Hall; 1999.

56. Schwarzer R. Life and death of health behaviour theories. *Health Psych Rev.* 2014;8:1, 53-56. doi: 10.1080 /17437199.2013.810959.

57. Head KJ, Noar SM. Facilitating progress in health behavior theory development and modification: the reasoned action approach as a case study. *Health Psych Rev.* 2014;8:1, 34–52. doi: 10.1080/17437199.2013.778165.

58. Hannawa AF, Kreps GL, Paek HJ, Schulz PJ, Smith S, Street RL Jr. Emerging issues and future directions of the field of health communication. *Health Comm.* 2014;29:10, 955–961. doi: 10.1080/10410236.2013.814959.

59. National Cancer Institute. Grid-Enabled Measures Database. https://www.gem-measures.org/public/Home.aspx? cat=0. Accessed January 10, 2016.

60. U.S. Department of Health and Human Services. http:// grants.nih.gov/grants/guide/rfa-files/RFA-RM-14-020 .html. Accessed January 10, 2016.

Appendix 8

Programmatic Research in Health Communication Campaigns

Nancy Grant Harrington, Philip C. Palmgreen, and **Lewis Donohew**

This entry reviews a program of research that focuses on ways to increase the effectiveness of televised antidrug public service announcements (PSAs). Spanning more than two decades, the research was based on principles of audience targeting and theory-based message design, using formative research, laboratory-based research, and field research. For a more comprehensive review of this work, its theoretic foundation, and its impact on policy and practice, readers should refer to Harrington, Palmgreen, and Donohew;[1] Donohew, Lorch, and Palmgreen;[2] and Palmgreen and Donohew.[3]

Audience Targeting

In our research, the target audience is high sensation-seeking adolescents and young adults. Sensation seeking is defined as "the seeking of varied, novel, complex, and intense sensations and experiences, and the willingness to take physical, social, legal, and financial risks for the sake of such experience."[4] There is a strong correlation between sensation seeking and substance use (see Zuckerman[4] for a review), with high sensation seekers (HSS) being more likely to start using drugs at a younger age and to use a greater variety and quantity of drugs than low sensation seekers (LSS). Therefore, sensation seeking offers an excellent audience segmentation variable.

Theory-Based Message Design

The activation model of information exposure[5] guides our approach to designing antidrug messages for our target audience. According to this model, attention to a message is partly the result of how much stimulation an audience member needs and partly the result of how much stimulation the message provides. If audience members do not reach and maintain an "optimal level of arousal" from watching a message—if it is too boring or too overwhelming—they probably will stop watching and look for something more suited to their needs. If the message does meet their needs for arousal, however, they probably will stick with it.[5,6] Because HSS prefer intensity, novelty, and high arousal, whereas LSS prefer the opposite, we can deduce that HSS and LSS should prefer messages that are more or less arousing, respectively.

The construct that captures a message's arousal potential is called message sensation value (MSV). MSV is defined as a message's ability to elicit sensory, affective, and arousal responses in audience members.[7] High sensation value (HSV) messages should be novel, creative, intense, ambiguous, and suspenseful; low sensation value (LSV) messages should be more familiar, predictable, and clear. We developed these definitions through extensive focus group research with HSS and LSS young adults who evaluated numerous commercial advertisements and PSAs, telling us what they liked/disliked about the messages and why they felt that way.

There are two approaches to measuring MSV. The subjective 17-item perceived message sensation value scale (PMSV) measures how emotionally arousing, dramatic, and novel people perceive a message to be.[7] The more objective 11-category MSV coding system assesses visual (e.g., number of cuts), audio (e.g., presence of music), and content (e.g., surprise/twist ending).[8] There is a moderate correlation between MSV and PMSV ($r = .46$).

Designing and Evaluating Messages Through Formative and Laboratory Research

We used formative research to develop messages to test in two laboratory-based studies. The purpose of these studies was to see if HSV and LSV antidrug messages would appeal differentially to HSS and LSS young adults. According to the activation model, HSS should be more responsive to HSV messages, and LSS should be more responsive to LSV messages.

After testing various message concepts with focus and reaction groups, the research team settled on one that depicted a pinball game as a metaphor for "the game of life." A professional producer then created 30-second HSV and LSV televised PSA versions of the message for use in the laboratory research; the messages showed the negative consequences of drug use and encouraged viewers to call a toll-free anti-drug hotline. The first laboratory study used a forced-attention design, which involved showing small groups of randomly assigned HSS and LSS participants (total $n = 207$) about 20 minutes' worth of a television show with a commercial break that included one version of the PSA. We defined message effectiveness in this study as participants' intentions to call the toll-free hotline. Results showed that LSS were more persuaded by the LSV PSA, whereas HSS tended to be more persuaded by the HSV PSA.[9] The second laboratory study used a simulated living room setting and ran 318 participants through the study one at a time, showing them 30 minutes of HSV or LSV television programming with commercial breaks that included one version of the PSA. Participants could watch TV, read a magazine, or even just rest on the sofa. We defined message effectiveness in this study as attention to the television screen, which we assessed through observation. Results showed that HSS paid more attention to PSAs in HSV programming and LSS paid more attention to PSAs in LSV programming, but LSS watched HSV PSAs almost as much as HSS did.[10] We concluded that designing HSV PSAs and scheduling them to appear during HSV programming would be crucial to attracting our campaign target audience of HSS viewers and that these messages could provide reinforcement to LSS viewers as well.

Evaluating Messages in Field Research

Finding that messages are effective in a laboratory setting is one thing; finding that they have a positive impact outside the laboratory is quite different. To see if our principles of message design and targeting worked in the "real world," we designed a campaign to run in Lexington, Kentucky. Our target audience was HSS young adults. We conducted more formative research to develop five new televised HSV PSAs for the campaign; the PSAs encouraged the audience to call a hotline to learn about exciting alternatives to drug use in the Lexington area. Over a five-month period, the PSAs ran a total of 1502 times; a media buyer ensured they were placed in HSV television programming. Callers to the hotline received a 20-page booklet called *A Thrillseeker's Guide to the Bluegrass*. The booklet described sensation seeking and how it is related to drug use, and it offered a long list of exciting activities to pursue in the area (e.g., places to go rock climbing, to take karate lessons, to go skydiving).

The evaluation was designed to determine if our audience targeting worked. It had three parts: (1) pre- and post-campaign surveys of a random sample of Lexington residents 16 to 25 years old conducted face-to-face, (2) four telephone surveys of random samples of 16- to 25-year-old Lexington residents conducted during the campaign, and (3) a survey of 18- to 25-year-olds who called the hotline and agreed to participate in the study. The number of telephone calls to the hotline and results across the surveys suggested the campaign was effective.[11] More than 2100 people made calls to the hotline, and the vast majority was in the 16 to 25 year old age group. Hotline callers were much more likely to be HSS and much more likely to use drugs than the random sample of pre-campaign survey participants. All of this indicated that the campaign was reaching its target audience. In addition, data from the four telephone surveys showed that HSS were more likely to recall campaign PSAs than other antidrug PSAs being aired in the Lexington market, but LSS were more likely to recall other antidrug PSAs than campaign PSAs. Post-campaign survey results showed that HSS drug users were most likely to say they had seen our campaign PSAs and LSS non-users were least likely to say so.

The televised PSA campaign, therefore, successfully encouraged HSS young adults to call a hotline designed to appeal to them. The next field study used a controlled interrupted time-series design to test the effectiveness of a televised campaign, with the more ambitious goal of actually reducing marijuana use among HSS adolescents.[12] The researchers ran the campaign in Lexington, Kentucky, and Knoxville, Tennessee, and collected data from random samples of 100 adolescents in each city each month for 32 months. They ran the campaign twice in Lexington and once in Knoxville. Results showed that each campaign reversed developmental trends in 30-day marijuana use among HSS adolescents. Palmgreen, Lorch, Stephenson,

Hoyle, and Donohew replicated these results in a similar study that evaluated the effects of the HSV "Marijuana Initiative" put into effect in 2002 as part of the Office of National Drug Control Policy's (ONDCP) National Youth Anti-Drug Media Campaign.[13]

Impact of the Programmatic Research

This step-by-step program of research culminated in a strategic approach to designing communication campaigns for HSS audiences. Called SENTAR (for SENsation seeking TARgeting),[3,14] the approach is based on four principles:

- Employ the sensation-seeking trait as a major audience segmentation variable

- Design HSV prevention messages to reach HSS
- Conduct formative research with members of the HSS target audience
- Place prevention messages in high-sensation-value contexts

Palmgreen and Donohew note that "SENTAR has evolved beyond the sphere of scientific research to guide policy and large-scale prevention interventions."[14(p609)] Indeed, the Society for Prevention Research presented the University of Kentucky SENTAR research group with its 2007 Prevention Science Award. The award recognizes a large body of scientific research that has tested preventive interventions or policies. In effect, it also recognizes the importance of programmatic research in health communication.

References

1. Harrington NG, Palmgreen P, Donohew L. Programmatic research to increase the effectiveness of health communication campaigns. *J Health Comm.* 2014; 19: 1472–1480.

2. Donohew L, Lorch EP, Palmgreen P. Sensation seeking and targeting of televised anti-drug PSAs. In: Donohew L, Sypher HE, Bukoski *WJ, eds. Persuasive Communication and Drug Abuse Prevention.* Hillsdale, NJ: Lawrence Erlbaum; 1991:209–226.

3. Palmgreen P, Donohew L. Effective mass media strategies for drug abuse prevention campaigns. In: Sloboda Z, Bukoski WJ, eds. *Handbook of Drug Abuse Prevention: Theory, Science and Practice.* New York, NY: Kluwer/ Plenum; 2003:27–43.

4. Zuckerman M. *Behavioral Expressions and Biosocial Bases of Sensation Seeking.* Cambridge, UK: Cambridge University Press; 1994:27.

5. Donohew L, Lorch EP, Palmgreen P. (1998). Applications of a theoretic model of information exposure to health interventions. *Hum Comm Res.* 1998;24:454–468.

6. Donohew L, Palmgreen P, Lorch EP. (1994). Attention, need for sensation, and health communication campaigns. *Am Behav Sci.* 1994;38:310–322.

7. Palmgreen P, Stephenson MT, Everett MW, Baseheart JR, Francies R. Perceived message sensation value (PMSV) and the dimensions and validation of a PMSV scale. *Health Comm.* 2002;14:403–428.

8. Morgan SE, Palmgreen P, Stephenson MT, Hoyle R, Lorch EP. Associations between message features and subjective evaluations of the sensation value of antidrug public service announcements. *J Comm.* 2003;53:512–526.

9. Palmgreen P, Donohew L, Lorch EP, Rogus M, Helm D, Grant N. Sensation seeking, message sensation value, and drug use as mediators of PSA effectiveness. *Health Comm.* 1991;3:217–227.

10. Lorch EP, Palmgreen P, Donohew L, Helm D, Baer SA, Dsilva MU. Program context, sensation seeking, and attention to televised anti-drug public service announcements. *Hum Comm Res.* 1994;20:390–412.

11. Palmgreen P, Lorch EP, Donohew L, Harrington NG, Dsilva M, Helm D. Reaching at-risk populations in a mass media drug abuse prevention campaign: sensation seeking as a targeting variable. *Drugs & Society.* 1995;8:29–45.

12. Palmgreen P, Donohew L, Lorch EP, Hoyle R, Stephenson MT. Television campaigns and adolescent marijuana use: tests of sensation seeking targeting. *Am J Public Health.* 2001;91:292–296.

13. Palmgreen P, Lorch EP, Stephenson MT, Hoyle RH, Donohew L. Effects of the Office of National Drug Control Policy's marijuana initiative campaign on high-sensation-seeking adolescents. *Am J Public Health.* 2007;97:1644–1649.

14. Palmgreen P, Donohew L. Impact of SENTAR on prevention campaign policy and practice. *Health Comm.* 2010;25:609–610.

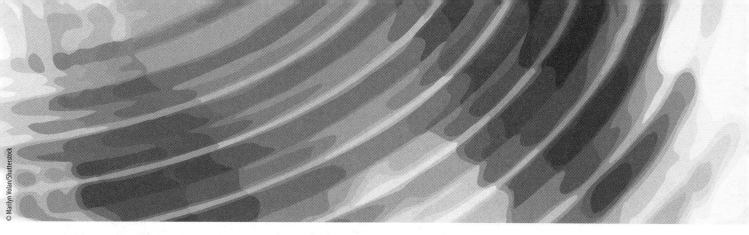

CHAPTER 9

Formative Research

Claudia Parvanta

LEARNING OBJECTIVES

By the end of this chapter, the reader will be able to:

- Describe the scope of formative research.
- Identify useful sources of secondary research.
- Use social marketing to organize primary research.
- Conduct a doer/non-doer study.
- Describe audience segments, profiles, and personas.
- Plan a customer journey mapping activity.
- Describe key qualitative and quantitative methods used in formative research.

▶ The Scope of Formative Research

Formative research is the collection and analysis of information to guide an intervention. Having defined a health problem, a population of interest, and the social, cultural, environmental, and behavioral factors involved, the next steps include the following activities:

- Bringing stakeholders together to plan the intervention
- Investigating what has already been done
- Carrying out primary audience research

Lefebvre makes the point that formative research for strategy development differs from scientific hypothesis development and testing in several ways. Chief among these is that meaningful behavior-change programs must be built upon a platform of understanding and empathy. Formative research can provide us with audience insights, empathy, and creative inspiration.[a]

Depending on what is known about the intended beneficiaries of the behavior-change program, their world, and the problem at hand, formative research can include the following phases:

1. Exploratory research to develop intervention concepts, an audience segmentation strategy, and audience profiles or personas.

---

a. Paraphrased from Lefebvre RC. *Social Marketing and Social Change.* San Francisco, CA: John Wiley & Sons, Jossey-Bass; 2013: location 3844 in the online Kindle edition.

2. Concept testing, in which the behavioral components, theoretical constructs, and message concepts are tested with diverse audience segments. Message framing research and media channel matching may occur during this phase.

3. Pretesting, in which first drafts or semi-produced "rough cuts" of content and media delivery options are exposed to intended users.

We will describe and provide examples of exploratory research and concept testing in this chapter. Pretesting is discussed elsewhere in this text.

In our experience, formative research can be a great catalyst to kick off the "forming, storming, norming, and performing" process of stakeholder group dynamics.[1] When stakeholders are proactively involved, they can become a source of research participants, perform specific data collection tasks, and help with collective analysis and interpretation of findings. Once stakeholders are meaningfully engaged in formative research, particularly if the beneficiaries whom they serve are involved, they generally become committed to seeing the program through to completion.

Reviewing and Analyzing Existing Information

Before rushing out to conduct focus groups (or whatever primary data collection method is appropriate), it is important to check out what others have done. As the U.K.-based National Social Marketing Center puts it, "Knowledge may be stored in reports, databases, journals and books, or held in the memories of people involved."[2] The way forward requires assembling existing knowledge and information about both the target audiences and the factors influencing their behaviors.

Begin by finding out "what works." Investigate comparative effectiveness trials, such as those done through the Patient Centered Outcomes Research Institute (PCORI).[b] Check out meta-analytic resources, such as the Guide to Community Preventive Services[c] and the Cochrane Reviews.[d] Finally, look for relevant topic-focused sites, such as Cancer Control PLANET,[e] What Works for Women and Girls (to prevent HIV),[f] or the National Diabetes Education Program,[g] to name a few.

Qualitative studies to gather audience insights can be voluminous and are difficult to publish. In the private sector, they are considered proprietary data and their results are closely held. The Centers for Disease Control and Prevention (CDC) publishes synthesized profiles of audience insights derived from numerous interventions.[3] Much audience research exists in the unpublished world of programmatic "gray literature." It is worthwhile to contact the Communications Office, division, or program at CDC, National Cancer Institute (NCI), or other government agencies to find out if relevant audience research reports are available for review. These studies are part of the public domain, but may require a Freedom of Information Act (FOIA) request to access them due to some restrictions on privacy related to the study's institutional review board (IRB) requirements.

For example, Nowak and colleagues from the CDC and Oak Ridge Institute for Science and Education (ORISE) published a qualitative meta-analysis of studies conducted between 2000 and 2013 by the CDC on influenza (flu) and seasonal flu vaccine.[4] By analyzing 29 unpublished reports, they identified "a wealth of information concerning the knowledge, attitudes and beliefs of the general public, specific sub-populations within the public, and health care providers and professionals, when it comes to seasonal influenza vaccination."[4] One application of their work was the development of the SHARE (Share, Highlight, Address, Remind, Explain) framework for healthcare provider communication (**FIGURE 9-1**). Future efforts may take many design cues from this study, particularly in the area of patient education.

Another way to obtain existing data is to contact funded researchers working on a similar topic or with similar target audiences. The National Institutes of Health (NIH) Research Portfolio Online Reporting Tool facilitates this process,[h] as do the websites of many philanthropic foundations. Some (but not all) researchers are willing to share preliminary findings, research instruments, and other insights ahead of publication with like-minded scientists. In addition, many publish study protocols per current reporting guidelines. (See, for example, Weymann et al.'s protocol for comparing tailored interactive health communication applications.[5])

Finally, government-funded Centers of Excellence provide message and media production resources that

---

b. http://www.pcori.org/

c. http://www.thecommunityguide.org/

d. http://www.cochranelibrary.com/

e. http://cancercontrolplanet.cancer.gov/

f. http://www.whatworksforwomen.org/

g. http://ndep.nih.gov/index.aspx

h. http://report.nih.gov/

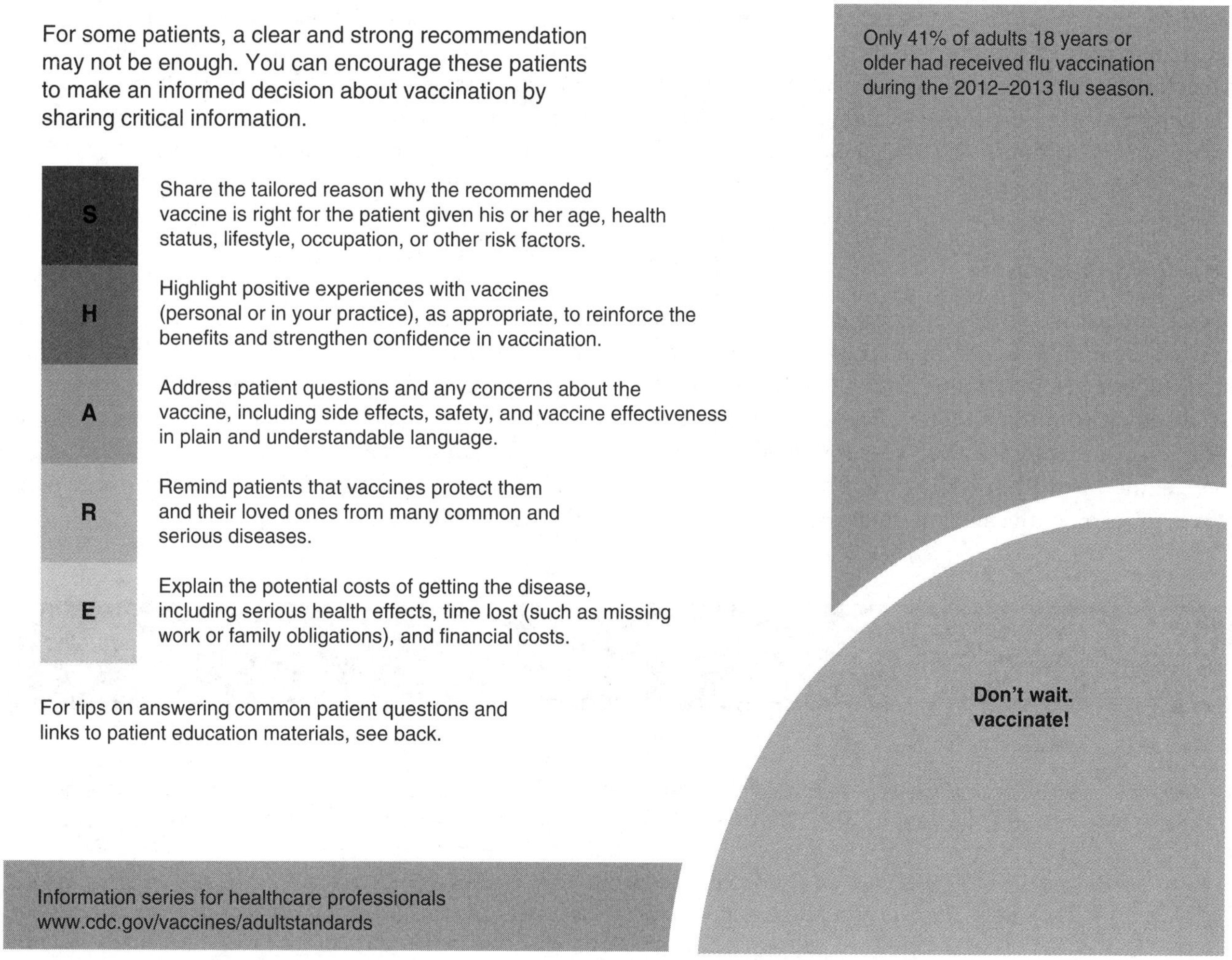

For some patients, a clear and strong recommendation may not be enough. You can encourage these patients to make an informed decision about vaccination by sharing critical information.

S Share the tailored reason why the recommended vaccine is right for the patient given his or her age, health status, lifestyle, occupation, or other risk factors.

H Highlight positive experiences with vaccines (personal or in your practice), as appropriate, to reinforce the benefits and strengthen confidence in vaccination.

A Address patient questions and any concerns about the vaccine, including side effects, safety, and vaccine effectiveness in plain and understandable language.

R Remind patients that vaccines protect them and their loved ones from many common and serious diseases.

E Explain the potential costs of getting the disease, including serious health effects, time lost (such as missing work or family obligations), and financial costs.

For tips on answering common patient questions and links to patient education materials, see back.

Only 41% of adults 18 years or older had received flu vaccination during the 2012–2013 flu season.

Don't wait. vaccinate!

Information series for healthcare professionals
www.cdc.gov/vaccines/adultstandards

FIGURE 9-1 SHARE Framework
http://www.cdc.gov/vaccines/hcp/adults/for-practice/standards/recommend.html.

can be adapted to fit a specific health communication intervention. These secondary data sources are discussed in the chapter on pretesting.

If evidence of what works, audience profiles, research frameworks, instruments, suggested messages, and customizable graphic materials are sufficient, the formative research might be complete and allow you to move on to pretesting or, for very well-understood problems and audiences, to disseminate of low-cost media messages. For problems and audiences that require more or new investigation, the rest of this chapter provides guidance on how to proceed.

▶ Exploratory Research Processes

Marketing as an Organizing Framework

In commercial marketing, developers learn everything they can about product categories and their customers. Using hair care products as an example, the myriad brands and types of shampoos, conditioners, and styling products are the result of market research that identifies "needs and wants" in different market segments, and the development of products to satisfy those needs. Once the tangible product is created, the rest of the marketing package—that is, price, placement, and promotional strategy—is worked out to position the new product to be a competitive offering in its category. Key decisions include the packaging, merchant selection (e.g., drug stores or beauty salons), shelf placement, media choices, and promotional content. While the product formulations may differ in small ways, most of the brand decisions are based on customer/audience insights. For example, Suave hair care products are positioned as "smart choices" for a value-based shopper, while the Oribe line consists of top-shelf products for the "hair obsessed." For the L'Oreal line, the slogan has alternated between "Because I'm worth it" and "Because you're worth it" over the past few years. Suave shampoo costs less than $3 per bottle, a L'Oreal product is approximately $7, and Oribe products cost more than $20 each (in luxury stores and salons). Each of these shampoo brands corresponds to a different market segment, yet unlike much of the research in communication or behavioral science, we have mentioned nothing about the gender or ethnicity of their audiences. Only customer self-perceptions and value choices are involved in positioning these brands.

Social Marketing

Social marketing is the application of principles derived from commercial marketing to the development of interventions that address health and social issues, albeit with some caveats. Few social marketing programs start with the close attention paid by commercial marketers to specific groups of people, which serves to segment the audience into the niches served by specific brands. Rather, in the healthcare arena, nearly all initiatives begin with behaviors considered important to public health. As a result, health communicators will focus on audience behavior research when developing an intervention strategy.

An example of a well-done social marketing study appears in **BOX 9-1**, in which Huhman describes promoting health insurance enrollment to community college students. Her work is an example of how the "Four Ps" of social marketing—product, price, place, and promotional strategy—were assembled for this target audience. Huhman's research strategy was particularly appropriate for a behavior that had relatively few "early adopters." Next, we discuss how research can be completed more quickly when there is an early adopter pool to study.

BOX 9-1 "Get Covered. Stay Covered.": A Social Marketing Initiative to Promote Enrollment in Health Insurance Among Community College Students

Marian Huhman, PhD

Enrollment in insurance by the uninsured is a central aim of healthcare reform that is being implemented through the Patient Protection and Affordable Care Act (ACA) of 2010. After the first enrollment period ended in March 2014, more than 7.3 million Americans had signed up for insurance under the ACA.[1] Of the new enrollees only 28% were young adults—men and women 18 to 34 years of age.[1] Enrollment among young adults needs to approach 40% in order for the low healthcare costs of young people to balance the typically larger expenses of older adults not on Medicare who represent the majority of enrollees.[1-3] Achieving this "balanced risk pool" will help make the insurance market appealing to insurers and keep premiums from having to rise steeply.[4]

To bridge this gap, researchers at the University of Illinois at Urbana–Champaign implemented a social marketing campaign called "Get Covered. Stay Covered." from November 2014 to February 2015, which matched the national and state enrollment periods. Social marketing provided us with a framework to design the campaign and develop messages that would be persuasive to the young adult audience.[5] The behavior on which we focused was getting uninsured young people to sign up for health insurance and encouraging already-enrolled young people to stay insured, but to also explore new, possibly better and cheaper, options for them.

Here, we summarize the key social marketing principles used in the "Get Covered. Stay Covered." program:

- *Audience segmentation:* We focused on community college (CC) students because community colleges enroll many older workforce development or reentry students who may have been laid off or chosen to change careers—these adults may not have insurance for themselves and their families.[6] Community colleges offer a path to higher education for many minority, low-income, and first-generation college students,[6] and these student groups may lack the financial resources to purchase health insurance without the financial subsidies offered through ACA. Community college students may have greater need for insurance through ACA because community colleges—unlike four-year colleges and universities—usually do not offer their students health insurance. Also, young adults, up to the age of 26, can stay on their parents' insurance plan, but CC students may not have that option if their parents do not have insurance. We segmented CC students further by focusing on students at four community colleges in central Illinois, because an important partner in the project was the University Extension, which had established relationships with leaders at these rural community colleges and at the county health departments where many of the in-person assistants for enrollment would be located.
- *Formative research:* To understand the barriers and motivators for enrollment, as well as the competing messages and behaviors that could be obstacles for CC students, we conducted formative research with focus groups of CC students and surveyed more than 800 students at six community colleges in central Illinois. Through the colleges' email systems, we reached out to students to complete the 12-minute survey and sent a $10 gift card to survey completers. Open-ended questions about students' perceptions of the benefits of having insurance and the disadvantages they anticipated helped us to develop persuasive messages.

- *Customer orientation:* With the findings from the formative research, we designed a marketing plan that addressed the key barriers, motivators, and alternatives for the CC students: (1) beliefs that the process was too complex for them to complete, (2) concern that they would not be able to find a plan they could afford, (3) attitudes of "invincibility"—that they did not need insurance, (4) confusion about what was covered, and (5) availability of in-person help as a motivator. Many CC students had no awareness of the in-person help by trained assistants that was available in their communities. We also used resources from national groups that recommended message strategies to reach the young adult audience.[7]

Marketing Plan

- *Product:* The *core product* (benefits that the customer wants) focused on the emotional drivers of peace of mind, the availability of financial assistance that would enable students to afford a plan, and assurance that they could, with the in-person help, find a plan that worked for them. The *actual product* (the goods and services that we were offering) was in-person assistance from local navigators who could walk people through the process of signing up or exploring new options if they were already enrolled. Ideally, we would have had navigators available on the CC campuses, but this was not possible for cost reasons and because the state managed the placement of trained navigators. Instead, our actual product was a user-friendly and trustworthy (run by University Extension) website where students could find a local navigator, a calculator for estimating the cost of insurance, and links to the national healthcare.gov website where students could complete enrollment. As is sometimes the case with social marketing initiatives, we did not develop an *augmented product* to provide (additional help to do the behavior, such as a reminder card.

- *Place: Place* is where the target audience actually does the behavior or receives associated services.[8] In our case, place had three components. The primary place component could be either the location where CC students could sign up for insurance with the local navigator, or the healthcare.gov website, where individuals also could enroll. At selected community colleges, we trained students ("Knowledge Ambassadors") to answer questions about enrollment and direct their peers to a conveniently located navigator. A strong place strategy is one that is convenient, is appealing, and overcomes barriers. Although we could not control the location or the attributes of the places where students would sign up for healthcare insurance, we contacted navigators or their supervisors to tell them about our project and to notify them that we were directing CC students to them. We believed this personal connection would increase the likelihood of a positive student experience. The on-campus Knowledge Ambassadors program was designed to overcome barriers such as concern that the process was too complicated, belief that insurance under ACA was unaffordable, and lack of knowledge about the in-person assistance that was available through the navigators.

- *Price:* Key to our price strategy was convincing the students that the benefits of enrolling in an insurance plan (e.g., security, low cost because of subsidies, avoidance of a penalty) outweigh the costs (e.g., actual premium costs and the hassle and uncertainty of the process). Lee and Kotler have outlined six price strategies.[8] Among the price strategies we used were (1) decreasing the effort and psychological costs of doing the behavior by developing the Extension website and by helping students find a navigator more easily and (2) developing messages that informed students about the high costs of uninsured injury or illness, stressing the monetary benefits of signing up under ACA, from which 8 out of 10 enrollees were receiving subsidies.

- *Promotions:* We used traditional channels of paid radio advertising, press releases, posters at the community colleges, and brochures featuring testimonials of peers helped by ACA. We developed a social media presence with messages and videos on college Facebook pages and pushed messages out through Instagram, Twitter, and blogs. Every ad we produced had a call to action to go to the Extension website to find information and a local navigator. The Knowledge Ambassadors distributed the brochures and giveaway items with the "Get Covered. Stay Covered." campaign title and were an on-the-ground envoy for the key campaign messages.

Theoretical Framework

This initiative was grounded in the reasoned action approach.[9,10] The survey items were based on the constructs of attitudes, social norms, perceived behavior control, and intentions to enroll. The messages we developed to encourage enrollment corresponded to the findings from the formative research of both the focus groups and the survey.[11]

Intervention and Evaluation Design

Rather than implement the full marketing plan at each of the four community colleges, we used a quasi-experimental design to find the most powerful approaches to achieving our goal of increased enrollment. One college received the full marketing plan components (Knowledge Ambassadors, traditional media, social media), another received the Knowledge Ambassadors and radio ads, a third was exposed only to the radio ads, and a fourth received only social

(continues)

media messages. A fifth college served as the control population (comparison group). We conducted a baseline survey across all five colleges in the fall of 2014 and a follow up survey was conducted in March 2016 after the enrollment period ended.

Summary

Getting young adults to sign up for insurance is critical to the success of healthcare reform. To this end, we undertook a social marketing initiative to encourage the enrollment of students at four community colleges in central Illinois. Different components of the social marketing intervention were implemented across the four sites, but at all the sites, students were encouraged to visit the Extension website for information and help with finding a navigator, and were exposed to messages that addressed their motivators and barriers to do this important behavior.

References

1. Department of Health and Human Services Office of the Assistant Secretary for Planning and Evaluation. ASPE issue brief: Health insurance marketplace: summary enrollment report for the initial annual open enrollment period. May 1, 2014. http://aspe.hhs.gov/health/reports/2014/marketplaceenrollment/apr2014/ib_2014apr _enrollment.pdf. Accessed October 12, 2016.

2. Cunningham PJ, Bond AM. If the Price is Right, Most Uninsured – Even Young Invincibles – Likely to Consider New Health Insurance Marketplaces. Center for Studying Health System Change Research Brief. Washington, DC: Center for Studying Health System Change; September 2013;(28). http://www.hschange.com/CONTENT/1379/1379.pdf. Accessed October 12, 2016.

3. Undem T, Perry M. Informing Enroll America's campaign: findings from a national study. 2013. https:// s3.amazonaws.com/assets.enrollamerica.org/wp-content/uploads/2013/11/Informing-Enroll-America-Campaign .pdf. Accessed October 16, 2016.

4. Levitt C, Claxton G, Damico A. The numbers behind "Young Invincibles" and the Affordable Care Act. 2013. http:// kff.org/health-reform/perspective/the-numbers-behind-young-invincibles-and-the-affordable-care-act/. Accessed October 16, 2016.

5. Edgar TE, Volkman JE, Logan AMB. Social marketing: its meaning, use, and application for health communication. In Thompson TL, Parrott R, Nussbaum JF, eds. *The Routledge Handbook of Health Communication*, 2nd ed. New York, NY: Routledge; 2011:235-251.

6. American Association of Community Colleges. Students at community colleges. 2014. http://www.aacc.nche.edu /AboutCC/Trends/Pages/studentsatcommunitycolleges.aspx. Accessed October 16, 2016.

7. Enroll America. Messaging framework for the second open enrollment period. 2014. https://s3.amazonaws.com /assets.enrollamerica.org/wp-content/uploads/2014/08/OE2-Messaging-Framework.pdf. Accessed October 16, 2016.

8. Lee N, Kotler P. *Social Marketing: Influencing Behaviors for Good*. Thousand Oaks, CA: Sage; 2011.

9. Fishbein M, Ajzen I. *Predicting and Changing Behavior: The Reasoned Action Approach*. New York, NY: Psychology Press; 2010.

10. Yzer M. Reasoned action theory: persuasion as belief-based behavior change. In Dillard J, Shen L, eds. *The Sage Handbook of Persuasion: Developments in Theory And Practice*, 2nd ed. Thousand Oaks, CA: Sage; 2013:120-137.

11. Huhman M, Quick B, Payne L. Community college students' health insurance enrollment, maintenance, and talking with parents intentions: An application of the Reasoned Action Approach. *J. Health Commun.* 2016 May;21(5):487-495.

Differentiating Behavioral Doers from Non-Doers: A Positive Deviance Approach

Doer/non-doer analysis compares people who already use the desired product or perform the desired behavior to those who are not using the product or performing the behavior. While this is possible only if some people have adopted the healthy behavior, in most cases you can identify people who have become early adopters. The anthropological term for people who move early in a bell curve of behavior change is "positive deviance" (PD).[6]

As the term *deviance* implies, a population can be assumed to demonstrate some normative behavior.

Nevertheless, a small group of people may have found alternative ways of living that deviate from this norm. We tend to think of deviation in a negative light. *Positive* deviance, however, refers to situations where the norm is associated with negative consequences and the deviants are healthier. This kind of behavior may be displayed, for example, by the few youth who do not get involved in gang activities in a gang-dominated neighborhood, or older women who are physically active despite having few environmental, time, or economic resources to support their efforts. An entire international health approach has grown up around identifying healthy individuals (or parents with healthy children) and finding out what they are

doing right. The health communication strategy is then based on encouraging these healthy, and presumably (but not always) environmentally consistent, culturally appropriate behaviors in the larger population.

PD research can be initiated by looking at outcomes, such as body mass index (BMI) or high school completion, or at positive beliefs, attitudes, or readiness to adopt behaviors, that have been gathered through a population-level assessment. It is crucial to learn how doers found ways to perform the desired behavior and what motivates them to continue it, given the same constraints as those in the community at large. **BOX 9-2** describes a seven-step approach to doer/non-doer analysis.

BOX 9-2 Conducting a Doer/Non-Doer Study Within a Positive Deviance Framework

For a *positive deviance approach* to be successful, doers and non-doers must be nearly identical in terms of their socioeconomic and environmental conditions. It is also helpful to eliminate as many cultural differences as possible. Then, when you find out how the doers have come to adopt a behavior, the chances are good that the non-doers will be able to emulate them. We discuss the seven steps in this process in some detail and provide some measure of the importance we attach to it.

Seven Steps

1. Clarify the behavioral goal.
   Suppose the goal is to help middle-school-age children maintain a healthy weight. There are two ways to start this process: one based on behavioral doing and non-doing, and one based on having a healthy weight and having an unhealthy weight.
   * You might use a biological measure, such as body mass index (BMI) or weight for height, to identify middle school children who are in a healthy weight range for their age and height. Working with school authorities, and going through the proper research review procedures, you might request to speak to all parents and compare the responses of parents with children who have a healthy weight to those who do not. Based on this first analysis, you could develop a list of behaviors that seem to be associated with having a healthy weight. Suppose you find that middle schoolers who have a healthy weight eat fewer sugary snacks, watch less TV, participate in more physical activities and sports, and perhaps ride their bikes or walk to school. You might choose to focus on several or only one of these facilitating factors when comparing the two groups of children and their parents.

   * A second way to start this process is to begin with those behaviors and environmental conditions known to help middle schoolers maintain a healthy weight. These might include: having healthy choices available in the school cafeteria for lunch; limiting school vending machines to water, low-fat milk, and low-calorie beverages; maintaining a regular physical education program; and encouraging children to walk or ride a bike to school instead of riding in a car or bus. Three of these options are primarily under the control of the school administration—the cafeteria, the vending machines, and the physical education program. This suggests that advocacy may be the best intervention to promote healthy decisions in these areas. The last option—having more children walk or bike to school—is a decision that will be made at home by the parents and the children.

2. Define the behavior and the audience.
   The decision of walking or biking to school actually involves several people. First, the middle school student might not own a bike, might feel too "tired" to walk or ride a bike, or might be worried that either the bike or the act of walking will not be perceived as "cool" by his or her peers. Parents might worry that their child will be late for school or harmed by traffic, the bike will be stolen, or the child will be walking home in the dark. Which of these concerns are most valid in shaping a decision? In this case, we will start with the parents' concerns. We can narrow our behavioral objective to the following two: Parents will allow and encourage their child to walk or bike to school. The target audience is the parents of middle school children.

(continues)

You might want to focus on conditions where bike riding or walking is more of a challenge, such as in urban environments. Alternatively, you might want to work with a population that typically does not engage in the recommended behavior, and seems to have a more of a problem with child obesity—for example, urban African American or Hispanic families. We will assume that you decide that you need to speak to city-living African American parents of middle school students and find out how they feel about children walking to school or riding bikes.

3. Determine how you will distinguish the doers from the non-doers.

   The first question to ask at this stage might seem straightforward: "Do you allow your child to walk or ride a bike to school?" But this question is too vague, because it does not address the amount of walking or riding necessary to contribute to a child's physical fitness. More likely, a child needs to walk or bike to school at least three days each week to improve fitness. A doer would then be defined by the descriptors "always or almost always walks to school or rides his/her bike" or "rides his/her bike more than twice a week." Again, working with the school authorities and using appropriate research reviewed protocols, you might be able to send questions home with children, identify children as they arrive at or leave school as walkers and bikers, and then do a phone, online, or in-person survey with their parents. Parents who do allow their children to bike or walk to school three days a week or more will be doers of the behavior. In the inner-city environment, and among the African American population you have selected as the focus of the program, these parents represent a minority opinion. As such, they have "deviated" from the norm in a positive direction.

4. Develop the attitude questions.

   We have reviewed the most essential theories that guide behavior change communication. Now we focus on perceived consequences, self-efficacy (or enabling factors), and social norms. Begin by thinking how to phrase questions based on these concepts. You will want to ask doers why they do something, what positive feelings they have about it, and what makes it easier for them to do it. If they have encountered obstacles, what were they and how they were overcome. This personal story of change will likely be a cornerstone of your message strategy, particularly if you use a "role model" approach. In essence, you are asking the non-doers about what gets in the way now to their performing the behavior, but you also want to know what they think might help them take a step toward performing the behavior.

   Here are some suggested questions to get at **perceived consequences**:
   * What do you see as the advantages or good things that would happen if your child (*walked/rode a bike*) to school?
   * What do you see as the disadvantages or bad things that would happen if your child (*walked/rode a bike*) to school?

   Here is a probe for current doers:
   * Thinking back about your decision to let your child walk/bike to school, did you have any worries? Can you tell me about how you compared the benefits to the disadvantages?

   Here is a probe for current non-doers:
   * When you compare the good and bad aspects of walking to school, is there anything that would make you decide to let your child do it?

   Here are suggested questions to get at self-efficacy or enabling factors:
   * What makes it difficult or impossible for you to let your child (*walk/ride a bike*) to school?
   * What makes it easier for you to let your child (*walk/ride a bike*) to school?

   Here are suggested questions to get at **social norms**:
   * Who (individuals or groups) do you think would object or disapprove if you let your child (*walk/ride a bike*) to school?
   * Who (individual or groups) do you think would approve if you let your child (*walk/ride a bike*) to school?
   * Which of the individuals or groups in the preceding two questions is most important to you?

   For any of these constructs, you may use free listing, pile sorting, and comparative tasks to get respondents to rank-order the variables.

5. Organize the data collection.

   As suggested earlier, you will be preparing a short questionnaire to collect the data during your formative research. Our experience has shown that asking the attitudinal questions in the previously given order is helpful. You also need to avoid combining ideas—that is, do not ask, "Which good *and* bad things happen when…." People will answer only part of the question, usually the bad side.

During formative research it is not essential to have statistically significant sample. Still, you need a large enough number of respondents to differentiate the doer responses from those of the non-doers. If you contact approximately 300 members of the target audience (parents of middle school children), you will be lucky to get 100 respondents. If 20% of the group are doers, then you will have only 20 responders in the positive group to work with. This result is what you could anticipate in the way of a response from busy parents in a large city.

Keep the questions open ended, and record as much of what people say as you can. Use the behavior question as the initial screen. Once you have more than 20 parents in either group (doer, non-doer), you can seek out parents in the missing group until you have at least the same number. Continue then to ask either type of parent the questions in your survey until you feel you have heard the same answers repeatedly from either group—that is, when you have reached the point of **saturation** (as it is called in qualitative research).

If you are just looking for a general impression from the two groups, you may form groups of doers and groups of non-doers as part of your research design. A better way to do this study, however, is as previously described—with individual interviews.

6. Tabulate the results.

In this step, you review all the answers and then list and count the responses for each question. This step is facilitated by using a coding sheet. Organize the lists by doers and non-doers, with the most frequently mentioned answers appearing at the top of each list. In addition, make sure you have a way of collecting narratives of how a decision was made, how an obstacle was overcome, and which rewards were experienced immediately and possibly later on as a result of performing this activity. Some respondents may keep slipping back to their old behavior and then reinstating the new behavior; it is also important to collect these data.

7. Interpret your results.

In looking at the key differences between how doers answered the questions compared to non-doers, focus on the five biggest differences. Also, look at where their responses are similar.

Tips for Doer/Non-Doer Analysis

- If doers and non-doers have similar percentages for any item, that item is not a likely determinant of the behavior for this audience.
- When doers' responses are radically different from non-doers' responses, that item is very likely a determinant of the behavior for this audience.
- Because the technique used in this type of formative research is not a statistical analysis, differences between the groups of respondents need to be large to be useful. If your sample includes 100 or fewer respondents in total, you will want to see a difference of at least 10%.
- Focus on what the doers tell you in terms of how they came to adopt the behavior. The concept of positive deviance suggests that because these strategies were developed under similar pressures and constraints as those faced by the non-doers, the behavior should be possible for everyone. Why did the doers choose to take the step? Can the non-doers be persuaded to follow their lead?
- Make sure you have collected the first-person stories from the doers and non-doers. These stories can be developed into compelling accounts and provide the creative energy for your message strategy. They may also contain answers to questions you had not thought to ask.
- Consider how the doers and non-doers answered the questions about approval and disapproval. Sometimes it can help to reach out to a secondary audience (e.g., fitness experts, media, health workers, community groups) and enlist support for the behavior before focusing your attention on the parents you originally identified as your target audience.
- Your research might reveal that structural differences actually exist between the two groups of parents of doers and parents of non-doers. The parents of doers might live in safer environments; they might be more economically prosperous and can afford bikes, or transportation fees, for their children. Conversely, parents of non-doers might live in areas that do not provide school bus service and, therefore, have no choice but to have their children walk to school. In this case, you will need to address structural barriers before trying to promote individual behavior change through advocacy.

EPHC, pages 172-174. This section is adapted from Smith W. *Comparing Doers and Non-Doers. A Rapid Assessment Tool for Social Marketing Programs*. Washington, DC: Academy for Educational Development; 1998.

A positive deviance approach can also be applied to organizations. Klaiman has been using this approach to conduct systems-level analysis of public health departments across a range of services, such as maternal and child health and immunization.[7]

Audience Segments and "Personas"

Audience segmentation is central to a social marketing approach in health promotion. It is used to:

- Groups potential audiences by common experiences, attitudes, beliefs, or sociodemographic factors.
- Gathers greater insights from these segments.
- Identifies one or more segment as the intervention focus.
- Crafts messages that resonate best with this group.
- Identifies the best media channels for the segment.

Segmentation for national programs is done using "big data." In smaller-scale programs, segmentation strategies are built from secondary resources, complemented by local insights and research. For example, the CDC has created audience-segment profiles related to nutrition, physical activity, and weight control, describing the resulting groups as "energy balance audience segments." The underlying data were derived from the Porter Novelli (P/N) Styles database, which includes responses from multiple waves of health and lifestyle surveys reaching more than 20,000 respondents. P/N researchers used principal component analysis and cluster analysis to generate the audience segments, which are depicted in a two-dimensional framework in **FIGURE 9-2**. P/N then analyzed the data further to create specific audience profiles, as shown in **BOX 9-3**.

The CDC program suggested that state- or local-level planners could use these energy balance audience profiles in two ways:

- Conduct similar surveys in their geographic area to define multiple audience segments relative to energy balance.
- Select one segment for audience research and programmatic investment.

Profiles to Personas

When the CDC conducted this research in 2005, the term "persona" was not in common parlance, but "profile" was. **FIGURE 9-3** and **FIGURE 9-4** show two of the audience profiles to which the CDC researchers attached a visual representation. Today, these characterizations would likely be given names (e.g., "Betty"

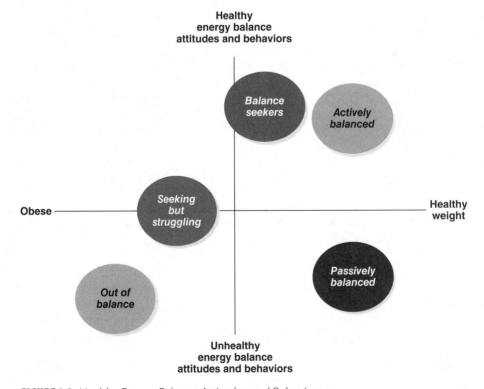

FIGURE 9-2 Healthy Energy Balance Attitudes and Behaviors.

Segmenting Audiences to Promote Energy Balance: Resource Guide for Public Health Professionals. Department of Health and Human Services Centers for Disease Control and Prevention Division of Nutrition, Physical Activity, and Obesity. Available at http://www.cdc.gov/nccdphp/dnpao/socialmarketing/pdf/audience_segmentation.pdf. 2005:9 _ (Figure 1).

BOX 9-3 CDC'S Energy Balance Audience Profiles

1. **Balance Seekers** (approximately 24% of population): This group is highly motivated. They are dissatisfied with their weight, actively trying to lose weight, and confident in their ability to engage in dietary and physical activity behaviors to achieve this goal. Well informed about healthy eating and physical activity behaviors, they have social support networks in place that help keep them motivated. Despite their motivation and confidence, 39% are overweight and 19% are obese.

2. **Seeking but Struggling** (approximately 23% of population): Approximately half of this segment is obese (53%) and another 35% are overweight. Members of this group are dissatisfied with their weight and recognize the threat to their health. They are trying to eat a healthy diet but often eat when they are stressed or upset. They do not like to exercise but are pleased with themselves when they do. Motivated to eat well and exercise more, they have confidence in their ability to engage in physical activity behaviors but have low self-efficacy for making dietary changes.

3. **Actively Balanced** (approximately 13% of study population): This audience is among the two segments with the highest proportion of participants with healthy weight according to body mass index measures (63%). Group members are generally satisfied with their weight and are not trying to lose weight. They actively engage in healthy eating behaviors and regular exercise. Health is a priority for them in making lifestyle choices.

4. **Out of Balance** (approximately 22% of population): More than half of the respondents in this segment are obese (56%), and approximately one-third are overweight (31%). They are dissatisfied with their weight and recognize the threat to their health. Unlike the *seeking but struggling* and *balance seeker* segments, they are not motivated to make healthy lifestyle changes. They are the least physically active group, do not get any satisfaction from physical activity, and have no intention to limit calorie intake to lose weight. They are not confident they can be more physically active, eat less, or lose weight, and they have less social support for these behaviors.

5. **Passively Balanced** (approximately 18% of population): This segment has the second highest proportion of persons with healthy weight (56%). Although they tend to be at a healthy weight, they make no conscious or active effort to maintain healthy weight. Unlike the members of the *actively balanced* audience, members of the *passively balanced* audience have low motivation and little interest in healthy eating habits. They are the most physically active group and are very confident they can stay thin or lose weight but are generally not trying to lose weight.

Segmenting Audiences to Promote Energy Balance: Resource Guide for Public Health Professionals. Department of Health and Human Services Centers for Disease Control and Prevention Division of Nutrition, Physical Activity, and Obesity. Available at http://www.cdc.gov/nccdphp/dnpao/socialmarketing/pdf/audience_segmentation.pdf. 2005:8. Accessed December 20, 2015.

or "Veronica") to go along with the image and descriptions. The section of the CDC profiles on "media habits" predates social media, but the descriptors for each persona are likely to still be quite valid. An approach such as customer journey mapping, described next, would then be used to add dimension to these characters and identify the best media channels through which to reach them.

Customer Journey Mapping

The Internet is awash in "customer experience" (CX) and customer journey (CJ) maps and mapping tools. From the *Harvard Business Review*[8] to Survey Monkey,[9] a multitude of tools and articles can be found on CX and customer journey mapping (CJM). Anthropologists and other social scientists have long promoted the idea of "walking a mile in someone else's shoes" to learn how another sees a challenge. CJM formalizes that process by analyzing an individual's trajectory in space and time as that person considers and adopts a product, service, or idea. CJM may be incredibly complex for what we would describe as a "high-involvement" decision, such as purchasing a car or health insurance. Simpler maps are appropriate for less-complicated decisions, such as buying toothpaste.

The point of CJM is that each *persona* is likely to follow a different path, and have different needs at each stage. At times, *persona* paths will vary significantly. For example, a young and healthy consumer follows a very different path when purchasing health insurance than does an older person with multiple chronic health conditions. Inevitably, as a *persona* moves through a decisional process, needs for information, encouragement, affirmation, and other positive reinforcement arise. CJM helps pinpoint critical opportunities for communication that can increase the likelihood of each *persona* having a positive experience. It can also identify points that were considered important by the provider, but to which the collective *persona* pays little attention.

Balance Seekers	
At a Glance	• Are actively trying to lose weight and are confident in their ability to eat less and be more physically activity to lose weight. • Are highly motivated, knowledgeable, and surrounded by a similarly motivated and supportive social network. • Weight profile: 41% normal/healthy weight, 39% overweight, 19% obese and 1% underweight.
Demographics	• Are similar to the general study population but slightly more likely to be women, be college-educated, have a higher household income, and be age 45 years or older.
Food and Diet	• Are actively trying to eat a healthy diet and prioritize health benefits in making food choice and managing weight. • Enjoy cooking, trying new foods and recipes, and are eating a healthy diet for personal reasons and set an example for others.
Physical Activity	• Enjoy getting regular exercise and get personal satisfaction from it. • Are the most physically active group and are among the more likely to belong to a health club or the YMCA.
Weight Loss	• Are the most likely group to be limiting calorie intake and trying various strategies to lose weight, such as exercising more and eating smaller food portions and less fat.
Social Support and Influence	• Are the most likely group to have friends who are also trying to eat a healthy diet, exercise regularly, and stay thin or lose weight. • Are more likely than the general study population to say people who matter most to them are pleased when they eat well and exercise regularly.
Health and Health Information	• Are in good health and want to look and feel healthy. • Believe being informed about health issues is important and make it a point to read and watch stories about health. • Have a good relationship with their physicians and rely on them, the web, and magazines for health information.
Media Habits	• Watch television less often than the general study population, read a newspaper more often and listen to the radio an average amount of time.

FIGURE 9-3 Balance Seekers.

Segmenting Audiences to Promote Energy Balance: Resource Guide for Public Health Professionals. Department of Health and Human Services Centers for Disease Control and Prevention Division of Nutrition, Physical Activity, and Obesity. Available at http://www.cdc.gov/nccdphp/dnpao/socialmarketing/pdf/audience_segmentation.pdf. 2005:10.

BOX 9-4 presents key steps in creating a CJM.[10] An example for purchasing health insurance appears in **FIGURE 9-5**.

▶ Research Tools

How is information to distinguish the doers from the non-doers, construct a *persona*, or map the customer journey collected? What are the most meaningful words and images to convey messages effectively? Why Facebook and not Twitter, or vice versa? Social and commercial marketers have many tools at their disposal for formative research. According to the

GreenBook Research Industry Trends Report (GRIT),[11] 69% of nearly 1500 major marketing research companies surveyed in 2015 used a combination of qualitative and quantitative research techniques, with 21% using qualitative exclusively and 10% using quantitative methods exclusively. GRIT surveys are based on approximately 1160 "suppliers" of market research and 330 "clients," of which 46% are located in North America. **FIGURE 9-6** presents GRIT's analysis of the most commonly used qualitative methods by their survey participants. Note that in-person focus groups and in-depth interviews (IDIs) outweigh their online equivalents by a 3 to 1 ratio. In contrast, GRIT's respondents said that most of their quantitative research was

Seeking but Struggling	
At a Glance	• Are actively trying to lose weight and are aware of the health threat overweight poses. • Are motivated to lose weight, have social support to do so but lack confidence in their to eat less food eat more healthfully. • Weight Profile: 12% healthy weight, 35% overweight, and 53% obese.
Demographics	• Are similar to the general study population but slightly more likely to be women and age 45 years older.
Food and Diet	• Are actively trying to eat a healthy diet but don't necessarily prefer healthy foods and are sometimes confused about which foods are healthy. • Eat when stressed or upset and are more likely than the general study population to eat high-fat foods and to prefer to eat on the go.
Physical Activity	• Do not enjoy getting regular exercise but get personal satisfaction from doing so. • Have levels of physical activity slightly lower than those of the general study population but are more likely to belong to a health club.
Weight Loss	• Are actively trying to lose weight but are not confident in their ability to do so. • View counting calories and eating a little less each day as somewhat difficult and are not confident in their ability to do so.
Social Support and Influence	• Have friends who are also trying to eat a healthy diet, exercise regularly, and lose weight, and say people who matter most to them are pleased when they eat well and exercise regularly.
Health and Health Information	• Are more likely than the general study population to have some health problems, such as high cholesterol and high blood pressure but report good-to-average health overall. • Are no more likely to be actively trying to prevent disease or stay healthy but are slighty more likely to want understand health risks and be informed about health issues. • Turn to sources of health information similar to those used by the general study population, such as physicians and the web.
Media Habits	• Are slightly more likely to read a newspaper, but watch television and listen to the radio an average amount of time.

FIGURE 9-4 Seeking but Struggling Segment

Segmenting Audiences to Promote Energy Balance: Resource Guide for Public Health Professionals. Department of Health and Human Services Centers for Disease Control and Prevention Division of Nutrition, Physical Activity, and Obesity. Available at http://www.cdc.gov/nccdphp/dnpao/socialmarketing/pdf/audience_segmentation.pdf. 2005:11.

BOX 9-4 Customer Journey Mapping Basics

1. *Stakeholder participation:* Bring together people within your organization or partner organizations who know the target audiences well and care about the mission, as well as representatives of the target audiences. You may conduct these activities sequentially, such as focus groups with audiences followed by workshops with staff and other stakeholders.

2. *Personas:* If your organization already has personas or customer profiles, lay them out. If they do not exist, look to create them as you do the research. Where do the participants differ? These differences are more likely to be behavioral or attitudinal than demographic. Different audience segments will have different journeys toward a behavior. Pull the data together to create well-defined profiles or personas.

3. *Outcomes:* What does the outcome behavior look like? Describe this for each of the personas with which you will work.

4. *Customer journey:* List all actions through which each persona typically passes through to reach the outcome. Typically, individuals who are planning a purchase move through four phases: awareness, research, choice reduction, and purchase. Some CJMs include a fifth phase—an advocacy phase that follows the purchase. Some of these actions are tangible steps of going somewhere and getting something; some involve seeking information online; some focus on discussing ideas with family or friends. Chart this activity on a horizontal line. Identify where

(continues)

BOX 9-4 Customer Journey Mapping Basics (continued)

the persona goes online or offline when seeking information, engagement, reinforcement, or other contact to solidify his or her decision or take a step.

5. *Touchpoints:* For every action of the persona, list the opportunities you have to engage with the persona either directly, through mediated messages, or via intermediaries. These are your windows of opportunity for persuasive communication. Highlight how different personas use different touch points.

6. *Moments of truth:* These are moments when the persona makes a decision based on what the individual encountered in the touchpoint. A touchpoint might correspond to a "stage" in the transtheoretical model, follow the precaution adoption process model (PAPM), or just be an "a-ha moment" for the individual. Imagine the various reactions a persona could have upon encountering the touchpoint. You want individuals to move forward: What could make them stop or go backward in their journey?

   Tincher defines moments of truth as "a point in the journey with a disproportional impact on the rest. For example, when a radiology patient gets lost in the hospital, it has a disproportionate impact on the rest of the journey. In sales-related journeys, it tends to be those moments when a customer makes a key decision to drop certain providers."

7. *Delivery:* At every touchpoint, what is the best way to deliver the encounter? How can you optimize this channel and content to assist the persona in moving forward?

8. *Emotional journey:* This is particularly important if the CJM is for a service—for example, bringing individuals in for immunizations or sexually transmitted disease (STD) prevention. How they feel upon encountering the service providers will be crucial to them in moving forward on the journey. Many people have been turned off early in their journey by rudeness or a lack of attention. The emotional journey is often the most critical outcome of CJM, because most organizations have become so accustomed to their work that they forget the powerful emotions experienced by their customers.

9. *Blueprint:* Most organizations have something on paper with a lot of sticky notes that is transformed into a workable document. Test it with the target personas. Use it to guide your channel, content. and message strategy.

10. *Improve and innovate:* Track your results. Know when you were right or wrong about any of the components: actions, touchpoints, moments of truth. Make modifications based on this feedback.

Example

Here is an example from CJM expert Jim Tincher:

I did a project with a hospital on understanding the advanced imaging journey, where the stakeholder workshop identified a clear problem. We ran two different stakeholder workshops simultaneously, and both had the same result—the biggest problem in the journey was in scheduling and registration. Customers hated waiting on hold and giving their information multiple times.

So as we left the workshop and headed back to the airport, we were already planning thoughts around an improved scheduling process. But we needed to research with patients to confirm the hypothesis study, beginning with a diary study with patients as they went through the process. How did they describe the "painful" scheduling process? Quick, easy, painless—the opposite of what the hospital leadership thought! Had we only done an internal workshop, they would have invested in new scheduling systems and processes, but not solved the true issues of the journey!

The true patient problem was that the hospital didn't help patients as they moved through the journey. The process was set up assuming a rational person who could calmly maneuver through the process. In reality, patients were incredibly anxious, and this caused them to have multiple problems throughout the process. One moment of truth was checking in at the hospital. More than 10% of the patients we talked to got lost in the hospital trying to find the radiology department. The hospital didn't send patients the information they needed—they just assumed they'd figure it out. But assuming a rational patient or customer is always a bad idea. (J. Tincher, personal communication, December 25, 2015)

Good Sources for Learning More About CJM

A. van Oosterom: http://www.mycustomer.com/experience/engagement/mapping-out-customer-experience-excellence-10-steps-to-customer-journey

Jim Tincher: http://www.heartofthecustomer.com/resources/

J. Tincher, personal communication, December 25, 2015.

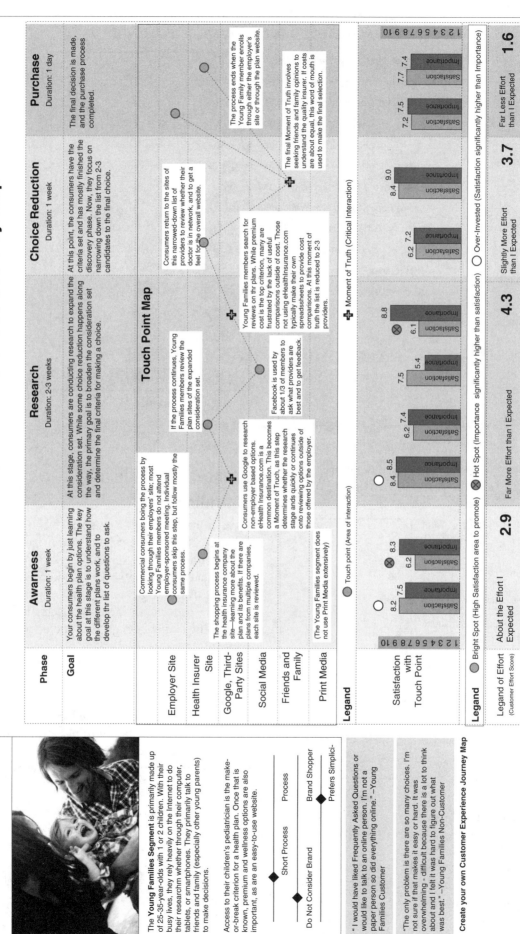

FIGURE 9-5 Health Insurance Purchase Journey Map.

WHICH OF THESE QUALITATIVE DATA COLLECTION METHODS
HAVE YOU USED MOST THIS YEAR? (SELECT UP TO FIVE)

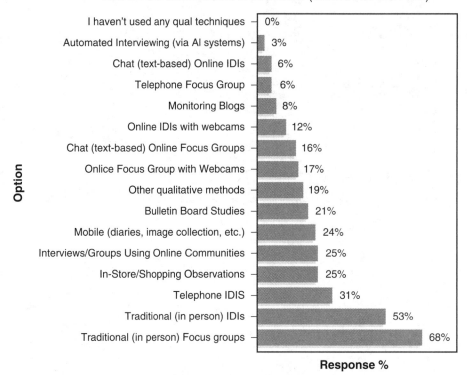

FIGURE 9-6 Qualitative Data Collection Method Usage.

GreenBook Research Industry Trends Report (GRIT). Available at http://www.greenbook.org/grit. Accessed December 12, 2015.

WHICH OF THESE QUANTITATIVE DATA
COLLECTION METHODS HAVE YOU USED MOST
THIS YEAR? (SELECT UP TO FIVE)

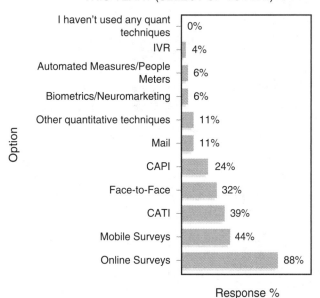

FIGURE 9-7 Quantitative Data Collection Method Usage.

Modified from GreenBook Research Industry Trends Report (GRIT). Available at http://www.greenbook.org/grit. Accessed December 12, 2015.

conducted via online or mobile surveys, as shown in **FIGURE 9-7**. Some of the most commonly used research methods are described next.

Quantitative Methods

Data Mining

Data mining applies statistical techniques such as exploratory data analysis, decision trees, clustering, classification and regression trees (CART), CHAID (Chi-square Automatic Interaction Detector), and other processes (e.g., neural networks, rule induction) to detect patterns in large data sets.[i] It is useful for identifying audience segments and attributes of those segments to create profiles and personas that, depending on the data set, may produce strong support for message strategies.

In recent years, the availability of several national, large-scale surveys and surveillance systems has led to increased use of data mining and analysis during the exploratory phase of formative research. A few key data sets that are intended for public use and open to researchers are highlighted here:

■ *The Annenberg National Health Communication Survey (ANHCS).* Between 2005 and 2012, ANHCS collected data monthly from a nationally representative sample of adults in the United States. It focused on trends related to health behavior and behavioral intentions after media exposure, health

i. See a really nice summary of data mining techniques here: http://www.thearling.com/text/dmtechniques/dmtechniques.htm

knowledge and beliefs, and policy preferences and beliefs. The survey made use of the Knowledge Networks online probability-based panel survey. While less useful for predicting future trends, this database is an excellent source of data for hypothesis generation and testing of media effects and related research. The data are archived publicly available through the ANHCS website: https://anhcs.asc.upenn.edu/index.aspx.

- *Behavioral Risk Factor Surveillance System (BRFSS) and Youth Risk Behavior Surveillance System (YRBSS).* These two large-scale surveillance systems, which are managed by the CDC, use different methodologies to gather data on behaviors related to disease control and prevention. The BRFSS is a phone-based survey that has been ongoing since 1984. It is based on more than 400,000 adult interviews annually, making it the largest continuously conducted telephone-based health survey system in the world. The YRBSS surveys 9th- to 12th-grade students in public and private schools in the United States. Students fill in machine-readable answer sheets while in class. The YRBSS sampling frame is complex, and the 2015 national sample produced 15,713 usable questionnaires. While neither of these surveys is all exclusive to health communication, each contains numerous items relevant to messaging and media options. The BRFSS data are available at http://www.cdc.gov/brfss/, and the YRBSS can be found at http://www.cdc.gov/healthyyouth/data/yrbs/index.htm.

- *Health Information National Trends Survey (HINTS).* In 2015, HINTS, which is managed by the National Cancer Institute, completed its fifth cycle of data collection and public release of those data. While focused primarily on attitudes and behaviors across the cancer continuum, HINTS asks numerous questions of a broad nature, such as those dealing with health information seeking, the impact of media on decision making, patient–provider communication, and more. These data are available to researchers to analyze changes in how adults use different communication channels to access and use health information for themselves and their loved ones, obtain information about how cancer risks are perceived, and to help create more effective health communication strategies across different populations. The website for HINTS is found at http://hints.cancer.gov/.

The websites for these data sets include information about how to access data, suggestions for cutting and analyzing data for custom reports, and publication links. In addition to these free sources, there are several marketing databases that charge a fee for use or to have their analysts run customized reports.

Developing Surveys

Surveys are the workhorses of audience research. While it is easy to use Survey Monkey[j] or Qualtrics to develop, disseminate, and analyze online surveys, the harder part is asking the right questions, getting the right people to respond, and getting enough completed surveys to use the results to make a decision. Each of these areas involves its own science and literature, which go far beyond the scope of this text. We will address the communication research techniques that are part of questionnaire development, making sure the question being asked is interpreted by the respondent as intended.

Cognitive Interviewing According to the Center for Aging at the University of California in San Francisco:

> **Cognitive interviews** can be used to revise or develop new items so that they are appropriate to respondents' cultural context and lifestyle… cognitive interview methods reflect a theoretical model of the survey response process that involves four stages: comprehension or interpretation, information retrieval, judgment formation, and response editing. In other words, the respondent must first understand the question, then recall information, then decide upon its relevance, and finally formulate an answer in the format provided by the interviewer.[12]

In 1985, the National Center for Health Statistics (NCHS) of the CDC established a cognitive testing laboratory, where it reviews and tests survey items for its own use and for collaborating agencies. NCHS has championed the use of two primary techniques in cognitive testing: think-aloud interviewing and verbal probing techniques.

Think-Aloud Interviewing In the think-aloud interviewing method, the research subject is asked to literally say what is on their mind. The interviewer reads a question to the subject and records

j. https://www.surveymonkey.com/
k. http://www.qualtrics.com/

BOX 9-5 Think-Aloud Example

Question: How many times have you talked to a doctor in the last 12 months?

SUBJECT: *I guess that depends on what you mean when you say "talked." I talk to my neighbor, who is a doctor, but you probably don't mean that. I go to my doctor about once a year, for a general check-up, so I would count that one. I've also probably been to some type of specialist a couple of more times in the past year—once to get a bad knee diagnosed, and I also saw an ENT about a chronic coughing thing, which I'm pretty sure was in the past year, although I wouldn't swear to it. I've also talked to doctors several times when I brought my kids in to the pediatrician—I might assume that you don't want that included, although I really can't be sure. Also, I saw a chiropractor, but I don't know if you'd consider that to be a doctor in the sense you mean. So, what I'm saying, overall, is that I guess I'm not sure what number to give you, mostly because I don't know what you want.*

By listening to how the respondent tries to answer this question, the interviewer might conclude that this question needs to be revised due to following:

- The subject has trouble remembering whether a specific event falls within the 12-month time period. This may be too long a period for accurate recall.
- The subject does not know (a) whether the question refers only to doctor contacts that pertain to his/her health and (b) the type of physician or other provider that is to be counted.
- The subject is not certain as to what level of health professional counts as a "doctor."

Based on: "Cognitive Interviewing and Questionnaire Design: A Training Manual," by Gordon Willis (Working Paper #7, National Center for Health Statistics, March 1994).

---

the subject's description of mental process used to arrive at the answer. The interviewer limits probes to general encouragement ("Please tell me what you're thinking") when the subject pauses. The example in **BOX 9-5** illustrates how a research participant reflects on what appears to be a straightforward question: "How often have you spoken to a doctor in the past 12 months?" After trying this question and alternative wording out with several respondents, the researchers would arrive at a better way to gather the information.

One significant problem with this seemingly easy-to-use method is that the research subjects may find it difficult to verbalize their thoughts. As a result, many researchers are moving to the more structured verbal probing approach.

Verbal Probing In the verbal probing method, the interviewer asks the survey question and allows the subject to provide a response. Then, the interviewer asks a set of questions that elicit how the subject understood the question and arrived at the answer. **BOX 9-6** provides some examples of the kinds of probes and questions.

Because formative research is conducted to generate concepts and messages that will be tested at a later stage, statistically significant sampling is not usually performed during the exploratory phase of research. Surveys, and increasingly online panels, are often used to pretest messages and materials, and certainly for evaluation.

BOX 9-6 Examples of Verbal Probing

Comprehension

"What does the term 'outpatient' mean to you?"

"Can you repeat the question I just asked in your own words?"

Confidence Judgment

"How *sure are you* that your health insurance covers this treatment?"

Recall probe

"You say you went to the doctor 5 times in the past year. *How do you remember* that number?"

Specific Probe

"*Why do you think* that cancer is the most serious health problem?"

General Probes (Similar to think-aloud probes)

"How did you arrive at that answer?"

"Was that easy or hard to answer?"

"I noticed that you hesitated—tell me what you were thinking."

Based on: "Cognitive Interviewing and Questionnaire Design: A Training Manual," by Gordon Willis (Working Paper #7, National Center for Health Statistics, March 1994). 2005.

Another reason why surveys are often avoided in public health formative research by federal agencies is the Paperwork Reduction Act (PRA) of 1995, which "requires that U.S. federal government agencies obtain Office of Management and Budget (OMB) approval before requesting or collecting most types of information from the public."[13] Despite its name, this regulation applies to online, telephone, and any other form of survey, and often causes lengthy delays in data collection and analysis. **BOX 9-7** lists the kinds of data collection not eligible for "fast track" approval by the OMB.

Perceptual Mapping Perceptual mapping relies on data collected using surveys in which participants respond to questions using a Likert-type scale. **BOX 9-8** provides an example of how this technique is being used by the Temple University Risk Communication Laboratory. In this perceptual mapping example, a 0- to 10-point scale is used by respondents to associate one item with another. Based on multidimensional scaling, perceptual mapping methods yield a graphic, three-dimensional, multicolored display indicating how respondents perceive the relationships among a set of elements.[14] This allows researchers to study how framing effects, perceptions of risks and benefits, attitudes toward risk, or other factors contribute to the cognitive and affective dimensions of decision making. The maps reflect how the decision elements are conceptualized relative to each other and relative to "self," a group average.

Survey Administration: Online or Offline? As indicated in the GRIT report, the vast majority of market researchers now conduct surveys online. This preference arises not only because of the difficulty of using random-digit dialing with mobile phones, the previous industry standard, but also because 89% of Americans now use the internet regularly. Of course, as the Pew Research Center notes, "89% is not 100%, and surveys that include only those who use the internet (and are willing to take surveys online) run the risk of producing biased results."[15] Online surveys are self-administered,

(continues)

BOX 9-8 Perceptual Mapping Example   *(continued)*

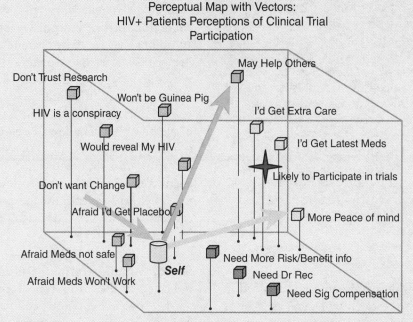

FIGURE 9-8 Perceptual Map with Vectors: HIV-Positive Patients' Perceptions of Clinical Trial Participation.

importance of different decision elements. For example, Figure 9-8 depicts how minority HIV-positive patients perceive participating in clinical research.

Once perceptual maps are developed, vector analytic procedures are applied to determine the best message strategy. To optimally position the target concept in the perceptual space, target vectors (dotted lines in Figure 9-8) are used to start the mathematical vector resolution process. By specifying the target vector and the number of concepts to be used in the final message, the software creates all possible vector resolutions, using the specified number of concepts, then rank-orders the solutions for best fit to the target vector. The vectors identify optimal message associations for moving respondents (the aggregated "self") within the model. These message strategies involve the dynamics of "pulling" concepts closer together by emphasizing their association, or "pushing" concepts further apart by emphasizing their differences. The final form of the message (i.e., content, wording, imagery, and format) is then constructed to include and illustrate the concepts identified as optimal for addressing the respondent's concerns, knowledge, and perceptions of the risks/benefits. For example, in Figure 9-8, the vectors indicate that to get this group to "move" in the space toward participating, a message strategy would have to focus on having "peace of mind" and participation benefiting others, and push away from negative perceptions of being afraid that the medications were not safe and mistrust of research. (For further details about use of the perceptual mapping approach, see http://cph.temple .edu/publichealth/research-centers-and-labs/risk-communication-laboratory-rcl.)

Researchers at the Risk Communication Laboratory have adapted these methods to a variety of public health behaviors and decision making, with their work focusing on a wide range of issues: colonoscopy decision making by low-literacy African American patients,[8,10,11] intended actions during a "dirty bomb" explosion for low-literacy urban residents,[12,13] smallpox vaccination decisions made by healthcare workers,[6] perceptions of avian flu,[14] attitudes of HIV healthcare providers,[15] and decisions related to participating in clinical trials made by HIV-positive minority patients.[16] This research has shown that perceptual mapping and vector modeling methods can be used to assess group perceptions; develop tailored messages and interventions; achieve changes in understanding, attitudes, and behaviors; and evaluate outcomes in a variety of public health situations.

References

1.   Borg I, Groenen P. *Modern Multidimensional Scaling: Theory and Applications.* New York, NY: Springer-Verlag; 1997.

2.   Herschfeld N, Gelman S. *Mapping the Mind: Domain Specificity in Cognition and Culture.* Cambridge, UK: Cambridge University Press; 1994.

3. Kitchin R, Freundschuh S, eds. *Cognitive Mapping: Past, Present, Future*. New York, NY: Routledge; 2000.

4. Barnett G, Boster F. *Progress in Communication Sciences: Attitude Change and Persuasion*. Norwood, NJ: Ablex; 1997.

5. Leventhal H, Halm E, Horowitz C, Leventhal EA, Ozakinci G. Living with chronic illness: a contextualized self-regulation approach. In: Sutton S, Baum A, Johnson M, eds. *Sage Handbook of Health Psychology*. London, UK: Sage; 2004:197-240.

6. Bass SB, Gordon TF, Ruzek SB, Hausman AJ. Mapping perceptions related to acceptance of smallpox vaccination by hospital emergency room personnel. *Biosecurity and Bioterrorism: Biodefense Strategy, Practice, and Science*. 2008;6:179-190.

7. Bass SB, Gordon TF, Ruzek SB, et al. Developing a computer touch-screen interactive colorectal screening decision aid for a low-literacy African American population: lessons learned. *Health Promot Pract*. 2012;14(4):589-598.

8. Ruggieri D, Bass SB, Rovito MJ, et al. Perceived colonoscopy barriers and facilitators among urban African American patients and their medical residents. *J Health Comm*. 2013;18(4):372-390.

9. Woelfel J, Fink EL. *The Measurement of Communication Processes: Galileo Theory and Method*. New York, NY: Academic Press; 1980.

10. Gordon TF, Bass SB, Ruzek SB, et al. Developing a typology of African Americans with limited literacy based on prevention practice orientation: implications for colorectal cancer screening strategies. *J Health Comm*. 2014;19(11):1259-77.

11. Bass S, Mora G, Ruggieri D, et al., eds. *Understanding of and Willingness to Comply with Recommendations in the Event of a "Dirty Bomb": Demographic Differences in Low-Literacy Urban Residents*. Washington, DC: American Public Health Association; November 2011.

12. Bass SB, Greener JR, Ruggieri D, et al. Attitudes and perceptions of urban African Americans of a "dirty bomb" radiological terror event: results of a qualitative study and implications for effective risk communication. *Disaster Med Public Health Prep*. 2015:1-10.

13. Bass SB, Ruzek SB, Ward S, et al. Predictors of quarantine compliance during a hypothetical avian influenza pandemic: results from a statewide survey. *Disaster Med Public Health Prepared*. 2010;4:1-10.

14. Matosky M, Terrell C, Gordon TF, Bass SB, Ruzek SB. *Using perceptual mapping to develop HIV medical case management*. Paper presented at the Annual Meeting of the American Public Health Association. San Diego, CA; 2008.

15. Wolak C, Bass SB, Tedaldi E, VanDenburg M, Rohrer C. Minority HIV patients' perceptions of barriers and facilitators to participation in clinical research. *Curr HIV Res*. 2012;10(4):348-355.

16. Bass SB. Wolak C, Greener J, Tedaldi E, Nanavati A, Rupert K, Gordon TF. Using perceptual mapping to understand gender differences in perceived barriers and benefits of clinical research participation in urban minority HIV+ patients. *AIDS Care*. 2015; Nov 17:1-9. doi:10.80/09540121.2015.1112352.

in contrast to respondents replying to a live interviewer. This aspect poses a number of challenges, particularly for those who may have lower literacy levels, limited English proficiency, or visual impairments. In contrast, self-administered surveys have a lower chance of creating "social desirability bias," in which respondents feel the need to present themselves, their neighborhoods, or their peers in a positive light to a live interviewer.

The Pew Research Center has compared its online and mail-based surveys (both of which involve self-reports) across hundreds of survey items and found a non-significant difference across most items. However, topics related to web and technology use, as well as those that skew with older age, rural location, lower family income, and less than a high school education, produced some significant differences, due to a higher proportion of these subpopulations being present in the mail-based response pool.[15]

Another consideration with online surveys and panels is how the panels are recruited. Some samples, such the American Trends Panel used by Pew, are probability-based panels for which respondents are selected from a previously conducted national landline and cell phone survey that included more than 10,000 respondents. Other organizations, particularly those using Amazon Mechanical Turk and other crowd-sourcing vendors, use all-volunteer "non-probability panels," also called "opt-in panels." Opt-in panels have come under criticism for data quality, given that many of the participants are professional survey takers who do not truly represent a typical audience segment. Leaders in this area, such as Callegaro at Google, have written extensively on this subject.[16]

We will say more about online research in the following discussion of qualitative methods. While some of the methods mentioned above, such as cognitive interviews, are also qualitative, they are used prior to development of research instruments that will be used with large survey samples. The qualitative methods described below are always used with small numbers of participants when depth and meaning are the research objective.

Qualitative Methods

Observation and Participation

All of the strategies to change behavior require understanding its practice *in situ*—that is, in its environmental and cultural setting. Anthropology gave the world the idea of "participant observation," in which social scientists live in a community for some length of time and learn about the community members' beliefs, attitudes, values, and practices through an immersion experience. Sending trained observers into homes and communities to watch what goes on, usually over several hours for several days sequentially, can help identify behavior patterns, alternative products, and obstacles to adopting new behaviors. It is important that the presence of the observer does not interfere with the routine behavior of the person or persons being watched. It can take a fairly long time for people to become comfortable with an outsider watching them. Even with the rash of reality television programs and video-cams documenting so much of what we do, the vast majority of people prefer their

privacy. For this reason, observations are usually limited to short stints of time or very specific interactions, at least in the United States.

In other countries, health communicators often work with observers who are local health workers or educated near-peers of the subjects to minimize the intrusiveness of observation. This rapid assessment process[17] has led to more participatory approaches in formative research. These strategies build strength in the community and tend to support buy-in for behavior changes. Many programs consider the time invested upfront to be justified given the more solid foundation for change that is established with this method.

PhotoVoice In the United States, a widely used participatory method is "PhotoVoice."[18] In this approach, communities are given the tools to document their own lives, problems, and possible solutions through photography. PhotoVoice has been used to put forward the words of individuals who usually go unnoticed, for advocacy purposes. It is also a legitimate way of gathering data on how an affected group of people view their own situation, and it can be the precursor to a very compelling intervention that enables them to change their circumstances for the better.

BOX 9-9 describes a PhotoVoice project conducted in the United States by a doctoral student from India. This researcher explored how his compatriots view the differences between health care in the

---

BOX 9-9 Photo-Voice Investigation of International Students' Perceptions of Health Care in the United States

- I see hordes of people lined up outside of CVS pharmacy outlets waiting to receive flu shots.
- CVS is **promoting that people receive flu shots** to avoid falling sick in the coming season.

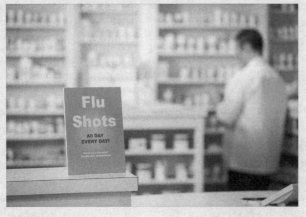

FIGURE 9-9

© Terry Vine/Getty Images.

- This is an **educational promotion**, where a pharmacy store is **advising people** to get their flu vaccine and stay healthy. **In India, we do not have any such activities** being conducted or promoted by pharmacies or hospitals.
- This situation exists in India because **people are not concerned** about such illnesses or vaccines, nor do insurance companies cover the cost of such vaccines.
- I would **want to create awareness** about such preventive activities in India and want people to be aware of methods to keep themselves healthy.
- I have captured pictures of the different kinds of milk available at a grocery store in the United States.

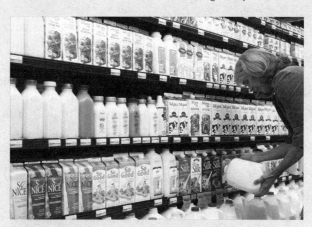

FIGURE 9-10

© Noel Hendrickson/Getty Images.

- The milk here in the U.S. is described by its fat content. There is reduced-fat milk and even fat-free milk. People who are allergic to dairy products often drink almond milk. I have also seen soy milk here in stores, but couldn't get a photograph of this type of milk.
- I would say this is because **people are aware of their own health** and in some way try to take care of themselves. They want to avoid fatty foods and take **precautions** against developing high cholesterol and other related problems, which is evident!
- In India, I have seen only cow's milk or buffalo's milk. I don't know if people are aware of fat-free milk or low-fat milk.
- **India should also have such options** available, as there are increased numbers of health problems due to high fat content in their daily diet.

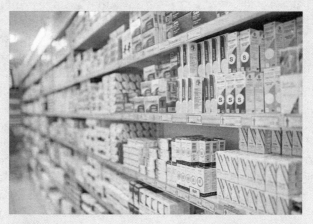

FIGURE 9-11

© PeopleImages/Shutterstock.

- All I mean with this photograph is to show the prices of medications and surgical accessories, such as bandages, in the U.S.
- In the U.S., 14 tablets of **omeprazole costs $12.49** if sold as a pharmaceutical company brand and $9.99 if it is a CVS brand. This amounts to **approximately 600-750 Indian rupees**.
- In **India, the cost of the same medication might range from 15-40 Indian rupees per 10 tablets**.
- In India, there are **many generic manufacturers that create a lot of competition** in the market, leading to **low costs for drugs**. Also, in India, **drug prices are regulated by a government authority**.
- The cost of **health care in the United States is high**, and one reason is **because of the drug prices**. There should be **proper regulations** for deciding drug prices in the United States.

United States and the health care they experienced back home in India. While visiting students were impressed by efforts made by pharmacies and even grocery stores to improve health, they found health care all but impossible to access and medications far more expensive compared to India. Lodaya used the findings from this small-scale project to advise his university about how to improve health services for foreign students.

Diagnostic Role Play Diagnostic role play (DRP) is another form of participatory formative research that is well described by the implementers of the Change Project, a behavior change program funded by United States Agency for International Development (USAID).[19] This method was created in the late 1980s by this chapter's first author and others working in development settings where it was unusual for rural community members to speak their minds easily. We observed village-level skits, and saw how the audiences for such performances got involved, suggesting changes in dialogue or even action: "You shouldn't speak to your wife like that. A real man would say, 'I will pay for my children's medicine.'" We started using role play to pretest concepts and materials, and eventually moved on to using it earlier in the formative research process to identify hidden behaviors and feelings.

Reported Behavior

In-Depth Interviews People are usually more comfortable talking about what they do than having someone watch them do it. In-depth interviews are sometimes used to discuss highly personal topics. The in-depth interview requires the interviewer to create a comfortable, nonjudgmental relationship with the person being interviewed. The researcher may use a topic guide to organize the interview or work from very open-ended questions.

Communications researchers typically conduct individual interviews either as a first step in the development of a focus group protocol (i.e., a group interview guide) or to interview **key informants**, such as gatekeepers. These informants work with members of the community or influence them in some way, and hence have a great deal of pertinent information to share.

An individual, in-depth interview is easier to arrange than a focus group, because it can be done in the respondent's home or office, or at a location of the interviewee's choosing (even on street corners for homeless respondents). At times, individual interviews are the only choice, especially when preservation of anonymity is paramount.

Focus Group Discussions Most social marketing researchers strongly prefer **focus group** discussions (FGDs) or interviews to collect information. By bringing together a group of 8 to 10 people who share certain characteristics together, they believe they can learn as much as if hundreds had been surveyed. At least, that is what qualitative researchers believe. Focus groups really give researchers a feeling for what people think, feel, and *say* they do. FGDs are useful in developing hypotheses, exploring broad topics, and producing a large number of ideas. A well-moderated group creates a casual environment that enables people to talk freely about their feelings, beliefs, and attitudes. Through such discussions, program planners and communicators become more sensitive to the values, concerns, and needs of their target audiences.

Because only a small sample of any target audience take part in focus group discussions, even if many are conducted, FGDs are exploratory and can only lead to hypothesis generation rather than hypothesis confirmation. Participants need to be recruited and screened carefully so that they are as representative as possible of the larger group to be studied. For example, if you are performing a doer/non-doer analysis, you need to recruit practitioners of the behavior in one group and non-practitioners in a second group. If you are interested in what young, Caucasian women have to say about a family planning product, your focus group should include only women meeting these criteria—not their mothers, not their boyfriends, and not people from other ethnic groups.

In the United States, the number of people invited for a casual dinner party is the ideal number for a focus group—no fewer than 6, and no more than 10, with 8 often considered a magic number. The group setting allows participants to question one another, and, while the moderator keeps the discussion on track, participants may bring up ideas that the researcher never considered. Perhaps it comes as a surprise, but participants often prefer discussing what might be considered embarrassing health topics with a group of people known to share their condition than discussing the same topics while alone with an individual investigator.

The FGD moderator must be able to create a comfortable environment in which everyone wants to participate. This trait—namely, being a good conversationalist—is probably more important than any formal training in research or even the topic itself. The best focus group moderators are recruited from near-peers of the target audience and trained in the technique and the topic guide.

While some researchers rely only on note taking, many more find it essential to record and transcribe focus group interviews. Computer qualitative analysis software can be used to code and analyze transcripts. It is important to record quotations exactly as spoken. When using one of the more creative, interpretive methods, creative teams might want to listen to voice recordings of respondents for inspiration. Again, it is critical that the informed consent procedure for the focus group tells the participants exactly who will listen to or review what they say, and ensures that they understand the nature of the analysis or use of the recording. Participants must be allowed to withdraw from the group if they are not willing to be recorded or have anyone listen to the recording. Anyone listening to or using the recording should go through human subjects training and be cleared for this purpose.

Many excellent resources on conducting focus group interviews are available.[1] The key elements are a quiet location, a good audio recorder, refreshments, compensation for the participants, and, of course, an expert moderator and excellent topic guide.

Intercept Interviews Perhaps even more than focus groups, some social marketing researchers rely on central-location **intercept interviews** to collect information from individuals. When this technique is used, the researcher goes to the location where the intended audience would encounter information about a behavior or acquire a product and then invites members of the audience to participate in an interview. Shopping malls are used extensively in the United States for this kind of research, but so are health clinics, supermarkets, and parks—anywhere the location plays a part in the consumer's decision. The high traffic volume in the intercept area allows the researcher to contact large numbers of respondents in a short period of time.

Intercept interviews can be used to collect either quantitative or qualitative data, depending on the form of the study. Intercepts are often performed when a concept is ready to be pretested on site. In addition, intercepts are useful for evaluating the readability and acceptability of print materials in an environment that is typical for the intended user. It is one thing to take people into a quiet testing site to review a brochure; it is quite another for people to try to read something in a supermarket aisle. The rule of thumb here is a simple one: If the supermarket is where the target audience will encounter the information, then test it in the supermarket.

The procedure for the intercept interview involves approaching individuals, asking a few screening questions to determine whether they match the characteristics of the target audience, and then bringing the participant over to a testing site. A variation of this theme is the "exit interview," in which participants who have already gone through an activity, such as a doctor's office visit or shopping trip, are invited to participate in the interview. While the advantage of this technique is the possibility of reaching a greater volume of respondents, many people do not want to be bothered. To overcome this kind of resistance, researchers almost always offer incentives, such as gift cards or cash rewards, for central-location intercepts.

Ethnolinguistic Techniques Ethnolinguistic techniques have been popularized by RAP (rapid assessment procedures, especially but not only for refugee populations) and other rapid ethnographic tools as a quick way of understanding how another group of people organizes their world into different cognitive categories.

- *Free listing:* In free listing, respondents are asked to list all the examples of a particular kind of thing that they know about—for example, appropriate foods for young children, important qualities in a spouse or partner, or common flu symptoms. The researcher records these items, usually on separate index cards. After a number of respondents are interviewed, the researcher should have a fairly large stack of cards. (If the respondents cannot read, use pictures or find another way of representing their ideas.) Not all topics are suitable to free listing, however. People are often unaware of what they know or do not know, are not accustomed to analyzing their own behavior, and may be unable to call up their "reasons" for doing something or not.
- *Pile sorting:* In pile sorting, individual items are printed on separate cards, with the item on the front and a number on the back. The researcher then asks respondents to sort the cards into piles. Often, it is helpful to begin by asking respondents to generate the categories themselves. For example,

---

1. For example, see Krueger RA, Casey MA. *Focus Groups: A Practical Guide for Applied Research.* 5th ed. Thousand Oaks, CA: Sage Publications, Inc.;2015.

if respondents were given a stack of cards with pictures of food and asked to put them in piles, many U.S. students would sort them into "foods I like" and "foods I don't like," then possibly into the learned categories of "good for you" and "not good for you," or the original four or five food groups. Other people might sort the foods into those appropriate for breakfast, lunch, or dinner. Still others might divide them up according to another medical system, such as "hot and cold" foods in a humoral medical system. Once the researcher has a sufficient number of categories, the respondents can be asked to sort the individual items by category.

- *Ranking:* The researcher may also ask people to **rank order** the individual items in a category. For example, flu symptoms can be ranked from most unpleasant to least unpleasant, life partner qualities from most important to least important, and breakfast foods from most favorite to least favorite.

A benefit of ethnolinguistic methods is that most people enjoy doing these activities, particularly if they get to work with illustrations and not words. Such research can be done quickly, and it can produce some interesting results in terms of which items are connected in a subject's mind and which are not. Simple statistics are sufficient to determine the relevancy of categories and ranking of item. More sophisticated multidimensional scaling analyses can assess the strength and weakness of associations and relationships among different categories and rankings.

Online Qualitative Research Much like central-location interviews, specific websites or communities can be used to identify specific participants at a virtual location, called "market research online communities". MROCs can be used to listen to specific audience segment representatives and explore some topics in depth, much as in a live focus group. Advantages of using MROCs include greater convenience for the participants, engagement over longer periods of time, and possibly greater anonymity if only audio or text responses are used. **BOX 9-10** provides a perspective from Parvanta *et al.* on using MROCs for formative research.

▶ Conclusion

Exploratory research is a creative process that can make or break any communication intervention. Most programs use a combination of qualitative and quantitative techniques, or mixed methods, to develop content such as concepts, images, and messages for further pretesting. Keep in mind that the purpose of exploratory research is not just to develop hypotheses about what might prompt behavior change, but to inspire creativity in writers and visual designers.

Appendix 9A presents a case by Kirby and Robinson of "message framing" research undertaken by the CDC and its partners. The research team used secondary and primary techniques in this order: a brief literature review and environmental scan, qualitative message framing assessments, key informant cognitive interviews, and an online survey with members of the public and health professionals. This case illustrates mixed methods formative research on a sensitive and often controversial public health topic.

BOX 9-10 Market Research Online Communities (MROCs)

An organization may establish a MROC as a password-protected website where a specific group of people are recruited to take part in daily, weekly, or monthly research activities around a shared topic of interest. The researcher could easily engage different audience segments by factors as such gender, language, and health concerns through different online communities. If you already have a social media site, such as a Facebook page or Twitter following, or an online site where, for example, new mothers or persons living with a specific illness interact, you have a way of recruiting individuals into an MROC. Alternatively, you can work with a vendor to do the recruiting, hosting, and management on your behalf.

Like focus groups, MROCs allow hosts to have a conversation with the participants and explore topics in depth. As with consumer panels, hosts are able to go back to the same people repeatedly over a specific period of time. An MROC project can have 50 to 500 participants and be accomplished in a week, if desired. The cost for running an online research community through a vendor for one month is about $5000.

Reprinted with permission from Sage Publications. Parvanta, C., Roth, Y., & Keller, H. (2013). Crowdsourcing 101: A Few Basics to Make You the Leader of the Pack. Health Promotion Practice. doi:10.1177/1524839912470654.

Wrap-Up

Chapter Questions

1. What is the purpose of formative research?
2. Describe and provide an example of exploratory research and concept testing.
3. Identify and describe two types of secondary research and one useful source for each type.
4. How would you use a positive deviance approach to distinguish the doers from the non-doers? for a behavior?
5. Why is audience segmentation central to a social marketing approach in health promotion?
6. How does the idea of "walking a mile in someone else's shoes" apply to customer journey mapping?
7. Compare and contrast qualitative and quantitative methods used in formative research.
8. Why do market researchers love intercept interviews?

References

1. Tuckman BW. Developmental sequence in small groups. *Psychol Bull.* 1965;63:384–399.
2. Social Marketing Gateway for the National Social Marketing Centre. The social marketing planning guide and toolkit: reviewing existing knowledge and current practice. http://www.socialmarketing-toolbox.com/content/reviewing-existing-knowledge-and-current-practice-0. Accessed December 12, 2015.
3. Centers for Disease Control and Prevention. Gateway to health communication and social marketing practice. June 26, 2012. http://www.cdc.gov/healthcommunication/audience/index.html. Accessed December 12, 2015.
4. Nowak GJ, Sheedy K, Bursey K, Smith TM, Basket M. Promoting influenza vaccination: insights from a qualitative meta-analysis of 14 years of influenza-related communications research by U.S. Centers for Disease Control and Prevention. *Vaccine.* 2015;33(24):2741–2756.
5. Weymann N, Härter M, Dirmaier J. A tailored, interactive health communication application for patients with type 2 diabetes: study protocol of a randomised controlled trial. *BMC Med Informatics Decision Making.* 2013;13:24. doi: 10.1186/1472-6947-13-24.
6. World Vision International. Positive Deviance/Hearth. http://www.wvi.org/health/publication/positive-deviance hearth. Accessed December 12, 2015.
7. Klaiman, T, Pantazis A, Bekemeier B. A method for identifying positive deviant local health departments in maternal and child health. *Front Public Health Serv Syst Res.* 2014;3(2): Article 5.
8. Managing the complete customer journey. *Harvard Business Rev.* November 5, 2013. https://hbr.org/2013/11/managing-the-complete-customer-journey/. Accessed December 12, 2015.
9. Sorman A. The best way to map the customer journey: take a walk in their shoes. *Survey Monkey Blog.* March 21, 2014. https://www.surveymonkey.com/blog/2014/03/21/map-customer-journey-keep-customers-happy/. Accessed December 12, 2015.
10. van Oosterom A. Mapping out customer experience excellence: 10 steps to customer journey mapping. March 12, 2010. http://www.mycustomer.com/experience/engagement/mapping-out-customer-experience-excellence-10-steps-to-customer-journey. Accessed December 12, 2015.
11. GreenBook Research Industry Trends Report (GRIT). http://www.greenbook.org/grit. Accessed December 12, 2015.
12. Measurement and Methods Core of the Center for Aging in Diverse Communities, University of California San Francisco. Using cognitive interviews to develop structured surveys: introduction. University of San Francisco Department of Medicine; 2007. http://dgim.ucsf.edu/cadc/cores/measurement/CognitiveInterviews.pdf. Accessed December 12, 2015.
13. U.S. Department of Health and Human Services. Information Collection and Paperwork Reduction Act (PRA) overview. http://www.usability.gov/how-to-and-tools/guidance/pra-overview.html. Accessed December 29, 2015.
14. Cox TF, Cox MA. *Multidimensional Scaling.* 2nd ed. Boca Raton, FL: CRC Press; September 28, 2000.
15. Keeter S, McGeeney K, Weisel R. Coverage error in Internet surveys: who web-only surveys miss and how that affects results. Pew Research Center; September 22, 2015. http://www.pewresearch.org/files/2015/09/2015-09-22_coverage-error-in-internet-surveys.pdf. Accessed December 29, 2015.
16. DiSogra C, Callegaro M. Metrics and design tool for building and evaluating probability-based online panels. *Soc Sci Comput Rev.* 2015:1–15. http://ssc.sagepub.com/content/early/2015/03/24/0894439315573925.full.pdf+html. Accessed December 29, 2015.
17. Scrimshaw N, Gleason G, eds. Rapid assessment procedures. In: *Qualitative Methodologies for Planning and Evaluation of Health Related Programmes.* Boston, MA: International Nutrition Foundation for Developing Countries; 1992. http://www.unu.edu/unupress/food2/UIN08E/uin08e00.htm.
18. Ankit L. PhotoVoice. https://photovoice.org/. Accessed December 29, 2015.
19. CHANGE Project, with Save the Children/Malawi. Guide to diagnostic role play. May 2002:1–17. http://pdf.usaid.gov/pdf_docs/Pnacw513.pdf. Accessed December 29, 2015.

Appendix 9

Framing Messages About Sexual Health: Research for Engaging All Stakeholders

Susan D. Kirby and **Susan J. Robinson**

▶ Overview

This case study presents an example of "message framing" research undertaken by the Centers for Disease Control and Prevention (CDC) and its partners. The research team combined data gathered through four connected lines of research: a brief literature review and environmental scan, message framing assessments, key informant cognitive interviews, and an online survey of members of the public and health professionals. The team identified two message frames that serve the widest range of stakeholders: (1) the importance of protecting health along the road of life by supporting good choices, and (2) bolstering traditional disease prevention and control with health promotion. This case illustrates mixed methods communication research on a sensitive and often controversial public health topic.

▶ Introduction and Problem Statement

For most public health issues, communication plays a critical role in garnering support for taking action based on the best evidence available.[1] Sexual health was defined by the World Health Organization (WHO) in 2002 as "a state of physical, emotional, mental, and social well-being in relation to sexuality; it is not merely the absence of disease, dysfunction, or infirmity. Sexual health requires a positive and respectful approach to sexuality and sexual relationships, as well as the possibility of having pleasurable and safe sexual experiences, free of coercion, discrimination, and violence."[2(p5)] Unhealthy or otherwise uninformed sexual behaviors or attitudes can lead to significant poor health outcomes, including HIV and other sexually transmitted infections (STIs), unintended pregnancies, coercive or violent behavior, and associated assaults to mental and physical well-being. Like many public health challenges, solutions depend on actions across multiple levels of the ecological model. But this requires engaging stakeholders in communities, or larger societal groupings, in which it is difficult to find consensus of opinion on sexual health matters. The purpose of our research was to develop a framework for communicating about sexual health issues and potential solutions in ways that signal openness to participation by all stakeholders.

▶ Theoretical Basis

We were guided by the work of Entman,[3] who described "dominant frames of reference" as cultural frames that are held by most individuals. Because these frames are more widely shared they have a higher "probability of being noticed, processed, and accepted by the most people."[3(p56)] Entman suggests that communication that violates these dominant frames will be less effective.

For example, Coca-Cola's 1971 iconic multi-ethnic advertisement "I'd like to teach the world to sing…" evoked hope, love, and world harmony at a time of civil strife. The next line of lyrics proclaimed, "I'd like to buy the world a Coke and keep it company; that's the real thing." There is nothing about a Coke that would have solved the political problems at the time. But Coca-Cola tapped into a widespread cultural value—a desire for harmony, to move past the bitterness of civil rights struggles and the Vietnam War, and move onto something sweeter, what Coke called "real."

When stakeholders hail from different political or cultural backgrounds, their different worldviews are associated with different frames of reference. Can messages about a controversial topic be framed so that they are received as intended by all or most stakeholders? Framing research suggests that communication research can identify common dominant frames that can engage multiple stakeholders. But dominant frames are often hidden in our subconscious. However, research techniques using metaphors and visual stimuli can be used to help respondents identify and articulate those frames to researchers.[4,5] Work by Lakoff[6,7] is foundational to these techniques, in which he addressed differences of opinion among stakeholders by identifying underlying values they shared in common, using indirect prompts to elicit qualitative information from stakeholders. We achieved this through a "red, green, yellow light" exercise, described in our methods section.

▸ Literature Review and Environmental Scan

Our research began with an environmental scan and a brief literature review. The team conducted the environmental scan to identify current messages in circulation on the topic and the types of dialogue found in networks of people interested in sexual health. The scan included national print and broadcast media, top daily newspapers through the United States, major weekly publications, major radio networks, and specialized media—for example, gay and conservative press, women's magazines, major African American and Hispanic/Latino newspapers and magazines, and influential blogs and advocate websites. The goal of the literature review was to understand efforts under way by national nonprofit, academic, and other institutions working on sexual health issues and the framing of the work. The literature review included both published research findings and gray literature such as program reports.

Search terms used in these activities included words related to audiences, behaviors, interventions, diseases, and health conditions, such as "LGBTQ," "adolescent," "sex," "sexual," "contraception," "HIV," "STD," and

"pregnancy." Between the national media scan and the literature review, the team used a total of 11 databases: Academic Search Premier, Cochrane Library, EBSCO, HSRProj (Health Services Research Projects in Progress), JSTOR Data for Research, Nexis, Psychology and Behavioral Sciences Collection, Reuters, PsycINFO, PubMed, and SocINDEX. **FIGURE 9A-1** shows the search process.

The team reviewed the final list of articles and abstracts for key themes, topics, tone, and audiences. Two sample analyses give a flavor of the diversity of publications considered in the media scan and literature review. The first is an article from a Christian media publication, summarized as follows: "A Christian woman's struggle with pornography addiction is briefly chronicled and her growing support group, Dirty Girl Ministries, is introduced. The general idea is that men are not alone in their addiction to porn; addiction affects women too and because it is taboo, they are forced into isolation when they need help"— positive tone. An example from the academic literature is a publication discussing several desirable social values of men that attract women, such as "62 undergrad couples found that when men's actions and values were consistent, girlfriends were more likely to behave in ways that benefited the relationship"—positive tone.

While both of these examples feature positive tones toward sexual health topics, much of the media content the team analyzed featured negative consequences of sexual diseases, such as the overall problem of HIV infections, as well as problems such as prostitution, pornography, and having sex at too young an age. Other themes included discussions of responsibility versus irresponsibility, sexual health as a choice, and, on the positive side, how having "good sex" contributed to well-being and happier lives. While the idea of increasing knowledge through sexual health education was associated with power and self-empowerment, often mentioned in the same context were issues of threats and the need to protect children and oneself from such threats, such as promiscuity as a "threat to society." But even conservative voices more than once drew parallels between sexual health education (including abstinence education) and other health education efforts, such as nutrition programs.

The literature review indicated that any messages around sexual health topics should be culturally tailored and appropriate to the intended audience—a daunting

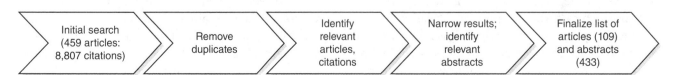

FIGURE 9A-1 Article Search and Selection Process.

task considering that informational needs vary greatly depending on age, gender, and circumstances. Eighty-seven percent of the articles reviewed had a focus on specific audiences, either by age (e.g., adolescents, college students), gender and sexual orientation, demographics, or other aspects, such as role (e.g., prison inmates, parents). In most articles, authors provided insights into approaches for research, different types of audiences, relevant frameworks and theories, and message evaluation strategies, and proposed interventions for communicating with the public, such as encouraging increased health provider–patient education.

The media scan and literature review helped investigators understand the existing dialogue on sexual health. This information also helped us develop the most promising and plausible sexual *health* messages that could supplement the current landscape of sexual *disease* messages.

▶ Message Framing Assessments

Our message development process was informed by the Zaltman Metaphor Elicitation Technique.[5] We asked the external stakeholder group to bring images of their work and to tell us stories about their work in sexual health. Our group elicitation process helped us build rapport and understanding within the group and between them and CDC staff members. As individuals spoke, the notes taken reflected important concepts. These concepts and perspectives were naturally reinforced when these individuals rated the draft frame messages described in the Red, Yellow, Green Light exercise below. Our team also reviewed the key concepts of this process during our final message selection for interviews and online testing to ensure we had a diverse set of messages for testing.

We constructed draft message frames based on the literature review findings as well as those reported in a publication by the Robert Wood Johnson Foundation (2010) entitled *A New Way to Talk About the Social Determinants of Health*.[8] These frames were embedded into six unstructured paragraphs [see **BOX 9A-1** for an example]. The research team used an independent facilitator to work first with six representatives from national groups, and next with 10 stakeholders from various CDC units, all involved in sexual or reproductive health issues.

Red, Yellow, Green Light

We asked each group of participants to review the material with highlighters in hand. They marked what they liked in green; words or phrases about which they were neutral, or found to be unclear, in yellow; and words or phrases they did not like, had issues with, or evoked a strong negative reaction, in red. We discussed their responses collectively, but did not seek any consensus. However, we did note if there was widespread agreement on specific points of green, yellow, or red

---

BOX 9A-1 Unstructured Paragraph for Red, Yellow, Green Light Exercise

Humans are intelligent, self-aware, and innately sexual. Sexuality is part of the human experience across the life span. Curiosity about our sexuality peaks during the teen years as children begin to mature into adults. We want to protect our youth by ensuring they know how to drive and have a license before they are allowed to drive a car alone. Likewise, we want to protect our youth from becoming sexually active before they know how to have and are able to sustain a healthy sexual relationship. Teens seldom understand that society pays a price when they do things that cause themselves and one another physical, mental, or emotional harm. They may not see how we all benefit when we act in ways that are responsible toward one another and ourselves. Fostering loving and committed relationships is good for us all. The United States is a diverse nation with people from many backgrounds and cultures and religious faiths, all of which shape our understanding and expression of sexuality. Because of this diversity, perspectives on appropriate sexual relationships range widely from abstaining from sexual activity until marriage to exploring casual relationships with one or multiple sexual partners. But most Americans agree on the following underlying principles or moral values regarding sexuality. First, sexual involvement should be based on love and respect for each other, which means there is no coercion, force, or physical or emotional harm. Second, sexual expression is most meaningful in a loving, committed relationship. Achieving those goals requires self-control, open communication, honesty, and trust (sentence underlined). Unfortunately, adolescents do not know and practice these skills all the time. We must protect the valuable futures of our youth by providing education about the moral values and responsibility of sexuality as well as the joyful unions it creates. To do that we need strong role models and age-appropriate education. Teens are seldom able to implement these tools effectively if they do not have the self-esteem, confidence, and social support for making the best choices for themselves. Helping young adults make the right choices regarding sexual activity requires a protective but positive and supportive environment that addresses all aspects of adolescent development, not just sexuality.

highlights. These findings helped reduce the number of frames and refine the message framing for the next step of research: cognitive interviews.

▶ Message Development

Four specific, dominant, high-level frames were selected for further testing. Each of these four ideas had from two or four message statements created for testing purposes. **TABLE 9A-1** shows the four frames and their message statements.

We also generated 18 "supporting message" statements on three key themes. **TABLE 9A-2** shows the themes and statements. Our intention with these message frames and supporting statements was to examine if specific word choices prompted positive, neutral, or negative reactions among reviewers with different political, religious, and other socially determined viewpoints.

TABLE 9A-1 Framing Messages from Cognitive Interviews	
A. Working Together	1. We all must work together — individuals, couples, families, and communities — to ensure that all of us have the opportunity to be sexually healthy. 2. As a society, we have the responsibility to help all Americans make healthy sexual choices.
B. Fair Chance/Fair Opportunity	3. All Americans need to have a fair opportunity to be free from sexually transmitted disease, sexual violence, and unintended pregnancy. 4. All people need to have a fair chance to make informed choices about their sexual health. 5. Everyone needs to have a fair opportunity to be sexually healthy.
C. Navigating a Journey/Protection	6. Life is a series of choices, including sexual choices. Throughout their lives, all people need information and skills to make healthy sexual choices that reflect their own values and deeply held beliefs. 7. Throughout life, we all make choices, including sexual choices. Along the way, Americans need the information, knowledge, and skills that will help them make sexual choices that protect their health and future partners. 8. Throughout life, we all make choices, including sexual choices. Along the way, all of us need the information, knowledge, and skills that will help us make sexual choices that protect us from the risks and dangers of unhealthy sexual activity. 9. If all people have the information, knowledge, and skills to help them make healthy sexual choices, this will help to reduce health costs.
D. Health Promotion/ Wellness	10. Living a healthy lifestyle is important to good health and this includes sexual health, too. It's time we focused on promoting and encouraging the behaviors that improve the emotional, social, spiritual, and physical aspects of sexuality. 11. Until the recent past, Americans focused on treating diseases like heart disease and cancer, not on preventing these diseases or promoting healthy lifestyles. Now, an emphasis on prevention and wellness promotes healthy lifestyles. In the same way, encouraging behaviors that improve sexual health, including the emotional, social, spiritual, and physical aspects of sexuality, would lead to better health for all Americans. 12. Today most us know that being healthy or well is more than just "not being sick." Being healthy is about making the most of your health, feeling good, and participating fully in life. In a similar way, being sexually healthy is more than just avoiding diseases. Changing how we think and talk about sexuality to a *wellness approach* could inspire more of us to behave in sexually healthy ways.

Robinson SJ, Stellato A, Stephens J, Kirby S, Forsythe A, Ivankovich MB. On the road to well-being: the development of a communication framework for sexual health. Public Health Rep. 2013 Mar-Apr;128 Suppl 1:43–52.

TABLE 9A-2 Supporting Statement Messages from Cognitive Interviews

E. About Sexual Health	13. Sexuality is a fundamental part of human life.
	14. Sexual health is an important part of a person's overall health.
	15. A person's sexual health affects their overall physical, emotional, mental, social, and spiritual health.
	16. Sexual health includes physical, emotional, mental, social, and spiritual dimensions.
	17. Promoting sexual heath means promoting responsible sexual behavior and healthy relationships to help prevent disease, unintended pregnancies, and sexual violence.
F. Role of Individuals	18. Talking about sexuality and sexual health can be difficult, but we benefit from open and honest conversations about these topics.
	19. Having appropriate, straightforward conversations about sex and sexuality help us to be sexually healthier.
	20. When we can have appropriate, straightforward conversations about sex and sexuality in our families, communities, and schools, we will all be sexually healthier.
	21. As young people become adults, they need accurate information in order to have respectful relationships that include honest conversations about sexuality.
	22. To be sexually healthy, Americans must take responsibility for the consequences of their sexual choices and their impact on themselves, their partners, their families, and their communities.
G. Role of Communities (1)	23. As a society, we need to teach young people about the nature of sexual relationships and how they can impact self-worth, personal development, and future life choices.
	24. We need to do a better job of promoting an understanding of healthy sexuality and healthy relationships.
	25. Communities must ensure that individuals have access to medically accurate, age-appropriate, and culturally appropriate information about sexuality and sexual health.
	26. Attitudes of secrecy around sexuality can lead to poor sexual health outcomes for individuals and communities.
H. Role of Communities (2)	27. Different communities require different approaches to achieving sexual health; what works in some communities may not work in others because of differences in what people believe and do.
	28. America contains diverse values and beliefs about sexuality and sexual health and we must all respect that diversity.
	29. Using a wellness approach to sexuality would mean some communities work to prevent stigma and discrimination regarding sexuality.
	30. An effective approach to improving sexual health includes engaging communities, bringing diverse groups together in partnerships, and implementing culturally appropriate and proven programs.

Robinson SJ, Stellato A, Stephens J, Kirby S, Forsythe A, Ivankovich MB. On the road to well-being: the development of a communication framework for sexual health. Public Health Rep. 2013 Mar-Apr;128 Suppl 1:43–52.

▶ Phone-Based Cognitive Interviews

We recruited 26 professionals representing health care, community organizations, and academia, policy makers, and opinion leaders (epidemiologists and health educators) in the field, beginning with recommendations from CDC. We also used a snowball sampling technique to expand the sample, taking care to include respondents with differing viewpoints on

sexual health and political outlook. A trained professional interviewed respondents by phone. We rotated the order of the messages to avoid any order bias. Interviewees were asked to identify their preferred message statement for each frame and supporting category. They were asked if there were words or phrases that were difficult to understand or could be better phrased, and finally to give alternate language, and provide rationale for their opinions.

For example, seven of interviewees selected the statement number 12 from the "Wellness Approach" frame (Table 9A-1). The original statement used the phrase "health-based outlook" where statement 12 now shows the phrase "wellness approach" in italics. Interviewees stated that the phrase "health-based outlook" was unclear to them. We learned a great deal about word choices, inclusivity, and perceptions of proof from varying stakeholders as the interviews continued. But, perhaps surprisingly, there were few differences in frame statement preference or supporting statement preferences by type of audience or respondent characteristics.

A few key message findings were instructional as we began to determine if any message statements needed to be refined. These findings included:

- The most effective messages are direct, actionable, and provide details.
- Many interviewees found the messages too vague and wanted additional detail.
- Many interviewees suggested framing sexual health positively.
- Several interviewees stated that responsibility for sexual health must be carefully framed.
- Several interviewees suggested tailoring the messages to particular audiences.

▶ Online Surveys with Diverse Public and Professional Participants

Next, we conducted a survey to identify the most effective frames that also contained attention-grabbing messages that were convincing, trustworthy, and personally relevant. Our final research step was to conduct online surveys with a vendor that maintained a standing panel of diverse consumer participants, $n = 240$. We used random sampling with over-sampling of certain types of participants to achieve a balance of attributes of interest. The vendor assessed these variables prior to including a panel participant in the survey. **TABLE 9A-3** shows the online survey sample classified by variables of interest to our study.

We supplemented the public online survey with 70 additional professional respondents who worked in health-related fields. We recruited these professionals using a snowball sampling technique, with referrals coming from our previous telephone interviewees. We attempted to achieve parity with the descriptive variables used in the consumer survey, but we did not pre-recruit on this basis. Instead, we used six questions in the survey to categorize respondents as

conservative, independent, or liberal in their views of sexual health and behavior. **TABLE 9A-4** shows the sample classified by variables of interest to our study.

The survey used questions from CDC's Health Message Testing System, approved by the Office of Management and Budget, following institutional review board (IRB) approval. Communication-relevant questions included items measuring how effective, attention-grabbing, convincing, trustworthy, and important the respondent felt each message statement was.

The web-based survey was programmed to ensure that respondents would not be overwhelmed by the amount of feedback requested, to avoid information overload, to collect additional detail on the reasons for selection of a particular message, and to prevent ordering bias.

▶ Online Survey Results

Respondents were asked to select the (1) most effective, (2) least effective, and (3) most attention-grabbing message frames for choices A through D in Table 9A-1. After selecting the most effective *frame*, they were then asked to select the most attention-grabbing *message* in the whole of Table 9A-1, regardless of frame. We used "attention grabbing" as our indicator because we wanted to learn more about messages that would likely cut through media clutter. The follow-up questions assessed if the attention-grabbing messages were also convincing, trustworthy, or personally relevant, or told the participant something new. Specifically, we needed to know if these attention-grabbing messages might have any negative aspects for specific audiences. For example, we would not want to recommend an attention-grabbing message that scored low on being "convincing." Overall, the most attention-grabbing messages were also scored as trustworthy, personally relevant, and convincing. Few respondents chose "learning something new" as a characteristic associated with the most attention-grabbing messages.

▶ Most Effective and Attention-Grabbing Frame

Each respondent selected a "best of the best" message regardless of frame. We then rolled these up to the frame level. For example, if 120 of the 240 participants selected *any* of the three Health Promotion/Wellness frame messages, we reasoned that 50% of the overall sample preferred the Health Promotion/Wellness frame.

TABLE 9A-3 Consumer Respondent Characteristics for the Online Survey

Characteristic	Categories	Respondents (n=240) N (percent)[a]
Target audience[b]	Young adults (aged 18–34 years)	96 (40)
	Adults (aged ≥ 35 years)	144 (60)
	Parents of adolescents	60 (25)
Social outlook	Conservative	79 (33)
	Liberal	67 (28)
	Moderate	94 (39)
Political party	Democrat	110 (46)
	Republican	65 (27)
	Independent	65 (27)
Religiosity (how often attend religious services)	Daily or weekly	87 (36)
	A few times a month/about once a month	33 (14)
	Less than once a month	120 (50)
Sexual orientation	Homosexual or "gay" or same gender loving/bisexual or two-spirited	32 (13)
	Heterosexual or "straight"	204 (85)
	Other, specify	0 (0)
	Don't know	0 (0)
	Decline to answer	4 (2)
Race/ethnicity[b]	Hispanic/Latino	36 (15)
	Caucasian	159 (66)
	African American	37 (15)
	Asian (non-Pacific Islander)/Central Asian/other	37 (15)
Gender	Male	115 (48)
	Female	124 (52)

(continues)

TABLE 9A-3 Consumer Respondent Characteristics for the Online Survey   *(continued)*

Characteristic	Categories	Respondents (*n*=240) N (percent)[a]
Education level	Less than high school	3 (1)
	High school graduate	28 (12)
	Some college or university	101 (44)
	College graduate with a two-year degree	71 (31)
	College graduate with a four-year degree	26 (11)
	Other	2 (1)
Geographic location	West	52 (22)
	Southwest	13 (5)
	Midwest	43 (18)
	Northeast	24 (10)
	Southeast	90 (38)
	Other	17 (7)
Region density	Rural/small town	10 (4)
	Micropolitan (large rural town) - population of 10,000–49,999	22 (9)
	Metropolitan (urban) - population ≥ 50,000	205 (87)

[a] Some categories do not total 240 due to missing responses. Percentages are based on total number of responses in each category and do not necessarily total to 100% due to rounding.

[b] The categories in these characteristics are not mutually exclusive.

Robinson SJ, Stellato A, Stephens J, Kirby S, Forsythe A, Ivankovich MB. On the road to well-being: the development of a communication framework for sexual health. Public Health Rep. 2013 Mar-Apr;128 Suppl 1:43–52.

As can be seen in **FIGURE 9A-2**, respondents most frequently selected messages from the Health Promotion/Wellness and Navigating a Journey/Protection frames as effective and also as the most attention grabbing. We found that liberals' results mirrored the results above. Conservatives tended to equally favor both the Health Promotion/Wellness and Navigating a Journey/Protection frames. Conservatives found the Health Promotion/Wellness frame more attention grabbing, but voted the Navigating a Journey Protection frame more frequently as an effective message.

In summary, the results indicate that messages that focus on the Health Promotion and Wellness frame will be effective *and* attention-grabbing with liberal audiences. Conservative audiences may find messages from the Wellness frame more attention grabbing, while messages that reflect the Journey frame may be more effective.

The Working Together and Fair Chance frames did not perform well across audiences in the "best of the best" message comparison.

Health Promotion/Wellness Theme

The three messages tested as part of the Wellness frame tested equally well on communication measures, with message number 12 being slightly more

TABLE 9A-4 Professional Respondent Characteristics for the Online Survey

Characteristic	Categories	Respondents (*n*=70) N (percent)
Target Audience*	(a) Community Based Organization	9 (13)
	(b) Physician	18 (26)
	(a) Other Health Care Provider	14 (20)
	(b) Policymaker	2 (3)
	(c) Other Key Opinion Leaders	32 (46)
Political outlook	(a) Conservative	12 (17)
	(b) Liberal	39 (56)
	(c) Moderate	19 (27)
Gender	(a) Male	14 (20)
	(b) Female	56 (80)
Geographic location	(a) West	6 (9)
	(b) Southwest	6 (9)
	(c) Midwest	9 (13)
	(d) Northeast	17 (24)
	(e) Southeast	21 (30)
	(f) Unknown	11 (16)
Region density	(a) Rural/Small Town	1 (1)
	(b) Micropolitan (Large Rural Town) = population between 10,000 and 49,999	2 (2)
	(c) Metropolitan (Urban) = population ≥ 50,000	54 (77)
	(a) Unknown	13 (19)

*The categories in these characteristics are not mutually exclusive.

Robinson SJ, Stellato A, Stephens J, Kirby S, Forsythe A, Ivankovich MB. On the road to well-being: the development of a communication framework for sexual health. Public Health Rep. 2013 Mar-Apr;128 Suppl 1:43–52.

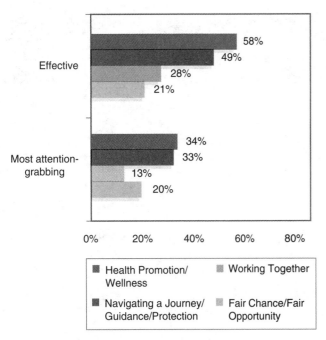

FIGURE 9A-2 Most Effective and Attention-Grabbing Frames.

Robinson SJ, Stellato A, Stephens J, Kirby S, Forsythe A, Ivankovich MB. On the road to well-being: the development of a communication framework for sexual health. Public Health Rep. 2013 Mar-Apr;128 Suppl 1:43–52.

effective than numbers 10 and 11 (**FIGURE 9A-3**). There was a statistically significant difference of opinion between liberal and conservative respondents, as only 35% of conservative respondents thought this message was effective, compared to 65% of liberal respondents ($p < 0.05$.).

Navigating a Journey/Protection Theme

Of the four messages tested as part of the Journey theme, two were selected as effective at the same rate, with a third message selected as effective just slightly less often. Slightly more than half of respondents selected the fourth message as the least effective message (**FIGURE 9A-4**).

We found a significant difference in effective message choices across different political outlooks in the message choices for this frame. More moderate (51%) and liberal (48%) respondents selected the message 8 as effective, whereas only 34% of conservative respondents thought this message was effective (chi-square $p < 0.05$).

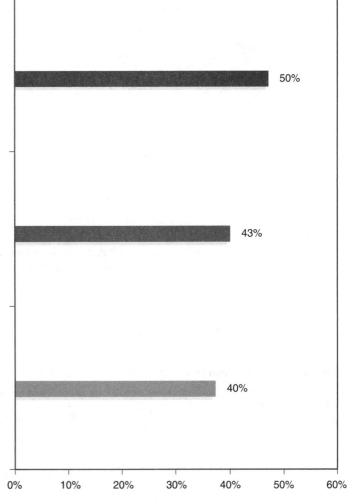

Message #12

Today most us know that being healthy or well is more than just "not being sick." Being healthy is about making the most of your health, feeling good, and participating fully in life. In a similar way, being sexually healthy is more...

50%

Message #10

Living a healthy lifestyle is important to good health and this includes sexual health, too. It's time we focused on promoting and encouraging the behaviors that improve the emotional, social, spiritual, and physical aspects of sexuality.

43%

Message #11

Until the recent past, Americans focused on treating diseases like heart disease and cancer, not on preventing these diseases or promoting healthy lifestyles. Now, an emphasis on prevention and wellness promotes healthy lifestyles...

40%

FIGURE 9A-3 Wellness Frame: Most Effective Message Across All Stakeholders.

Robinson SJ, Stellato A, Stephens J, Kirby S, Forsythe A, Ivankovich MB. On the road to well-being: the development of a communication framework for sexual health. Public Health Rep. 2013 Mar-Apr;128 Suppl 1:43–52.

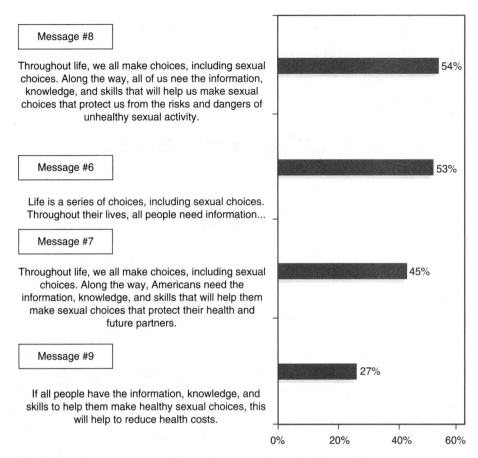

FIGURE 9A-4 Journey Frame: Effective Messages Across All Stakeholders.

Robinson SJ, Stellato A, Stephens J, Kirby S, Forsythe A, Ivankovich MB. On the road to well-being: the development of a communication framework for sexual health. Public Health Rep. 2013 Mar-Apr;128 Suppl 1:43–52.

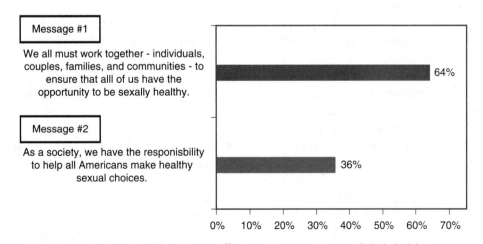

FIGURE 9A-5 Working Together Frame: Effective Messages Across All Stakeholders.

Robinson SJ, Stellato A, Stephens J, Kirby S, Forsythe A, Ivankovich MB. On the road to well-being: the development of a communication framework for sexual health. Public Health Rep. 2013 Mar-Apr;128 Suppl 1:43–52.

Working Together Theme

Under the Working Together theme, message 1 was much more frequently selected as the most effective message compared to message 2 (**FIGURE 9A-5**). There were no significant differences in effective message choices across any of the key respondent characteristics.

Fair Chance/Fair Opportunity Theme

Of the three messages tested as part of the Fair Chance frame, message 3 was most frequently found to be effective, followed closely by message 4 (**FIGURE 9A-6**). We found a significant difference in effective message choices across different ethnicity groups in response

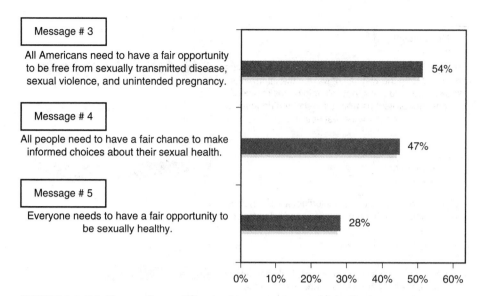

FIGURE 9A-6 Fair Chance Frame: Effective Messages Across All Audiences.

Robinson SJ, Stellato A, Stephens J, Kirby S, Forsythe A, Ivankovich MB. On the road to well-being: the development of a communication framework for sexual health. Public Health Rep. 2013 Mar-Apr;128 Suppl 1:43–52.

to message 5: "Everyone needs to have a fair opportunity to be sexually healthy." Thirty-nine percent of the Hispanic respondents selected this message as most effective, whereas only 25% of the non-Hispanic respondents selected this message as most effective (chi-square $p < 0.05$).

Supporting Statements

The 18 supporting statements were tested at the same time as the frame messages. Respondents were asked to select the most effective, least effective, and most attention-grabbing statements from each of the three sets of supporting statements (Table 9-2, E-H). All respondents evaluated the set of supporting statements About Sexual Health (Category E). However, due to a limited amount time, each respondent was randomly assigned to view and respond to only one of the following sets of supporting statements: Role of Individuals, Role of Communities 1, or Role of Communities 2 (F-H). Therefore, the percentages for these three sets of supporting statements are based on only a portion of the survey sample.

The supporting statements were nearly all effective and can be used to support either of the two recommended themes. However, across all of the audiences, we found some of the supporting statements to be particularly effective, as shown in **TABLE 9A-5**.

In addition, there were a number of specific message findings by audience characteristic that effective health communicators should consider, based on our research on sexual health. These findings result from audience-specific findings in this research. These recommendations are specific to tailoring messages to an audience when the opportunity arises.

- Messages intended for **policy makers**.
  Example: *If Americans have the information, knowledge, and skills to help them make healthy sexual choices, this will help to reduce health costs.*
- Messages using the word "community" and an emphasis on access to care for audiences in **rural or less densely populated regions of the country**.
  Example: *Communities must ensure that individuals have access to medically accurate, age-appropriate, and culturally appropriate information about sexuality and sexual health.*
- Messages that use the word "Americans" should be used sparingly to ensure that a **wider audience** is reached (e.g., immigrants, racial/ethnic minorities).
- Communicating with **gender-specific professional audiences**.
  Professional females: *Life is a series of choices, including sexual choices. Throughout their lives, all people need information and skills to make healthy sexual choices that reflect their own values and deeply held beliefs.*
  Professional males: *Throughout life, we all make choices, including sexual choices. Along the way, Americans need the information, knowledge, and skills that will help them make sexual choices that protect their health and future partners.*
- Messages intended for and about **youth**.
  Example: *As young people become adults, they need accurate information in order to have respectful relationships that include honest conversations about sexuality.*

TABLE 9A-5 Supporting Statement Preferences

Supporting Statement Category	Supporting Statements
About Sexual Health	A person's sexual health affects their overall physical, emotional, mental, social, and spiritual health.
Role of Individuals	Talking about sexuality and sexual health can be difficult, but we benefit from open and honest conversations about these topics.
	As young people become adults, they need accurate information in order to have respectful relationships that include honest conversations about sexuality.
Role of Communities	As a society, we need to teach young people about the nature of sexual relationships and how they can impact self-worth, personal development, and future life choices.
	Communities must ensure that individuals have access to medically accurate, age-appropriate, and culturally-appropriate information about sexuality and sexual health.
	Different communities require different approaches to achieving sexual health; what works in some communities may not work in others because of differences in what people believe and do.
	An effective approach to improving sexual health includes engaging communities, bringing diverse groups together in partnerships, and implementing culturally appropriate and proven programs.

Robinson SJ, Stellato A, Stephens J, Kirby S, Forsythe A, Ivankovich MB. On the road to well-being: the development of a communication framework for sexual health. Public Health Rep. 2013 Mar-Apr;128 Suppl 1:43–52.

■ Messages supporting diverse values and beliefs **for homosexual and bisexual audiences**.

Example: *America contains diverse values and beliefs about sexuality and sexual health and we must all respect that diversity.*

▶ Discussion

Public health communicators must remain sensitive to human perspectives across cultural, social, and political boundaries to engage stakeholders with public health messages and to mitigate concerns as new approaches and policies are introduced. In the field of public health, one can find varying attitudes among program planners regarding the usefulness of including perspectives that may be differ from those strictly informed by scientific studies.[1] However, as long as the public is part of public health,

communicators must understand diverse stakeholder perspectives to communicate scientific findings and policy decisions effectively.

We have described in this case study methods and findings from a study aimed at developing messages to engage stakeholders with diverse perspectives and values in a socially charged public health issue, sexual health. The key to success was to use mixed-methods research systematically to identify common values held by stakeholders and to translate these values into messages for use in improving communication. One can apply the techniques described here to many public health issues, but these will be particularly helpful to communicators working on health issues that may invoke debate. We have learned through other studies on different public health issues that underlying values found in stakeholder groups vary according to the issue. There is a great need for additional framing research on a myriad of public health topics.

References

1. Choi BC, Pang T, Lin V, et al. Can scientists and policy makers work together? *J Epidemiol Community Health.* 2005;59:632-637. doi: 10.1136/jech.2004.031765.

2. World Health Organization. *Defining Sexual Health: Report of a Technical Consultation on Sexual Health, 28–31 January 2002.* Geneva, Switzerland: World Health Organization; 2006.

3. Entman R. Framing: clarification of a fractured paradigm. *J Comm.* 1993;43(4):51-58.

4. Christensen G, Olson J. Mapping consumers' mental models with ZMET. *Psychol Market.* 2002;19:477-502.

5. Zaltman G. *How Customers Think: Essential Insights into the Mind of the Market.* Boston, MA: Harvard Business Review Press; 2003.

6. Lakoff G. *Moral Politics: What Conservatives Know That Liberals Don't.* Chicago, IL: University of Chicago Press; 1996.

7. Lakoff G. *Don't Think of an Elephant!: Know Your Values and Frame the Debate.* White River Junction, VT: Chelsea Green Publishing; 2014.

8. Christiano, A., Westen, D., Carger, E. (2010). *A new way to talk about the social determinants of health.* Princeton, NJ: Robert Wood Johnson Foundation.

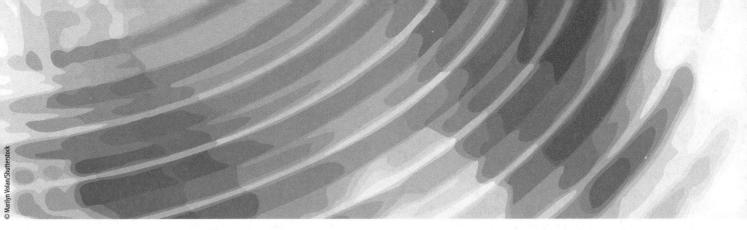

CHAPTER 10

Media Vehicles, Platforms, and Channels

Claudia Parvanta

LEARNING OBJECTIVES

By the end of this chapter, the reader will be able to:

- Identify sources of data on media use.
- Define a spectrum of media options available to health communicators.
- Use the "theory-informed media selection" framework to identify media channels for audiences.
- Describe customer-centric and content management approaches for selecting media channels and formats.
- Compare features and best practices for various media options.
- Cite examples of focused media and transmedia strategies used in public health.

▶ Introduction

As Nedra Kline Weinreich asserts:

> We live in a transmedia world, seamlessly moving from mobile phone to computer to television—often all at the same time. Audiences encounter many different types of media throughout the course of a day. In addition to spreading your messages and interventions across multiple media or platforms, you need to find a way to grab their attention through the clutter.[1]

Health communicators need to use multiple media to attract different audiences not only at different times of day and different locales, but also at different stages of life or moments in a behavior change journey. From broadcast mass media to individual text messages, the array of media options is almost overwhelming. Our goal in this chapter is to provide a reasonable approach to developing a multimedia strategy that will allow you to reach—and then engage, inform, or persuade—your intended audience. These decisions will flow from the theory and intervention model you have adopted for your particular communication purpose.

A Word About Terminology

Words associated with media get thrown around a lot without too much precision. For example, in common usage, the term "media" often refers to news journalism, and the term "media relations" to the process of interacting with reporters, agents, bloggers, and others who publicize a story through "mass media." Mass media are, in fact, channels that convey vehicles to audiences in the form of print, radio, television, the Internet, mobile networks, and so on. As an analogy, you can think of channels as the roads that carry motor vehicles, with each vehicle carrying passengers, which are the messages. Media vehicles, like automobiles, vary in their appearance and features. Generically, we refer to these messages as "content," which is what a communicator writes, illustrates, captures, and edits in video and/or sound. The creative talent producing the content will use specific tools depending on the format required, be it sound recordings, videos, or graphic renderings.

Some of this work is done for a specific platform, such as Twitter, HTML, Internet video, "Wordpress" (for blogs), a game, an Android app, or—here it gets confusing—Facebook. According to photographer and digital asset manager Peter Krogh,

> You need to be much more careful about the services you use as a platform compared to those which are simply channels…. For example, if you use Facebook's email system to communicate with your [audience], and you use Facebook's servers to store your portfolio, then you are using it like a Platform. It becomes a foundation of your marketing efforts. The longer it goes on, the more "married" you are to the platform. It may be difficult or impossible to disentangle yourself from the platform if the service goes away, or becomes objectionable. You could also use Facebook more like a Channel. You could use your own email address, and upload your photos to your own website and then link them to your Facebook page. This strategy takes advantage of Facebook as a great viral marketing tool, without giving the company so much leverage over your business.[2]

You should not be overly concerned with keeping this terminology straight. It will generally be understood within the context in which you are working. We begin our discussion of who uses which media (and here we mean channels) next.

▶ An Overview of Media Use in the United States

Sources

When starting a journey with media, take advantage of the information available at resources such as the Pew Research Center,[a] DigitalGov[b] (a federal cross-agency support site), the *Journal of Medical Internet Research*, and the International Association for the Measurement and Evaluation of Communication (AMEC).[c] Research companies such as Forrester,[d] Neilsen,[e] and the data compiler Statista[f] sell data and analyses relating to specific media markets or business applications, and provide some overarching reports for free. This chapter has made generous use of these resources in addition to some private-sector blogs and postings, as indicated.

The Big Picture

According to the Pew Research Center, 85% of all American adults were using the Internet and 67% were using smartphones in 2015.[3] Nearly all were using television (TV) and radio. The general trend in the United States is to replace set-time broadcasts (TV, radio) and print media with digital versions that can be accessed on demand through personal devices. Nevertheless, this trend varies by demographics and time of day. **TABLE 10-1** shows Nielsen's analysis of a "Week in the Life" for different segments of the population by hours and minutes of time spent with various media devices and channels in the second quarter of 2015. **FIGURE 10-1** shows Nielsen's data for average platform use throughout a weekday by numbers of users.

As can be seen from the Nielsen data, broadcast media provide the most powerful channels to reach large numbers of viewers quickly. Digital and interactive media channels allow for customization and the ability to reach specific segments interactively. Together, broadcast and interactive media provide a wide array of

a. http://www.pewresearch.org/
b. https://www.digitalgov.gov
c. http://amecorg.com
d. http://www.forrester.com
e. http://www.nielsen.com/us/en.html
f. http://www.statista.com

TABLE 10.1 A Week in the Life Q2, 2015

(A) Kids and Teens

	Kids (Ages 2-11) Hours:Minutes	Teenagers (Ages 12-17) Hours:Minutes
Live + DVR/Time-shifted TV	20:46	16:32
DVR/Time-shifted TV	2:12	1:35
AM/FM Radio	n/a	7:02
DVD/Blu-Ray Device	1:36	0:55
Game Console	2:37	4:13
Multimedia Device	1:15	0:57
Internet on a PC	0:17	0:43
Video on a PC	0:22	0:29
App/Wed on a Smartphone	n/a	n/a
Video on a Smartphone	n/a	n/a

(B) Adults

	Ages 18-24 Hours:Minutes	Ages 25-34 Hours:Minutes	Ages 35-49 Hours:Minutes	Ages 50-64 Hours:Minutes	Ages 65+ Hours:Minutes
Live + DVR/Time-shifted TV	16:26	22:09	29:17	39:55	48:02
DVR/Time-shifted TV	1:31	2:58	3:53	4:07	3:40
AM/FM Radio	10:02	11:20	13;27	14:51	11:58
DVD/Blu-Ray Device	0:45	0:59	0:59	0:57	0:37
Game Console	4:15	2:54	1:10	0:22	0:07
Multimedia Device	1:22	1:45	1:13	0:43	0:29
Internet on a PC	3:58	5:49	6:13	5:41	3:01
Video on a PC	1:47	2:08	1:50	1:20	0:31
App/Wed on a Smartphone	10:56	10:07	9:43	7:12	1:35
Video on a Smartphone	0:36	0:24	0:16	0:09	IFR

Note: IFR represents data that is insufficient for reporting due to small sample sizes. n/a represents data unavailability.

Data from The Total Audience Report Q2 2015; p.10, Table 1A- Weekly time spent in hours:minutes by age for US population. Copyright 2015 The Nielsen Company.

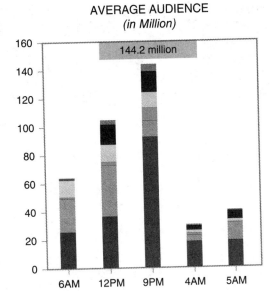

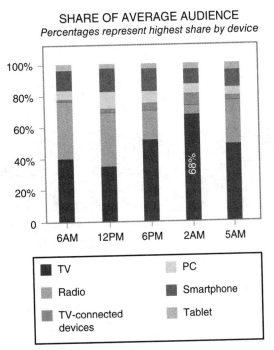

FIGURE 10-1 Media Use During the Day in Millions and by Percent Share by Device According to Nielsen, Second Quarter 2015.

Data from The Total Audience Report Q2 2015; p.3, Weekday (M-F) Overall media usage: P18+ May 2015. Copyright 2015 The Nielsen Company.

outlets from which health communicators can choose those most appropriate for disseminating their health intervention messages. The final mix will depend on the communication objectives, tempered by organizational limitations of budget and staffing.

Broadcast Media Channels

Television According to the Nielsen Company, there are 116.4 million TV-equipped homes in

the United States, and 296.8 million people age 2 years or older were living in these homes for the 2015–2016 TV season.[4] While Americans spend an average of nearly 30 hours each week tuned into the TV, this number varies greatly by demographic group. In 2015, those persons classifying themselves as "Asian American" averaged a low of 16 hours, and those self-identifying as aged 65 or older averaged a weekly 48 hours of TV viewing.[5] The good news for health communicators is that half of all people living in a community watch their local news on the TV. These media buys (purchases of time on paid media) are much less expensive than national network programming.

Radio Radio remains the most popularly consumed media channel, with 91% of surveyed Americans tuning in at least once a week.[6] Listening formats vary greatly by market (geographic location), making radio one of the most customizable mass media available. In 2014, the "Country" music format attracted 15.2% of all listenership and surpassed the listenership of "News, talk, information" segment (10.6%) for the first time, a continuing trend. All other music forms—for example, adult contemporary, rock, classics, and urban—had single-digit percentages of listeners. Of course, even those single digits represent millions of people tuning in every day.

Radio personalities can be extremely influential in their media markets. The Incite media company provides a dramatic case study of an HIV prevention activity to reach men who have sex with men led by radio personalities in Los Angeles and New York City (**APPENDIX 10A**).

Print Media/Magazines According to the Pew Research Center, newspaper readership has been steadily declining since 2000, with fewer than 20% of Americans 18 to 24 years old and fewer than 60% of those 65 and older reading a daily newspaper in 2014.[7] If this were the end of the story, we could kiss newspapers goodbye. But, while only 56% read the print version of a newspaper, the rest of us use other platforms—including the Internet, mobile, and print—to read the same content.

Magazines have also found a new life with digital audiences. According to Mediamark Research & Intelligence (MRI), readership for general-interest print magazines has declined substantially in the past few years, including readership for the publications as diverse as the *National Enquirer* and the *Reader's Digest*.[8] Conversely, digital readership has increased, for those magazines that attract and measure specific audiences across multiple platforms, including print, digital, web, mobile, video, and social media.[8] Such magazines have highly targeted, curated content and faithful audiences. Health communicators should take notice.

▶ Media Channel Selection

When planning a multimedia strategy, the objective—to inform, persuade, or engage—is paramount. Some media channels and formats are best for conveying "information," while others are more suited to "entertainment education." This section provides some guidance on how to select media channels and vehicles depending on the overarching approach.

Theory-Informed Media Selection Framework

The USAID-funded Health Communication Capacity Collaborative (HC3) created the Theory-Informed Media Selection (TIMS) framework to guide demand generation for reproductive health products in resource-poor countries.[9] This framework combines media richness theory (MRT) and uses and gratifications theory (UGT).

Media Richness Theory

According to HC3, richer communication media, such as face-to-face communication and some emerging technologies, tend to be more effective for conveying ambiguous messages because they allow for discussion and immediate feedback, transmission of both verbal and visual information, and greater personalization. Important "richness" factors include the following:

- Interactivity/feedback: the ability of communicators to interact directly and rapidly with each other
- Language variety: the ability to support natural (conversational or vernacular) language as distinct from more formal language (e.g., formalized business language) or abstract language (e.g., mathematical symbols)
- Tailoring: the ability to modify the message based on the needs of the recipient in real time
- Affect: the ability to transmit feeling and emotion

Uses and Gratifications Theory

UGT considers why and how people use specific media and channels to achieve their own ends—for

example, for information, consensus building, entertainment, or connecting. For the general public, Facebook is primarily a means of interpersonal communication, a form of entertainment, and a source of information. In contrast, healthcare professionals prefer professional meetings, professional association sites, peer-reviewed journals, ResearchGate, and similar sites for connecting, and the National Institutes of Health (NIH) and Centers for Disease Control and Prevention (CDC) websites for their information. Few healthcare professionals would regard a posting on Facebook as a credible, authoritative source (unless the page was managed by a trusted, respected colleague or institution).

FIGURE 10-2 illustrates the TIMS framework's basic idea of choosing your media dissemination strategy according to these two principles. TIMS is applied following these steps:

1. Use the MRT criteria (without taking current use or resource availability into consideration) to identify which medium or combination of media can support the necessary level of communication richness. (How complex or ambiguous is the information?)
2. Use the UGT criteria (without considering their specific media richness) to identify the media channels used by the intended audience for the intended type of communication (e.g., information, entertainment, engagement).
3. Prefer media identified by both MRT and UGT. With no overlap, consider using multiple channels to disseminate less rich media.

If the overall approach is to inform the audience, content needs to appear in those media channels in which consumers have faith. A good indicator for making this determination is where the consumers get their news. If the overall approach is to engage the audience, select channels that the audience presently uses to engage with specific communities. The same is true for entertainment strategies. The next consideration is where and when to present your content.

Person-, Place-, and Time-Mediated Touchpoints in the Customer Journey

The customer journey (CJ) is an individual's experience that begins with *becoming aware* of an offering—be it an idea, a product, or a service—and continues through *actions taken*. The journey may end with

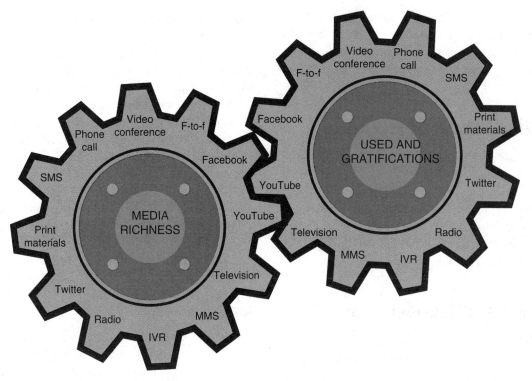

FIGURE 10-2 The TIMS Framework.

The Health Communication Capacity Collaborative HC3. A theory-based framework for media selection in demand generation programs. Baltimore: Johns Hopkins Bloomberg School of Public Health Center for Communication Programs; 2014.

adoption of the idea or purchase of the product, or it might continue on to include post-purchase or adoption advocacy. For those instances when customers are dissatisfied with an offering, it might include post-purchase or -adoption criticism, mostly through social media. The opportunities for an organization promoting an idea, product, or service to engage with the customer are referred to as "touchpoints." Touchpoints can be tangible structures or services normally associated with branding, including buildings, signage, staff clothing, packaging, and products—but they are also every communication interaction. Whether it is a live phone call, a billboard, a TV ad, or a tweet, you should choose a media channel because of its potential to deliver the right kind of touch at the right place and time for the intended recipient.

We have selected a healthcare example to illustrate the process of matching mediated touchpoints to a CJ, using patients as the customers. **FIGURE 10-3** traces a patient journey from the home community, through the hospital, and back out. In this case, the health communication objective is to minimize hospital-acquired infections, and almost all of the touchpoints are interpersonal, or make use of print and small media. As with the example that addresses preventing healthcare-associated infections (HCAIs), the patient journey is quite literally the trip in and out of the hospital, and the touchpoints are almost literal as well.

A map for a less literal journey requires more investigation of the customers' needs and desires. Is the customer seeking information, encouragement, validation, a sense of community, a reward, or something else? A media map for a CJ can be fairly complex, particularly if there are several audiences, or *personae* in the plan. Even so, it boils down to answering the "who, what, where, when, and how questions," just as we always have, for specific audiences and behavior change goals. **FIGURE 10-4** shows a generic CJ and mediated touchpoints. (CJs and media selection are discussed elsewhere in this text in the context of implementation.)

Media Management Framework

A final consideration in selecting media is how much control your organization exercises over each channel. In general, there is a trade-off between cost and control. Following are descriptions of the various types of media modified from G. Dietrich's blog "Spin Sucks":

- *Paid media*: Channels you pay to leverage, including print and outdoor advertising, commercial spots on TV and radio, as well as paid search leads, display ads, social media advertising, and email marketing.
- *Earned media*: Where public relations (PR) used to live—"free" coverage in news or trade

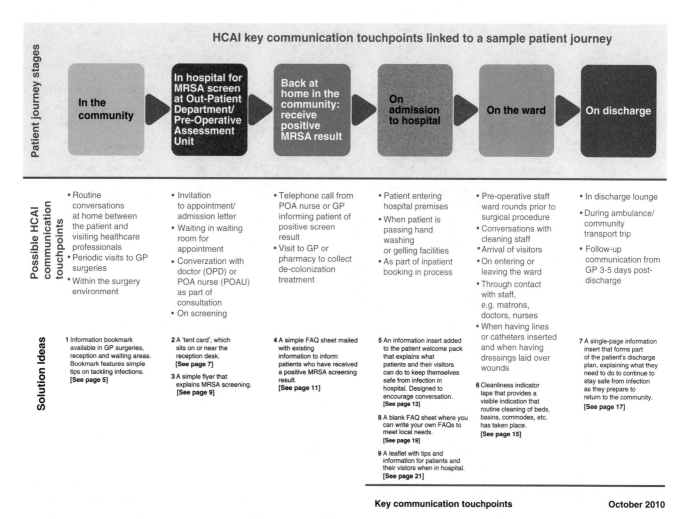

FIGURE 10-3 Reducing Healthcare-Associated Infections: Key Communication Touchpoints Linked to a Sample Patient Journey.

NHS Institute for Innovation and Improvement. Key Communication Touchpoints; Example patient journey diagram. October 2010. Available at http://www.institute.nhs.uk/images//documents/Tackling_infections/Updates/Example_patient_journey.pdf.

publications. This was achieved mostly by creating events, inviting the press to briefings, new product releases, and the like.

- *Shared media*: The new frontier for PR—other people talk about "you" through social media

channels. In essence, your users and/or fans produce or "curate" content about you, such as blogs, tweets, YouTube videos, and the original "word of mouth." The jackpot standard here is "going viral."

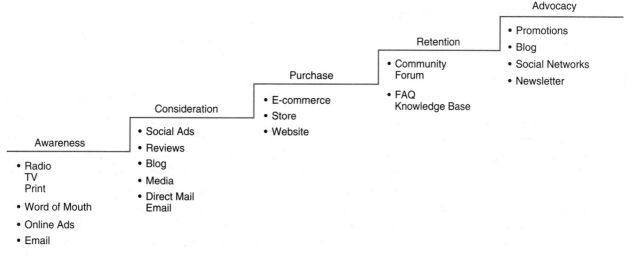

FIGURE 10-4 Customer Journey Life Cycle.

Data from https://www.clickz.com/clickz/column/2191650/optimizing-social-media-across-the-customer-lifecycle#. Lee Odden, Social Media Smarts blog post published July 16, 2012

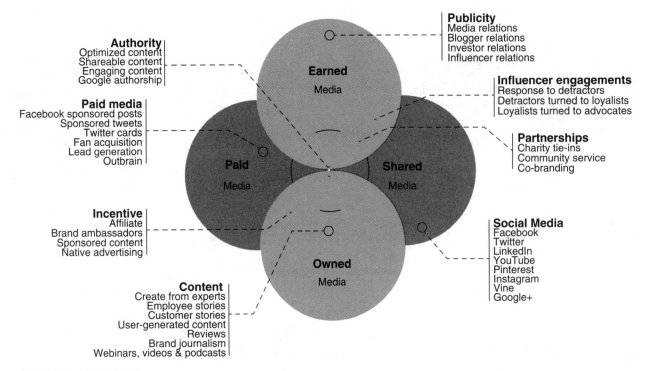

FIGURE 10-5 PESO Model.

■ *Owned media*: The content you produce yourself. It lives on your website, the editorial content on your TV or radio station, your print publications, and your blog. You control the messaging and tell the story your way.

The combination of paid, earned, shared, and owned media is referred to as the "PESO" model. **FIGURE 10-5** shows an array of media options in a PESO model.

We will now discuss various media channels keeping these frameworks in mind.

▶ "Inform Me": The Search for Information

Media You Earn: News

Two studies conducted recently by the American Press Institute and the Associated Press–NORC Center for Public Affairs Research (at the University of Chicago) indicate that three-fourths of Americans get news at least daily, including 60% of adults younger than age thirty.[10(p12)] **BOX 10-1** and **FIGURE 10-6** provide some highlights from the surveys conducted in 2014 among U.S. adults older than age 18, and among "Millennials" (born between 1982 and 2002).

The surveys found that respondents were most likely to *trust* local TV news, newswires, radio news

organizations, national network news, 24-hour TV news channels, and magazines *more than online only* sources.[10] If people are particularly interested in a topic, particularly those in the Millennial generation, 57% say they will go online through a search engine, or use a news site (23%) to learn more. Fewer than 10% will go to Facebook, and fewer than 5% to Twitter or a blog.[11] According to one respondent:

> [If] I'm on social media and I see people are posting about something, then I'm like, is this really factual information or is it possibly fictional information? And it triggers a domino effect for me to look at multiple other sites because I get curious sometimes. Then I can interpret things for myself. [A] lot of it starts at social media.[11(p19)]

Media You Own: Your Website or Blog

Your organization's website—that is, a collection of electronic pages at a single address—is entirely under your control. Anyone can have a blog, which is a chronological collection of content you post with the expectation that others will comment on what you have said. Websites may contain blogs, or blogs may link to websites. Determining how these forums are managed is mostly a matter of organizational policy and size. In public health communication (apart from any brick and mortar sites you run,

BOX 10-1 What About News? It's All Media All the Time

- Americans follow the news on a wide variety of devices,… television, radio, print,… newspapers and magazines, computers, cell phones, tablets, e-readers, and devices such as an Xbox or PlayStation that link the Internet to a television.
- Americans on average reported that, during the past week, they followed the news using four different devices or technologies. The most frequently utilized devices include television (87%), laptops/computers (69%), radio (65%), and print newspapers or magazines (61%). Figure 10-6 shows the preferred source of news among survey participants.
- Local TV news stations are the most popular source for news about crime and public safety (40%), traffic and weather (32%), and health and medicine (12%).
- People also turn to specialized news sources for some topics, ahead of traditional sources. Specialty news sources are the most commonly mentioned source for news about sports (38%), entertainment (22%), lifestyle news (14%), and science and technology (10%).
- Twenty-four-hour news sources are most popular for news about foreign or international issues (31%), national government and politics (28%), social issues (24%), and business and the economy (21%). Some people simply cite television as a source, not mentioning whether they mean cable, local, or network.

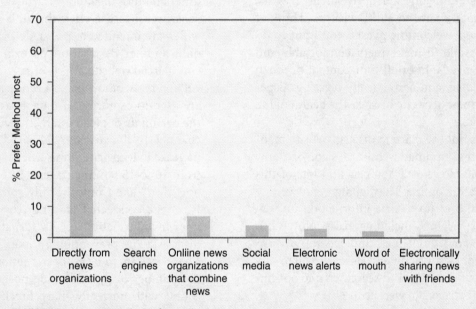

FIGURE 10-6 How People Prefer to Find News.

Copyright 2014. The Media Insight Project. American Press Institute and Associated Press. The Personal News Cycle: How Americans choose to get their news. http://www.american pressinstitute.org/wp-content/uploads/2014/03/The_Media_Insight_Project_The_Personal_News_Cycle_Final.pdf. Published March 17, 2014. Accessed December 20, 2015.

e.g., health centers, pharmacies, hospitals), websites and blogs are the primary channels through which you create and maintain your identity, brand, and credibility. These channels will become the primary locations for keeping your content together in a way that it can be easily found by your intended audiences.

Following some initial activation trigger, which could be word of mouth or a social media contact, almost every customer journey today begins with online exploration. Most Americans use browsers and search engines (such as Google, Bing, Yahoo, or nontracking browsers like DuckDuckGo) to find information on the web. Ideally, you want your website or blog to show up at the top of a search, preferably without paying for that ranking.

Search Engine Optimization

What moves you to the top of the page, short of paying for it, in a search engine? Searchengineland.com has created a "periodic table" of **search engine optimization (SEO)**, which is available to view at http://search engineland.com/seotable. This table covers just about every aspect of how search terms can lead to your online content. It is clear that quality of content, the ease of navigating the site, and the reputation of the organization based on several factors all contribute to it moving to the top – not only the use of 'key words', which still matters as well.

Inbound Marketing

When a viewer gets to your website, whether by accident or by design of SEO, you want that person to stay a while, look at your content, and take some action. An essential difference between media you own, such as websites or blogs, and broadcast or social media channels is that the consumer *is coming to you to look for something*. This type of interaction, which is referred to as **inbound marketing**, relies on luring visitors because they want to come to the site, rather than depending on interruptive media (tweets, pop-up ads, email spam) to attract visitors. Think of yourself as a host welcoming guests. You want to do everything possible to make them comfortable and attend to their needs. In brief, your content needs to be useful, findable, and aesthetically pleasing. Especially, it needs to be accurate because the health of the public is at stake.

This text is not the place to discuss website management systems, optimal website design, or "how to write an epic blog post." You can find lots of this kind of information online. The digitalgov.gov website contains a wealth of up-to-date information on web design, user experiences including accessibility (also see section508.gov) guidelines, and federal government policies for posting content. Here, we will briefly discuss content marketing and search engine optimization, the main drivers of website use.

Content Marketing: Size Does Matter   Per HubSpot's 2015 survey of marketing benchmarks from more than 7000 businesses, there is a relationship between the number of website pages, landing pages, blog posts, and other features and the volume of traffic to these pages.[12] Here are a few highlights from this organization's survey:

- Organizations with 51 to 100 webpages generate 48% more traffic than those with 1 to 50 pages. Organizations with more than 1000 pages see five times the amount of traffic as those with fewer than 51 pages.

- The more **landing pages**, the more "leads." A landing page is how you get to a website. For most websites, it is the home page, but there are reasons to have multiple landing pages (not necessarily connected to the main website) to attract different kinds of audiences from other platforms. Most websites use **click-through** landing pages, which are intended to persuade the user to move onto another destination page in the site. In a commercial website, this is often a "shopping basket" or registration page. Lead-generation pages are used to capture user data so as to connect to the person through an interactive communication channel. In the commercial world, there is a big increase in lead generation when a website moves from 10 to 15 landing pages.[13] **BOX 10-2** describes how the "Take Control Philly" program used its Facebook-connected landing page to guide visitors to information on its sexually transmitted disease (STD) prevention program.

- There appears to be a linear relationship between the number of monthly blog posts and inbound traffic, with no really sharp break in this trend. Companies that post more than 15 times a month will see five times more traffic than companies that do not blog.

BOX 10-2 Take Control Philly STDs

Matt Prior, MPH

The Philadelphia Department of Public Health's STD Control Program (PDPH STD) is tasked with preventing and controlling the spread of STDs in the fifth largest city in the United States. Philadelphia has a high burden of STDs, ranking 11th for number of reported syphilis cases, third for number of reported gonorrhea cases, and fourth for number of reported chlamydia cases among U.S. cities; it also has an HIV incidence rate five times the national average. The city's adolescents bear a disproportionate burden of STDs, with rates 3.5 and 3 times the national rates for gonorrhea and chlamydia, respectively. In 2010, PDPH STD saw a 38% increase in gonorrhea cases and a 7.2% increase in chlamydia cases, with 1 in 8 teen girls being diagnosed with an STD. Clearly, STDs were at epidemic levels in Philadelphia at that time.

   In late 2010, the adolescent STD epidemic was established as a top priority by the Health Commissioner of the City of Philadelphia, which gave rise to the Adolescent STD/HIV Prevention Project (ASHPP). ASHPP was designed around the goal of increasing the availability, accessibility, and acceptability of condoms among youth in Philadelphia, and decreasing the rates of STDs among young people in Philadelphia. In April 2011, a sexual health website for teens, www.TakeControlPhilly.org, and a Philadelphia-branded condom, called the Freedom Condom, were launched through the early efforts of ASHPP. The Take Control Philly website provides STD education, links to services, a map locating all teen-friendly condom distribution sites in the city, and a nationally unique condom mailing program that mails condoms directly to adolescents' (ages 13 to 19 years) homes. A corresponding Facebook page, www.facebook.com/TakeControlPHL, was launched simultaneously with the idea of connecting youth to TakeControlPhilly.org and its services. The hope for this Facebook page was that "if we build it, they will come"—but after a few months it was apparent that this page was not reaching the population it sought, and had only 196 page followers.

Social media have become the normal and routine way that teens communicate with one another. A 2011 STD survey conducted by PDHD reported 88% of the 300 high school students surveyed used Facebook, similar to the national average of 71% reported by the Pew Research Institute.[1] In September 2011, after limited success at reaching young people in Philadelphia through social media, PDHD launched its first Facebook advertising campaign with the hope of reaching young people where they congregate—online. In response to dwindling interest in ASHPP, which was made evident by decreases in condom orders and interactions on social media, the first Facebook advertising campaign, which was initiated in September 2011, had the goal of boosting the number of followers of the page and driving the condom mailing program.

The first campaign, entitled "Mail Me Condoms," ran for two weeks and cost $3000; every campaign since then has used the same time and pricing model. It was unclear who PDHD would reach with the campaign, but an increase of 2500 new Facebook followers was observed and nearly 7000 condoms were mailed to young people in Philadelphia. PDHD saw a clear link between Facebook ads and young people in Philadelphia taking action on behalf of their own sexual health—namely, ordering condoms to be delivered to their house. A clear pattern was established of teens seeing the ad, clicking on the page, liking the page, and then going on to order condoms. At that time, however, it was unclear whether these outcomes would be repeatable.

In December 2011, in an effort to replicate the first campaign, another "Mail Me Condoms" ad campaign was launched. Similar results were seen, with more than 2500 page follows, 20,000 website views, and 8000 condoms mailed to teens in Philadelphia. After that campaign, Facebook analytics reported that more than 95% of the page followers were teens living in Philadelphia, the campaign's target audience.

Clearly, this was proving a useful method for reaching young people in Philadelphia. Between September 2011 and February 2012, eight Facebook campaigns were run, resulting in a Facebook page with 17,000 followers, 96% of whom are teens living in Philadelphia. The condom mailing program sent out nearly 25,000 condom orders (250,000 condoms) during the same period of time. This fan base can now be reached easily with posts about their sexual health.

Social media, such as Facebook, can be successfully utilized as tools to disseminate health promotional materials or interventions. Based on PDHD's experiences, Facebook advertisements are measurable, targeted to a specific demographic, and reasonably priced when compared to the cost of traditional media. Using social media ads and posts, teens can be directly linked to a website where taking a positive health action—namely, ordering condoms—is as easy as a few clicks on their computers.

The full potential of social media has yet to be explored in the realm of public health. It should be noted that although the PDHD's campaign reached its goal of increasing availability and accessibility of condoms among youth in Philadelphia, in lieu of research that correlates actual condom usage with the campaign, it cannot be definitively determined that receiving condoms by mail led to an increase in condom usage. However, in just two weeks the program managers could glimpse the possibilities of using one particular social media platform to promote the condom distribution program and safer sex messages among adolescents, and have continued to do so with subsequent campaigns. A strength of Facebook and other social media platforms is that you can immediately see the reactions of your followers and alter your approaches to reaching them accordingly. The Philadelphia program treated its ad campaigns like a real-time focus group, and applied the lessons learned from each campaign to subsequent campaigns. As Facebook is currently the largest social media platform, PDHD STD decided to use this platform to promote condom availability, condom use, and prevention messaging directly to adolescent users. Based on the positive results of the PDPH program evaluation, local health departments, community-based organizations, and other nonprofit organizations would be well advised to examine the effectiveness and net benefits over harms of social media marketing as means to promote their services, interventions, and health campaigns in their jurisdictions.

Reference

1.   Lenhart A. *Teens, social media & technology overview 2015*. Pew Research Institute; April 9, 2015. http://www
.pewinternet.org/2015/04/09/teens-social-media-technology-2015/.

▶ "Engage Me": Social Media

Heldman et al. define social media as "digital channels and tools… that facilitate engagement—the interactive, synchronous communication and collaboration among numerous participants via technology."[14(p2)] In this text, we focus on digitally enabled social media. Just as not all social media are digital (remember handwritten love notes?), so not all digital communications are social. Preprogrammed health applications (**apps**), of which there were more than 165,000 available to consumers in 2015, are digital and interactive, but are not considered "social."[15] Many public health organizations continue to use digital media in the same way that they use mass media—namely, to disseminate messages and materials.

Increasingly, however, public health organizations are also engaging and interacting with specific audiences through social media. To paraphrase Schein et al., "It is the process of engaging users to co-create, rate, and comment on content, that is perceived to give a heightened authenticity to messages."[16(p3)] The adoption of social media by leading public health organizations reflects a widespread sense that these tools are necessary to reach demographic groups that are abandoning traditional broadcast technologies (e.g., telephones, television) and a significant portion of the public that is transforming the manner in which they interact with experts.

Which Social Media Predominate?

FIGURE 10-7 shows an infographic of the leading social media platforms in use in 2015. Facebook was leading at 1.4 billion monthly active mobile users (in September 2015), followed by LinkedIn (380 million), a tie between Google+ (300 million) and Instagram (300 million), Twitter close behind (289 million), and Pinterest (70 million).

Demographic Breakdown

Nearly two-thirds of American adults (65%) used social networking sites, with 90% of young adults (18 to 29 years) and 35% of those older than age 65 saying they did. There were relatively small differences, if any, by gender (68% women, 62% men), or ethnicity (65% white, 65% Hispanic, 56% African American). However, persons living in rural areas (58%) were less likely to use social media sites than their urban (64%) or suburban (68%) counterparts.[17] **FIGURE 10-8** shows the leading sites by demographic breakdown in 2015.

In another 2015 Pew survey of teens (aged 13 to 17 years), the authors reported that "92% of those surveyed go online daily—including 24% who say they are online almost constantly." They found that 85% of African American teens have access to a smartphone, compared with 71% of both white and Hispanic teens.[18(p8)]

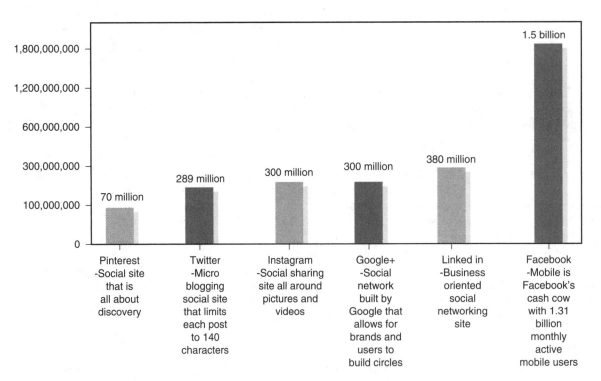

FIGURE 10-7 Marketing Industry Report of Social Media Platform Use in 2015.

Data from Leverage Media. Retrieved from: www.leveragenewmedia.com.

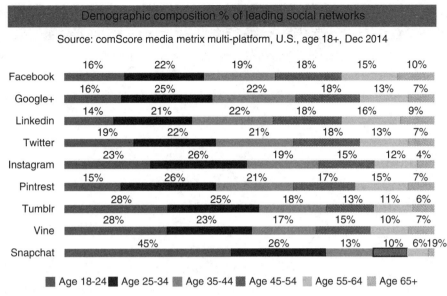

FIGURE 10-8 Demographic Composition of Leading Social Networks.
Courtesy of comSource.

A Sampling of Social Media Tools by Function and Use

Cell Phone Texting

Texting, also known as short message service (SMS), is both the most ubiquitous and the most studied social media used in public health communication interventions. Hall *et al.*'s systematic review of 15 high-quality systematic reviews of text message interventions (TMIs), which encompassed 89 individual studies conducted between 2009 and 2014, reported:

> Consistent evidence that TMIs generally resulted in significant positive benefits in the areas of diabetes self-management, physical activity, weight loss, smoking cessation, and medication adherence for ART (antiretroviral therapy). Greater effects were associated with text messages on ART adherence that were sent less frequently than daily (such as weekly) and that used bidirectionality, personalization,

and tailoring to clinical needs... However, caution toward unintended consequences of TMIs should be considered before applying them to other health areas.[19(p12-13)]

In their article, Hall *et al.* were mindful of the uptick in mobile messaging applications (e.g., WhatsApp) as well as use of image-based messaging (e.g., Snapchat). In 2015, the Pew Research Center included the use of messaging apps in its survey and found that 36% of smartphone owners reported using apps such as WhatsApp, Kik, or iMessage, and 17% used apps that automatically delete sent messages, such as Snapchat or Wickr. Nearly half of the 18- to 29-year-old age group used these messaging apps, which are free when the user is connected to WiFi, and hence do not count against their cell phone data use plans.[20]

BOX 10-3 provides a great example (and linked resource) of how Seattle and King County Department of Public Health uses texting in emergency communication and health promotion.

BOX 10-3 Texting for Public Health: Emergency Communication, Health Promotion, and Beyond[1]

Hilary N. Karasz, PhD, and Lindsay Bosslet, MPH

Introduction: Texting and Health Agencies

Public health agencies communicate with many different audiences, including residents, advocacy groups, the media, elected officials, and other stakeholders. Television, radio, newspapers, and the Internet cast a large net, but these outlets lack a personal touch and often fail to reach vulnerable populations. Text messages, also known as short message service (SMS), can help bridge the communications gap between mass media, social media, and one-on-one consultation, allowing agencies to share customized messages with thousands of individuals.

(continues)

BOX 10-3 Texting for Public Health: Emergency Communication, Health Promotion, and Beyond   *(continued)*

While most of us are familiar with text messaging to friends or family, public health text message programs demand a strategic approach. A good texting program requires the consideration of following components:

- Technology and cost
- Audience research
- Getting subscribers and marketing
- Crafting text messages
- An evaluation plan
- Legal and security issues

Why Use the Mobile Phone to Reach Your Audience?

Cell phones are ubiquitous, and texting is a popular mode of communication. According to the Pew Research Center, as of January 2014, 90% of American adults owned cell phones, 97% of people ages 18 to 29 sent text messages, and 81% of American cell phone owners sent or received text messages.[2] Texting may be particularly useful for reaching some low-income communities of color, who text most frequently[3] and who often suffer from disproportionate rates of adverse health conditions.[4] Costs rarely pose a barrier for text message program enrollment, because many people have unlimited texting plans.[5] Perhaps most importantly, people are highly engaged with their phones. In 2013, mobile users in Europe, Asia, and the United States checked their phones an average of 150 times per day.[6] Stanford University innovator B. J. Fogg described cell phones as "a heart, a wristwatch, and a magic wand" because people are emotionally attached (or "addicted") to their phones, because they carry them all the time, and because they are literally tiny supercomputers.[7]

Given that more than 2 trillion texts were sent in the United States in 2011, it is clear that this mode of communication presents a great opportunity for public health agencies.[8] When they ignore its potential, agencies miss opportunities to provide medication reminders, emergency notification or alerts, appointment reminders, and customized health promotion. Yet, to really reach people's hearts (or their cell phones), practitioners must gain people's trust and offer them a valuable service through personalized messages and content. Without apparent value, the end user (text message recipient) may quit the texting program.

Technology and Costs

Sending Mass Text Messages

Web-based platforms can send messages to many people at once, schedule messages in advance, and track messages. Web-based SMS vendors, such as Voxiva and Mobile Commons, provide the interface for a fee and also track message delivery. Given the hundreds of vendors that offer these capabilities, it is important to ask potential vendors questions about the service they provide.[9]

Web-based interfaces typically rely on short codes, which are dedicated "phone numbers" that are used to transfer messages. People use these codes to enroll in text message programs. For instance, a person might text "ENROLL" to 85443 to sign up for a program. In this case, 85443 is the short code. Short codes are owned and regulated by cell phone carriers. SMS vendors can help you gain access to a code for a fee. Short codes are often used to opt in subscribers to your messaging service.

What Are the Variables in Cost for a Texting Program?

Texting programs can vary wildly in their approach. As with most things in life, the bigger and better they are, the more expensive they are. The following factors influence cost:

- Vendor
- Staff time
- Equipment
- Marketing
- Length of project
- Number of messages you plan to send
- Whether the program uses one-way or two-way texting (One-way programs allow you to send messages in bulk with no expectation of response from your recipients. Two-way programs enable back-and-forth communication with a program manager and a recipient, which is more time and resource-intensive, but also more personal.)
- Web-based platform type

To avoid wasteful spending, choose vendors and platforms that can be used for more than one project and for a long time. The nearby table illustrates the different types of texting platforms available, from those with the fewest features and lowest cost ($50/month) to those with the most features and highest cost ($1000/month). Many of these features are invisible to the end user but make your program more efficient by automating or allowing multiple administrators to share the day-to-day work needed for a successful initiative. Phone-to-phone texting may allow an administrator to send a text message from "anywhere," freeing him or her from a desktop computer. Scheduling texts adds to the convenience for the administrator, and reporting features can be very useful in documentation and evaluation. Other features, such as two-way texting, allow programs to be more personalized, which can be helpful for the end user.[10]

Cost	$	$$	$$$	$$$$	$$$$$
Technology platform	Phone-to-phone texting only	Web-based interface	Web-based interface	Web-based interface	Web-based interface
Create subscriber list(s)		Single	Single	Multiple	Multiple
Schedule texts		✓	✓	✓	✓
Two-way texting			✓	✓	✓
Reporting				Basic	Advanced
Multiple administrators		✓	✓	✓	✓
Database integration					✓
Security systems					✓
Focus on reliability and throughput					✓

Audience Research

All good communication efforts start with researching the targeted audience. Effective messages must fit the end user's wants and needs. Gathering information about the audience will help establish the program's tone, frequency, and content. Most importantly, it will indicate whether the audience will even be interested in signing up for a text message program. Focus groups, key informant interviews, and distributing and analyzing a brief survey may all help answer key questions about the audience:

- Whether audience members use cell phones
- Whether they send and receive text messages
- How often they send and receive text messages
- Why they send text messages
- Whether they would trust messages from your agency
- Which types of messages they want (e.g., entertaining, informative, cues to action)
- Which type of content they would like to receive
- Which languages they prefer

Note that some carriers don't support non-English characters, including accents on Latin-language letters. Thus, messages may need to written to avoid characters that are not supported.

Using Q Methodology,[12] a research method that ascertains subjective viewpoints by asking people to sort statements based on preference, researchers at Public Health—Seattle and King County (PHSKC) identified four main "types" of texters in the general population. These profiles provide a framework for understanding some audiences, but are not a comprehensive analysis of all possible audiences.

- On-the-go texters are characterized by their busy lifestyles. To them, texting is a means for quickly organizing, planning, and managing all facets of their lives.
- Strategic texters are characterized by their use of texting exclusively as a tool for quick, specific communications. They prefer other forms of communication for long conversations, but find it efficient for short exchanges.

(continues)

BOX 10-3   Texting for Public Health: Emergency Communication, Health Promotion, and Beyond   *(continued)*

- Intimate texters use texting to maintain relationships with close friends and family members. Although they will use texting for some practical reasons, they think of it as a tool to use with a tight-knit circle of close people.
- Security texters appreciate the texting's privacy and reliability, and it offers them peace of mind. It is used for physical protection, in cases of social emergencies, and when they feel personally threatened.

These types of texters might be considered when developing a marketing campaign for text message program enrollment.

Getting Subscribers and Marketing

Unlike billboards, newspapers, and radio ads, text messages sent from groups and organizations (using a short code) require "opt in" from the end user. Some agencies may develop programs that do not require a short code, but elective enrollment is still a best practice. Because people who receive text messages must actively participate in the program, strategic marketing is essential.

When developing a marketing campaign for a text message program, think about the types of marketing messages that might appeal to different types of texters. On-the-go texters will want to know how this program will save them time and keep them organized. Strategic texters might want to understand how this program will give them information that is useful and succinct. Intimate texters may be more interested in the program if it will empower them to help friends and family. Security texters may find the most value in a program that keeps them safe and can be employed in case of emergency.

How to Appeal to Different Types of Texters

Marketing materials should reflect the different characteristics of the group the program is trying to reach. Consider the types of texters identified earlier who might use a hypothetical emergency alert program being offered by a health agency to the public:

- *On-the-go texters*: "Sign up for emergency message service. It's quick & easy to get updated information. Best of all, texting fits right into your busy lifestyle."
- *Strategic texters*: "Sign up for emergency message service. Texts will be short and to the point, allowing you to follow up only on the information that interests you."
- *Intimate texters*: "Sign up for emergency message service. Make sure you have the information your close friends and family need in the event of an emergency."
- *Security texters*: "Sign up for emergency message service. Have information at your fingertips in case of a dangerous situation."

Real-World Examples

As with any marketing effort, "place" (one of the many "marketing Ps") is critical. In collaboration with a community-based organization serving gay Latino men, PHSKC investigators developed and pre-tested a texting program for HIV prevention. After careful planning, the team decided to market the program by interacting with the target audience at a gay bar, but very few people signed up. Investigators concluded that, even though people might be interested in the program, they were not in the right frame of mind to hear about it at a bar. The marketing team should have performed audience research to figure out where people are willing and able to make decisions about signing up for a health-related text message program.

What Is Opting In?

To opt into a program, a user must do one of the following:

- *Sign up via short code*. End users text a key word (e.g., "enroll") to a number. In response, they receive information about terms and what to expect from the program.
- *Sign up online*. End users fill out a form and accept terms such as that standard text messaging rates apply.
- *Manual enrollment*. End users fill out a hard-copy form agreeing to terms, and a program administrator adds their information to a web-based system or, if an individual phone, to the cell phone address book.

Crafting Text Messages

Texts are limited to 160 characters (including spaces) and must be engaging and helpful. Follow these best practices:

1. Offer immediate value.
2. Avoid abbreviations or "textease." Use proper grammar and punctuation where possible.
3. Use a link shortener such as bit.ly or tinyURL.com to make room for other important information.
4. Use engaging writing devices, such as questions, facts and figures, and even humor, when appropriate.

The following example shows how to craft messages about an emergency preparedness program, and are aimed at each type of texter discussed earlier. Notice how the same information is delivered differently for each end user.

- *On-the-go texter*: "Stock up on canned goods during your next trip to the grocery store. It saves time and hassle during an emergency."
- *Strategic texter*: "Plan ahead! Stock up on canned goods before an emergency happens."
- *Intimate texter*: "Remind your friends and family to stock up on food before disaster strikes. Ask them to remind you!"
- *Security texter*: "Better safe than sorry! Stock up on canned goods today."

How to Personalize Text Messages

The key to a successful texting program is personalization. Distinguishing factors may include:

- Location
- Answers to previous questions/preferences
- Age (provided by end user)
- Time of enrollment
- Method of enrollment (direct/via short code, online, manual)
- Time since last office visit

When creating your text messaging program, remember these best practices:

- Write clear messages.
- Test messages before sending them.
- Do not spam your audience—know how often they want to receive messages.
- Customize your messages to your audience's needs.
- Send texts that are interesting and provide value-added information.
- Remind your audience that they can opt out and provide specific instructions for doing so.
- Avoid sending protected health information.

Legal and Security Issues

Using text messaging to send protected health information (PHI) requires analysis of federal (and sometimes state) laws that govern the protection of electronic health information. "Covered entities" (usually, but not always, healthcare providers) are subject to the federal Health Insurance Portability and Accountability Act (HIPAA).

HIPAA's Privacy and Security Rules and Texting

HIPAA's Privacy Rule refers to a patient's right to decide what happens with his or her medical records: "The Rule requires appropriate safeguards to protect the privacy of PHI and sets limits and conditions on the uses and disclosures that may be made of such information without patient authorization."[12] Thus, a piece of protected health information (such as a test result) potentially may be delivered via text message if the patient has given the healthcare provider permission to do so, but significant security issues must be considered first.

HIPAA's Security Rule governs how electronic health information is protected: "The Security Rule requires appropriate administrative, physical, and technical safeguards to ensure the confidentiality, integrity, and security of electronic protected health information."[13] These requirements put an additional burden on the covered entity to ensure that electronic PHI is protected in a way that minimizes the potential for breach, even if a patient has given permission to text him or her. A breach could be unauthorized viewing of a text message by someone for whom the text message is not intended.

Text messaging PHI is possible through two approaches: (1) restructuring text messages to remove personal health information or (2) retaining personal health information in the message, but first conducting a risk analysis and satisfying other requirements to meet the Security Rule.[14,15] Organizations should start by determining the scope of the risk analysis, which may include the following elements:

- Evaluation of the potential threats and vulnerabilities in proposed messages that contained protected heath information
- Assessment of current security measures that would apply to SMS
- Determination of the likelihood of a breach occurring
- Assessment of the potential impact on the individual and the organization if a breach occurred in which protected health information was intercepted by an unauthorized person.

(continues)

BOX 10-3 Texting for Public Health: Emergency Communication, Health Promotion, and Beyond *(continued)*

- Identification of mitigation strategies to minimize a breach
- Documentation of the process
- Creation of policies to guide employees who want to use text messaging to reach the public and their clients

Ultimately, while clients may demand information via text that includes protected health information, health agencies that are covered entities must thoroughly vet this process and manage their risks. Compliance offices and risk management programs are critical to this work, and should be consulted early on in a texting program's development.

Real-World Example: Flu Vaccine Reminders

During a flu outbreak, Public Health—Seattle and King County held a mass flu vaccination clinic for children and adults. Some children needed a second dose of vaccine to be fully protected, and parents were offered the opportunity to sign up for SMS reminders to bring in their child for a second dose. In creating the text message reminders, the PHSKC team encountered federal Privacy and Security Rule issues. With the help of PHSKC's compliance office, messages were analyzed to determine if they contained protected health information; subsequently the PHSKC decided to eliminate protected health information from the messages.

The first message written and reviewed was "It's time for [child's name]'s second dose of seasonal flu vaccine. Visit a pharmacy or clinic today for the booster to keep your child protected." This message was rejected because the team determined that the first-dose information constituted protected health information, and a person who was unauthorized to see the message could infer from the message that the child had a first dose of vaccine. The compliance team's analysis was that this would constitute a breach.

The second draft eliminated the child's name: "It's time for your child's second dose of seasonal flu vaccine. Visit a pharmacy or clinic today for the booster to keep your child protected." This message was also rejected because if the unauthorized viewer knew to whom the phone belonged, he or she could infer the child's name and the fact that the child had received flu vaccine.

The third attempt was also rejected: "If it's been 30 days since a first flu shot, then it's time for some children to get a 2nd dose of flu vaccine. Call a doctor or pharmacy to schedule an appointment." While this did not contain protected health information, the team thought it was inappropriately vague.

At the end of the review process, the team decided to send two messages, moments apart. The first message cued parents to think about flu vaccine and their child: "Keep your child protected against the flu. Some kids need a second dose 30 days after they receive their first flu shot." The second message cued the parents that they had asked to receive a reminder about flu vaccine: "Do you remember asking for a text message reminder for flu vaccine? It's time! Call a doctor or pharmacy to schedule an appointment." As neither of these messages contained any protected health information, the PHSKC analysis was that it met the requirements of the Security and Privacy Rules.

Evaluation

Process evaluation is important to improve texting programs. Through user satisfaction ratings and utilization statistics, such as opt-in and opt-out rates, evaluating your SMS program can help evolve the program to be easier to administer, better for the client, and more targeted. A short survey, focus group, or direct output metrics are a few examples of how you can collect data and valuable qualitative feedback without complex research and statistics..

Here are some sample questions to use on pre-test and post-test surveys:

- How did you hear about this program?
- Was this program useful?
- Would you recommend this program to a friend?
- What would you change about this program?
- Did this program encourage you to behave differently?

The following metrics might also be considered:

- The number of subscribers
- How long the subscribers stayed in your program
- Whether they responded to texts/surveys
- Peaks in enrollment following specific marketing pushes
- Location and other demographic descriptors associated with enrollment
- The cost of your program relative to other programs
- The amount of time spent by staff implementing the program

Real-World Example: Results of Evaluation of Second Dose Study

As mentioned earlier, PHSKC investigators developed a pilot text message program to see if people would like to receive vaccine reminders via text. During a mass flu vaccination exercise, PHSKC asked parents of children who needed two doses of flu vaccine if they would like to receive a text message reminding them when it was time for their child's second dose of vaccine.

The scope of this project did not include evaluating whether text message recipients were more likely to get their children a second dose of vaccine than parents who did not receive a reminder text, but studies show that these kinds of reminders can be effective.[16] Rather, the PHSKC investigators were interested in parents' willingness to sign up for the reminders. In the first year of the pilot program, 84% of parents whose children needed two doses of vaccine opted in to receive text messages, and in the second year of the pilot program, 95% of eligible parents opted in.

Real-World Example: Results of Evaluation of Employee Emergency Texting Program

PHSKC designed an emergency preparedness texting program that allowed employees to receive texts during emergency situations.[17] The program was tested during a 2012 snowstorm. Fifteen messages were sent over the course of five days, alerting employees to late workday starts, site closures, and commuting reminders. In the week following the snowstorm, 180 employees (36% of subscribers) responded to an online survey evaluating employee satisfaction with the texting program.

- Sixty-three percent of survey respondents thought the text messages were very relevant and helpful, 20% thought they were fairly relevant and helpful, and 12% thought they were somewhat relevant and helpful. Only 5% of those surveyed thought the texts were annoying.
- Eighty-three percent of survey respondents thought PHSKC sent about the right number of texts, 15% felt they sent too few, and only 2% thought PHSKC sent too many texts.

This information suggested that, by and large, the emergency texting program was useful and appreciated by employees. It continued to exclusively send emergency messages.

Conclusion

Text messaging has the potential to be a powerful new way for public health agencies to improve communication with audiences, but there are many considerations to address before an agency invests in a texting program. These considerations include taking enough time to understand the various texting technologies and their associated costs, the audience needs, ways to market to the audience to build a subscriber base, the creation of messages, evaluation of the program, and potential security and privacy pitfalls. With millions of texters in the United States and hundreds of millions across the globe, public health should use this ubiquitous technology to help achieve its communication goals.

Acknowledgments

Some of this work was supported by the Centers for Disease Control and Prevention, Grant no. 5P01TP000297. Its contents are solely the responsibility of the authors and do not necessarily represent the official views of the Centers for Disease Control and Prevention.

Additional Resources

Public Health—Seattle and King County: Texting for Public Health Communication: http://www.kingcounty.gov/healthservices/health/preparedness/texting.aspx

Public Health—Seattle: http://www.nwcphp.org/docs/sms-toolkit/index.htm

References

1. Public Health—Seattle and King County. Texting for public health: emergency communication, health promotion, and beyond. http://www.nwcphp.org/docs/sms-toolkit/index.htm. Accessed December 30, 2015.

2. Pew Research Center. Mobile technology fact sheet. 2015. http://www.pewinternet.org/fact-sheets/mobile-technology-fact-sheet/. Accessed December 24, 2015.

3. Smith A. How Americans use text messaging. Pew Research Center; 2015. http://www.pewinternet.org/2011/09/19/how-americans-use-text-messaging/. Accessed December 30, 2015.

4. Meyer P, Yoon PW, Kaufmann RB. Introduction: CDC health disparities and inequalities report—United States, 2013. *MMWR*. 2013;62(3):3-5. http://www.cdc.gov/mmwr/preview/mmwrhtml/su6203a2.htm?s_cid=su6203a2_w. Accessed December 30, 2015.

(continues)

BOX 10-3 Texting for Public Health: Emergency Communication, Health Promotion, and Beyond *(continued)*

5. Reardon M. AT&T and Verizon deny price-fixing accusations. *CNET*. http://www.cnet.com/news/at-t-and-verizon-deny-price-fixing-accusations/. Accessed December 30, 2015.

6. Kleiner, Perkins, Caufield & Byers. 2013 Internet trends. May 29, 2013. http://www.kpcb.com/blog/2013-internet-trends. Accessed December 30, 2015.

7. Fogg, BJ. Why texting 4 health? In: Fogg BJ and Adler, eds. *Texting 4 Health: A Simple, Powerful Way to Improve Lives*. Stanford, CA: Stanford Captology Media; 2009: 3-8.

8. O'Grady M. *SMS usage remains strong in the US: 6 billion SMS messages are sent each day*. Forrester Research; June 19, 2012. http://blogs.forrester.com/michael_ogrady/12-06-19-sms_usage_remains_strong_in_the_us_6_billion_sms_messages_are_sent_each_day. Accessed December 30, 2015.

9. Public Health—Seattle and King County. Considerations when selecting a text messaging vendor. http://www.kingcounty.gov/depts/health/emergency-preparedness/text-messaging/~/media/depts/health/emergency-preparedness/documents/ChoosingVendors.ashx. Accessed December 30, 2015.

10. Public Health—Seattle and King County. SMS text messaging for public health communication. http://www.kingcounty.gov/healthservices/health/preparedness/texting.aspx. Accessed December 30, 2015.

11. Brown SR. A primer on Q methodology. *Operant Subjectivity*. 1993;16:91-138.

12. U.S. Department of Health and Human Services. The HIPAA Privacy Rule. http://www.hhs.gov/hipaa/for-professionals/privacy/index.html. Accessed December 24, 2015.

13. U.S. Department of Health and Human Services. The Security Rule. http://www.hhs.gov/hipaa/for-professionals/security/index.html. Accessed December 24, 2015.

14. Karasz H, Eiden A, Bogan S. Text messaging to communicate with public health audiences: how the HIPAA Security Rule affects practice. *Am J Public Health*. 2013;103(4):617-622. doi: 10.2105/AJPH.2012.300999.

15. Health IT. Security risk assessment. May 2, 2014. http://www.healthit.gov/providers-professionals/security-risk-assessment. Accessed December 24, 2015.

16. Kalan R, Wiysonge CS, Ramafuthole T, et al. Mobile phone text messaging for improving the uptake of vaccinations: a systematic review protocol. *BMJ Open*. 2014;4:e005130. doi: 10.1136/bmjopen-2014-005130.

17. Karasz H, Bogan S, Bosslet L. Communicating with the workforce during emergencies: developing an employee text messaging program in a local public health setting. *Public Health Rep*. 2014;129(suppl 4):61-66.

Social Networking Sites: Facebook and Friends

There are many online sites and services that allow users to create personal profiles, post content, and invite friends, colleagues, or strangers to interact with this content. Different sites tend to attract different followers, and the popularity of sites and their features can be fleeting. Major sites in use at this writing are profiled in this section.

Facebook leads the social networking world, with the most users and functions. Of special interest to international public health practitioners, 84% of Facebook's daily active users are outside of the United States and Canada.[21] Facebook dominated the field in a recent meta-analysis of social networking sites (SNS) used in behavior change interventions.[22] This study found a positive effect of SNS interventions on health behavior change, but considerable heterogeneity was observed and only 12 studies were included in the analysis. Facebook continues

to serve, in reality, as a blog for those of us who are too (fill in the blank) to start our own blogs, because it allows users to share or not share posted content with enrolled friends or the public at their discretion.

BOX 10-4 shows CDC's best practice guidelines for using Facebook in public health communication. Facebook also offers its own guidance for nonprofit organizations.[23]

BOX 10-5 continues the case study of the Tips From Former Smokers campaign. The CDC uses Facebook as the primary social media channel to connect smokers to other helpful sites.

Another social media site, LinkedIn (https://www.linkedin.com), functions as a professional networking site. Individuals post individual profiles equivalent to curriculum vita (CV) and receive lots of job announcements. Recruiters use LinkedIn for initial candidate screening. Organizations use LinkedIn to share information about conferences, post links to research and publications, and hold discussions. The *Journal of Health Communication*, the American Academy

BOX 10-4 CDC's Recommendations for Using Facebook

1. **Become familiar with other Facebook sites**. There are several public health–related social network sites available, which have different targets, purposes, and functions. Visiting other sites will help you gain an understanding of the participants, the culture, and the functionality. It is important to note the difference between a Facebook page and an individual Facebook profile. Facebook pages are utilized by organizations and businesses, whereas Facebook profiles are for individuals. Unlike profiles, pages are moderated by page administrators who log on to post content or monitor comments; they do not receive notifications when users take action.

2. **Consider the overall communications strategy and objectives**. Before launching a page, make sure your social networking activities mesh with your overall communication strategy and objectives. Once a target audience has been identified, it is essential to determine if a social networking site such as Facebook is an appropriate channel for disseminating your messages. Facebook is a public platform that reaches the general public. Specifically targeted Facebook pages can be developed to address healthcare providers, public health professionals, and others. CDC's "Parents are the Key to Safe Teen Drivers" is an example of a Facebook page that targets parents of teenagers.

3. **Be thoughtful about resources**. Ensure that adequate resources (time and staff) are available to support the ongoing maintenance of the page to keep content fresh and fans engaged.

4. **Provide engaging posts and communication material on the site**. Incorporate videos, quizzes, widgets, games, applications, images, and other materials to actively and repeatedly engage users.

5. **Create a comment policy**. Develop a policy that covers the response to inappropriate or derogatory comments. Refer to CDC's "Social Networking Comment Policy" for an example: http://www.cdc.gov/SocialMedia/Tools /CommentPolicy.html.

6. **Consider associations with partner content**. It is possible to display "featured likes," "likes," or comments on partner status updates, and to share partner content. When considering promotion of a partner's page or engagement with the partner's content, it is important to determine the advantages of this activity to ensure that your organization's brand will benefit from its association with a particular organization, agency, or group. Additional information can be found in CDC's "Facebook Guideline and Best Practices."

7. **Collect and store comments**. Develop a system to archive comments.

8. **Develop a promotion plan**. Establish a promotion plan before launching the page; encourage fans to share and cross-promote using other social media channels and webpages.

9. **Develop an evaluation plan**. Have an evaluation and metrics plan in place prior to launch to determine if efforts are successful. For example, it will be helpful to:

   - Determine how participation will be measured. Evaluation can include simple measures of user engagement (e.g., How many followers/fans/friends does the account have? How many users commented on recent posts?)
   - Take advantage of the analytic packages available on the social networking sites. These can be utilized to determine the number of people ("fans") participating in the activity and to observe how users engage with the site. For example, Facebook Insights are available to users (administrators) who maintain a page for an organization. Facebook Insights allow the administrator to see demographic information and fan interactions with the page over time.
   - Consider tracking the amount of traffic being driven to a website from an organization's Facebook page. If using an analytics tool for a website (such as Google Analytics or WebTrends), that tool will show the source of traffic to a page, and the number of users who are visitors coming via a link on the Facebook page.
   - Plan to evaluate the Facebook-based program with an online survey (through a tool such as SurveyMonkey) to measure user satisfaction, increases in knowledge due to the social networking page, or changes in behavior or attitudes.

For more information, see CDC's Facebook Guidance and Best Practices: http://www.cdc.gov/SocialMedia/Tools /guidelines/pdf/FacebookGuidelines.pdf.

CDC's Facebook Guidance and Best Practices: http://www.cdc.gov/SocialMedia/Tools/guidelines/pdf/FacebookGuidelines.pdf

BOX 10-5 Case Study: Using Web, Social Media, and Mobile Platforms in the "Tips From Former Smokers" Campaign

Since the inception of the Tips From Former Smokers campaign, CDC has used social and digital media platforms to amplify the campaign's messages. The campaign has used digital assets, like the *Tips* website and YouTube page; paid digital media, including banners and video on websites; and social media as means to communicate with various audiences. Digital efforts have become a year-round activity, which has helped maintain awareness of the *Tips* brand during the times when campaign is off air.

At the center of the campaign's digital media activity, the *Tips* website was developed to support the campaign by providing information about the health conditions and ad participants who were featured, resources for smokers looking to quit, and tools for partners to help support and engage with the campaign. The website also offers access to the campaign's online and social media channels, such as CDC's Tobacco Free Facebook, Twitter, and YouTube forums, for those people who want to connect with others about the campaign. Paid advertising methods, such as digital videos, web banners, and search engine marketing, drive users directly to the *Tips* campaign page. In 2013, 2.8 million unique additional visitors went to the website during the time the campaign was on air. [1] These activities allow the *Tips* site to operate as a central hub for digital media activity and enable all of CDC's assets to work in concert with each other.

To provide support for smokers looking to quit because of seeing the ads, CDC syndicated cessation content from smokefree.gov onto its *Tips* webpages. Thanks to third-party ad tagging (code added to the site to track users paths), CDC could determine whether people who clicked on a *Tips* ad later looked at cessation content on the website, and which types of cessation content users were interested in. In 2013, the data produced by the ad tagging showed that among all visitors who were exposed to the *Tips* digital ads and went to the primary "Quit Smoking" page, 69% took a secondary action (such as viewing another page). This demonstrated that this audience had a strong interest in seeking content to assist them with cessation (e.g., influence behavior change). Additionally, "Quit Buttons" were added to most *Tips* pages; clicking the buttons took users to the *Tips* "Quit Smoking" section of the site. Given that the primary goal of the campaign is to promote quitting, this action ensured that visitors to the site had access to quitting resources no matter where they were on the site.

The Tips From Former Smokers campaign has also used social media as a multifaceted tool to provide support and encouragement for smokers trying to quit, educate audiences about new diseases linked to smoking, and provide resources for nonsmokers to help them encourage others to quit. CDC identified Facebook as the main driver for much of the social media activity, based on the rationale that Facebook is built around people and their connections. CDC developed a monthly calendar and posted content almost every day. The first step in bolstering the influence of the *Tips* social media was to acquire fans through "like" ads. By incorporating a variety of ads that appealed to different groups of people, the CDC Tobacco Free page grew from 2000 fans to more than 107,000 fans in slightly more than two years.

For a relatively small investment, CDC used Facebook's targeting capabilities to deliver content to people with similar connections and interests as the target audience. For example, people with interests in video games, certain television and music genres, and fast food were identified and served *Tips* ads on Facebook. Using this strategy enabled CDC to reach many more people than it would have without the paid placement.

Mobile media have also played an increasingly important role in *Tips* digital communications. In 2014, time spent with mobile apps in the United States surpassed the amount of time spent accessing the web on desktops or laptops.[2] To keep up with the rapid growth of mobile usage among the general population, CDC created mobile websites in 2013, both in English and in Spanish, with core content from the main *Tips* site. Ads specifically targeting mobile users were purchased to drive and differentiate traffic to both the English and Spanish mobile sites by targeting the language settings of a user's device.

CDC has found that digital media channels can be a strong vehicle for providing cessation content to help motivate smokers who are considering quitting. The evolution of the digital media activities around the Tips From Former Smokers campaign has emphasized the need for continuous year-round support and analysis to engage with audiences, especially those who are seeking information and exploring behavioral changes, such as smoking cessation.

References

1. Centers for Disease Control and Prevention. Impact of national tobacco campaign on weekly numbers of quitline calls and website visitors—United States—March 4–June 23, 2013. *MMWR*. 2013;62(37):763-767.

2. Comscore. *US Mobile App Report*. August 2014. http://www.ella.net/pdfs/comScore-US-Mobile-App-Report-2014.pdf. Accessed October 14, 2016.

for Communication in Healthcare, *Social Marketing Quarterly*, and other organizations for healthcare communicators maintain active LinkedIn presences.

Pinterest (https://www.pinterest.com) serves as an online bulletin board where individuals collect and "pin" media from other online sources. Users create thematic boards that are searchable by the public. Women outnumber men by 3 to 1 on the site, which trends toward commercial products and resources. Pinterest is a good source for infographics and design ideas.

Twitter: Micro Blogging

Twitter is a real-time information network that enables millions of users to send and read messages of 140 or fewer characters called tweets. Tweets can be posted to Twitter via text message, mobile websites, or a variety of mobile and web applications. According to Twitter:

> "Reading Tweets and discovering new information" is how one finds the most value on Twitter… This is done by finding and following other interesting Twitter accounts. Messages from those you follow will show up in a readable stream on a Twitter homepage, called a "Timeline."… Click hashtagged keywords (#) to view all Tweets about that topic.[24]

By following Twitter's simple guidelines for how the world uses Twitter, public health and corporate entities have found multiple ways to both use Twitter to share information and, perhaps more importantly, to collect information from tweets.

Using Twitter to Share Information According to Bartlet and Wurtz:

> Twitter's main public health role to date has been to educate and inform people about health issues; health departments have tweeted information

about diabetes management, tobacco cessation, immunizations, and prenatal health, among other topics. Twitter offers a way to overcome the digital divide. Because Twitter is an Internet platform, it inserts this accessibility into the pocket of anyone with a smartphone.[25(p379)]

On an almost daily basis, someone posts new ideas on how to get more out of Twitter. Some advice is very simple, such as keeping tweets short (62 characters instead of 140), adding pictures or videos, tweeting after lunch (since everyone else is rushing to do it in the morning), and using hashtags (#) links to specific topics wisely and abstemiously. In addition to sending basic messages, CDC recommends using other Twitter-based activities as part of health communication:

- Twitter Chats—scheduled events that allow organizations or programs to communicate with their followers. Chats include free-flowing discussions, question-and-answer sessions, and dissemination of information to a large audience through sharing or retweeting of content
- Twitterview—a type of interview in which the interviewer and the interviewee are limited to short-from responses of 140 characters per message.
- Twitter Town Hall—a scheduled forum that allows followers to submit questions on a specific topic. Responses can be delivered through live tweets, video, or live streaming.
- Live Tweeting—tweets from an event to highlight key points of a presentation, audience engagement and comments, and play-by-play moments, often used to allow conferences non-attendees to follow the events.

BOX 10-6 presents CDC's current best practices for using Twitter.

BOX 10-6 CDC's Best Practices for Twitter

1. **Clearly define your objectives**. It is important to have clearly defined objectives before participating in Twitter. Do you want to highlight content, spark action, or encourage awareness of an issue? Clearly defined objectives will help you to determine if Twitter can help you in meeting your larger communication goals.
2. **Know your target audience(s)**. As with any communications activity, it is important to define your intended target audience(s) so that you can develop and communicate messages that resonate with your audience and prompt them to take action.
3. **Determine resource needs**. Determine whether you have the appropriate staffing resources to create content and manage a Twitter profile. It is important to designate a channel manager to serve as the point of contact for Twitter activities and ensure that content is posted on a regular basis.
4. **Keep your content short and simple**. Although the maximum character limit for a tweet is 140 characters, CDC recommends using 120 characters (including URLs, punctuation, and spaces) to make it easy for followers to

BOX 10-6 CDC's Best Practices for Twitter *(continued)*

retweet the message without having to edit it. It is appropriate to use abbreviations and shorten URLs in a Twitter message to save characters.

5. **Determine the schedule and frequency of your Twitter posts**. It is important to set a posting schedule that defines a frequency for posts per week. Setting a regular schedule helps to ensure that the account is active and encourages engaged followers. Consider posting weekly at a minimum.

6. **Conduct promotion activities**. Ongoing promotion of your Twitter profile is strongly recommended. Promotion tips include cross-promoting your account on other CDC social media and web channels. For example, you might leverage the existing CDC Twitter profiles and Facebook pages with similar audiences and/or content to promote your own Twitter activities. Consider Twitter advertising to increase the number of Twitter followers. It is recommended that you determine your budget, target audience, and objective before beginning a Twitter advertising initiative.

7. **Determine your approach for engaging with Twitter followers**. In addition to being a channel for health information dissemination, Twitter should be used to engage your target audience in two-way interactions and communication. Two examples of engagement activities on Twitter are the development of criteria for whom to follow on Twitter and the identification of relevant partners, influencers, and federal, state, and local agencies who are involved in and interested in your specific health topic(s).

8. **Share relevant partner and follower Twitter content on your Twitter profile**. Develop a strategy for identifying and retweeting or replying to posts from partners and followers. Consider holding Twitter events. Twitter events encourage followers to participate in conversations about your priority health topics.

9. **Evaluate your Twitter activities**. Evaluation is an integral component of all social media activities, including Twitter. Evaluation approaches for Twitter may include reviewing metrics, identifying lessons learned, and determining whether the social media effort successfully met project goals. Regularly monitor your Twitter account to review the number of followers, updates, retweets, and mentions in Twitter. You might also consider monitoring the increases in traffic to your website as well as the mentions outside of Twitter on blogs, websites, or articles. Examples of Twitter metrics that can be collected include the number of retweets a post receives, the number of click-throughs from a Twitter post to your webpage, and the number of @replies. Adobe SiteCatalyst, for example, can be used to determine the number of click-throughs from a tweet to a website. Automated metrics reports can be established for programs.

10. **Establish a records management system**. Set up a system to keep track of your Twitter posts, @replies, retweets, and mentions to comply with federal guidelines for records management and archiving.

Social Media at CDC: Twitter Guidelines & Best Practices.' Available at https://www.cdc.gov/socialmedia/tools/guidelines/twitter.html.

Using Twitter to "Listen" The opposite side of tweeting is reading ("listening") to tweets. Researchers have published several articles analyzing tweets as an alternative form of syndromic (symptom cluster) surveillance (sometimes referred to as "infodemiology" or "infosurveillance". See the work by Eysenbach[26] and by Paul and Dredze[27]) for early illness identification. According to Aslam and colleagues, algorithm-based filtering and machine learning programs have improved the correlations between Twitter data—for influenza reports at least—and the data collected from sentinel public health sites.[28] This area of bioinformatics is important but lies outside the primary scope of this text.

Other researchers have studied the wording of tweets (other than "I'm sick #flu"). The brevity of tweets, their impromptu nature, and the fact that senders usually tweet from a "naturalistic setting" (in contrast to sitting in a focus group, for example) make them ideal for capturing top-of-mind reactions to a public health campaign or stimulus in real time. Whereas the corporate world has the resources to implement large-scale computer-based sentiment analysis (called opinion mining; see Bing Liu[29] and others), most public health projects employ people to do the coding. **BOX 10-7** describes a notable case in which Twitter data were analyzed to gauge the public (and pseudo-public) response to a policy initiative.

Using Social Media Effectively in Public Health Communication

An early adopter, CDC conceptualized social media in this manner (paraphrased from Heldman et al.[14]):

- Social media should be integrated with traditional public health communication channels.
- Social media afford users a way to reach specific, diverse audiences with targeted messaging.
- Social media bring health information into new, non-health-related spaces.

BOX 10-7   Use of Twitter to Gauge Response to a Public Health Policy Initiative

In January 2014, the Chicago City Council scheduled a vote on local regulation of electronic cigarettes as tobacco products. One week prior to the vote, the Chicago Department of Public Health (CDPH) released a series of messages about electronic cigarettes (e-cigarettes) through its Twitter account. Shortly after the messages, or tweets, were released, the department's Twitter account became the target of a "Twitter bomb" by Twitter users sending more than 600 tweets in one week against the proposed regulation. [From the abstract]

The authors collected and analyzed the tweets. They found that 89.2% were against the proposed policy. More than half suggested the use of e-cigarettes as a healthier alternative to combustible cigarettes. About a third of anti-policy tweets said the health department was lying or disseminating propaganda. And, 14% of the tweets used an account or included elements consistent with "astroturfing," a strategy employed to suggest a sense of consensus around an idea where none exists. Finally, most of the (predominantly negative) tweets came from outside the Chicago area; tweets from Chicago were significantly more likely to support the policy.

This article casts doubt on the reliability of tweet data to gauge community reactions to an upcoming policy initiative, unless all of the potentially confounding factors are recognized and considered.

Synthesis and interpretation of: Harris JK, Moreland-Russell S, Choucair B, Mansour R, Staub M, Simmons K. Tweeting for and Against Public Health Policy: Response to the Chicago Department of Public Health's Electronic Cigarette Twitter Campaign. J Med Internet Res 2014;16(10).

- Social media provide qualitative ways of "listening" to audiences as well as gathering quantitative data about online behaviors.
- Social media provide channels for direct engagement with specific groups, such as patients with specific conditions, or self-identified communities.

The first four points demonstrate this federal agency's enthusiasm for how social media might allow health communicators to do more—essentially with less financial cost—than was possible through conventional media. The last point, direct engagement, has been a double-edged sword, however. Engagement allows for two-way social and emotional communication with specific groups formed around a condition, a persona, or an intervention. Such two-way connections require constant review of user-generated content (USG) to prevent inaccurate or distorted information from appearing to be sanctioned by a government or private source. Maintaining a timely presence and oversight can be daunting.[14]

By 2013, most federal agencies used some form of social media, but Harris et al. found that only 24% of local health departments had Facebook accounts, 8% had Twitter accounts, and 7% had both.[30] The private sector's use of social media was then, and continues to be, multiplatform and nearly universal.[31,32]

Freeman *et al.* compared nine case studies of successful corporate and international campaigns that used social media, and provide a few organizing principles for moving forward:[33]

- Use *simple, familiar social media tools* to encourage participation and collect data. Use functions familiar to social media users, such as photo tagging and retweeting. Complex third-party tools or requests for personal data dissuade participation and engagement.
- Build online communities by *tapping into existing networks*. Site managers should routinely and explicitly ask all members and followers to help build the community, as it leads to not only more followers, but more highly engaged followers.
- Develop *engaging content* with a clear call to action. The action that is sought can be a personal behavior change to a social sharing tactic.
- Provide *incentives* to participate. Participants enjoy interacting on social media because they can be both anonymous and personal. Rewards for participating can range from tangible items to a personalized "thank you" for sharing content.
- An *ongoing strategy* is necessary—you cannot depend on your content "going viral." Successful campaigns often recruit large numbers of motivated volunteer "seeders" who leverage their personal social media connections. This approach works better than impersonal advertisements.
- Social media are low in cost compared to traditional media, but labor intensive. *Reducing complexity* and running simple, low-tech, low-cost campaigns can be highly effective when they are conducted through the appropriate channels.
- Diligent and timely *moderation and monitoring* of social media pages is necessary. Multilayered approval processes for public communications can certainly impede moving at the speed that social media require. This is an acknowledged

challenge that many public health agencies have somewhat resolved through clear policies, extension of staffing, or use of partner organizations to manage their social media accounts.

In **APPENDIX 10B**, Schroeder and colleagues present a case study using predominantly social and online media to reach out to Hispanic audiences to encourage enrollment in health insurance plans as part of the Patient Protection and Affordable Care Act.

▶ "Entertain Me"

Cross-Channel or Transmedia Storytelling

Many of the media channels discussed earlier are used extensively for entertainment as well as sharing information—particularly television, radio, and the Internet. In **BOX 10-8**, Weinreich describes "transmedia storytelling" and its use to engage Hispanic young adults and enable their interaction with a risk-reduction storyline.

Virtual Worlds and Gaming

According to Shegog (whose work appears elsewhere in this text), 97% of American teens play computer, web, console, or mobile games. Of these, 31% of teen gamers play games every day and another 21% play games three to five days per week.[34] Gaming provides a highly customizable format for reaching adolescents through young adults with health-related content. Within the realm of gaming, virtual worlds provide an immersive experience that enables the user to enact decisions and experience consequences, albeit on a fantasy or dramatic plane. Cowdery and Ahn provide an extensive description and examples of using virtual worlds and gaming in **BOX 10-9**.

BOX 10-8 Transmedia Storytelling for Health Communication

Nedra Kline Weinreich

What Is Transmedia Storytelling?

Transmedia storytelling takes advantage of your target population's media habits by spreading different parts of a story across multiple communication channels and allowing the audience to become participants in integrating the pieces. Putting the story where the people you want to reach are already spending their time—whether on Twitter, Facebook, YouTube, mobile phones, flyers on school bulletin boards, or elsewhere—creates an immersive experience. When it feels like a story is unfolding around them, and especially when they have spent enough time with the characters to care what happens to them, they are primed to pay attention.

The transmedia approach has been used extensively by Hollywood movies and television shows, as well as commercial brands, to draw people into their story, on whatever platform the audience happens to be using. Shows such as *Heroes*, *Game of Thrones*, and *Mad Men*; movies such as *The Hunger Games*, *District 9*, and *Prometheus*; and brands such as Audi, Coca-Cola, and Lego purposefully seed different narrative elements across media to draw people into the story from various starting points. For example, a transmedia story might have some of the characters posting to Twitter between episodes, writing blog posts, uploading short videos to YouTube, or sending text messages to participants; it might create a faux website for a key company in the story world, distribute business cards directing people to that website, put on a live event, or offer an online game that provides clues to get to the next part of the story. The project can also be built around nonfiction stories about real people, whether selected strategically or crowdsourced.

Why Use Transmedia Storytelling for Health Communication?

By combining the transmedia approach with the research-proven entertainment education model, the potential for influencing knowledge, attitudes, and behaviors is heightened. Entertainment education-based social marketing has traditionally focused on "product placement" of content related to health and social issues within the plotlines of television shows, radio serials, movies, video games, and other media. Transmedia storytelling for behavior change involves designing a story across these platforms to create an immersive experience for the audience that leads them to take some kind of action.

When someone is emotionally invested in the plotline of a show, and has the experience of being mentally "transported" into the story, that person is more likely to remember information delivered during the program and to desire to act on it. By vicariously experiencing another's challenges, the audience learns by seeing the consequences—both positive and negative—of how the character tries to resolve his or her problems. Stories can also establish or reinforce social norms that support the behavior you are promoting; if the characters make healthy food choices or use sunscreen in the story, it can create the feeling that this is just what people do and so they should, too. This approach is especially effective when the audience feels that the characters are very similar to themselves.

When we make the different parts of the story appear where our audience spends its time, the characters can start to feel like trusted friends, and we can provide opportunities for interaction and participation. Social media are an optimal place to do this, with character tweets showing up in the audience's Twitter stream, videos posted on their Facebook pages, and even things like a LinkedIn page that provides some backstory for a character or a Pinterest board that highlights characters' interests and rounds them out to make them seem more real.

Elements of Effective Transmedia Storytelling for Change

Transmedia storytelling makes use of an entertainment education approach, particularly the Immersive Engagement for Change Model.[1] The elements that use transmedia storytelling are (1) making use of a behavior change model, (2) having a good story with compelling characters, (3) using media platforms and channels frequented by the audience, (4) providing opportunities to participate (mostly through social media), and (5) suggesting applications in the "real world," such as products, services, or behaviors to "try at home."

Case Study: *East Los High*

East Los High is a multiple-season video series on Hulu beginning in 2013. The show seeks to address health and social issues affecting Latino teens, such as teen pregnancy, risky sexual behaviors, nutrition, fitness, domestic violence, and more. Developed by the Population Media Center and produced by Wise Entertainment, the series was built on a firm foundation of research with the target population and advised by more than 15 public health organizations with expertise in the areas addressed by the show.

East Los High centers on a group of students at a fictional high school in East Los Angeles, with friendship and romantic relationship dramas, as well as depictions of sexual and reproductive health issues that arise for them. The show consists of a series of half-hour video episodes, with additional transmedia elements that extend the storyline and provide more insights into the characters. In the first season, these included the school newspaper, which has online articles and information about what is going on in the school, a video "column" by one of the male characters answering guys' questions about sex, a video blog by a pregnant character, a healthy cooking series featuring two main characters who work in a restaurant together, instructional dance videos to learn the school dance team's routine, and other short video clips. The series also includes Facebook pages for the characters and a Twitter account with updates about the show.

This series incorporates all of the elements of the Immersive Engagement Model. The project identified the health-related objectives and built the storyline around them, drawing on the Sabido method (a method for creating engagement for social change that was developed by Miguel Sabido in Mexico in the 1970s), is based on communication theory, and uses carefully crafted, long-running soap operas to reach large populations) and other behavior change models. Focus groups with the target audience, a youth advisory committee, and additional extensive research drove the ongoing development of the program. The producers ensured engaging storytelling by bringing in experienced Latino writers from East Los Angeles who understood the audience. Knowing that their teen Latino audience spends a lot of its time watching online video and interacting via social media, the transmedia production team focused its efforts on creating content for these channels. The audience had opportunities to participate by interacting with the characters on social media, "auditioning" for the dance team, and submitting questions to "Ask Paulie." Finally, the issues depicted in the series were brought into the real world through the show's website, which provided resources on all the topics addressed in the storyline and even directed users to the nearest Planned Parenthood clinic.

The evaluation of the first season of *East Los High* showed that the show had an impact.[2] A viewer survey found that, in addition to being emotionally engaged with the characters and storyline, approximately 40% to 50% of the participants learned information about correct use of condoms that they did not know before. Close to one-third learned something new about birth control and emergency contraception. After watching the show, almost all of them reported being willing to get tested for sexually transmitted diseases themselves and to recommend the service to others. A lab experiment found that knowledge about condom use was significantly higher among those who had been exposed to the transmedia version of the story, as opposed to those who watched the online dramatic version of the show without the transmedia elements and those who read the script. The series also

(continues)

BOX 10-8 Transmedia Storytelling for Health Communication *(continued)*

drove web traffic to its nonprofit partners, with Stayteen.org receiving 566,000 visits during the first month after its premiere on Hulu; Planned Parenthood's website received more than 57,000 visits in the first 5 months. Preliminary results from season 2 showed additional significant changes in knowledge, attitudes, and behavioral intentions among viewers.[3]

References

1. Weinreich NK. The Immersive Engagement Model: transmedia storytelling for social change. 2014. http://social-marketing .com/immersive-engagement.html. Accessed October 14, 2016.

2. Wang H, Singhal A. *Assessment of* East Los High (Season 1): *Using Transmedia Storytelling to Promote Safe Sex and Teen Pregnancy Prevention among Latino Communities in the U.S.* Internal evaluation report: an integrated research report submitted to Population Media Center; January 2015.

3. Rosenthal EL, Zavahir Y, Backes KL, Folb KL. *Streaming Sexual Health: Entertainment Education on Hulu's East Los High.* In preparation.

BOX 10-9 The Use of Virtual Worlds in Health Promotion

Joan E. Cowdery, PhD, and Sun Joo (Grace) Ahn, PhD

Virtual Reality Technology

Virtual reality technology can refer to a variety of applications but typically consists of some type of immersive 3-D experience for the user. Virtual reality environments are created by digital devices that simulate multiple layers of sensory information so that users are able to see, hear, and feel as if they are in the real world[1] and give the user the perception of existing in an alternate space. Depending on the purpose of the application, these spaces can mimic the real world or be highly fantasized, as is the case in many gaming environments. Early virtual reality applications such as flight simulators have expanded into many areas of health care, including surgery simulations and trainings.

While the initial application of virtual reality technology and the development of virtual worlds took place in the gaming realm, more recent applications have included social networking, education and training, and health care. One of the defining characteristics of virtual worlds is that they generate simultaneously shared spaces.[2] In addition to fostering real-time social interaction, virtual worlds allow users to have a physical presence in these shared spaces. Users exist and interact in these computer-simulated environments where participants create what is commonly known as an avatar, a digitally constructed form of virtual representation that marks a user's entity.[3]

Publicly Available Spaces

Unlike previous gaming applications that required additional equipment, current virtual technologies are readily available to anyone with a computer and an Internet connection. There is a plethora of publicly available spaces where one can interact with others for a variety of reasons for little to no cost. Many are game-specific and targeted toward specific age groups—for example, Virtual Worlds for Teens (http://virtualworldsforteens.com/), Twinity (http://www .twinity.com), and 3Dchat (http://www.3dchat.com). The list of online virtual worlds continues to grow, so any attempt to provide a current list would be instantly outdated.

One of the oldest, largest, and most active virtual world is Linden Labs' Second Life (http://www.secondlife.com). Current estimates indicate the site has approximately 1 million regular monthly users, with 70,000 concurrent users. In Second Life, residents can shop, attend business meetings, take classes, participate in trainings, swim, ski, watch a live concert, and do just about anything that they could do in real life.

The geography of Second Life is organized as Islands. One of the most popular and frequently visited is Health Info Island (http://maps.secondlife.com/secondlife/Healthinfo%20Island/172/222/27). Created and funded by a grant from the National Library of Medicine, HealthInfo Island has grown from a resource for health information to include more than 120 support groups for patients and caregivers, as well as mental health simulations and an area for individuals with disabilities called Virtual Ability Island (http://slurl.com/secondlife/Virtual+Ability/132/165/25).

An increasing number of real-world health-related institutions and organizations have begun to promote the use of virtual worlds and have created virtual world presences. For example, the National Institutes of Health has suggested the use of virtual reality technology for research and education on diabetes and obesity because of the potential to engage patients in interventions that focus on healthy eating and physical activity.[4] Given that interactive technologies have been used to facilitate the delivery of health information and interaction between patients, caregivers, and health professionals, the application for health behavior change interventions seems plausible.

Use of Virtual World Technology in Public Health and Health Promotion Research

Virtually Experiencing the Consequences of Negative Health Behaviors

Virtual worlds offer novel media characteristics that allow researchers and healthcare practitioners to implement new strategies in approaching health behavior change that may have been difficult or impossible to achieve with traditional tools and media platforms. One such characteristic is the virtual acceleration of time,[5] wherein users can transcend the temporal boundaries of the physical world by experiencing digitally depicted events of the past or the future in the virtual worlds. For instance, with the help of simulated sensory information via digital devices, users may be able to virtually experience the negative future consequences of present problematic health behaviors, allowing users to construe the health risks as personally relevant[6] and temporally imminent.[5] The increased sense of relevance and urgency through the virtual experience encourages individuals to reduce problematic health behaviors.

The virtual acceleration of time would be particularly useful for healthcare issues because one of the greatest challenges of communicating health risks is the large temporal gap that exists between present health behaviors and future negative health consequences. This gap explains why individuals tend to have a more "rosy" view of distant futures[7]; it may be that individuals are unaware of how imminent the health risk may be. For example, smoking a cigarette is unlikely to lead to immediate illness or fatality. The length of time it takes for emergence of negative health outcomes makes the causal relationship between the present cause (smoking) and the future outcomes (e.g., lung cancer) abstract and difficult to grasp. Relatedly, earlier research demonstrates that when health messages can present a negative health consequence as an immediate risk, they are more effective at behavioral modification.

Virtual Selves

Another novel characteristic of virtual worlds is a by-product of the plasticity of avatar creation. With the development of advanced digital technology, users may now easily create photorealistic avatars that share realistic physical feature similarities with the self. For example, if a health pamphlet features a virtual entity that really looks like you, rather than a typical but unfamiliar person, you are more likely to pay attention and accept the associated message as personally relevant.[8] Moreover, once the photorealistic virtual self is created, computer software is easily able to manipulate its appearance—the virtual self may be aged to make you look like you are in your 60s, or its physique may be altered so that it looks like the virtual self has gained weight. These virtual selves may be used to present health messages that allow individuals to realize that the health risk applies to them, not just someone else.

In one such study, the effects of virtual experiences that incorporate virtual acceleration in time and photorealistic virtual selves on health attitudes and behaviors in the physical world were explored in the context of soft-drink consumption.[5] In this study, different groups of participants were exposed to four experimental conditions in a 2×2 between-subjects design. Participants either saw only the pamphlet, which was tailored to the self or untailored, or were exposed to both the pamphlet and the virtual depiction of it. The six-page, full-color pamphlet provided specific information on the health risks of soft drinks, with an emphasis on weight gain and obesity. In the virtual experience, participants wore a head-mounted display, a set of goggles that provides three-dimensional perception through stereoscopic views of the virtual world, and observed either a virtual self or an unfamiliar, generic virtual human (i.e., virtual other). During the two-minute virtual experience, participants saw the virtual self or virtual other imbibe a soft drink and continue to gain weight. Two years in the physical world were depicted in two minutes in the virtual world. Self-reported soft-drink consumption intentions were assessed immediately following the experimental treatment, and actual soft-drink consumption was measured one week following experimental treatment.

Results indicated that immediately following the experimental treatment, the effect of tailoring significantly affected intentions to consume soft drinks in the future. The messages, regardless of whether they were presented in a pamphlet or in the virtual world, led to shorter perceived distance between the self and the health risk and, in turn, to higher involvement. The increased involvement ultimately led to lower intentions to consume soft drinks than were produced by the untailored messages.

Interestingly, the effect of the tailoring seemed to dissipate over time. One week following the experimental treatment, only the effect of medium was significant. The participants who were given the pamphlet coupled with the virtual experience perceived a shorter temporal distance between their present health behaviors and future health

(continues)

BOX 10-9 The Use of Virtual Worlds in Health Promotion   *(continued)*

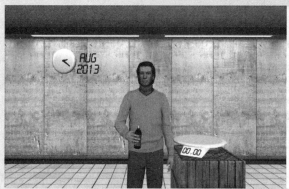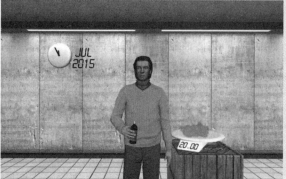

Participants entered the virtual world and saw either a virtual self or a virtual other (left panel). As time in the virtual world progressed at an accelerated speed, the virtual human continued to drink the soft drink. In two minutes in the virtual world, two years in the physical world was depicted to have passed, with the virtual human gaining 20 pounds in weight as a result of drinking soft drinks (right panel).

outcomes, which led to greater perceived imminence of the risks related to soft-drink consumption. The increased risk then resulted in significantly lower soft-drink consumption than was found among participants who only saw the pamphlet. This experiment provided strong preliminary evidence for the potential of incorporating virtual experiences as a part of multicomponent and multimedia health promotion campaigns.

In another study, Ahn and colleagues demonstrated that not all virtual representations used to promote health behaviors are required to take on human forms.[9] A virtual pet system was developed guided by the framework of social cognitive theory,[10] with the goal of systematically promoting physical activity in children through goal setting, vicarious experiences, and positive reinforcement. A kiosk was built to present the virtual pet system, using a laptop and a flat-screen television stationed on top of a rolling cart. A Microsoft Kinect for Windows device with motion-detecting capabilities was mounted on top of the television.

In the study, children's physical activity was measured with an activity monitor and synchronized with a unique pet so that the child would interact with this personalized pet for the duration of the intervention. The integration of the activity monitor with the virtual pet system allowed children to use this system with minimal or no technical expertise; they simply had to plug the activity monitor into the computer, and the system would automatically synchronize the activity data with the child's unique virtual pet and update the system as necessary.

The interaction cycle was a repetition of goal-setting, evaluation, and reinforcement processes. Upon first engaging with the virtual pet, children were asked to personalize their pets (e.g., select the collar color, select the tag color, name the pet). The virtual pet then asked children to establish their own physical activity goals to promote self-efficacy by way of mastery experiences. That is, by setting and meeting goals for behavior change and recognizing their ability to overcome challenges along the way, the children were expected to gain confidence in their capacity to engage in that particular behavior.[11] Similarly, the goal-setting feature in the virtual pet was designed to allow children to repeatedly engage in the experience of setting and meeting physical activity goals to promote mastery experiences.

Once the goal was set, children engaged in physical activity away from the kiosk, wearing the physical activity monitor. When children believed that they had met their physical activity goal, they returned to the kiosk and plugged the activity monitor into the computer. The computer then automatically synchronized the unique identifier chip embedded in the activity monitor to the child's unique virtual pet and brought the pet up on the screen while also evaluating the physical activity recorded on the child's activity monitor. If the child was unable to meet the goal, the virtual pet verbally informed the child that he or she had failed to meet the physical activity goal and encouraged the child to go back to engaging in physical activity. If the child did meet the goal, the virtual pet invited him or her to teach it a trick using verbal and gesture commands detected by the Kinect for Windows device. For instance, the child could verbally command, "Fetch!" and see a virtual ball appear on the screen. He or she could then make a throwing motion toward the Kinect, and the ball would fly into the

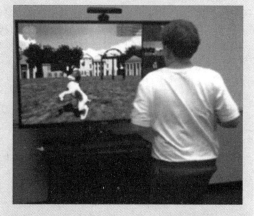

The virtual pet kiosk, created with consumer-grade digital devices.

virtual world, following the trajectory of the child's physical arm. The virtual pet would then chase after the ball and bring it back. Because the underlying assumption was that the virtual pet would be engaging in physical activity in the virtual world while children stayed physically active in the physical world, the tricks began with simpler ones (e.g., sit, stay) and eventually more sophisticated ones as children met more goals and the virtual pet became more fit (e.g., fetch, moonwalk). Once the child taught the virtual pet one trick, the pet asked the child to set a new physical activity goal, and the cycle would repeat.

This virtual pet system was compared against a computer system that offered the same goal-setting, evaluating, and reinforcing features without the virtual pet. The study took place for three full days at a local summer camp with children between the ages of 9 and 12. Compared with children in the control group who were given an identical computer system with the same functionalities but without the virtual dog, children who interacted with the virtual dog engaged in approximately 1.09 more hours of physical activity daily. Self-report survey data revealed that interacting with the virtual dog led children to feel confident about their abilities to set and meet physical activity goals, which in turn heightened their beliefs that physical activity is good for them. The increase in physical activity belief ultimately led to an increase in physical activity.

When virtual worlds are established using highly mobile setups such as the one in this study, they can be used in health promotion campaigns outside of the laboratory. For instance, this virtual pet system may be set up anywhere that children are, including classrooms, doctor's offices, or health centers, as a highly translatable and scalable solution for using virtual worlds in public health promotion efforts.

Promoting Health in a Virtual World

To examine the use of an online virtual world for the delivery of health communication messages designed to encourage healthy behavior change regarding physical activity and nutrition, a study was conducted entirely within the virtual world of Second Life.[12]

Participants included 40 undergraduate students with little to no prior experience with Second Life. During an initial orientation session, participants were assisted in creating their avatars and in learning how to navigate and communicate in world. In Second Life, participants can customize their avatars in many ways, including gender, physical attributes, clothing, accessories, and even whether to be human, animal, or an object. Most participants in this study chose to be represented by human-looking avatars.

The study consisted of a brief intervention delivered by a trained health educator avatar in a common area of a teaching parcel. Participants were sent a link to the location and upon logging in, were instructed to travel (teleport) there. The geography of Second Life is set up as a series of Islands divided into parcels of land. Our intervention was conducted in a common area on a teaching parcel where our university had a virtual presence. The program was designed as a traditional lecture followed by a question-and-answer session held in an open-air amphitheater. The space included rows of bench seats facing a stage with a podium and overhead interactive signs. The intervention consisted of approximately 15 minutes of information about physical activity and nutrition, including recommended guidelines and on- and off-campus resources. The program was developed by trained health educators and was delivered by a health education graduate student. Her avatar was intentionally designed to present a conservative, somewhat authoritarian image.

Second Life allows participants to communicate in several different ways. For this study, the health educator and the participants could speak to each other using the chat feature. Interactive signs were designed so that participants could click on them to receive additional information.

Qualitative and quantitative data were collected on a multitude of variables, including usability, participant satisfaction, changes in theoretical constructs of health behavior change (readiness to change, motivation, self-efficacy, intention), and the relationship between participant body mass index (BMI) and participant body ratings of self and avatar. Quantitative data were collected with pre-test and post-test surveys, while qualitative data were collected with a series of four focus groups, three of which were held in Second Life.

Results showed that although all participants had less than three months' experience with Second Life, the majority thought the program was easy to use (87.5%) and would be interested in experiencing other health-related programs in Second Life (82.5%). Furthermore, 80% found the information useful in helping them think about changing their health behaviors, while 92.5% found the information easy to understand and personally relevant.[12]

Given that this was a brief intervention, the pre-test and post-test data collection occurred during the same session. Therefore, only the theoretical constructs related to behavior change could be assessed rather than actual behavior-change outcomes. Although increases were observed in motivation, intention, and self-efficacy to make healthy behavior changes regarding physical activity and diet, only participants' rating of self-efficacy regarding physical activity was statistically significant ($p = 0.039$).[13]

One of the concerns regarding the delivery of health information in a virtual world is whether the information is perceived and processed as our real-world selves or as our in-world avatars. In Second Life, before users customize their

(continues)

BOX 10-9 The Use of Virtual Worlds in Health Promotion *(continued)*

avatars, the default human avatars tend to be attractive and typically normal to underweight. It was therefore of interest to us to explore how the participants processed, received, and applied the health information as their real-life selves. Both survey and focus group data from this study show that most participants received and processed the information as their real-world selves. Additionally, more than 50% of those in our study reported that they designed their avatar to look like themselves. Only 5% stated that they sometimes appeared in Second Life as the opposite gender and 2.5% as an animal.[12]

Previous research has indicated that Second Life users prefer to create avatars that represent an idealized self. Users who create an idealized avatar tend to have a high attachment to their avatar, and people with high BMIs tend to create idealized avatars more so than other users.[14] It has also been found that avatars generally resemble their owner's *body image* more than their owner's *actual body*, and that virtual world users' perceptions of their avatar's body influence their perceptions of their own body.[15] To explore these relationships in our study, we collected data on participants' BMI (from self-reported height and weight), ratings of self and avatar body weight, and avatar appearance and attractiveness compared to participants' ratings of their own real-life attractiveness. Our results showed that based on BMI, 42.5% of participants were overweight or obese—the same percentage that rated themselves as slightly or markedly overweight. In contrast, only 12.5% rated their avatars as slightly or markedly overweight. With regard to attractiveness, 40% rated their avatar appearance as more attractive than their real-life appearance.[13]

Overall, the results of this study support the approach of using a virtual world as a feasible and potentially effective way to accomplish health promotion objectives regarding physical activity and nutrition. Participants were receptive to receiving health information in this virtual-world setting and to using the Internet in general to access health information. Web 2.0 technologies are continuing to provide opportunities for patients and caregivers to share information and support as well as for individuals to engage in behavior change efforts. The anonymity of web-based interactions, including those occurring in Second Life, can also potentially contribute to the engagement of hard-to-reach populations and to addressing particularly sensitive subjects such as drug use and sexual behavior.

Designing Virtual Reality Technology for Research

Novel virtual technologies allow researchers to conduct laboratory experiments that optimize ecological validity without compromising experimental control. There are several advantages to using virtual technologies in social and behavioral science studies. First, virtual worlds allow researchers to create experimental situations with more mundane realism compared to the rigidly controlled traditional laboratory settings, potentially eliciting more genuine participant reactions to stimuli.[16] For example, rather than invoking fear by asking participants to imagine developing lung cancer as a result of smoking or giving them a traditional pamphlet with details on lung cancer, virtual worlds allow participants to perceptually experience lung cancer through vivid and realistic simulations. This contributes to high external validity.

Despite this freedom to construct any environment or stimulus of the researcher's desire, with his or her imagination being the only limit, virtual worlds still allow researchers to tightly control every element down to the millisecond and millimeter. For instance, once virtual humans are created, researchers may control and manipulate minute details.[17] If researchers were to study the effect of body posture on perceptions of a speaker's credibility, they must deal with several confounding cues in the real world, such as the speaker's natural facial expressions, head movements, and gestures. By using virtual humans, these cues can be removed or neutralized to allow researchers to examine the specific cue of interest "in a vacuum." Furthermore, the exact same stimulus can be replicated and shared with other researchers almost flawlessly for countless iterations of experiments, eliminating variance that may impact outcomes.[16] This contributes to high internal validity.

Thanks to the incorporation of sensitive tracking devices, researchers can go above and beyond traditional means to measure user's naturalistic responses in virtual worlds.[16,18] For instance, virtual worlds may be programmed to automatically record data regarding the user's movements, gaze, and gestures,[19] thereby eliminating the subjective and often painful process of having coders review videotape and follow coding schemes. These functions also gather data almost continuously, reporting at fractions of a second that are too minute for human coders to make distinctions. The level of detail presented in the behavioral data can serve as meaningful supplements to surveys and self-report questionnaires that are open to multitude of errors and misrepresentations. These affordances make virtual worlds ideal environments in which to study human cognition and behavior.

Strategies, Challenges, and Implications for Future Use

Although virtual technologies offer a multitude of health promotion opportunities, they are not without challenges. Although widely available and accessible, virtual worlds such as Second Life can be transient, as can the resources and programs contained within them. It is therefore incumbent upon health promotion program planners to be diligent in confirming their availability before recommending these virtual worlds to clients or program participants, and in updating materials frequently.

Future areas of research inquiry should include the examination of how people create and interact with online personas and how such interactions might translate to real-world behavior changes. The creation and use of avatars presents a unique dynamic for exploration regarding the receptivity to health messages. Understanding how participants process health information relevant to the needs of their real-world selves versus the perceived needs of their in-world avatars is crucial. Future research should also consider how our experiences in virtual worlds change with long-term participation.

Finally, virtual systems are becoming more accessible and affordable through gaming platforms and consumer-grade devices. Soon it may be possible to send tailored health promotion messages directly to individuals' homes through the existing infrastructures of virtual worlds. For instance, the Microsoft Kinect Xbox console is one of the fastest-selling consumer electronics products, with more than 24 million units sold since its launch in late 2010.[20] Sophisticated head-mounted displays, similar to the ones used in the studies discussed here, are now available for a few hundred dollars and easily incorporated into everyday computing systems as a plug-and-play device. Moreover, large companies, including Samsung, Facebook, Apple, and Sony, are vying to create the most sophisticated, yet affordable head-mounted display for consumers, signaling a virtual revolution in the near future. Like the Internet mobile revolutions, the virtual revolution is likely to transform traditional patterns of health communication and health promotion campaigns.

References

1. Blascovich J, Bailenson JN. *Infinite Reality: Avatars, Eternal Life, New Worlds, and the Dawn of the Virtual Revolution*. New York, NY: William Morrow; 2011.

2. Ondrejka C. Education unleashed: Participatory culture, education, and innovation in Second Life. In: Salen K, ed. *The Ecology of Games: Connecting Youth, Games, and Learning*. Cambridge, MA: MIT Press; 2008:229-251.

3. Ahn SJ, Fox J, Bailenson JN. Avatars. In Bainbridge WS, ed. *Leadership in Science and Technology: A Reference Handbook*. Thousand Oaks, CA: Sage; 2011:695-702.

4. Ershow AG, Peterson CM, Riley WT, Rizzo, A, Wansink B. Virtual reality technologies for research and education in obesity and diabetes: research needs and opportunities. *J Diabetes Sci Technol*. 2011;5(2):212-224.

5. Ahn SJ. Incorporating immersive virtual environments in health promotion campaigns: A construal-level theory approach. *Health Communication*. 2015;30(6):545-556.

6. Ahn SJ, Fox J, Hahm JM. Using virtual doppelgängers to increase personal relevance of health risk communication. *Lect Notes Comput Sci*. 2014;8637:1-12.

7. Trope Y, Liberman N, Wakslak C. Construal levels and psychological distance: effects on representation, prediction, evaluation, and behavior. *J Consumer Psychol*. 2007;17:83-95.

8. Ahn SJ, Bailenson J N. Self-endorsing versus other-endorsing in virtual environments: the effect on brand attitude and purchase intention. *J Advertising*. 2011;40(2):93-106.

9. Ahn SJ, Johnsen K, Robertson T, et al. Using virtual pets to promote physical activity in children: an application of the youth physical activity promotion model. *J Health Comm*. 2015;20(7):807-815.

10. Bandura A. *Social Learning Theory*. Englewood Cliffs: NJ: Prentice-Hall; 1976.

11. Bandura A. Self-efficacy: toward a unifying theory of behavioral change. *Psychol Rev*. 1977;84(2):191-215.

12. Cowdery JE, Kindred J, Michalakis A, Suggs LS. Promoting health in a virtual world: impressions of health communication messages delivered in Second Life. *First Monday*. 2011;16(9). http://firstmonday.org/htbin/cgiwrap/bin/ojs/index.php/fm/article/viewArticle/2857/3048. Accessed October 14, 2016.

13. Kindred J, Cowdery JE. Using a virtual world to encourage healthy lifestyle choices among college students. *Cases Public Health Comm Market*. 2012;6:3-20.

14. Ducheneaut N, Wen MH, Yee N, Wadley G. Body and mind: a study of avatar personalization in three virtual worlds. *Proceedings of the 27th International Conference on Human Factors in Computing Systems, CHI 2009*; Boston, MA; April 4–9. 2009.

15. Chandler J, Konrath S, Schwarz N. Online and on my mind: temporary and chronic accessibility moderate the influence of media Figures. *Media Psychol*. 2009;12:210-226.

(continues)

BOX 10-9 The Use of Virtual Worlds in Health Promotion *(continued)*

16. Blascovich J, Loomis JM, Beall AC, Swinth K, Hoyt C, Bailenson JN. Immersive virtual environment technology as a methodological tool for social psychology. *Psychol Inquiry*. 2002;13:103-124.

17. Bailenson JN, Blascovich J, Beall AC, Loomis JM. Equilibrium revisited: mutual gaze and personal space in virtual environments. *PRESENCE: Teleoperators and Virtual Environments*. 2001;10:583-598.

18. Loomis JM, Blascovich J, Beall AC. Immersive virtual environments as a basic research tool in psychology. *Behav Res Methods Instruments Computers*. 1999;31:557-564.

19. Yee N, Harris H, Jabon M, Bailenson JN. The expression of personality in virtual worlds. *Soc Psychol Personality Sci*. 2011;2(1):5-12.

20. Epstein Z. Microsoft says Xbox 360 sales have surpassed 76 million units, Kinect sales top 24 million. http://bgr.com/2013/02/12/microsoft-xbox-360-sales-2013-325481/. Accessed June 11, 2013.

▶ Conclusion

There are a dizzying number of channels available for health communication. The last decade has seen the rise of social media as a powerful set of tools to reach and interact with not only a selected audience but individuals as well. New opportunities for communicating personal health information and persuasion have developed and will continue to do so. The challenge for health communication is to keep up with the new methods and integrate them with the established ones.

Wrap-Up

Chapter Questions

1. Define the five elements of effective transmedia storytelling for behavior change.
2. List three "on the page" and three "off the page" factors that can significantly contribute to search engine optimization.
3. What does the phrase "not all social media are digital, not all digital communications are social" refer to? How does this relate to how public health organizations use digital media?
4. What does the widespread adoption of social media by leading public health organizations indicate, and which process appears to give messages shared via social media heightened authority?
5. Briefly summarize Hall *et al*.'s findings in their systematic review of text message interventions.[19]
6. Describe the differences and similarities in how public health organizations use Facebook and Twitter.
7. Describe, with examples from the chapter, two ways that health communicators can integrate new methods with established media channels.

References

1. Weinreich NK. The immersive engagement model: transmedia storytelling for social change. 2014. http://social-marketing.com/immersive-engagement.html.

2. Krogh P. Platforms and channels. *Strictly Business Blog*. October 10, 2013. https://www.asmp.org/strictlybusiness/2013/10/platforms-and-channels. Accessed January 23, 2016.

3. Duggan M, Pew Research Center. Mobile messaging and social media 2015. August 19, 2015. http://www.pewinternet.org/files/2015/08/Social-Media-Update-2015-FINAL2.pdf. Accessed October 9, 2015.

4. Nielsen Company. Nielsen estimates 116.4 million TV homes in the U.S. for the 2015-16 TV season. August 28, 2015. http://www.nielsen.com/us/en/insights/news/2015/nielsen-estimates-116-4-million-tv-homes-in-the-us-for-the-2015-16-tv-season.html. Accessed November 9, 2015.

5. Nielsen Company. The total audience report Q2 2015. *Total Audience Series*. http://www.nielsen.com/content/dam/corporate/us/en/reports-downloads/2015-reports/total-audience-report-q22015.pdf. Accessed November 9, 2015.

6. Nielsen Company. All things considered: comparable metrics offer a solid line of sight for the industry. June 23, 2015. http://www.nielsen.com/us/en/insights/news/2015/all-things

-considered-comparable-metrics-offer-a-solid-line-of-sight-for-the-industry.html. Accessed November 9, 2015.

7. Newspapers: daily readership by age. Nielsen Scarborough USA+ 1999–2014, Release 1. Pew Research Center Media and News Indicators Database. http://www.journalism.org/media-indicators/newspapers-daily-readership-by-age/. Accessed November 9, 2015.

8. Association of Magazine Media. Magazine media factbook 2015. http://www.magazine.org/magazine-media-factbook-2015. Accessed November 11, 2015.

9. Health Communication Capacity Collaborative. *A Theory-Based Framework for Media Selection in Demand Generation Programs.* Baltimore, MD: Johns Hopkins Bloomberg School of Public Health Center for Communication Programs; 2014.

10. American Press Institute and Associated Press, Media Insight Project 2014. The personal news cycle: how Americans choose to get their news. March 17, 2014. http://www.americanpressinstitute.org/wp-content/uploads/2014/03/The_Media_Insight_Project_The_Personal_News_Cycle_Final.pdf. Accessed December 20, 2015.

11. American Press Institute and Associated Press, Media Insight Project 2015. How millennials get news: paying for content. 2015:19. http://www.mediainsight.org/PDFs/Millennials/Millennials%20Report%20FINAL.pdf. Accessed December 9, 2015.

12. HubSpot. Marketing benchmarks from 7,000+ businesses. http://www.hubspot.com/. 2015. Accessed December 9, 2015.

13. Unbounce. What is a landing page? http://unbounce.com/landing-page-articles/what-is-a-landing-page/. Accessed December 9, 2015.

14. Heldman AB, Schindelar J, Weaver JB. Social media engagement and public health communication: implications for public health organizations being truly "social." *Public Health Rev.* 2013;35(1):1-18.

15. IMS Institute for Healthcare Informatics. *Patient Adoption of mHealth.* September 2015. Parsippany, NJ: IMS Health.

16. Schein R, Kumanan W, Keelan J. Literature review on effectiveness of the use of social media: a report for Peel Public Health. http://www.peelregion.ca/health/resources/pdf/socialmedia.pdf.

17. Perrin A. *Social networking usage: 2005–2015.* Pew Research Center: October 2015. http://www.pewinternet.org/2015/10/08/2015/Social-Networking-Usage-2005-2015. Accessed November 11, 2015.

18. Lenhart A. *Teen, social media and technology overview 2015.* Pew Research Center; April 9, 2015. http://www.pewinternet.org/files/2015/04/PI_TeensandTech_Update2015_0409151.pdf. Accessed November 11, 2015.

19. Hall AK, Cole-Lewis H, Bernhardt JM. Mobile text messaging for health: a systematic review of reviews. *Annu Rev Public Health.* 2015;36:393-415.

20. Duggan M. *Mobile messaging and social media 2015.* Pew Research Center; August 2015. http://www.pewinternet.org/2015/08/19/mobile-messaging-and-social-media-2015/. Accessed November 9, 2015.

21. Facebook company info. https://newsroom.fb.com/company-info/. Accessed November 9, 2015.

22. Laranjo L, Arguel A, Leves AL, et al. The influence of social networking sites on health behavior change: a systematic review and meta-analysis. *Am Med Inform Assoc.* 2015;22:243-256.

23. Meet the people who'll love your organization: a nonprofit's guide to Facebook pages and ads. https://fbhost.promotw.com/fbpages/img/non_profit_resources/GCD_NPGuide_20140602_v3_JR.pdf. Accessed November 9, 2015.

24. Getting started with Twitter. Twitter Help Center. https://support.twitter.com/articles/215585. Accessed November 5, 2015.

25. Bartlett C, Wurtz R. Twitter and public health. *J Public Health Manag Pract.* 2015;21(4):375-383.

26. Eysenbach G. Infodemiology and infoveillance tracking online health information and cyberbehavior for public health. *Am J Prev Med.* 2011;40(5 suppl 2):S154-S158.

27. Paul MJ, Dredze M. You are what you tweet: analyzing Twitter for public health. *Proceedings of the Fifth International AAAI Conference on Weblogs and Social Media.* Association for the Advancement of Artificial Intelligence; 2011.

28. Aslam AA, Tsou M-H, Spitzberg BH, et al. The reliability of tweets as a supplementary method of seasonal influenza surveillance. *J Med Internet Res.* 2014;16(11):e250.

29. Liu B. *Sentiment Analysis and Opinion Mining: Synthesis Lectures on Human Language Technologies.* Morgan and Claypool Publishers, University of Illinois at Chicago; May 2012;5(1):1-167. doi: 10.2200/S00416ED1V01Y201204HLT016.

30. Harris JK, Mueller NL, Snider D. Social media adoption in local health departments nationwide. *Am J Public Health.* 2013;103(9):1700-1707.

31. Stelzner M. Social media marketing industry report for 2015. http://www.socialmediaexaminer.com/social-media-marketing-industry-report-2015/. Accessed November 9, 2015.

32. Wright DK, Hinson MD. Examining social and emerging media use in public relations practice: a ten-year longitudinal analysis. *PR J.* September 2015;9. https://www.prsa.org/Intelligence/PRJournal/Documents/2015v09n02WrightHinson.pdf. Accessed October 14, 2015.

33. Freeman B, Potente S, Rock V, McIver J. Social media campaigns that make a difference: what can public health learn from the corporate sector and other social change marketers? *Public Health Res Pract.* 2015;25(2):e2521517.

34. Shegog R, Peskin MF, Markham CM, et al. "It's your game-tech": toward sexual health in the digital age. *Creative Educ.* 2014;5(special ed):1428-1447.

Appendix 10A

Harnessing the Power of Radio to Raise HIV Testing Rates

Jeremy Smith and **Matthew Scelza**

▶ Introduction

For the past two years, Incite has been working closely with the AIDS Healthcare Foundation (AHF), the largest provider of HIV/AIDS medical care in the United States. Their shared goal: to increase HIV awareness and testing rates, specifically among difficult-to-reach populations in Los Angeles and New York.

As a group, men who have sex with men (MSM) have disproportionately high rates of HIV/AIDS. There are several reasons that men engage in sex with other men: identifying as gay or bisexual, adhering to societal or cultural norms, because of environmental factors (such as prisoners), or for income purposes (prostitution). Within this group, the African American MSM population is particularly vulnerable to contracting HIV. This is due to a myriad of social attitudes and circumstances, ranging from risky behavior and practices to insufficient tools such as resources, role models, and self-esteem. Furthermore, intentional secretive practices concerning lifestyle choices and sexual preferences can discourage HIV testing.[1] Because of these factors, the MSM population is a priority audience to which AHF provides HIV testing and outreach services.

▶ Los Angeles

Los Angeles radio station Power 106 has been influencing hip-hop culture for more than 25 years. Reaching nearly 3 million people weekly, the station's audience comprises predominantly black and Hispanic young people in southern California. Beyond this significant reach, many Power 106 listeners have grown up on hip-hop, engaging with the music and interacting with disc jockeys (DJs) to such a degree that Power 106 has become influential in shaping attitudes and behavior.

Working with Incite and Power 106, AHF's goals were to increase testing rates and drive people to www.FreeSTDCheck.org. Using radio ads, DJ endorsements, mobile-targeted ads, digital ads on Power106.com, event-based marketing, social media posts, and grassroots activation, AHF and Incite utilized the Power 106 reach and relevance to engage people who identified with the hip-hop lifestyle. To change people's views of testing, the AHF campaign used attention-grabbing creative elements, including the theme "Check Your Wiener" (**FIGURE 10A-1**).

Popular Power 106 personality Louie G endorsed the message on air during a weekly morning show feature, "Smash-a-Lot Fridays," encouraging listeners to take responsibility for their sexual health entering the weekend. Louie G also demonstrated the quick and simple process of getting tested and encouraged people to get tested via a recorded video vignette—all leading into National HIV Testing Day (**FIGURE 10A-2**).

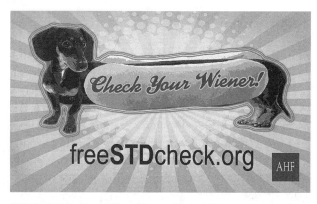

FIGURE 10A-1 *Check Your Wiener* Digital Advertisement.
Courtesy of AIDS Healthcare Foundation / Incite.

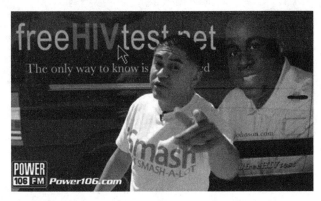

FIGURE 10A-2 Louie G Gets a Rapid HIV Test.

Courtesy of AIDS Healthcare Foundation / Incite.

These activities directed people to take action by going to www.FreeSTDCheck.org. From there, users could learn more about safe sexual health practices and receive information about local testing facilities. The campaign resulted in more than 1300 people signing up for information, more than 140 people being tested for HIV, and one newly diagnosed individual who was immediately directed to appropriate medical care.

Power 106 continued the "Check Your Wiener" effort leading up to Valentine's Day. Louie G took a humorous approach to sharing sexual health information by becoming the "STD Fairy" and reminding couples to always "Check Your Wiener." In keeping with the behavior-change marketing theory of "meeting people where they are," Incite and AHF brought the "Check Your Wiener" campaign to Power 106's Valentine's Crush concert, where they interacted with 18,000 people by distributing condoms and providing sexual health information to concertgoers. During the concert, audiences were exposed to campaign ads on the venue marquee and interacted with the "smash cam" showing couples kissing on the Jumbo Tron. The concert activation resulted in an additional 115 people getting tested for HIV.

▶ New York City

Building on the success of the Los Angeles–based campaigns, Incite partnered with AHF to increase testing rates in New York City around the opening of AHF's new testing facility in Brooklyn. In contrast to the orchestrated media campaign executed in Los Angeles around major concerts and existing testing events, Incite and AHF were able to take advantage of a timely media story to share a public health message through a powerful endorser.

In September 2013, Mister Cee, a popular DJ for New York hip-hop radio station HOT 97, found himself in a difficult situation when it was revealed

that he was engaging in MSM practices. His long-standing relationship with the hip-hop community was challenged by its general sentiment regarding MSM behavior. In response, Incite and AHF worked with HOT 97 and Mister Cee to launch "The Living Truth" campaign. Audiences were directed to the HOT 97 and AHF websites to view a video revealing Mister Cee's sexual health story (**FIGURE 10A-3**). The first-of-its-kind video served as a personal plea and intentional call to action from a male hip-hop celebrity to his peers, especially young people, to live their truth and know their status.

"The Living Truth" online video campaign resulted in more than 47 million media impressions and 57,000 YouTube video views. It drove more traffic to the AHF website in a 48-hour period than the website had received in the previous three years.

▶ Impact

Media and celebrity influencers are powerful driving forces that, when utilized timely and effectively, can serve as powerful catalysts for public health and behavior change.

Through its partnership with Incite, AHF has reached nearly 30,000 individuals on site at events and distributed more than 12,500 condoms. Incite's social marketing efforts drove more than 10,000 page views of FreeSTDCheck.org. Viewed more than 57,000 times, Mister Cee's "The Living Truth" video began a conversation in the hip-hop community that was long overdue. Perhaps most importantly, AHF tested more than 250 people on site at entertainment venues.

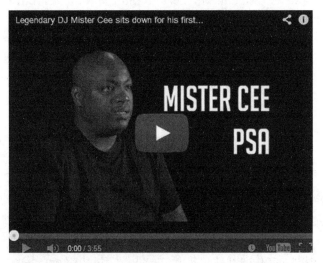

FIGURE 10A-3 Mister Cee's "The Living Truth" Video Testimonial.

Courtesy of AIDS Healthcare Foundation / Incite.

This case study highlights the strategic use of entertainment and media to improve public health outcomes. Used effectively, entertainment and media channels meet people where they are, influence attitudes and beliefs, and encourage people to act for their personal health, which improves the public health. Furthermore, culturally relevant personalities—because of their ongoing reach and trusted influence with large communities—can be effectively used to inspire target audiences that would not otherwise consider positive sexual health messages and behaviors.

Reference

1. Malebranche D. The truth about the "down low." April 2011. http://www.apa.org/pi/aids/resources/exchange/2011/04/down-low.aspx.

▶ About the Authors and Incite (Emmis Communications)

Jeremy Smith is National Director of Business, Incite. Matthew Scelza is Director, Incite Los Angeles. Dedicated to using media to inspire positive action, Incite is a cause marketing firm within Emmis Communications—a multimedia company operating radio stations throughout the country.

Appendix 10B

Health Communication Strategies for Hispanic Enrollment into the Affordable Care Act Health Insurance Exchanges: A Case Study

Dirk G. Schroeder, ScD, MPH, **Gloria P. Giraldo**, MPH, and **Brianna Keefe-Oates**, MPH

▶ Introduction

U.S. Hispanics have historically had the highest rates of uninsurance of any racial or ethnic group. At the time the Patient Protection and Affordable Care Act (ACA) was signed in 2010, 30% of Hispanics lacked health insurance, compared to 18% for blacks and 13% for non-Hispanic whites.[2] Under the ACA law, 10.2 million uninsured Hispanics who are U.S. citizens or legally reside in the United States, or nearly 8 in 10 uninsured Latinos, were given the opportunity to obtain affordable healthcare coverage through Medicaid, Children's Health Insurance Program (CHIP), or lower monthly premiums through the Health Insurance Marketplaces.[3] Not only did Hispanics have a great deal to gain by signing up for health insurance through the Marketplace, but the country would also benefit by enrolling the mostly young and generally healthy population that Hispanics represent.[4] In 2013, it was estimated that half of all uninsured Hispanics were between the ages of 18 and 35.[3] Enrolling this younger population was and remains crucial to financial sustainability of the ACA, since younger members tend to offset the costs of older, typically sicker people.[5]

Although the importance of assuring that Hispanics would sign up for health insurance through the Marketplace was widely understood among policy makers, exactly how to go about achieving this goal was less clear. Officials responsible for the state-based exchanges, the federal government, and organizations such as Enroll America knew that

there would be many challenges to educating and motivating Hispanics to enroll in health insurance under the ACA. These challenges included language barriers, cultural differences in health beliefs and behaviors, and fear of government programs, especially among Hispanic families that contained family members who were undocumented.[6] In anticipation of these challenges, state and local groups began laying the groundwork for reaching out to this important demographic audience long before the first open enrollment period began. Preparations included translating materials, training bilingual call center staff, and recruiting community-based health educators for outreach.[3] Once these foundational elements were in place, a wide range of approaches were then used to try to educate Hispanics about the ACA, including online/digital messaging and advertising; traditional marketing methods such as TV, direct mailings, billboards, and radio; and field outreach consisting of trained individuals implementing events and reaching out in person to those who might qualify to help them understand what the ACA was and why it was important to enroll.[7]

The objective of this case study is to share insights into what worked and what did not work during the first two years of educating and enrolling Hispanics in the ACA Marketplaces. We draw on HolaDoctor's experiences educating Hispanic consumers directly through its Spanish-language health website as well as the experiences gained through collaborations with health plans, state and federal agencies, and nonprofit organizations.

▸ HolaDoctor: Putting Experience in Hispanic Health Communications to Work for the ACA

HolaDoctor, Inc., is a health communications firm that has been designing and delivering Hispanic-focused campaigns since 1999. It owns and operates the largest Spanish-language network of health websites on the Internet, in partnership with the Interactive Division of Univision.

This case study is predominately based on the work we did in collaboration with health plans and local community organizations in California, New York, Georgia, and Colorado. We compare and contrast these experiences with those of some governmental agencies, such as Covered California, that were also working to educate Hispanics about the ACA at the same time.

Market Research to Understand the Target Audience

HolaDoctor and its health plan partners used a variety of approaches to understand the target audience, including (1) literature and web reviews, (2) demographic analyses for geographic targeting, and (3) original research using focus groups and online surveys.

Hispanics/Latinos in the United States

According to U.S. Census Bureau population estimates, as of July 1, 2013, Hispanic/Latinos living in the United States represented approximately 17% of the U.S. total population (54 million), making people of Hispanic origin the nation's largest ethnic or racial minority. This is the second largest population of Hispanic/Latinos in the Americas, exceeded only by Mexico, population 120 million.[9]

Hispanics traditionally have been concentrated in Arizona, California, Colorado, Florida, Illinois, New Jersey, New York, and Texas. However, as of the latest census estimates, Hispanics are the largest minority group in 22 states. Hispanics trace their origins to many countries and to diverse sociopolitical configurations. Hispanics of Mexican descent account for 63% of the population overall, but Cubans dominate the population in Florida and Puerto Ricans are the Hispanic majority in the Northeast (**FIGURE 10B-1**).[10]

Demographic Analyses

Population data from sources such as the Census and the Pew Hispanic Research Center were used to locate uninsured Hispanics who would qualify for subsidies through the Marketplace. These demographic data were converted into visual "heat maps" that clearly show the highest areas of need were,down to the zip code and block-level. The resulting heat maps show the counties near Tampa Florida with the largest number of subsidy-eligible Hispanics.

Health Insurance Literacy

Before the Marketplaces opened, HolaDoctor conducted multiple focus groups in three states to understand perceptions of the new healthcare law, the level of understanding that Hispanics had about the ACA and health insurance in general, and which messages were important to them. Focus group questions included "How do you use your insurance?", "Why is it important to you to have health insurance?", and "What do you want to know about the new health reform law?"

BOX 10B-1 Hispanic or Latino?

Both *Hispanic* and *Latino* are terms used by the U.S. federal government to describe individuals who self-identify as having cultural and linguistic roots in Latin America or Spain. Many organizations use the terms interchangeably. The Pew Hispanic Research Center has found that Hispanics themselves are ambivalent about the two terms. Half (50%) say they have no preference, and the rest prefer "Hispanic" over "Latino" by a margin of about 2 to 1, depending on the region of the country.[8]

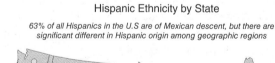

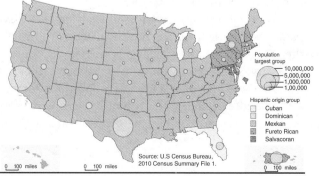

FIGURE 10B-1 Hispanic Enrollment in the ACA Case Study.

After the Marketplaces opened, HolaDoctor conducted online surveys with its community of more than 1 million Hispanics to understand which parts of the law were clear, which were not clear, and why people were or were not enrolling in the ACA. The online community was very responsive and could provide quick insights during the course of the campaigns. For example, in February 2014, near the end of the first open enrollment period, we conducted an online survey targeting adult Hispanics and received more than 1000 completed surveys within 24 hours. Even so, we found that more than 50% of Hispanics still were unaware that financial assistance was available to help pay for health insurance through the ACA.

These research projects provided important insights into Hispanics' previous experiences with health insurance, their evolving level of knowledge about the ACA, and the kind of information that would be important to communicate prior to the first open enrollment period.

Developing and Testing Concepts, Messages, and Materials

Given the very low knowledge and understanding among the entire U.S. population about the Patient Protection and Affordable Care Act, the key messages that were chosen for the start of the first open enrollment period (2013–2014) contained only basic information about the law, the Marketplaces, enrollment qualifications, and enrollment dates. These messages were tested in the field both prior and during the open enrollment period and often changed or tweaked immediately depending on the community's responses. During the second year of the ACA implementation of the Marketplaces, the messaging strategy shifted significantly, as Hispanic consumers became better informed and began focusing on more specific aspects of their options, such as how close geographically a Spanish-speaking doctor was in their network. **TABLE 10B-1** summarizes how the

TABLE 10B-1 Evolution of Messages Targeting Hispanics During the First Two Years of the Health Insurance Marketplaces

Stage (Time Period)	Purpose of Message	Messages Crafted to Answer the Following Questions
Pre-enrollment I (June 2013–August 2013)	Create basic familiarity with the new law	What is ACA?
		Is ACA the same as Obamacare?
		"Is this for real?"
Pre-enrollment II (September 2013)	Setting expectations and the need to enroll	Do I really need to buy health insurance?
First phase of first enrollment period (October 2013–December 2013)	Preparing to enroll	How much does a plan cost?
		Will I receive financial assistance
		What are the due dates?
Second phase of first enrollment period (January 2014–March 2014)	Tangible assistance to enroll	How do I enroll?
		Who can help me enroll?
		What happens if I don't enroll?
Post-enrollment (April 2014–November 2014)	Assistance with new health insurance	Where is my health insurance card?
		How do I find a doctor?
Second enrollment period (November 2014–February 2015)	Assistance to re-enroll	What do I need to do to re-enroll? What does this new tax form means?
	Assistance to first-time enrollers	I just got a penalty from the IRS—what do I do?
		How do I avoid a second penalty?
Special enrollment period	Assistance to those who were "laggards" or have resisted enrolling	How do I avoid a second penalty?

Field notes compiled by G. Giraldo

purpose of the messaging evolved and offers some specific examples over the first two years of the ACA open enrollments.

Messaging Mishaps with Hispanics

Although California has in many ways led the country in its implementation of ACA, early communications that targeted Latinos seemed to lack cultural and linguistic appropriateness. During the early stage of the campaign, Covered California, the state's health insurance marketplace, ran a "welcome" campaign. The ads featured a series of people looking into the camera saying in Spanish, "Welcome to a new state of health. Welcome to Covered California." This message was confusing to Hispanics because it required a deeper understanding of the basics such as the fact that a new entity (Covered California) had been formed to run "Obamacare" in the state of California. Instead of clarifying or making a connection with ACA or Obamacare, it created more confusion, especially at the early pre-enrollment stage. Additionally, some advertising experts noted that the literal translation from the English ad was grammatically correct but did not have the same nuanced connotation it had in English.

A second issue arose in a series of messages that highlighted the fact that the ACA prohibited denial of insurance due to a preexisting condition. That benefit did not resonate with the uninsured Latinos whom the ad was trying to influence, because the vast majority had no previous experience trying to buy health insurance and, therefore, had never been denied in the past. Latinos had not "felt the pain" of being denied; in fact, they were not very clear about the concept of "preexisting conditions" at all.

Finally, early ads touted the Covered California website (whose Spanish-language version was delayed) and did not recognize that although Hispanics may use the web to obtain health information, most like to make final purchases in person.

These three errors in messaging reflected an inadequate understanding of the target population and a rushed effort to get communications out under very tight timelines.[11] As the campaign progressed, Covered California made course corrections in response to research and feedback. Additionally, Covered California reoriented its marketing campaign to highlight the availability of free, confidential, local, and in-person enrollment assistance until the end of the open enrollment.[12]

Implementing the Integrated Solution

Using the findings from the market research and HolaDoctor's previous experiences in health communications, HolaDoctor designed and implemented a Hispanic education, qualification, and enrollment campaign in collaboration with its health plan clients. The multifaceted program incorporated digital, field, and phone techniques that were crafted with a specific focus on gaining trust and ensuring that Hispanic consumers had the information they needed to enroll. HolaDoctor partnered with local nonprofit organizations in each of the states of California, Georgia, and Colorado to train and deploy *promotores de salud* (health promoters) through grassroots field outreach tactics to educate about the ACA.[a] In addition, HolaDoctor built digital educational content that was featured on the Holadoctor.com and Salud.Univision.com websites. When it was discovered that Hispanics needed much more guidance enrolling in the Health Insurance Marketplace, HolaDoctor opened a call center staffed with trained bilingual agents.

Throughout the project, feedback and data were constantly gathered in the field, online, and through the call center to assess the process and success of the program. We also monitored the national and state contexts in which the outreach was being carried out, and sought out best practices that other organizations were identifying in reaching out to Hispanics.

The implementation of HolaDoctor's Hispanic outreach strategy began in June 2013, about five months ahead of the first open enrollment period. More detailed descriptions of the key components of the integrated outreach program are presented next.

Hispanics: Digital, Social, and Mobile

Like the rest of the U.S. population, Hispanics are going online and using mobile devices more than ever. The "digital divide," in which Hispanics and other minority groups lacked access to the Internet, has effectively been closed. Most Hispanics are going online through their (Internet-accessible) smartphones. In 2013, more than 75% of HolaDoctor's traffic on its Spanish-language health websites came through desktop computers, and 25% through mobile devices. In 2015, this situation was almost totally reversed: 70% of Hispanics accessed the web through their mobile phones or tablets and just 30% through a desktop or laptop. For health communications practitioners, the implication

---

a. The nonprofit organizations that partnered with HolaDoctor were Latino Health Access (Santa Ana, California), CREA Results (Denver, Colorado), and Hispanic Health Coalition of Georgia (Atlanta, Georgia).

of this tremendous shift is clear: Any and all campaigns targeting Hispanics simply *must* be optimized for mobile devices and have a clear, mobile-based strategy.

The other major trend associated with online Hispanics and health is the growing importance of social media. Many Hispanics are, by nature, very social. They choose to keep close contact with family and friends—and traditionally have had a lot of both. In this collectivistic culture, group activities are dominant, responsibility is shared, and accountability is collective. Because of the emphasis on collectivity, harmony and cooperation among the group tend to be emphasized more than individual function and responsibility.[13] These cultural characteristics translate into a very high use of social media for obtaining information about health and making decisions about healthcare providers and health insurance options.

A May 2014 study by PwC examined the use of digital and social media among Hispanics and concluded that both are key for marketing healthcare insurance to Hispanics. Hispanics both search the Internet for health insurers and use social media to learn about health care and health plans (**FIGURE 10B-2**).[14]

HolaDoctor incorporated these trends in digital, social media, and mobile usage within its campaigns to educate Hispanics about the ACA. Almost as soon as the legislation was passed in 2010, HolaDoctor began building an online, Interactive Health Insurance Center (IHIC) that would help Hispanics understand the ACA and how and why to enroll. The IHIC was designed not by medical professionals, but rather by experienced journalists, many of whom had decades of experience writing stories for Hispanic audiences. These journalists took the very complex concepts of the ACA, subsidies, tax credits, and even just insurance itself, and developed engaging, interactive games, quizzes, videos, and tools that allowed people to learn the concepts in fun and easy ways.

The IHIC was extremely popular during the first two years of the ACA and was recognized as uniquely suited for the Hispanic audience it was designed to serve. In 2014, HolaDoctor's lead writer for the IHIC was awarded the highly prestigious "Maggie" award from the Planned Parenthood Federation of America for excellence in online reporting and for "her extremely informative coverage of the Affordable Care Act through the enrollment period and her efforts to educate the Latino community on the benefits of the ACA."[15]

Promotores de Salud

A key component of HolaDoctor's enrollment strategy was the use of *promotores de salud. Promotores* often share common life experiences, culture, beliefs, and norms with the community members whom they serve, so they can more easily build trust and rapport and more effectively engage community members in their care.[16] *Promotores* are community experts; they are immersed in the communities and have extensive knowledge about real-time attitudes and knowledge. In the case of the ACA, well-trained *promotores* were keenly aware of people's reservations, fears, concerns, and feelings of confusion during the period that preceded the full implementation of the ACA's individual mandate. *Promotores* were also well aware of the sensitivity of the topics that health insurance would bring up for many Latino families. Conversations about health insurance could quickly become highly sensitive because the enrollment process touches on highly personal and sensitive areas such as immigration status, income, and taxes. HolaDoctor identified the leading community-based organizations in each

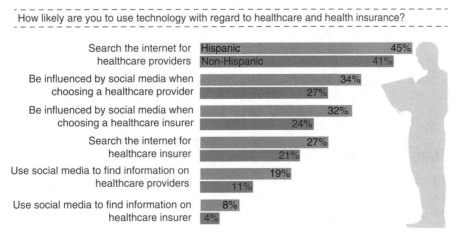

FIGURE 10B-2 Hispanic Enrollment in the ACA.
Courtesy of PwC Health Research Institute. EMC Hispanic consumer survey, 2014

state and worked closely with them to prepare a cadre of highly prepared *promotores* for the field.

Bilingual Call Center

HolaDoctor also staffed a bilingual call center located in Latin America to field calls about the ACA from Hispanics. The representatives at the call center were fully bilingual and extensively trained on the U.S. healthcare system, health insurance, the ACA, the subsidies and the Health Insurance Marketplaces. Hispanics could call the call center anytime for free using a toll-free number that was widely disseminated online and by the *promotores*.

This call center was extremely popular with Hispanics, especially during the first open enrollment period. In total, the center has fielded more than 100,000 inbound and outbound calls, with the most common calls focusing on where and how to purchase health insurance through the Marketplaces. The high volume was due, in part, to the fact that the call center was run by objective, trusted entities (i.e., HolaDoctor and Univision), and not by a health insurance company.

Determining Need and Developing One-on-One Relationships

Through each of the outreach channels described previously, we offered a number of ways that Hispanics could get additional support. In the online and social media environments, we provided "web forms" that Hispanics could fill in to get more information and subscribe to a Spanish-language health eNewsletter. The *promotores* used paper "opt-in" cards that functioned in the same way. One of the most actionable approaches was the use of mobile phone–based banners that allowed people to "click-to-call" and speak directly to the call center or someone who would help them purchase insurance right then.

How It All Fits Together

We have described each of the planning components of the Hispanic education, qualification, and enrollment campaign. The most effective messages were simple, direct, and consistent across multiple channels.

Evaluation and Improvement

Since the health insurance exchanges were an entirely new concept to most people in the United States, there was a very steep learning curve during the first year of the ACA's implementation. Those responsible for education and outreach were forced to "test and learn,"

seek feedback quickly, and refine their messages based on the feedback they were receiving. HolaDoctor used two main approaches to do this.

Qualitative Feedback from the Field

HolaDoctor's teams of *promotores de salud* that were working in four different states provided on the ground outreach and education about the ACA and were integral in the feedback process. They were trained to actively seek out insights into whether the messages and tactics were working with the low-income Hispanics to whom they were talking on a daily basis. The *promotores* reported their successes and failures in qualitative and quantitative reports on a weekly basis to HolaDoctor. Program managers also met with HolaDoctor teams to provide feedback on what they were seeing in the field. This feedback was critical, as the level of knowledge of the target population increased over time, and in turn the messaging had to be refined and modified as time went on.

Promotores' Field Reports

On a regular basis, the *promotores de salud* reported the results of their field activities so that the team could analyze the best locations and logistics for outreach. The success of each of the field activities was measured by attendance, the number of people who conversed with *promotores de salud*, and the number of individuals who shared their contact information for follow-up. Following analysis of these real-time data sources, HolaDoctor worked to refine and target the most important messages in the campaign as time progressed.

Lessons Learned

Ten of the key lessons learned in helping Hispanics enroll in the ACA health insurance exchanges are presented in this section. We have framed these insights to be most helpful for health communicators working with Hispanics in health-related areas and others striving to educate hard-to-reach groups about health insurance and access.

Establishing Trust with the Target Population Is Key

Enrolling in the ACA Health Insurance Marketplace touches on a range of highly sensitive areas, including documentation status, income, and taxes. If the Hispanic audience we were trying to influence did not trust us, the specific messaging or channels used would not matter. We gained audience trust in two main ways: (1) by partnering with local nonprofit, *promotores* organizations that had been working with the target communities for many years (and in some cases, many decades) and (2) by leveraging the Univision brand, which has been documented as the most trusted brand for Hispanics. This combination of very local, face-to-face contact, overlaid with web, social media, and TV broadcast messaging delivered in partnership with Univision, was very effective is garnering trust with the target audience.

A word of caution is in order about partnering with local community-based organizations. These partnerships need to be based on genuine intent and mutual benefit. Community members and community leaders can readily perceive when they are being used. Thus, when deciding to form a partnership, it is important to have a long-term vision and commitment to mutual benefit to prevent the partnership from backfiring.

Deliver Education in Small Doses to Small Groups and Through One-on-One Conversations

Outreach activities were key to reach the Hispanic community. Small-group meetings, presentations, "campouts,"[b] and one-on-one conversations proved to be very successful to provide information to this population. During the first year, when education and awareness levels were very low, it was especially important to reach people where they were because they were not actively seeking information. We invested considerable time in seeking entry into community fairs and events, as well as clinics, churches, stores (e.g., *carnicerías, panaderías*), and other social services agencies that work with Latinos. This time was very well spent and proved integral to reaching the target population.

Use Culturally and Linguistically Optimized Messages and Tools

Though many Hispanic families speak and understand both Spanish and English, a 2012 survey found that 73.9% of Hispanics age 5 and older reported speaking Spanish at home.[17] Given the fact that many Hispanics live in multigenerational families whose family members have varying degrees of English proficiency, an even better approach is to provide materials and tools that are in both Spanish and English. Materials that were originally created in Spanish, rather than being translated, were much better understood and more culturally competent. Materials developed in Spanish and then translated into English were more effective than trying to culturally adapt English materials for a Hispanic audience.

It Is Important to Provide a Call Center to Answer Additional Questions

Many individuals had questions or doubts about the law, especially regarding their eligibility and the enrollment process. Providing them with a toll-free phone number allowed them to continue learning more and provided additional contacts with our program. The call center also proved a useful resource to continue educating others through word of mouth. Individuals often referred their friends and family members to the call center line so they could also learn more.

Coordinated Multiple Channels Are Better Than Isolated Single Channels

The times when the educational activities were coordinated and had the same messaging through all channels (e.g., digital content, the *promotores*, and TV) proved more effective in generating interest than if the messages were delivered through a single channel. We measured this effect, in part, through digital metrics and the fill rate in an online web form to request more information about health insurance. For example, the fill rate of this online form was much higher during the weeks when the messages were also being promoted over other channels at same time.

Hispanics Are More Likely to Respond to Mobile and Social Media Channels

Mobile phone usage is higher among Hispanics in the United States than among the general U.S. population. Click-through rates (CTRs) among mobile users were higher than CTRs for those Hispanics using desktop methods to access information. Use of mobile-based messaging, apps, and responsive website design (so that websites look good on a mobile device) are absolutely essential for any communications campaign with Hispanics.

---

b. "Campouts" was the term used during the campaign for one or two *promotores* manning a table in front of a supermarket, church, or other location frequented by Hispanics who most likely to be part of the target audience.

Social media were found to be very effective in generating deep online discussions about the ACA and health care, increasing interest in call center marathons, and driving Hispanics from the online world to specific community education and enrollment events. Without a doubt, the power of social media to educate, influence perceptions, and drive specific actions was one of the key takeaways from all of the efforts.

Direct Messages Work Best

We found Hispanics wanted to hear direct messages and know how the law would affect their specific situation. On the HolaDoctor website, for example, banners with clear and direct calls to action had better CTRs than more softly worded messages. Banners offering help through articles or phone numbers had better CTRs than more general education. Once Hispanic consumers understood that the law *required* them to have health insurance, they were direct and to the point about getting guidance for their own specific situation. The most common questions that health promoters and the call center received were about how the ACA would directly affect them individually: "Will I have to pay a fine?" "Do I qualify?" "How exactly do I sign up?"

Health Insurance Is Boring: Pairing Various Health Topics with ACA Messages Increases Interest

On the one hand, Hispanics were more responsive to ACA health insurance education when it was paired with other health topics. On the other hand, banners that were placed on pages that focused on health and insurance topics had higher CTRs and longer pageview times than those displayed on digital entertainment and news channels. Field educational activities had higher turnouts if they included other services such as health screenings.

Here are the top three articles viewed on the health insurance page of *Univision Salud con HolaDoctor*:

1. 25 Key Words to Understand Better Your Health Insurance
2. Key Things for the Registration in the Marketplace
3. How Does the Marketplace Work

Cost Matters

It is important to acknowledge that cost proved to be a very important determinant of whether Hispanics actually enrolled and which plan they picked. The majority of Hispanics were concerned about how much the health insurance would cost them, even with the subsidies. Many Hispanics who qualified for the subsidized, lowest-cost health insurance through the Health Insurance Marketplaces were on a very limited budget and simply did not think they could afford health insurance. Others, fearing a fine but also considering their budget, had purchased inexpensive plans, only to realize later that those plans had limited provider networks and high deductibles. Some individuals reported that if they had known more about the system, they might have chosen another insurance plan. Others canceled these plans because they did not think they were worth the monthly premium.

Helping Hispanics Enroll Is One Thing— Keeping Them Insured Is Another

Heading into the third year of the ACA Health Insurance Marketplaces, a lesson we are learning now is that it is one thing to enroll Hispanics in the health insurance marketplace, but a whole other challenge to assure that they stay covered by paying their monthly premiums on time. Making it easy for them to pay, assuring they clearly understand what their benefits are, and providing access to Spanish-speaking, culturally competent doctors can help. Addressing some of the common complaints among Hispanics is critical to ensure they are satisfied with their plans and that these high levels of satisfaction can be incorporated into future health communications strategies and campaigns.

▶ Conclusion

With the advent of ACA, it was clear from the beginning that Hispanics would be an important demographic who would benefit greatly from the ACA, and that a disproportionate number of Hispanics would qualify to buy health insurance through the Health Insurance Marketplaces. Additional barriers, such as language, suspicion of the government, lack of experience with health insurance, and cultural differences in healthcare usage, impeded enrollment. Practitioners worked in tandem with health insurers, government agencies, and community-based organizations to craft appropriate strategies guided by social marketing principles to increase enrollment of Hispanics into the Health Insurance Marketplace. One of the most important lessons learned from working with the ACA and its programs was that constant feedback, assessment, and research are needed to improve and refine messaging for a new audience and program.

References

1. Senate Passes Health Care Overhaul on Party-Line Vote. *New York Times.* December 25, 2009. http://www.nytimes.com/2009/12/25/health/policy/25health.html?_r=2&hp&. Accessed March 6, 2015.

2. *Health insurance coverage status: American Community Survey 2008–2013 five year estimates.* U.S. Census Bureau; 2013. http://factfinder.census.gov/bkmk/table/1.0/en/ACS/13_5YR/S2701. Accessed April 2, 2015.

3. Department of Health and Human Services. The ACA is Working for the Latino Community. http://www.hhs.gov/healthcare/facts-and-features/fact-sheets/aca-working-latino-community/index.html#. Accessed October 14, 2016.

4. Enroll America. National coalition of organizations launch unprecedented effort to enroll Latinos in new health care options under Affordable Care Act. 2014. http://www.enrollamerica.org/press-releases/2014/02/national-coalition-of-organizations-launch-unprecedented-effort-to-enroll-latinos-in-new-health-care-options-under-affordable-care-act/. Accessed April 2, 2015.

5. Goodwin L. Latinos remain wary of Obamacare as deadline looms. *Yahoo! News.* 2014. http://news.yahoo.com/latinos-remain-wary-of-obamacare-as-deadline-looms-165314855.html. Accessed May 2, 2014.

6. Contreras J. *Best practice for outreach in Latino communities.* Centers for Medicare and Medicaid Services; 2013. https://marketplace.cms.gov/technical-assistance-resources/outreach-latino-communities.pdf. Accessed April 2, 2015.

7. Enroll America. State of enrollment: lessons learned from connecting America to coverage, 2013–2014. 2014. https://s3.amazonaws.com/assets.getcoveredamerica.org/20140613_SOEReportPDFlr.pdf. Accessed May 7, 2015.

8. Taylor P, Hugo Lopez M, Martinez J, Velasco G. *When labels don't fit: Hispanics and their views of identity.* Pew Research Center Hispanic Trends; 2014. http://www.pewhispanic.org/2012/04/04/when-labels-dont-fit-hispanics-and-their-views-of-identity/. Accessed April 2, 2015.

9. U.S. Census Bureau. Facts for figures: Hispanic Heritage Month 2014: Sept. 15–Oct. 15. 2014. http://www.census.gov/newsroom/facts-for-features/2014/cb14-ff22.html. Accessed May 7, 2015.

10. Ennis SR, Rios-Vargos M, Albert NG. The Hispanic Population: 2010. *2010 Census Briefs.* U.S. Census Bureau; May 2011. http://www.census.gov/prod/cen2010/briefs/c2010br-04.pdf. Accessed May 14, 2015.

11. Dembowsky A. Selling health care to California's Latinos got lost in translation. *National Public Radio.* March 6, 2014. http://www.npr.org/blogs/health/2014/03/06/286226698/selling-health-care-to-californias-latinos-got-lost-in-translation. Accessed May 7, 2015.

12. *Covered California open enrollment 2013–2014: lessons learned.* Covered California; 2014. https://www.coveredca.com/PDFs/10-14-2014-Lessons-Learned-final.pdf. Accessed April 16, 2015.

13. Gudykunst W. *Bridging Differences.* Newbury Park, CA: Sage; 1991.

14. Hispanics: a growing force in the new health economy. PwC's Health Research Institute; 2014. http://www.pwc.com/en_US/us/health-industries/publications/assets/hri-hispanic-study-chart-pack.pdf. Accessed May 7, 2015.

15. Planned Parenthood. PPFA Maggie Awards for media excellence: Planned Parenthood. 2014. http://www.plannedparenthood.org/about-us/newsroom/ppfa-maggie-awards-for-media-excellence. Accessed May 7, 2015.

16. Broderick A, Barnett K. *Community health workers in California: sharpening our focus on strategies to expand engagement.* Public Health Institute; 2015. http://www.phi.org/uploads/application/files/2rapr38zarzdgvycgqnizf7o8ftv03ie3mdnioede1ou6s1cv3.pdf. Accessed May 7, 2015.

17. U.S. Census Bureau. Nativity by language spoken at home by ability to speak English for the population 5 years and over (Hispanic or Latino). 2013. http://factfinder.census.gov/bkmk/table/1.0/en/ACS/13_5YR/B16005I. Accessed May 7, 2015.

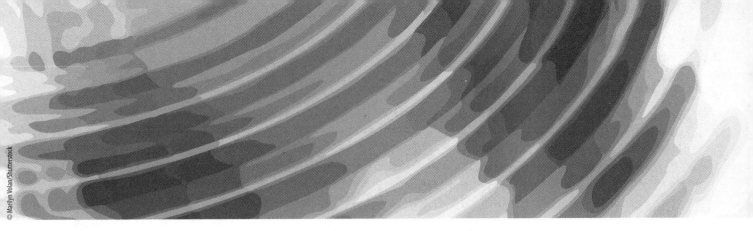

CHAPTER 11

Implementing a Communication Intervention

Claudia Parvanta

LEARNING OBJECTIVES

By the end of this chapter, the reader will be able to:

- Follow RE-AIM criteria for planning.
- Prepare SMART objectives from formative research.
- Prepare a creative brief.
- Pre-test concepts and messages using a range of low-cost methods.
- Describe physiological and neuromarketing techniques used in high-tech audience testing.
- Describe workflow and quality factors necessary for a content strategy.
- Draft a timetable, budget, and work plan for a health communication program.
- Develop metrics to monitor elements of a health communication program.
- Assemble the components of the total health communication plan.

▶ Introduction: Are You Ready?

After having completed the initial planning, done formative research, and considered the various media options, a health communication planner is ready to develop the intervention. This step transforms the logic model and creative concepts into messages, content, and media dissemination plans. It is also time to prepare an operational plan that includes a timeline, budget, and assignment of responsibilities. Finally, this phase of the program development is when you set up the criteria by which you will judge whether your program is working. Using these tools in a school or community project will help you acquire the competencies needed to use them on a larger scale. But before moving forward with the "fun" part of your health communication journey, we need to take a moment to "check the tires."

▶ Planning Tools—Again

Based on your preparatory research, the logic model for your program will suggest that certain activities will lead to specific outcomes and, in turn, to the projected results. Before moving forward, two tools are particularly helpful in refining and finalizing the objectives for your specific intervention; RE-AIM and SMART.

RE-AIM

RE-AIM is now in its second decade of publication and use, and has been used to guide the planning and evaluation of scores of evidence-based interventions.[1] RE-AIM refers to the following criteria:

- **R**each: The absolute number, proportion, and representativeness of individuals who are willing to participate in a given initiative, intervention, or program.
- **E**ffectiveness: The impact of an intervention on important outcomes, including potential negative effects, quality of life, and economic outcomes.

- **A**doption: The absolute number, proportion, and representativeness of settings and intervention agents (people who deliver the program) who are willing to initiate a program. (For site-based interventions, this is an institutional-level criterion.)
- **I**mplementation: At the setting level, the intervention agents' fidelity to the various elements of an intervention's protocol, including consistency of delivery as intended and the time and cost of the intervention. At the individual level, implementation refers to clients' use of the intervention strategies.
- **M**aintenance[2]: The extent to which a program or policy becomes institutionalized or part of the routine organizational practices and policies. At the individual level, maintenance has been defined as the long-term effects of a program on outcomes occurring 6 or more months after the most recent intervention contact. **BOX 11-1** provides a RE-AIM planning tool[3] that you can use before moving forward.

BOX 11-1 RE-AIM Planning Tool

The RE-AIM Planning Tool is intended as a series of "thought questions," which serve as a checklist, for key issues that should be considered when planning an intervention. The best way to use this section would be to think about the issues raised, their pertinence to your intervention(s) and to help you make any relevant changes before launching the intervention. The questions listed are generalized and meant as self-checks, so don't worry about not answering the ones that are not relevant to your unique program and situation.

Planning Checklist
Questions to Improve REACH

1. Do you hope to reach all members of your target population? If yes, provide a number or estimate for your target population. If no (due to large size of the target population or budget constraints), provide the proportion of the target population that you want to reach ideally given constraints. _____

2. What is the breakdown of the demographics of your target population in terms of race/ethnicity, gender, age, and socioeconomic status?

3. How confident are you that your program will successfully attract all members of your target population regardless of age, race/ethnicity, gender, socioeconomic status and other important characteristics, such as health literacy?

1 2 3 4 5 6 7 8 9 10

(where 1 = not at all confident, 5 = somewhat confident, and 10 = completely confident)

4. What are the barriers you foresee that will limit your ability to successfully reach your intended target population?

5. How do you hope to overcome these barriers?

6. Rate how confident you are that you can overcome these barriers?

1 2 3 4 5 6 7 8 9 10
(where 1 = not at all confident, 5 = somewhat confident, and 10 = completely confident)

Questions to Improve EFFECTIVENESS

1. Would you categorize your intervention as evidence-based or a new innovation?

2. Why did you choose this intervention and its components?

3. What are the strengths of your intervention?

4. Have you come to agreement with key stakeholders about how you will define and measure "success"?

5. List the measurable objectives that you wish to achieve in order to accomplish your goal.

6. What are the potential unintended consequences that may result from this program?

7. Are you confident that your intervention will achieve effectiveness across different subgroups, including those most at risk and having the fewest resources? If no, what can be done to increase the changes of success for these groups?

8. Rate your confidence that this intervention will lead to your planned outcome?
1 2 3 4 5 6 7 8 9 10
(where 1 = not at all confident, 5 = somewhat confident, and 10 = completely confident)

Questions to Improve ADOPTION

1. What percent of other organizations such as yours will be willing and able to offer this program after you are done testing?

2. How confident are you that your program will be adopted by those settings and staff who provide services for people in your target population who have the greatest need?

1 2 3 4 5 6 7 8 9 10
(where 1 = not at all confident, 5 = somewhat confident, and 10 = completely confident)

(continues)

BOX 11-1 RE-AIM Planning Tool *(continued)*

3. What do you think will be the greatest barriers to other sites or organizations adopting this program? Do you have a system in place for overcoming these barriers?

4. What percent of your organization (e.g., departments, relevant staff, etc.) will be involved in supporting or delivering this program?

Questions to Improve IMPLEMENTATION

1. How confident are you that the program can be consistently delivered as intended?

1 2 3 4 5 6 7 8 9 10
(where 1 = not at all confident, 5 = somewhat confident, and 10 = completely confident)

2. How confident are you that the program can be delivered by staff representing a variety of positions, levels and expertise/experience of the organization?

1 2 3 4 5 6 7 8 9 10
(where 1 = not at all confident, 5 = somewhat confident, and 10 = completely confident)

3. Is your program flexible (while maintaining fidelity to the original design) to changes or corrections that may be required midcourse?

4. Do you have a system in place to document and track the progress of the program and effect of changes made during the course of the program?

5. What is the greatest threat to consistent implementation and how will you deal with it?

Questions to Improve MAINTENANCE (individual)

1. What evidence is available to suggest the intervention effects will be maintained six or more months after it is completed?

2. How confident are you that the program will produce lasting benefits for the participants?

1 2 3 4 5 6 7 8 9 10
(where 1 = not at all confident, 5 = somewhat confident, and 10 = completely confident)

3. What do you plan to do to support initial success and prevent or deal with relapse of participants?

4. What resources are available to provide long-term support to program participants?

Questions to Improve MAINTENANCE (community)

1. How confident are you that your program will be sustained in your setting a year after the grant is over and/or a year after it has been implemented?

1 2 3 4 5 6 7 8 9 10

(where 1 = not at all confident, 5 = somewhat confident, and 10 = completely confident)

2. What do you see as the greatest challenges to the organizations continuing their support of the program?

3. What are your plans for intervention sustainability? Will additional funding be needed?

4. Do you have key stakeholder commitment to continue the program if it is successful?

5. How will the intervention be integrated into the regular practice of the delivery organization?

Reproduced from: Gaglio B, Shoup JA, Glasgow RE. The RE-AIM Framework: A Systematic Review of Use Over Time. *Am J Public Health* 2013;103(6):e38–e46.

SMART

RE-AIM can serve as a platform for crafting SMART objectives, which are used extensively in planning any program. SMART is an acronym for **S**pecific, **M**easurable, **A**chievable, **R**elevant (or **R**ealistic), and **T**ime bound. There is debate about SMART's origins, but many associate SMART goals or objectives with the work of management guru Peter Drucker. What do these terms mean?

- *Specific.* Exactly which result are we expecting to see? The "specific" part of an objective tells us who and what will change in concrete terms.
- *Measurable.* Objectives must have detectable, quantifiable indicators that we can measure, using the resources at hand. If we are prompting adoption of a new behavior, for example, we need clear criteria to detect whether such adoption has occurred and at what rate.
- *Attainable/Achievable.* Can the target population demonstrate this change within the proposed time frame? Do we have the resources available to

prompt this level of change? There are two parts to this parameter: (1) Are there sufficient resources to support sufficient reach and frequency of communication interventions and (2) is there adequate time for the target audience(s) to adopt and demonstrate the proposed change? Studies have shown that unless at least 50% of the target audience is aware of a message, it is unlikely that higher-order responses (e.g., contemplation, trial, maintenance) will occur.

- *Realistic/Relevant.* Will this objective have a measurable effect on the desired health goal? Is it reasonable to expect this level of change? If the "effect size" of the intervention is relatively small, then it is better to set correspondingly small change goals within a short duration of time. As groups begin to change, larger goals can be set.
- *Time Bound.* When will this objective be accomplished? We need an ambitious, but reasonable time frame for the behavioral objective. If our resources are limited in terms of penetration of the target audience, we need to allow for more

time for the desired outcome to occur. Cyclical and environmental constraints on the behavior in question may require more time to reach criteria for adoption.

The Kenya hand washing campaign carried out by Botta *et al.* provides a good example of how generic goals can be transformed into SMART objectives after the program developers complete their formative research (see Appendix 11A). For example, instead of the generic goal "Increase frequency of proper hand hygiene practices within the community," Botta et al. developed several objectives related to proper hand hygiene, including "Increase frequency of hand washing with soap at 5 (specified) key times by 10% in the community within 6 months of starting the campaign."

Effect Size

You need some numbers to develop SMART objectives. Starting with your own baseline survey or relevant estimates for the population, and using what you know about the effect size of your intervention on a specific behavior, you can estimate a result that makes sense. For example, Noar and colleagues found a mean effect size of 0.074 for tailoring interventions on a range of behaviors, amounting to slightly less than 1 standard deviation (SD) of change.[4] Snyder *et al.*'s earlier meta analysis found effects ranging from 0.15 for seat belt use (a good level of change) to 0.04 for sexual behavior change (almost no change).[5] Thus, from your measured baseline, for the same population and behavior, you could reasonably project an intervention-induced behavior change ranging from approximately 0.5 SD to 1.5 SD within the time limits of the intervention (not too long after the intervention occurs). Overly optimistic behavior change objectives that go far beyond the estimated effect size are not likely to be achievable. Conversely, overly conservative objectives are not relevant to the problem—they are not worth doing.

BOX 11-2 presents the objectives developed for the Tobacco Free Alachua (TFA) campaign against e-cigarette use. TFA is a community health partnership

---

BOX 11-2 Goals and Objectives of Program[*]

Background: Demographic, Geographic, and Psychographic Information

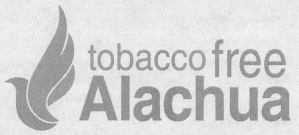

Courtesy of Tobacco Free Alachua

The primary target audience for Tobacco Free Alachua's messaging is the Alachua County municipality, which consists of the Florida cities of Alachua, Archer, Gainesville, Hawthorne, High Springs, Newberry, Waldo, LaCrosse, and Micanopy. More specifically, Tobacco Free Alachua is initially concerned about reaching the commissioners and leadership within the county. The secondary audience for Tobacco Free Alachua is the residents of these municipalities, specifically those who can lend their support with current and future policy goals.

According to the U.S. Census Bureau (2010), Alachua County is made up of the following populations[1]:

- Total population: 247,336
  - Males: 119,786
  - Females: 127,550
- Population aged 10–24 years: 76,773

- Major race/ethnic groups:
  - White: 172,156
  - Black or African American: 50,282
  - Hispanic or Latino: 20,752

Campaign Purpose

Public engagement campaigns "focus on the public's responsibility to create the supportive environment that will allow or promote a desired behavior change."[2] Therefore, the purpose of this campaign was to expose the discovered message strategies of e-cigarette advertising and advance the mission of Tobacco Free Alachua through active education of, and engagement with, Alachua County community members so as to legitimize the concerns surrounding e-cigarettes and advocate for local public policy regarding the marketing of e-cigarettes online. Through strategic application of grounded theory, this campaign aimed to attract the target audiences' attention, communicate compelling messages, divulge specific skills, and provide motivation for behavior change in conjunction with reinforcing environmental change.

Goal

To educate and inform the Alachua County parents, educators, and legislators about e-cigarettes, e-cigarette features, and the six prominent themes found in online e-cigarette advertising, creating an increase in awareness by 40% over a measured baseline by the end of the campaign.

Objectives

Process

1. To estimate how many Alachua County residents are aware of what e-cigarettes are by creating and distributing an online survey to the community by June 1, 2014.
2. To create at least five press materials to distribute to local media organizations to be disseminated by May 1, 2015.
3. Host 10 events at local middle schools, high schools, nonprofit organizations, and other local community and civic organizations to create awareness of the underlying message strategies (e.g., *satisfaction, reducing anxieties, convenience, innovation*, and *affordability*) used by e-cigarette companies in online advertisements by May 1, 2015.

Outcome

1. To increase awareness about e-cigarettes in the Alachua County community through means of an online social platform by gaining 1000 new followers on Facebook by May 1, 2015.
2. To achieve a minimum of 50 people in attendance at each public meeting or event each quarter.

References

1. U.S. Census Bureau. Census demographic profile data for Florida. http://edr.state.fl.us/Content/population-demographics/2010-census/data/index.cfm. Accessed January 27, 2014.
2. Coffman J. *Public Communication Campaign Evaluation: An Environmental Scan of Challenges, Criticisms, Practice, and Opportunities*. Cambridge, MA: Harvard Family Research Project; April 2002.

---

* This and all material presented from Tobacco Free Alachua is abstracted from the full plan, available at this text's website, with the permission of the authors.

Belva N, Hojnacki R, Justice A., Rodriguez S, Susock S. 2014. Proposed public health communications campaign for tobacco free Alachua. Presented in partial fulfillment of the requirements for the degree of Master of Arts in Mass Communication, University of Florida.

supported by the Health Policy Program of the Florida Department of Health in Alachua.

▶ The Creative Brief

The term *creative brief* comes from the advertising field, and describes a short document prepared by the agency account manager, in consultation with the client, to brief the creative team on the issues to be considered. Yes, we did just say "agency account manager" and "client," because working without a professional communications agency (be it marketing, advertising, or public relations) is somewhat akin to being your own lawyer in a court trial. If you do not have

the resources to hire an agency, or get the help of an expert in this field on a *pro bono* basis, then you will simply need to "make it work," to quote Tim Gunn.[a]

The basic form of the creative brief used in public health communication and social marketing has evolved little since it was first introduced in the 1970s. It is impossible to specify all the elements of a creative brief without taking the communication channel, activity, or medium into consideration. If you plan to work with healthcare providers and give them materials and training to communicate more effectively with patients, your creative brief and your entire strategy will be different than if you plan to use social media or a radio serial drama with the public, for example. Clear thinking produces a clear creative brief—and

---

a Esteemed fashion design mentor on *Project Runway*.

the opposite is also true. Although some agencies and organizations use different elements, the following outline reflects the general consensus of what a creative brief should contain.

Elements of a Creative Brief

1. *Overview of project.* This is a short summary of the overall goals of the project and its importance to the organization(s) involved.
2. *Target audience segment/persona.* This should be a clear and detailed description of one unique segment or persona. It might include a demographic description, behavioral readiness "stage," literacy level, lifestyle information, or role in the overall communication strategy (e.g., primary audience, secondary audience). You may include more information here, as necessary.
3. *Objectives.* Which specific behavior or behavioral antecedent do you want the target audiences to perform as a result of this communication? This outcome is often phrased in terms of what you want the audience members to think, feel, or do, and may be referred to as the "call to action."
4. *Obstacles.* What structural barriers, beliefs, cultural practices, social pressure, or misinformation are barriers to your audience taking this step? Is there an audience that must be approached first to free your intended audience to act as desired?
5. *Benefit/key promise.* What is the single most important reward (from the audience's point of view) that will result from doing the desired behavior? Is there a secondary reward? Which is more immediate, and which will take longer to achieve? From the audience perspective, "What's in it for me?"
6. *Support statements/reasons.* This section explains why the target audience should believe the promise of the key benefit. This evidence may take the form of data from quantitative scientific studies, qualitative findings obtained from a relatively small number of individuals (e.g., emotions), or information drawn from the experience of others whom the target audience admires or can relate to. Support statements should also provide solutions to the obstacles raised earlier.
7. *Tone.* What feeling or personality should your message or medium have? The tone set by the communication materials will influence how the target audience feels after interacting with the communications. Examples of tones include authoritative, family-oriented, funny, loving, modern, preachy, rural, scary, sad, and so on.
8. *Distribution opportunities.* What venues, seasons, or events increase the likelihood of your communication reaching the target audiences? In which other ways might this material be used? Are different versions needed to reach audiences in different settings?
9. *Creative considerations.* What else should the writers and designers keep in mind during development? What is the intended medium and channel for this product? Which style of presentation is likely to resonate more strongly with the selected target audiences: conversational, testimonial, informational, emotional, or instructional? Will the material need to be prepared in more than one language? Will known spokespersons be involved, such as political figures or entertainers? Are there special words or phrases to use or avoid?
10. *Other elements.* These might include routing of concepts to key individuals for approval, timelines, and just about anything else that is needed to reach management consensus before beginning creative development.

BOX 11-3A provides an example of the creative brief for the original folic acid campaign developed by the Centers for Disease Control and Prevention (CDC) and the March of Dimes. **BOX 11-3B** is a sample creative brief for tobacco control.

Use Feedback from Early Pre-testing

The health communicator uses a creative brief to organize planning ideas before moving on to the concept, message, and materials production phases of communication. When working with a creative team, either in-house (e.g., you, your friend, or your organization) or with a hired agency, it is essential to keep the artists "on message" and "on strategy." It is extremely easy to let a great creative idea steal the show. The creative brief, however, helps you ensure the quality of the program. Because people are often moved by truly inspirational stories and creative content, there is a time and place for letting the creative aspects drive the bus.

The next step of pre-testing is determining how and when to make that decision.

BOX 11-3A Creative Brief: Folic Acid First Campaign

Target Audience 1

- *Primary audience: pregnancy contemplators:* Women of childbearing age, 18 to 35 years old, who were planning to get pregnant in the next year. Some of these women took a multivitamin; others did not.
- *Secondary audiences*: The health/support systems for these women: friends, mothers, health professionals, and so on. Two campaigns were implemented here, one for a general audience and one for a Hispanic audience.

Objectives

Convince women that they must start taking a multivitamin with folic acid (or a folic supplement) before they get pregnant.

Obstacles

- *Regarding folic acid:* Only 16% of women knew that folic acid prevented birth defects, and 9% understood that it must be taken before conception to be effective.
- *Regarding multivitamin (and folic acid) supplements:* Some women did not feel that they needed a multivitamin supplement. They perceived themselves as young, healthy, and not in need of any "supplementing." Most recognized the need for prenatal vitamins during pregnancy, but not the need for folic acid before conception. This group thought that their regular diet contained everything needed for good health.
- *Additional concerns:* Objection to taking pills, in general; fear of weight gain; inability to remember to take vitamins; fear of excessive cost.

Key Promise

If you take a multivitamin with folic acid every day before you get pregnant, you will reduce the risk of your baby being born with birth defects.

Support Statements/Reasons

- As many as 75% of birth defects of the spine and head (neural tube defects) can be prevented by taking an adequate amount of folic acid before becoming pregnant.
- Folic acid is essential for the body to make cells duringthe very first stage of a baby's development.
- Folic acid should be taken daily for at least one month prior to conception.
- Vitamin supplements are the easiest way to get the required amount of folic acid.
- Multivitamins cost as little as 3 cents per day; folic acid supplements cost as little as 1 cent per day.
- Folic acid is an essential B vitamin.

Tone

It was necessary that the communication convey a sense of good health, warmth, and energy, because that is how this audience saw itself. In addition, a sense of importance and urgency was needed to motivate these women to overcome their own obstacles to behavioral change.

Media

Television, radio, and print.

Creative Considerations

Spots were produced in English and Spanish so as to recognize and reach diverse populations.

Target Audience 2

Pregnancy non-contemplators: Women of childbearing age, 18 to 24 years old, who could become pregnant. These women were, or could have been been, sexually active and able to conceive. They were not planning a pregnancy in the near future and were unlikely to be taking a vitamin supplement with folic acid. However, because this group accounted for a significant percentage of pregnancies, most of which were unplanned, there was still a need for these women to take a folic acid supplement.

Objectives

To raise awareness among young women that taking a multivitamin or folic acid supplement is necessary, regardless of whether they are planning to become pregnant.

(continues)

BOX 11-3A   Creative Brief: Folic Acid First Campaign   *(continued)*

Obstacles

- *Regarding pregnancy/birth defect messages:* If a pregnancy was not planned, there was an assumption that a pregnancy would not occur. Concern over birth defects, therefore, was not a priority.
- *Regarding multivitamin/folic acid supplements:* There was the belief among audience members that a multivitamin supplement was unnecessary, a belief reinforced by their self-images as young, healthy people who did not need special supplements. Key nutrients were thought to be received through diet and there was a perception that only "old people" took supplements.
- *Additional concerns:* Fear of weight gain, aversion to large pills, disruption of daily routine, cost.
- *Regarding folic acid:* Lack of knowledge of existence of folic acid, when to take it, and relevance in lifestyle.

Key Promise

If I take folic acid every day, I will look and feel better, as well as reduce the risk of my baby being born with birth defects.

Support Statements/Reasons

- Folic acid is necessary for healthy cells, and most women do not get enough of it.
- If taken in sufficient amounts, folic acid can eliminate as many as 75% of the most commonly disabling birth defects if taken before pregnancy and through the first month of pregnancy.
- Folic acid is an essential B vitamin.

Tone

This campaign was geared toward a younger audience and addressed them on their level—hip, youthful, and energetic. A tone that conveyed a sense of good health and vibrancy was chosen because that was how this audience perceived themselves.

Media

Television, radio, and print public service announcements (PSAs).

Creative Considerations

Spots had to recognize a diverse population.

BOX 11-3B   Creative Brief: Tobacco Counter-Marketing

Project Description and Background

- Develop comprehensive introductory advertising for a new program designed to reduce exposure to secondhand smoke.
- Develop a public education campaign designed to spur individual and community action to reduce young people's access to tobacco products, especially by building support for local enforcement efforts.

The assignment might also be as specific as the following:

- Develop a new television advertising execution (sometimes called a "pool-out") for a campaign in progress.
- Create ads for billboards to supplement existing TV and print ads.

Description of the Target Audience

Examples of primary audiences include the following:

- Restaurant owners who smoke
- 11- to 15-year-old nonsmokers
- African American adult male smokers

Secondary audiences:

- Family members of smokers
- Policy makers

Target Audience Insights

Descriptive details about the target audience should include specific information about demographics, lifestyles, psychographics, and other characteristics of the target audience that will help the creative team develop materials appropriate for this audience. Creative materials are most persuasive when based on one or more insights into the target audience's beliefs or practices related to the concept, product, attitude, or behavior being addressed. These target audience insights can be positive or negative. They are the foundation for building the content of communications materials.

One example of a target audience belief that might influence the creation of advertising executions encouraging youth not to smoke is that youth are more afraid of living a life of pain and physical problems as a result of smoking than they are afraid of dying from smoking, because their perception of death is vague and abstract.

Goals

What do you want the target audience to do as a result of hearing, watching, reading, or experiencing the communication? Examples include the following:

- Increase knowledge about tobacco industry marketing practices
- Change attitudes about exposing other people to secondhand smoke
- Support policies restricting smoking in public buildings
- Enter a smoking cessation program

Obstacles

Obstacles are beliefs, attitudes, values, behaviors, or environmental factors that prevent the target audience from adopting the desired attitude or behavior. Obstacles stand between the audience and the desired attitude or behavior. Examples include the following:

- Lack of knowledge of the harmful effects of secondhand smoke
- The belief that smoking is not harmful if one smokes only occasionally in social settings
- The tobacco industry's financial support of community organizations
- Smokers' belief that they must quit on their own without getting help

Key Promise/Key Benefits

Statement of the key benefits or rewards (including emotional benefits, if appropriate) that the audience will experience by adopting the desired attitudes or behavior. The key benefit is something that will make changing to the desired attitude or behavior worth it for the audience. Examples include the following:

- Ability to live long enough to see one's children grow up
- Saving oneself from great pain and suffering caused by smoking-related disease/illness
- Being a good parent by protecting one's children from secondhand smoke

Statements of Support or Reasons to Believe

A statement of support, a reason to believe, or evidence that adopting the desired attitudes or behavior will result in gaining the key benefits should be compelling enough to overcome the obstacles. Examples include the following:

- Sharing the fact that smokers who quit live an average of 15 years longer than smokers who continue smoking throughout their lives, and showing middle-aged and older nonsmokers enjoying life with their children and grandchildren.
- Showing a credible portrayal of someone who became ill from smoking and revealing how difficult that smoker's life became. [This idea became the basis of the "Tips from Former Smokers" campaign.]
- Persuasively communicating the fact that children in households where smoking occurs inhale the same poisons as the smoker.

Brand Character

The description of the brand's image or qualities should be designed to appeal to the target audience (e.g., nurturing and helpful, strong and powerful, credible and trustworthy, or rebellious and independent). Because many tobacco counter-marketing campaigns are not based on a brand, this section is often not included in a creative brief.

(continues)

BOX 11-3B Creative Brief: Tobacco Counter-Marketing *(continued)*

Copy Strategy

A short paragraph should be developed to succinctly summarize what the advertising needs to achieve, including to whom the advertising is directed, which action is desired, the key benefit(s) of taking that action, the reason(s) to believe that benefit will be realized if the action is taken, and the brand character (if relevant). The format of a copy strategy might be something like this: "The television ad will convince A (target audience) to do B (desired action) because they will believe that doing so will provide them with C (key benefit). The reason to believe will be D."

Centers for Disease Control and Prevention. Designing and Implementing an Effective Tobacco Counter-Marketing Campaign. Atlanta, Georgia: U.S. Department of Health and Human Services, Centers for Disease Control and Prevention, National Center for Chronic Disease Prevention and Health Promotion, Office on Smoking and Health, First Edition October 2003.

From the Creative Brief to Concepts

One of the most fascinating exchanges in health communication takes place when project managers meet with a creative team to discuss what is needed for the communication materials. Working through the creative brief, the managers will describe the project's overall purpose and provide all the information they have available about the intended audience. Next, they will relay the objectives of this specific communication campaign or material.

Before strategic communication became widespread, project managers focused on a few key ideas that they framed as **messages**.[b] The message was actually the final, intended behavior sought from the target audiences. It might be "Wash your hands after going to the bathroom" or "Don't send your children to school when they are sick." The exact words used to describe the behavior, in fact, might not be what we say to a target audience. Instead, the desired behavior—together with all the other information gathered about the audience—generates a **concept**. The concept is a creative interpretation of the information provided by the project managers about the objectives, the obstacles, the key benefits, the support statements, the tone, and the intended media channels—as well as anything else included in the creative brief.

Concepts are gestalt interpretations—that is, they try to grab the main idea and give it a personality. From social marketing, we have learned that the core of the concept is the most compelling benefit, which should be surrounded by the supporting information. The concept should appeal to both the head and the heart, and it must communicate how this idea fits into the lives of the target audience. Does it make their life easier? Is it fun? Will it seem to be a popular thing to do?[c]

BOX 11-4A shows the first set of concepts developed in response to the folic acid creative brief. **BOX 11-4B** describes the development of concepts for the CDC's Tips from Former Smokers campaign.

The folic acid and smoking cessation examples demonstrate some general ideas that need to be considered during the concept testing phase. Overall, we want to identify which words and images help the target audience understand and want to act on the issue. If a series of concepts is presented, then we try to find out:

- Which have the most appeal?
- Which prompt a reaction to think, feel, or do (the intended response)?
- Which are easy to understand?
- Which are memorable?
- Which are credible?
- Which are inoffensive?
- Which are culturally appropriate?

We will elaborate on these factors when we discuss pre-testing messages and materials. Another important goal of concept testing is to learn which other ideas the target audience might have, whom they see as credible spokespersons, and which media channels they feel are most appropriate for the message.

Most often concepts are tested in focus group settings, with online versions of focus groups becoming increasingly popular. You may also pre-test concepts with individuals, or in a theater-type testing setup. In the latter cases, audiences view images on screen while the moderator speaks to them. Their collective reactions are gathered using an anonymous response system (i.e., clickers) to tally up how many people select a particular answer to a question.

---

b UNICEF's Facts for Life uses this form of message to simplify the communication process for a global audience of health promotion managers.

c To paraphrase Bill Smith.

BOX 11-4A Concepts for Original CDC/March of Dimes Folic Acid Campaign

Nine concepts were developed: Four were specifically designed to appeal to women hoping to become pregnant in the next year; four were for women who were not yet planning a pregnancy; and one was intended to test its appeal to both groups.

CDC used focus groups to test the concepts. A total of 79 women participated in nine groups. The focus groups were used to determine if women could identify the main idea of each concept and if the concepts motivated the target audience to increase their folic acid consumption. Five focus groups included women of different racial and ethnic backgrounds, and the remaining four groups were exclusively Hispanic women.

Concepts Developed for Pregnancy Contemplators

1. "The Fetus" depicted a fetus with the text, "Even before you realize you're pregnant, her little body is growing a spine. Begin taking folic acid when you stop taking birth control." The concept was developed in response to exploratory focus group research that indicated women were unfamiliar with the importance of folic acid before conception.
2. "Brussels Sprouts" displayed a picture of many Brussels sprouts with the text, "To protect your unborn child from birth defects, you would need to eat this many Brussels sprouts every day. Or, take one of these. Folic Acid. It needs to start when birth control stops." The main idea of this concept was to show women how hard it was to consume enough folic acid from naturally occurring dietary folate, because women had previously stated their well-balanced diets provided them with enough folic acid.
3. "Fooling Around" depicted a man and a woman laughing with each other, while the text printed above them stated, "And you thought all you needed to do was 'fool around.'" At the bottom of the concept, the text stated, "Folic Acid. The pill to take when you're planning." This concept was designed to inform women that folic acid must be taken before conception.
4. "Pill Pack" depicted a pack of birth control pills at the top, and a bottle of folic acid supplements below it. The text accompanying the pictures stated, "When you stop taking these [picture of birth control pack], start taking these [picture of the folic acid bottle]. Folic acid. The other pill." This concept's main idea was that when a woman is ready and able to become pregnant, she needs to start taking folic acid.
5. "Sanitary Napkin" featured a sanitary napkin with the text, "You may not be planning a pregnancy, but your body's been preparing for many years" written on top. Underneath the sanitary napkin, additional text stated, "Folic acid today. So your body's ready when you are." This concept was supposed to convey the idea that as soon as the body is capable of becoming pregnant, folic acid is needed.

Important Findings from the Concept Testing with Women Planning to Become Pregnant

1. "The Fetus" was well received as attention-getting and informative. Several women associated the image of a fetus with anti-abortion campaigns. Additionally, the image of a fetus conflicted with the idea that folic acid should be taken before conception. The image should suggest, and reinforce, the importance of taking folic acid before pregnancy—an important focus in this campaign.
2. "Brussels Sprouts" was problematic because some Hispanic women did not recognize the vegetable as something they would eat.
3. "Fooling Around" confused women because it seemed to imply that folic acid was an alternative to birth control or improved fertility.
4. "Pill Pack" was also confusing to women because it implied that folic acid was an alternative to the birth control pill. That was not the intended message.
5. "Sanitary Napkin" shocked participants, but they clearly understood the message. A different image to display the same message was suggested. It involved showing a young girl through the different stages of maturity.

Concepts Developed for Women Not Thinking About Pregnancy

1. "Folic Female" (version 1) was designed to convey the benefits of folic acid in promoting good health in general. An African American woman was shown sitting in a grassy meadow with the text at the top: "Folic Acid. It brings out the best in you." At the bottom of the picture, additional text asked the reader, "Are you a folic female?"
2. "Folic Female" (version 2) showed a smiling woman who was white, but could be Hispanic or any other Caucasian ethnic group with dark hair. The words "The Folic Female" were printed at the top of the concept and the text, "Folic

(continues)

Acid. It brings out the best in you," was printed at the bottom of the picture. These two concepts were developed in response to a large number of women in the focus groups reporting that they would be motivated to take a multivitamin with folic acid daily if it made them feel their best.

3. "Penny" featured a penny as the main visual. The headline stated, "Bring out your inner beauty for a penny a day," and the tag lines said, "Folic acid. The beauty supplement we can all afford." This concept was designed to address the concern that taking a multivitamin every day can be costly.

4. "Life happens" focused on the benefits of folic acid in preventing birth defects in future or unplanned pregnancies. The concept showed a teenager/young adult looking surprised with the caption, "Life. It's what happens to you when you're making other plans. Folic Acid. It's what prevents birth defects in babies." This concept intended to convey the main idea that girls/women need to be prepared for an unplanned pregnancy.

5. "Sanitary Napkin" was the same concept as tested for the pregnancy contemplators.

Important Findings from Concept Testing with Women Not Contemplating a Pregnancy

1. "Folic Female" concepts conveyed the message that folic acid promoted good health and beauty, but women did not like the phrase "folic female" when seen without additional text. The question, "Are you a folic female?" was well received, however, because it was not standing alone.

2. "Penny" did not convince women that folic acid was an inexpensive beauty supplement.

3. "Life Happens" clearly illustrated that women should be prepared because an unplanned pregnancy could happen, but the women did not believe that they would have an unplanned pregnancy.

4. "Sanitary Napkin" was hard for women to see (the graphic of the sanitary pad) but communicated the message most clearly. Women not planning a pregnancy both understood the message and felt it was directed to them.

Test of Concepts with Individuals Affected by Spina Bifida Births

To guard against offending persons who had children with spina bifida (the primary birth defect resulting from folic acid insufficiency), the concepts were also tested with a group of mothers willing to view the materials and make comments.

1. "Sanitary Napkin": While most participants felt that the concept was powerful, some were concerned that the explicit image (the sanitary napkin) used in the example would be offensive and unappealing. It was suggested that showing someone purchasing sanitary napkins would be a gentler way of depicting the same message.

2. "Penny": Focus group members were not offended or alienated by a message focusing on beauty instead of birth defects. They felt the CDC should do whatever it took to convince people to consume folic acid.

Other Important Findings from Concept Testing with This Group

1. Campaign messages needed to emphasize the purpose of preventing birth defects, not saying the people born with birth defects could have been avoided.

2. Messages needed to avoid making parents of children with spina bifida feel guilty. Materials had to make it clear that in addition to folic acid, genetics and other factors also play a role in neural tube defects (NTDs).

3. Depictions of individuals with spina bifida (e.g., in a wheelchair or on crutches) were acceptable, if the individual was not portrayed as pathetic. It was also recommended that a range of severity levels be depicted.

4. Materials should make it clear that while folic acid greatly reduces the risk of having a baby with neural tube defects, it does not eliminate the risk altogether. Furthermore, materials should not specify a date when the association between folic acid and NTDs became known.

5. The campaign should include scientific evidence supporting folic acid and birth defects research. Emphasis should be placed on the idea that folic acid is needed one month prior to conception to reduce the risk of having a baby with an NTD.

6. It was important to test campaign materials with adolescents affected by spina bifida, because they may have been particularly sensitive to images and messages.

Findings from these groups were particularly revelatory for the Division of Birth Defects at CDC. In focus groups, most women said that they would want to see what the birth defect looked like,[a] and that women in general needed to see the extent of the defects to know their seriousness. At the same time, CDC was sensitive to how mothers of children with neural tube defects might feel about having their children portrayed as "what you are trying to avoid." Hence, a key challenge of the campaign was finding the balance between presenting difficult scientific information and the sensitivities of the already affected population. A decision was made to limit the more graphic images of neural tube defects to materials that would be used by physicians or other medical personal to counsel women contemplating a pregnancy.

---

[a]In fact, neural tube defects can be among the most frightening birth defects, with some children not surviving birth, or living only a moment or two, because they lack a fully formed brain or head. Other neonates have an opening in the back that must be surgically repaired, but this defect is almost always survivable in the United States.

BOX 11-4B Creating Concepts for the *Tips from Former Smokers* Campaign

In 2011, CDC was provided with funding from the Prevention and Public Health Fund (part of the Patient Protection and Affordable Care Act) to develop, implement, and evaluate a hard-hitting, national tobacco education campaign with strong messaging about the health consequences of tobacco use to reduce cigarette smoking among adults. To measure how the campaign would resonate with the target audience and what the emotional impact would be, formative research was conducted.[1] CDC used a rigorous process, including message platform testing, creative concept development, and focus group testing to optimize the impact of the campaign.

Following a review of the literature, the development phase of the Tips from Former Smokers campaign began with message platform testing. Ten messages were developed across four categories based on scientific evidence on smoking and health. The messages that most resonated with the target audience were (1) the high risk of developing serious, debilitating diseases from smoking, (2) the immediate damage that smoking does to the body, and (3) the impact of secondhand smoke on children.

Once a message platform was selected, a creative brief was developed to ensure that the messages were conveyed to the advertising agency's creative team both emotionally and conceptually. During the development of the brief, the advertising agency began developing "creative concepts." Using the creative brief as a guide, the creative team developed multiple executions that included draft storyboards of television advertisements; initial layouts of print, outdoor, and digital advertisements; and draft radio scripts.

Next, three potential "creative concepts" were tested in a focus group setting: "What Happens," "Known For," and "Tips." The overall theme of each campaign was the health consequences of tobacco exposure (either active or passive), and they all featured testimonials from people who were living with a tobacco-related disease. Each ad presented a graphic representation of the damaging effects of tobacco, such as living with a stoma hole in the throat after a laryngectomy, suffering the loss of movement and mobility from a stroke, or losing a child from an asthma attack brought on by exposure to secondhand smoke.

Each of the three creative concepts presented this information in a different way. "What Happens" featured people describing in straightforward language what exactly has happened to their bodies as a result of smoking tobacco. (For example, a man who lost his jaw to cancer describes how the cancerous cells that develop as a result of tobacco exposure are frequently not detectable until it is too late to fight them). "Known For" featured people describing how other people now view them only through the lens of their tobacco-related disease. "Tips" featured people suffering the results of tobacco-related disease offering suggestions to others that foreshadowed disabilities to come.

The focus groups evaluated each of the three creative concepts, the draft storyboards, and other materials produced to ascertain the following:

- Participants' reactions to draft storyboards to determine whether these concepts were effective in communicating campaign messages as intended
- Whether the key messages were understood
- Participants' emotional reaction to the tone of the materials
- Participants' changed perceptions about health consequences from tobacco and secondhand smoke at the end of the session

(continues)

BOX 11-4B   Creating Concepts for the *Tips from Former Smokers* Campaign   *(continued)*

The "Tips" creative concept was selected for development following the focus group research. This concept gave participants insight into living with a tobacco-related disease in a way that was emotionally evocative and meaningful for the participant. The focus group participants were moved by the plight of the people in the storyboards, and they could see beyond the reasons for the victim's suffering (i.e., because they smoked) to comprehend how much a tobacco-related disease can affect one's life. They also responded to the graphic nature of the ads, with many people commenting that although the images were difficult to watch, they felt that it was important for people to see the true impact of tobacco use. Respondents also appreciated the testimonial aspect of the ads, and they said they felt the ads were more compelling because the stories were from real victims of tobacco-related disease.

In the "Tips" creative concept testing, the key finding was that people are more afraid of living with a tobacco-related disease than death due to a tobacco-related disease. This finding has formed the foundation of the Tips from Former Smokers campaign advertisements since 2012.

Reference

1. Centers for Disease Control and Prevention. *Best Practices for Comprehensive Tobacco Control Programs—2014*. Atlanta, GA: U.S. Department of Health and Human Services, Centers for Disease Control and Prevention, National Center for Chronic Disease Prevention and Health Promotion, Office on Smoking and Health; 2014.

Audiences and **gatekeepers**, meaning the people who have some control over dissemination or interpretation of messages at the community or larger social level,[d] need to be invited to **pre-test** concepts before moving onto final messages and to see messages and draft materials before final production. Sometimes the entire package has to be seen *in situ*—that is, in the exact setting where it will be aired or used—to judge its appropriateness and effectiveness.

In addition to gatekeepers, it is important to consider who else might be sensitive to the ideas being put forward by a health communication campaign. When we think about how many things we try to "prevent" in public health, we have to be mindful of the people who already suffer from these conditions. Perhaps that condition is HIV infection. Or perhaps it is a preventable birth defect or a chronic disease. Health communicators must consider how these people, or their loved ones, will feel if their condition is portrayed as something to avoid at all costs. Consequently, pre-testing with persons who represent this audience of affected individuals is also advised.

"Fail early, fail small" is an aphorism from marketing that provides a useful caution for health communicators. Some of what you think are your best ideas may not work with the intended audience, may outrage the gatekeepers, or may offend audience members who currently have the condition or behavior. Data obtained from audience pre-testing can be useful in overcoming gatekeeper resistance to a message or

media concept—or a creative person's love affair with his or her work. It is essential to find out if the idea is not working by testing it with a small group of people at any early stage (concept, message, or even materials testing), rather than waiting until a fully developed multimedia campaign has been released to the public to discover that it is a failure.

BOX 11-5 shows the methodology and questions used in pre-testing the concepts for the CDC's original folic acid campaign.

From Concepts to Messages and Materials

Having tested your concepts, you can now build on that foundation to create bundles of words, images, and/or sounds that carry your idea to the hearts and minds of your intended recipients. The channels and activities carrying your content will determine the format for production, not the reverse. For example, to design an effective and persuasive Internet-delivered video, it helps to know if the majority of the audience will view it on the small screen of a smartphone. Similarly, materials designed for healthcare providers to use in counseling patients are likely to be too complex to display on top of pharmacy counters or in grocery stores. Different versions will be necessary.

More often than not, the actual words chosen for the message will come from your exploratory concept testing, when participants describe a problem or solution in their own words. If you are using the

---

d Persons who are influential in the community, particularly concerning information meant for people whom they care about, are gatekeepers. These individuals might be health professionals, local government or religious officials, or other community leaders.

BOX 11-5 Methodological Overview of Concept Testing for a Folic Acid Campaign

Concept Testing for Folic Acid

Concepts are designed to be preliminary ideas, rather than actual campaign materials. In this case, a series of nine concepts were used to stimulate participants' thinking about words and pictures that would help them (and women like them) learn about folic acid and neural tube defects (NTDs) and motivate them to take folic acid daily. Concepts are not meant to stand alone. The concepts created for this campaign might be used, for example, on the cover of a brochure, or as part of other materials that would contain additional information about folic acid and NTDs.

Description of Focus Group Participants

The focus groups conducted for this concept-testing study included the following subgroups of women at risk:

- Women from various races/ethnicities, with specific emphasis on African American and Hispanic women (both English-speaking and Spanish-speaking)
- Women between the ages of 18 and 35 years
- Women in lower to middle income brackets (less than $50,000 annual household income, with emphasis given to women with annual household incomes less than $30,000)

Method

Welcome and Introductions

The welcome and introductions section was the same for each focus group. The female moderator put the participants at ease, introduced the topic area for the discussion, and explained how focus groups work. The moderator used the opening minutes of the group to:

- Thank participants for attending and to introduce herself
- Identify the purpose of the discussion and emphasize that the planned campaign was a public health campaign sponsored by CDC and not by a company trying to sell something
- Stress that comments would be kept confidential (names do not appear in any report) and there were no right or wrong answers
- Explain the presence and purpose of recording devices and observers seated behind the one-way mirror

Framing the Interview

The moderator started each discussion by displaying a foam core-mounted statement that gave participants some background information about the topic for discussion. For women planning a pregnancy, the moderator displayed the following scientific statement.

- Folic acid is a vitamin that can prevent birth defects.
- Most women don't get enough of this vitamin.
- CDC wants to talk with you about what might help convince you to take more folic acid.

This statement was chosen for women planning a pregnancy, because women who matched this profile in exploratory research said they would be motivated to take more folic acid if it would help prevent birth defects.

The statement was kept on display throughout the discussion so that participants could refer to it while viewing the potential campaign concepts. This was important so that the women could provide their opinions about whether the concepts conveyed the information presented in the scientific statement.

For women not planning to become pregnant, the moderator showed a different statement that exploratory research suggested might motivate women with this profile to take folic acid.

- Folic acid is a vitamin that everyone needs for good health.
- Your body is producing new cells all the time and folic acid is important for this development.

Three of the concepts tested for this group were developed around motivators of feeling and looking your best, not always eating right, and preventing long-term illnesses. This statement was also displayed throughout the group discussion so that participants could refer to it when discussing if the concepts conveyed the information presented in the statement. Next, this group was also exposed to the idea of preventing birth defects through folic acid, and shown the concepts created for women planning a pregnancy.

Showing and Discussing the Concept Boards

After showing each group the initial statements, the moderator proceeded by obtaining reactions to each concept, one by one. Each concept was printed in color and mounted on a large (20 by 30 inches) foam core board. Before

(continues)

BOX 11-5 Methodological Overview of Concept Testing for a Folic Acid Campaign *(continued)*

viewing the concepts, participants were told that the concepts were preliminary ideas, not finished words or artwork but might be used to develop materials for communicating the statement they had just seen. For each of the concepts, participants were asked the following questions:

- What is the main idea of the concept?
- What were your thoughts and opinions on the words and images used in each concept?
- Was there any personal relevance and motivational effect for the concept?
- How would you change the concept?

The moderator changed the order of the concepts, as well as the questions, in each group to guard against bias that might occur due to order effects.

Concept Ranking

After discussing the concepts collectively, participants were asked to rank order the concepts individually and anonymously. Each concept had a small label with a letter on it (A through E) that corresponded to the five letters listed on the sheet of paper. Participants were asked to write the number "1" next to the letter of the concept that would most motivate them to take folic acid, the number "2" next to the second most motivational concept, and so forth. Participants were also told that if none of the concepts motivated them, they should leave the sheet blank.

Wrap-Up Discussion of Logo and Channels

After a group discussion of their rankings, the moderator asked about whether it would be beneficial to display a logo on the materials, such as for the CDC, the National Task Force on Folic Acid, a charitable organization, or a pharmaceutical company. The group also suggested potential channels for disseminating the information.

Conclusions

The moderator thanked the women for their time and gave them information about obtaining their incentive money following the group. After all sessions, a subject-matter expert from the CDC or a local public health expert was available to answer any questions that participants had about folic acid or birth defects, and to hand out pamphlets on folic acid.

Analysis

At the time these groups were conducted, the research agency used group transcripts and notes taken during the groups to analyze themes and compare findings within and across groups. No computer-aided qualitative coding system was used, although it would be recommended now.

Abstracted from a research report prepared by Westat for the Birth Defects and Pediatric Genetics Branch (BDPG), Division of Birth Defects, Child Development, Disability and Health at the Centers for Disease Control and Prevention (CDC), 1998. Available in its entirety on CDCynergy, Webversion, www.cdc.gov.

entertainment education approach, then messages will emerge from role-plays, dialogues, or finished dramatic treatment. These words are then embedded in a narrative that is fully articulated with characters and context. In the 21st century, "viral" or "buzz" marketing techniques count heavily on the intelligence and often ironic worldview of the intended (usually youthful) audience and can sometimes succeed with an "anti-message" that communicates the opposite of the actual words. We will next discuss strategies for choosing the right media channels for your content.

▶ Matching Content to Media Channels

We have described the many forms of media you might choose to disseminate your content and engage

with audiences elsewhere in this text. Those discussions focused on the question, "All things being equal, what are the best choices of media to accomplish your objectives?" Now it is time to admit that all things are not equal—you have to make a realistic media plan in light of your objectives, budget, and staffing limitations.

Content Management and Strategy

Usability.gov[6] has embraced Melissa Rach's "quad" model of content management,[7] as follows:

Content-Focused Components

- Substance: Which kind of content do we need (e.g., topics, types, sources.), and which messages does content need to communicate to our audience?

■ Structure: How is content prioritized, organized, formatted, and displayed? (Structure can include communication planning, information architecture, metadata, data modeling, and linking strategies, among other things.)

People-Focused Components

■ Workflow: Which processes, tools, and human resources are required for content initiatives to launch successfully and maintain ongoing quality?

■ Governance: How are key decisions about content and content strategy made? How are changes initiated and communicated?[7]

In public health, the substance is your strategic health communication messages and all the media you create in the context of a specific campaign, or in response to specific needs. The structure will be determined by your creative and digital teams, and will depend on which media channels you will use, based on factors such as the customer journey (CJ), uses and gratifications theory (UGT), or more traditional audience/channel use measures. The workflow and personnel needed to manage digital and social media are often limiting factors in public health. Nevertheless, just as the "reach" of mass media underlies all other health communication objectives, we might say the "persistence" of social media channels is what makes them worth your while. Not only the quality of information, but also the frequency of blog, Facebook, or Twitter posts make a difference in user engagement. In addition, most public-sector organizations have "clearance" channels that manage their governance. The rules for posting to social media vary, for example. The federal government's rules are available on the Digital Communications Division's website.[e]

Production and Dissemination Factors

Some considerations are more important than others when producing media for public consumption. These include the overall quality of the content (you will hear the terms "high production values" and "low production values" used), the potential reach of the media channel, and the sustainability of the effort in terms of either budget or human resources, which boils down to the cost-effectiveness or return on investment (ROI) for the effort.

Production Value

Today, there is a trend in viral or buzz marketing to make media appear "home-made." Even these approaches, however, rely on professionals to produce their somewhat shaggy, messy appearance.[f] How many people toss the black-and-white, photocopied brochure in the trash as they exit a health clinic? If a four-color brochure on nice paper seems worth keeping, then it may be worth the added expense. (Pre-test this.) The same is true of effort and time expended. Anything worth doing—whether it is mass media, entertainment education, or counseling—is worth doing well. Quality communication can improve outcomes and raise the ROI despite the "I" cost being higher. The surest route to reaching multiple audiences with higher-quality media is to work with partners and share the expenses.

Reach and Scalability

Almost anything will work in a small community with loving care lavished on every detail. The real challenge, as the RE-AIM strategy makes clear, is to be effective at a scale that can have a genuine public health impact. In general, mass media are used to expand the scope of an intervention, because they are the least expensive way to reach a lot of people. However, the communication by such media goes in only one direction. More recently, channels have emerged that offer inexpensive ways of scaling up communications to allow for a two-way exchange of views.

Traditionally, the most costly interventions to bring to scale have been those involving trained counselors working with clients on behavior change (although this type of intervention can appear to be inexpensive in a pilot study). There are also ways of bringing interpersonal communication to scale by working with partners or widely spread networks of practitioners (e.g., pharmacists), but quality control of the intervention and the ability to tie results to inputs become more attenuated with such approaches. Online health coaching and use of social media to perform this function is expanding, but with undocumented results at this point in time.

Sustainability

A strategic health communication program matches partner organizations with intended audiences and spreads the costs of a campaign broadly. This enables an intervention to have a broader reach and be

---

e   https://www.digitalgov.gov
f   A quote that I love, attributed to Dolly Parton, expresses this concept: "You have no idea how much it costs to look this cheap."

something that each organization can afford. It is not pointless to do something really spectacular once, or even on an annual basis. Nevertheless, such an activity is not strategic unless it is worked into a longer-term schedule of public relations, partner counseling, or other ways of carrying the message beyond a single time and place.

Cost-Effectiveness

Public health interventions tend to have very limited budgets, certainly compared to competing commercial campaigns for products such as tobacco, soft drinks, and fast foods. When little money is spent on health communication interventions, assessing their cost-effectiveness is an academic exercise. For those organizations with adequate budgets, newer evaluation methods go beyond "costs per impression" (an older mass-media term referring to the number of times an advertisement is run on TV, radio, or print copy) to "costs per person reached." If a communication strategy can be linked to health outcomes—for example, an antismoking campaign examined over many years against deaths due to tobacco—then a measure of cost-effectiveness such as "costs per deaths averted" can be used. Whether the metric has a short or long time scale, strategic communication uses resources creatively and to best advantage based on audience research and process evaluation.

At this stage, you should have a idea of which media channels you intend to use for each of your kinds of content, and you can move on to pre-testing of your content as it will appear in a particular media channel. **BOX 11-6** shows the communication strategies and tactics proposed for Tobacco Free Alachua's campaign against e-cigarettes.[g]

BOX 11-6 Tobacco Free Alachua: Media Strategies and Tactics

Strategy 1: Organized Personal Communication

Personal communication is vital to the implementation of this campaign. To expose the message strategies that e-cigarette companies are utilizing in their advertisements, meetings and events will be held to personally demonstrate how e-cigarette companies are targeting youth through strategic appeals to adolescents' psychological needs, attracting minors by not including age disclaimers, and making or issuing unsupported health claims.

Given the opportunity to partner with the area universities, local middle and high schools, and other local nonprofits for conferences, meetings, and information sessions, relevant publics will be reached and will in turn be able to spread awareness and educate others. The aforementioned organizations will have a direct interest in e-cigarettes' future because of potential health effects and minors use of the product.

Key Messages and Channels

A messaging platform will be created and will include key messages exposing the message strategies of e-cigarette companies. It will include findings from the campaign research.

Materials will include graphs and statistics to help communicate findings to relevant publics. The following materials will be used to help communicate messages:

1. A phone call "pitch" to inform other organizations about our goals
2. A slide presentation
3. An outline/talking points for presentation
4. A brochure with facts about e-cigarettes, e-cigarette advertisements, and current e-cigarette studies, including our content analysis

Three key messages will run on various communications materials to create community awareness with lasting impact:

- "E-cigs. Unproven."
- "Do you know what you're inhaling?"
- "Don't let opinions guide your health decisions."

To reach attendance goals, educators and local organizations will be reached through personal emails and phone calls, posts on community bulletins, and Listervs with information about the time and location of meetings and conferences.

---

g Tobacco Free Alachua is not a division of the local health department (Florida Department of Health in Alachua County), but rather a separate community partnership that is supported by the health department's Health Policy Program.

Belva N, Hojnacki R, Justice A., Rodriguez S, Susock S. 2014. Proposed public health communications campaign for tobacco free Alachua. Presented in partial fulfillment of the requirements for the degree of Master of Arts in Mass Communication, University of Florida.

▶ Pre-testing Your Content

In-Person Pre-testing

Creative content is ideally tested in the format it will be used. In other words, if an individual is meant to see a commercial spot on the television, it should be tested as if it were being shown on TV. Likewise, if the ad will appear in a magazine, it should be tested as if it were a part of a magazine.

For decades, the most widespread form of pre-testing materials has been the focus group or individual interview setting. Here are two common scenarios:

Scenario 1

You are walking in a shopping mall, and a nice person with a clipboard approaches and asks if you can spare 15 to 20 minutes. You have been selected because, unbeknownst to you, you fit a particular profile. If you say yes, you are taken to an area you did not know existed, but is present in almost every large shopping mall in the United States—the research suite. You enter a cubicle with your facilitator, and he or she shows you materials or products and usually asks you to fill in a questionnaire yourself or to complete a brief interview with the moderator. You might be given a coupon for the product, if you liked it, or some other small compensation, and you are sent on your way.

Scenario 2

You are invited to attend a special event to test out a "pilot for a new television show." This event takes place in an office suite, or perhaps a small screening room. Anywhere from 50 to 100 people are present. After the preliminary introductions, you are given a brief survey to complete that, surprisingly (because it had nothing to do with a television show), asks you to select products from different categories that you might like to have if you could have them for free to take home after the

screening—that is, you are given the option of personalizing your gift for participation.

Next, you see several short segments for what seems to be a new TV show, with the various segments being separated by commercial advertisements. Usually there are several ads bookending each segment. At the end of the showing, you are given another brief survey to complete that asks you questions—maybe one or two about the TV show, but, again, about the products, many of which are advertised, but some of which are not.

You realize that you cannot recall if the "coffee being drunk" was actually part of the pilot television show or an advertisement. You cannot actually remember if you saw a spot for a laundry detergent or orange juice—gee, your memory is not as good as you thought. Also, you thought the show itself was rather banal. Finally, you are again asked to check off the products you would like to have in a shopping bag to take home. One lucky participant is selected to win his or her shopping bag, and the rest of you go home with some small prize and the thanks of the research company.

A variation of this scene would involve a higher-technology setting, where you would get to use an audience-response system (clickers) to respond to the interviewers' questions.

Standard focus groups where people sit around and speak about the materials are also used extensively to pre-test content. Their primary drawback is that individuals can influence one another with their interpretations and opinions about the materials. Unless the content is meant to be used by a group—such as in a game— the collective response is not used.

Market research online communities (MROCs, described elsewhere in this text in the context of formative research) are also asked to pre-test content. Again, if the content will be accessed online, it can be tested online through connections to private YouTube channels, websites, and the like. We will say more about pre-testing websites and other online materials in the later discussion of high-tech pre-testing.

Questions for Pre-testing Content

BOX 11-7 describes some sample questions that might be used when pre-testing a short piece such as a television or radio spot or a print piece.

You will notice that there is some redundancy in how we ask these questions. We also ask respondents to comment on how others would feel about the pieces being tested. These are deliberate attempts to get people to speak honestly. Respondents in pre-tests often do not want to offend the researcher and will try to give

what they believe are the "right answers," (i.e., pleasing). By asking them what others might say, there is a better chance that they might provide some negative feedback. Remember—there is no perfect draft material. If you come back with "No changes necessary," the pretest should be suspected of inadequate probing.

You might be surprised at how much ideas change when going from concepts to media materials. For example, there are now multiple spots for the "Tips from Former Smokers" campaign that are designed to appeal to different audiences and concerns.[h] **BOX 11-8** provides an example of pre-testing digital signage in a healthcare setting in British Columbia.

BOX 11-7 Questions for Pre-testing Draft Content

Comprehension

Does the target audience fully understand and interpret the materials in the way you intend? Some questions that assess comprehension include these examples:

- In your opinion, what is the message of this (television spot, radio spot, print piece)?
- Are there any words that you would change to make it easier for others to understand? Which ones?
- Please explain this message to your neighbor in your own words (have the respondents do so).
- (Indicate a particular image.) Can you tell me what this is and why it might be in this picture?

Attractiveness

Taste obviously varies a great deal and is related to cultural factors as well as the changing times. While you are testing a rough cut of material, you should strive to make it as close as possible to the finished piece. If it is a radio spot, have someone with a good voice do the recording. If it is a storyboard for a video, or a "home video" version of the script, still strive to be as professional as possible to prevent the low production value from distracting the audience. For print materials, you can probably produce a near-finished piece with today's simple graphics programs. Some questions that assess attractiveness include these examples:

- What do you like the most about this piece?
- What do you dislike?
- How would you change this piece?
- What do you think others in this community would say about this piece?

Acceptance

The acceptance factor has more to do with norms, attitudes, and beliefs of the target audience. Can they believe the information? Is it congruent with the community's norm? Does it require a major change of opinion to act on the information? Some questions that assess acceptance include these examples:

- Is there anything about this piece that you find objectionable?
- How about others in this community—what would they say?
- Do you know any people like this, or have you seen a situation like this?
- (Indicate a particular aspect of the piece.) Is this believable to you?
- Can you think of anyone else, such as a religious leader or important community leader, who we should show this to before distributing it widely?

Involvement

The target audience should be able to recognize themselves in the materials. Based on the elaboration likelihood model, if the target audience is already concerned about the issue, then it might not be necessary to match up the

---

h These can be seen at http://www.cdc.gov/tobacco/campaign/tips/

imagery with their stylistic preferences. If you need to first focus their attention on the fact that this information is meant for them, however, then featuring spokespersons and images that the target audience would like to see is important. Some questions that assess involvement include these examples:

- If using non-celebrities: Whom does this piece represent? Are these people like yourselves?
- If using celebrities: Who is this? What do you feel having [name] speak to you about [topic]?
- Do you feel that this piece is speaking to you? Why or why not?
- If this isn't meant for you, who do you think it is speaking to?

Inducement to Action

All materials need a "call for action." Because you have tried to identify a behavior, attitude, or change that you think is feasible for the target audience to embrace, now is the last chance to test whether this piece will prompt them to make it. Even if you are just trying to raise awareness of a problem, you want to prompt the audience to seek more information, or tell others about what they have learned. Some questions that assess call to action include these examples:

- What does this piece ask you to do?
- How do you feel about doing this?
- Would you need to do something else before you could do this?
- How would you explain this to a friend?
- How would they respond to this piece?

Modified from AED Toolbox, Question 18:19–21. http://www.globalhealthcommunication.org/tool_docs/29/a_tool_box_for_building_health_communication_capacity_-_question_18.pdf.

BOX 11-8 Pre-testing Digital Signage in Primary Care Settings: A Pilot Intervention in Langley, British Columbia

Andy S. L. Tan, Rachel Douglas, Victoria Lee, Ellen Peterson, Geoffrey Ramler, and Jeff Plante

Background

Digital signage is a term used to describe informational videos or still shots that are displayed in public areas (typically on television screens). From 2012 to 2014, the Department of Population and Public Health at the Fraser Health Authority in British Columbia (BC), Canada, partnered with the Langley Division of Family Practice (LDFP) to deliver prevention and health promotion messaging via digital signage in patient waiting areas at five primary care clinics. This case study of the digital signage pilot in Langley, B.C., describes the development and implementation of this intervention and summarizes key success factors and challenges.

Population

The community of Langley is in southwest British Columbia, some 25 km east of Vancouver, the province's most populous city. The community consists of slightly more than 140,000 people, divided into two regions: Langley City, which is home to more than 25,000 people, and the surrounding Township of Langley, where more than 104,000 reside.[1] A socioeconomic disparity exists between these two regions. For instance, average income in Langley Township ($36,645) is higher than the B.C. average of $33,758, and considerably higher than that of Langley City ($30,943). A higher proportion of residents in Langley Township received a high school diploma (91.6%) compared with the B.C. average (89.9%) or Langley City (88.2%). The digital signage locations were primarily in Langley City.

The initial subject matter focus for the digital signage was clinical prevention. Clinical prevention services include primary and early secondary prevention activities such as immunization, screening, preventive medication, and counseling. Clinical prevention services in British Columbia are underutilized in comparison to global best practices. For instance, the colorectal screening rate for adults older than 50 years in British Columbia (16.3%) is less than one-fourth the rate in Finland (71%).[2]

Objectives

The LDFP's and Fraser Health Authority's shared goals to foster informed, activated patients and improve population health in Langley formed the foundation for the digital signage partnership. The objectives for the pilot project were as follows:

1. Increase awareness of priority clinical prevention activities among patients and their family physicians.
2. Improve participation in clinical prevention activities among patients and their family physicians.

(continues)

BOX 11-8 Pre-testing Digital Signage in Primary Care Settings: A Pilot Intervention in Langley, British Columbia   *(continued)*

3. Increase the collaborative working relationship between the Division, Public Health, and participating clinics.
4. Conduct feasibility testing of a digital signage intervention.

Formative Research and Pilot Program

Step 1: Literature Review

The project team first conducted a review of digital health education interventions in public areas, including primary care waiting rooms, available through Medline and gray literature sources. They found that few studies used digital media displays to disseminate preventive health information. Instead, most programs used other channels, including television advertising, public notices, pamphlets, personalized letters, and educational seminars to encourage health behavior change. Examples were public signs encouraging the use of stairs at escalators in an airport, digital displays to promote hand washing in public restrooms, and print posters in clinics to promote road safety. Clinic physicians and staff recognized that waiting areas provided a venue to conduct opportunistic health promotion because of the presence of a "captive" audience. The digital signage project offered advantages in terms of its reach, impact on patient behaviors and the ability to present multiple health messages that could be changed at will.

Step 2: Identification of Priority Health Topics

Fraser Health Authority staff and clinician partners at LDFP adopted the top 10 clinical prevention services from the Lifetime Prevention Schedule as the initial focus area for digital signage. These are listed in **FIGURE 11-1**.

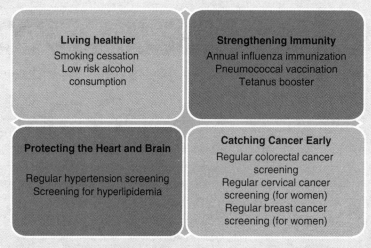

FIGURE 11-1 Four Main Themes of Health Topics for the Digital Signage Pilot Program

Step 3: Consultation with Stakeholders

Based on the International Association of Public Participation (IAP2) Framework,[3] there was continuous stakeholder consultation between Fraser Health Authority and practitioners in LDFP in the design and implementation of the pilot program.

Step 4: Implementation

Development and sourcing of the content for the digital library (infographics, videos, and static images) for the pilot program was completed between December 2012 and January 2013. The digital signage was launched at five partner clinics in April 2013 and ran for one year. Additional content was released in the fall of 2013. The criteria for selecting pilot sites were willingness of the clinic leadership to participate in the evaluation, absence of existing digital signage, presence of a wireless Internet connection, presence of LDFP members practicing in the clinic, and high patient traffic. Funding for this pilot program was provided by an Innovation Grant from the General Practice Services Committee of the Government of British Columbia and Doctors of BC.(www.gpscbc.ca)

Step 5: Evaluation

Baseline data were collected using focus-group discussions and surveys of physicians and staff in participating sites. A follow-up evaluation at one year post rollout was conducted, including focus-group discussions among clinic physicians and staff and site visits by an external clinician observer. Outcomes for the evaluation of the pilot program included clinician and patient awareness of the digital signage, perceived effectiveness among clinicians, and potential unintended consequences on clinical workflow. Additional evaluation activities will be included in the next phase of the program (i.e., utilization of preventive or cancer screening services).

Digital Signage Implementation

Examples of digital signage for healthy aging and colon cancer screening appear in **FIGURE 11-2**.[4]

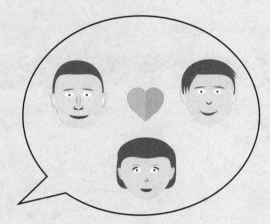
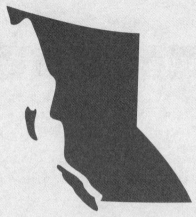

Let your family know you want to stay in your home as you age

Colorectal cancer is the second leading cause of **cancer death** in British Columbia

FIGURE 11-2 Examples of digital signage for healthy aging and colon cancer screening.

Summary of Focus-Group Discussions

Overall, the digital signage messages were viewed favorably by clinic staff and physicians, who found the messages relevant for their clinical practice. Two videos on sugar-sweetened beverages[5] and breast cancer prevention (Canadian Breast Cancer Foundation's ad titled "One New Thing"[6]) were the most highly rated by respondents. Clinic staff and clinicians observed positive impacts of the digital signage pilot program, including patients inquiring about preventive services (e.g., vaccinations, Pap tests for cervical cancer screening). They noted a few challenges, including the timeliness of some of the messages (e.g., flu vaccination videos were less relevant toward the end of flu season), noise-level restrictions limiting the use of audio-visual content, and inability to change the signage content more regularly. Suggested improvements included ability to customize signage material for each clinic, regular updates for the content, and content that coincided with significant events (e.g., Breast Cancer Awareness Month). Most participants agreed the digital signage program should be continued at their clinics and should be expanded to other primary care clinics. Selected verbatim quotes from respondents are included in **TABLE 11-1**.

TABLE 11-1 Focus Group Comments About Digital Signage Videos from Clinicians at Participating Clinics

Comments on sugar-sweetened beverage video:
- "Strong imagery, strong message, holds your attention."
- "Very informative, as I think a child seeing this clip would remember it."

Comment on One New Thing ad from Canadian Breast Cancer Foundation:
- "Well produced, visually strong, message well delivered"

Comment on Digital Signage Program in general:
- "Messages need punch. They need to be produced like a good TV ad, with strong, simple take-home messages, or they will be forgotten as soon as they leave the room."

(continues)

BOX 11-8 Pre-testing Digital Signage in Primary Care Settings: A Pilot Intervention in Langley, British Columbia *(continued)*

Field Notes from Participating Clinics

A family practitioner was invited to visit all five participating clinics and to provide qualitative feedback on the implementation of the digital signage across these clinics. The family practitioner observed that the individual setup at each clinic and the positioning of the digital signage influenced how much attention patients paid to the health messages. The presence of competing media such as magazines or television programs interfered with patients' engagement with the digital signage. Videos within the digital signage attracted more interest and sustained attention among patients in the waiting rooms. Selected verbatim quotes from this evaluation are highlighted in **TABLE 11-2**.

TABLE 11-2 Field Notes from Family Practitioner Evaluation

- "Even though the signage in each clinic has essentially the same information, its effectiveness in engaging patients varies enormously among clinics. The best clinic in terms of patient engagement may be Dr. A's clinic, but it has the advantage of having multiple monitors in patient rooms."

- "The waiting room setup determines whether the signage is reaching patients. I found that patients sitting about 8 feet in front of the signage are most likely to pay attention to it. Most clinics have about 3–5 seats that fall in this sweet spot."

- "The video segments are far more effective in getting attention than animated slides, which in turn are more effective than static texts. The patients may take a glance at the monitor and if they see mostly texts, they are more likely to lose interest and look for something else to do. If they see a video, they are more likely to pay attention until the video is finished."

Key Lessons Learned

Based on the team's experience in implementing the digital signage pilot, there were several important key lessons for the next phase of the program to expand digital signage to other clinics across region.

Lesson 1: Develop and Maintain Strong Partnerships

Significant time and resources were invested to develop and build strong partnerships between the stakeholders, including Fraser Health Authority, LDFP, and clinic staff at the conception of the program. Continued engagement between partners and clarification of the roles of each partner also were identified as important factors that aided the implementation of the pilot program.

Lesson 2: Keep Evaluation Plans Flexible

Initial plans for the pilot program involved various evaluation components, including a checklist to collect data from patients and reviewing of patients' electronic medical records to assess the proportion of patients who received one or more clinical prevention services in the pilot sites. However, these evaluation components were not implemented fully owing to constraints in terms of the clinic workflow and capacity of the staff at the pilot sites to collect these data. As an alternative, a focus group and engagement session with physicians and clinic staff were conducted to gather feedback on the first phase of implementation and plan for phase 2. Alternative mechanisms to collect reliable data with a reduced burden on staff will be considered for the next phase of implementation.

Lesson 3: Focus on Evidence-Informed Decision Making

The design and implementation of this pilot was based on an evidence-informed decision-making model as described by the National Collaborating Centre on Methods and Tools (NCCMT).[7] This means that the research evidence was considered in conjunction with other factors to make decisions about how to proceed in a way that was appropriate to the context. These other factors included community health issues and the local context; community and political preferences and actions; and available fiscal and human resources. More information on this model is available at http://www.nccmt.ca/eiph/index-eng.html.

In our context, a key element for consideration included valuing and incorporating clinician judgment for all aspects of design, including topic selection, content of the individual videos, and logistical mechanisms for implementation.

Clinicians were given opportunities to review content and retained decision-making power over which videos were displayed in their offices.

Limitations

There were some limitations to this pilot program, which would need to be addressed in subsequent phases of the digital signage program. The initial content for the digital signage was limited to the ten clinical prevention services. In addition, one clinician noted that certain messages may be less relevant in certain months of the year (e.g., messages to get flu vaccinations would not be relevant after the flu season is over). Another limitation was that static messages were viewed as less effective in attracting patients' attention compared with video messages. Additional resources will be necessary in future phases to ensure that the content library is updated with new messages regularly, includes seasonally relevant preventive health messages, and utilizes videos instead of static messages. Data to evaluate the impact of the digital signage on increasing patients' adoption of recommended clinical preventive services were not available in this pilot. In the next phase, supplementing clinic capacity to gather utilization data will enable quantifying the uptake of preventive care services following the implementation of digital signage.

Summary and Next Steps

This case study of the digital signage pilot in Langley, B.C., described the development and implementation of a health communication intervention within five primary care clinics. The pilot demonstrated the feasibility of implementing digital signage for disseminating clinical health prevention messages within waiting rooms and acceptability among clinicians, staff, and patients. Key success factors for the pilot and subsequent phases included establishing a strong partnership with stakeholders at the outset, continued engagement with the LDFP and clinic partners, in-depth understanding of the population health needs and priorities, and understanding each clinic's unique environment and work processes. The next step in the digital signage program involves completing and reporting evaluation findings of the pilot to clinicians and staff at the five sites. This will be followed by securing additional resources to expand the number of sites receiving the digital signage across British Columbia and rigorous evaluation of the impact of this program.

Notes

1. BC Stats. PEOPLE 2014 population projections. 2014. http://www.bcstats.gov.bc.ca/.
2. H. Krueger & Associates. *Establishing Priorities Among Effective Clinical Prevention Services in British Columbia: Summary and Technical Report*. British Columbia; 2008.
3. International Association for Public Participation. Foundations of public participation. http://www.iap2.org.
4. For more examples, visit https://www.youtube.com/playlist?list=PL8WdEvLZoZ4TKmFeblCdfLzLzP780HYnK.
5. http://youtu.be/xVujTlivtvY
6. https://youtu.be/dJYHJA3GBKM?list=PL8WdEvLZoZ4TKmFeblCdfLzLzP780HYnK
7. Cilisk D, Thomas H, Buffet C. An introduction to evidence-informed public health and a compendium of critical appraisal tools for public health practice. (2008). http://www.nccmt.ca/pubs/2008_07_IntroEIPH_compendiumENG.pdf.

Andy SL Tan, PhD MPH MBA MBBS, Harvard TH Chan School of Public Health, Boston, MA; Rachel Douglas, MPH, Fraser Health Authority, Surrey, BC; Victoria Lee, MD MPH MBA CCFP FRCPC, Fraser Health Authority, Surrey, BC; Ellen Peterson, MBA, Langley Division of Family Practice, Langley, BC; Geoffrey Ramler, BSc, Fraser Health Authority, Surrey, BC ; Jeff Plante, MD, Langley Division of Family Practice, Langley, BC.

Higher-Tech Pre-testing

Usability Testing

A lot of jargon is used in website development. Some of it corresponds closely to terms or concepts used in health communication, and the rest is unique to the information technology (IT) sector. Usability refers to how well an intended "user" (e.g., of a website, software program, or game) can learn and use the product to achieve his or her goals, as well as his or her satisfaction with the process. The central concept in usability testing is "user-centered design," which is similar to what we have been calling a focus on the intended audience, consumer, or patient. **BOX 11-9** provides explanations of what is measured in usability testing.

Physiological Effects Testing

There is increasing interest in the use of physiological measures, (such as galvanic skin response (lie detector test), heart rate, pupil dilation, eye tracking, and

Usability measures the quality of a user's experience with the product or system. It is a combination of factors, including the following:

- *Ease of learning:* How fast can a user who has never seen the user interface before learn it sufficiently well to accomplish basic tasks?
- *Efficiency of use:* Once an experienced user has learned to use the system, how fast can he or she accomplish tasks?
- *Memorability:* If a user has used the system before, can he or she remember enough to use it effectively the next time, or does the user have to start over again learning everything?
- *Error frequency and severity:* How often do users make errors while using the system, how serious are these errors, and how do users recover from these errors?
- *Subjective satisfaction:* How much does the user like using the system?

Usability Evaluation Basics. Available at: https://www.usability.gov/what-and-why/usability-evaluation.html.

even electroencephalographic (EEG) and functional magnetic resonance imaging (fMRI)) to evaluate responses from participants who are exposed to stimuli such as text, images, or videos. These techniques are used extensively by the private sector, but less so by public health organizations due to the costs involved in testing.

Galvanic Skin Response Popularized in crime shows as part of a polygraph lie detector procedure, or more recently as a biofeedback tool, the **galvanic skin response (GSR)** is a measure of the electrical current that passes along the surface of the skin. Because perspiration conducts electricity much better than dry skin, even a minute increase in perspiration resulting from an emotional response can be detected as an increase in electrical conductance. GSR is painless and can be measured easily using uncomplicated devices and computer display. In addition to its contribution to criminology, GSR has been used to gauge attention and emotional response to media-delivered messages. While an emotional response can be detected with GSR, remember that there is no way to know the nature of the actual underlying emotion without asking the subject.

Pupil Dilation and Eye Tracking Technology The eyes may not be "the windows of the soul," but they do give away the locus and level of our interest. **Eye tracking** is a measure of where and how long we gaze at an image (moving or still) or text. Pupillary dilatation is an innate response of the autonomic nervous system to stimuli such as excitement, danger, or arousal. Together with the blink rate (which also speeds up when we are aroused or experience fear), pupil dilation can be measured by photographic processes embedded in a computer screen. An industry leader in this area is the Danish company iMotions.

BOX 11-10 describes how one university-based group used eye tracking to assess how low-literacy readers responded to risk communication materials.

EEGs and fMRI A prevalent tool used in neuromarketing is high density **electroencephalography (EEG)**. When groups of neurons are activated in the brain, a small electrical charge is generated, resulting in an electrical field. By placing electrodes on a person's scalp (a painless procedure), the resulting EEG signals can be detected and amplified for analysis. Different brain waves measure different brain processes. Oddly enough, EEG was initially developed by a psychiatrist to analyze behavior, but it was never widely accepted in the medical field for this use. Today, the primary medical uses of EEG are for the diagnosis of epilepsy, sleep disorders, and cognitive disorders. In recent years, computerized EEG analysis and mapping have been increasingly used in research and specialized applications, including neuromarketing, and now hold promise for providing information about the nature, timing, and localization of cognitive processes.

Functional magnetic resonance imaging (fMRI) uses a much larger and more expensive device to visualize small regions of neuronal activity associated with brain functions. This technology provides a high-resolution, three-dimensional image of the brain's activity, including localized visual and cognitive responses to different products, stimuli, or situations.

According to Wilson, Gaines, and Hill:

… More than 90 private neuromarketing consulting firms currently operate in the United States. The media has sensationalized many of these investigations, alleging that marketers found the "buy button in your brain" and that the population is about to be "brain scammed (sic)". As a result, use of neuroscience in marketing has both advocates and critics.[8]

One firm, Sands Research, has shared some of its information with us for this text in **BOX 11-11**.

BOX 11-10 Use of Eye Tracking and Gaze Pattern Analysis to Test Health Messages in Low-Literacy Groups

Sarah Bauerle Bass

The Risk Communication Laboratory at Temple University is using eye tracking technology and gaze pattern analysis to understand how individuals with low literacy access and process health messages transmitted through visual, graphic, web, or textual message elements. Eye tracking assesses an individual's attention to visual content (e.g., print, video) by systematically monitoring eye-movement patterns with high-speed cameras that are either mounted on a flat, stable surface such as a desk, or worn by the participant (e.g., cameras mounted on a pair of glasses). New portable eye-tracking systems can also track eye movement on moving messages or video, such as when using a smartphone or tablet (**FIGURE 11-3**).

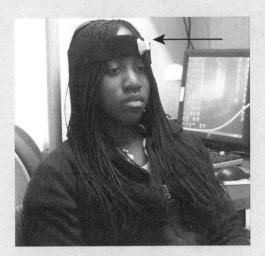

FIGURE 11-3 Portable Eye Tracker

Eye movements are a powerful indicator of interest, and provide an index of the input of information to a person's more complex processing or reasoning faculties.[1-5] As such, eye movement measures can provide valuable information for the design and refinement of health communication messages, particularly when those messages involve combinations of language processing and visual processing. Because of its ability to show interest, eye tracking has been primarily used in marketing to maximize product placement and message. This technology can be especially informative when working with low-literacy populations, but has not been used to an appreciable extent in this context to date. Eye tracking can produce vivid graphs of data that show not only gaze duration (gray dots—the size indicates the length of the gaze) but also gaze pattern (dark gray line). In research done at the Risk Communication Laboratory with adults with limited literacy, eye tracking results showed clear patterns of differential text use in a randomized pilot comparing a literacy-appropriate decision aid on "dirty bombs" (**FIGURE 11-4A**, right) to a higher-literacy-level aid from the CDC (**FIGURE 11-4B**, left).

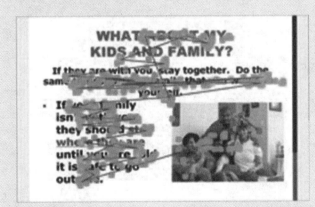

FIGURE 11-4 Eye Tracking of "Dirty Bomb" Study Participants with Limited Literacy

This study, funded by the National Institute of Biomedical Imaging and Bioengineering, was conducted to understand attention to a decision aid on "sheltering in place" during a radiologic terror event (e.g., "dirty bomb"). In this study, the decision aid was developed using formative evaluation (focus groups and surveys)[6,7] and then tested in a between-subjects pilot randomized controlled trial with low-literacy adults. Participants were shown either a CDC-authored set of "frequently asked questions" on dirty bombs (control condition) or a literacy-appropriate decision aid (experimental condition). Both conditions were presented on a computer screen as a series of slides. The experimental literacy-appropriate decision aid included visual cues, contained less information, and was written at a sixth-grade reading level. Subjects were recruited through community-based agencies (food bank, senior services, federal services, churches, community centers) and literacy screening occurred in-person using the Rapid Estimate of Adult Literacy in Medicine—Short Version (REALM-R)[8] or over the phone using the Single Item Literacy Screening (SILS).[9]

Fifty participants were randomized to the control and experimental conditions. The mean REALM-R score was 2.11 out of a possible 8 (range, 0 to 5), confirming the inclusion of low-literacy adults. Eye tracking was performed with an Applied Science Laboratory (ASL) stationary eye tracker (Eye Trac 6000), and the Eyenal software program was used for analysis. In addition, a 5-point subjective rating scale was developed and tested by the author to characterize gaze patterns. Interrater reliability was excellent, with coefficients for scores of participants' ability to accurately track written text of 0.90 [Pearson coefficient] and 0.99 [Spearman coefficient].

Overall, the ability to track information was higher in the experimental group than in the control condition for three of seven content-similar slides, with an additional two slides being close to statistical significance. The difficulty in attending to the relatively dense text that participants had in the control condition was reflected in significantly longer pupil fixation and gaze duration. Participants spent more time in the experimental condition looking at individual words (four of seven slides) and more time overall (all seven slides). As a consequence, participants in the experimental condition were also more likely to be "certain of what to do," had higher self-efficacy on their ability to protect themselves and their family, and were more likely to agree that they would stay home if a "dirty bomb" exploded. The results of this study clearly indicated the eye tracking is a viable and important method for understanding how low-literacy groups attend to health-related information and its association with comprehension.[10–12]

Eye tracking was thus found to be especially helpful in understanding how best to design materials for low-literacy groups, providing tangible evidence of how tracking of text is directly related to comprehension as well as intended or actual behavior. Eye tracking output can clearly differentiate whether an individual is reading text as expected or if he or she instead has to read and then reread sections because of literacy ability. If study participants are presented with material that is above their literacy and/or numeracy levels, eye tracking can be used to show areas where those individuals have difficulty accessing the content, which can then be related to other outcome measures. The Risk Communication Laboratory is continuing to use these methods as a method to test developed health communication messages to ensure that they meet the needs of individuals with all literacy abilities.

References

1. Beatty J. The papillary system. In: Coles G, Donchin E, Porges S, eds. *Psychophysiology: Systems, Process, and Applications*. New York, NY: Guilford Press; 1986:43-50.

2. Beatty J. Pupillometric signs of selective attention in man. *Neurophysiol Psychophysiol Exp Clin App*. 1988:138-143.

3. Granholm E, Asarnow RF, Sarkin AJ, Dykes KL. Pupillary responses index cognitive resource limitations. *Psychophysiology*. 1996;33(4):457-461.

4. Steinhauer S, Boller F, Zubin J, Pearlman S, eds. *Pupillary Dilation to Emotional Visual-Stimuli Revisited*. Washington, DC: Society for Psychophysiology Research; 1983.

5. Steinhauer S. Pupillary responses, cognitive psychophysiology and psychopathology. 2006. http://www.wpic.pitt.edu/research/biometrics/Publications/PupilWeb.htm.

6. Bass S, Mora G, Ruggieri D, et al., eds. *Understanding of and Willingness to Comply with Recommendations in the Event of a "Dirty Bomb": Demographic Differences in Low-Literacy Urban Residents*. Washington, DC: American Public Health Association; November 2011.

7. Bass SB, Greener JR, Ruggieri D, et al. Attitudes and perceptions of urban African Americans of a "dirty bomb" radiological terror event: results of a qualitative study and implications for effective risk communication. *Disaster Med Public Health Prep*. 2015:1-10.

8. Bass PF, Wilson JF, Griffith CH. A shortened instrument for literacy screening. *J Gen Intern Med*. 2003;18(12):1036-1038.

9. Chew LD, Griffin JM, Partin MR, et al. Validation of screening questions for limited health literacy in a large VA outpatient population. *J Gen Intern Med*. 2008;23(5):561-566.

10. Bass S, Gordon T, Parvanta C. *Final Program Report to the NIBIB: Developing Radiological Risk Communication Materials for Low-Literacy Populations*.

11. Bass S, Gordon TF, Parvanta C, eds. *Utilizing Gaze Patterns and EKG Methods to Test Health Messages: A Case Study with Low-Literacy Populations*. Amsterdam, Netherlands: International Communication in Health Care Conference; September 2014.

12. Bass S, Gordon T, Gordon R, et al. *Utilizing Marketing and Psychology Methods to Test Health Messages: A Case-Study of How Gaze Patterns and Psycho-Physiological Measures Can Be Used to Analyze Responses to a "Dirty Bomb" Decision Aid in People with Limited Literacy*. Bethesda, MD: National Health Literacy Research Conference; 2012.

BOX 11-11   EEG Neuromarketing Example from Sands Research

EEG data [are] sampled continuously throughout our in-lab and mobile studies.... When enough sensors are used, the data can be viewed in three dimensions and plotted onto a model brain.... When a test subject gazes for an extended period of time at a product, activated brain areas help determine if the gaze was due to confusion or interest. In addition to the insight gained from functional brain areas, the frequency of the EEG waveforms can provide information about attention states. A complete spectral analysis is performed on the EEG.

In hundreds of commercials with thousands of participants tested by Sands Research to date, we have seen that a good ad will always have a large spike in brain activity within the first 800 milliseconds of the ad and sustain a high plateau across the length of the commercial.

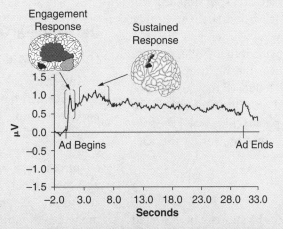

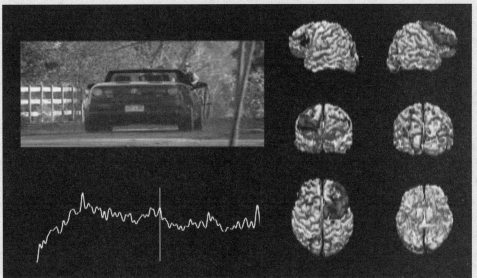

With Super Bowl advertising spots being sold for an average $2.6 to $2.7 million for 15 seconds, many companies are banking that neuromarketing pre-testing will pay off.

According to developer Steven Sands, a common question in behavioral and neuromarketing research is, "What is the appropriate number of subjects needed to obtain a reliable result?" Traditional methods of market research use large numbers of respondents, and there seems to be general consensus that approximately 150–200 participants or more (depending on research objectives) are needed to obtain consistent results. With electroencephalogram methodologies (EEG), a much smaller sample size is needed to achieve a similar statistical threshold. When the number of study participants is between 30 to 40 (per target demographic grouping), there is a less than 1% chance of error, and the associated Neuro-Engagement Factor (NEF) score portrays an accurate and significant rating for the media stimulus in question. Sands Research utilizes the less than 1% chance of error threshold for all studies. A larger sample size could be utilized to achieve an even smaller margin of error, say 0.25%, although that degree of threshold does not provide us with a significant amount of "new" knowledge about the stimulus, nor is it financially efficient.

Sands, S.F. White Paper: Sample Size Analysis for Brainwave Collection (EEG) Methodologies, October 2009. http://www.sandsresearch.com/.

Testing the Final Media Package
In-Situ Testing

Once we make changes based on this first round of materials testing, we move onto the real test: how the intended package performs in its "natural environment," which is a crowded media context. If we are testing a print piece intended to go in a magazine, we want to show it in a mock-up of a magazine. If we are testing a radio spot, we will play our spot along with others and some music. A television spot similarly will be sandwiched between a television show and other advertisements. Almost anyone will tell you they can remember a piece of advertising if that is all they have seen. But while driving down the highway, do they really think much about the billboard they just saw, or the message they just heard on drive-time radio? Do they get up and fetch some potato chips when the spot promoting healthy eating comes on during the televised ballgame?

Test Marketing

Exposing all the elements of the strategy in a limited number of locations to a limited audience for a limited time with social marketing evaluation is sometimes called a **pilot test**. Following the launch of a product in the testing phase, or an important behavior change campaign, researchers will conduct intercept interviews or day-after recall surveys (i.e., calling people on the phone to see if they heard or saw the information) to see how the trial is going. If a tangible product is being sold, then a longer period will be used to evaluate the sales data for the product, with varying degrees of promotion and other incentives (e.g., mailed coupons, media advertising) being applied to influence consumer behavior. The data collected from this trial are then used to adjust the final product, its packaging, its price, and its promotional campaign or, in some cases, to cancel it altogether. (Remember—"fail early, fail small.")

Pilot testing is typically used when a tangible product is close to its final form, or is being adapted to new market conditions. This technique is also used when there may be a need to obtain a success story that can be touted while conducting advocacy on behalf of the project among public- or private-sector partners.

▶ Preparing the Work Plan, Timetable, and Budget

Now you have a clear sense of what will make your health communication program more likely to succeed. How do you establish your stakeholders as true partners in the intervention? You do this by defining roles, specifying who will pay for what, and deciding how to share the credit.

Defining Partner Roles
International Partners

In international work, most major health communication interventions will be directed by the health agency or ministry of the country needing an intervention. As in the United States, the national government effort is often supplemented by support and resources from governmental and non-governmental agencies or organizations within subregions of a country (e.g., provinces). In low-income countries many health ministries place the financial and human resources from various sources (UNICEF, USAID, and other bilateral donors,[i] as well as the many nongovernmental organizations[j]) in different regions of the country to spread out the available technical assistance and material resources. Partner roles are often defined by this process.

When planning a health communication program with a national scope, there will be many partners with which to work. These partners may be eager to participate if the collaboration brings superior resources into their local area and helps them serve their constituencies, while not requiring an over-extension of their own resources.

The tricky part can be integrating each stakeholder's objectives into a unified plan so that the collective communication intervention supports individual organizational program needs. This level of negotiation could take many months (or even years) to accomplish, but it often determines whether a program will succeed or fail. In our experience, the best programs include several key organizations that underwrite the initial stages of an intervention, while transferring responsibilities, training, and material

---

i   International aid programs managed by France, Germany, Italy, Sweden, and Canada were prevalent in west Africa at the time. Other countries predominated in development aid elsewhere.

j   From the United States, Save the Children, CARE, Africare, and World Vision were highly visible in west Africa. Other nongovernmental organizations led efforts elsewhere.

assets down to smaller entities to continue the project on their own. This builds a level of sustainability into what otherwise might be a relatively short burst of mass media, or other communications, with little subsequent follow-up.

Partnering in the United States

Working in the United States is not that different, except that even a very few organizations working together can often come up with sufficient resources to mount an impressive intervention. For example, the key partners for the folic acid program were the CDC and the March of Dimes, which then recruited additional organizations into the National Council for Folic Acid. Allowing organizations to contribute based on their strengths is the most strategic way to plan an intervention. In the case of the folic program, CDC contributed most of the audience research as well as the epidemiologic data tracking. The March of Dimes provided advocacy. The costs to produce

the mass-media spots were shared, but air time was donated by media outlets because of federal policies pertaining to public service announcements (PSAs) at that time. None of the air time was paid for at the time. Print materials were initially covered by the National Council for Folic Acid, but eventually became available for partner distribution for the cost of production. CDC and the Council covered the costs of developing a partner resource guide to mount community and other small-scale interventions and, later, a media resource guide.[6] These tools, together with the website, have allowed the life of the folic program to extend well beyond the resources available to the CDC alone, by empowering any organization concerned about this issue with facts as well as outstanding communication assets.

For planning your program, **TABLE 11-3** provides a model partner asset worksheet to help you think about what different partners can contribute to implementing a large- or small-scale communication intervention.

TABLE 11-3 Partner Assets Worksheet

Organization: Partnering Role(s):		Task/Objective
Assets	**% Time or Yes**	
People		
Leadership		
Expert staff		
Administrative support		
Students/volunteers		
Expertise		
Research		
Regulatory		
Product		
Packaging		
Shipping		
Marketing		

Organization: Partnering Role(s):		Task/Objective
Assets	**% Time or Yes**	
Communication		
Marketing facilitation		
Training		
Others		
Relationships		
Our primary target audience		
Our secondary audience		
Donors		
Policy makers		
Community leaders/groups		
Media		
Suppliers		
Others		
Resources		
Information/data (capture)		
Public health		
Environmental		
Regulatory		
Marketing		
Public opinion		
Local knowledge		
Other		
Information (Dissemination)		
Electronic listservs/blogs/tweets		
Print/online publications		

(continues)

TABLE 11-3 Partner Assets Worksheet		*(continued)*
Organization: Partnering Role(s):		**Task/Objective**
Assets	**% Time or Yes**	
Paid advertising		
New outreach (public relations)		
Word of mouth		
Viral		
Tangibles/Products		
Food/beverage		
Ingredients		
Medicines		
Information technology		
Equipment		
Energy		
Transportation		
Advertising time		
Advertising creative		
Other		
Accommodations		
Meeting rooms (10–49 capacity)		
Meeting rooms (more than 50 capacity)		
Project office		
Individual office		
High-profile events		
Media setup		
Storage		

Data from: GAIN/International Business Leaders Forum, Partnering Toolbook, http://tpi.iblf.org/publications/Toolbooks/partneringtoolbookdownload.jsp

Budget

Popular guidebooks available today can tell you how to do health communication and social marketing "on a shoestring budget." If you want a good result (and there is no reason to do a campaign that will not be effective), you will need to trade off time for money—and you must create a budget. There is no reason that a dedicated group of students, for example, could not mount an effective health communication campaign using Internet-based media, live events, and potentially obtain coverage by local broadcast and print media for "nothing more" than the time and effort they devote to the campaign. Out-of-pocket expenses—such as professional talent, video and sound production, printing services, and paid placement—are what drive up costs.

Another major cost in health communication is salaries for any personnel with expertise that you cannot acquire for "free." For example, the salary of counselors or educators is what makes the interpersonal approach relatively expensive. Your budget should cover all the costs or expenses of the intervention activities. The following categories are normally reflected in health communication budgets.

Direct Costs

Direct costs are the part of the budget that contributes directly to a program's outputs. This line item is made up of personnel costs and out-of-pocket costs (those associated with products and services not obtained through a salaried employee).

- *Personnel costs.* These costs include the salaries and benefits, or portions thereof, for the people who will work on the project. Full-time employees who will work part-time on the project should be included at the appropriate percentage of time. For example, if a research assistant will spend 20 hours per week on the project for its first year, he or she should be budgeted for 50% of the total salary and 50% of the fringe benefits. (Fringe benefits include Social Security taxes, health insurance, dental insurance, and other benefits that your agency or organization provides.) Most organizations have a calculated fringe benefit rate that can be used when developing a budget; it is often in the range of 25% to 30% of the salary.
- *Out-of-pocket/non-personnel costs.* These expenses are connected to program outputs that are provided by vendors. Such costs may include production services, travel, equipment, office supplies, postage, telephone expenses, and other routine expenses. Some donors allow you to break out

facility rental, maintenance, and insurance in your non-personnel costs; others expect them to be covered by your overhead.

Indirect Costs

Also called "overhead," **indirect costs** are what it costs your agency to exist, but they are not tied directly to creating the program's outputs. Examples include office space, environmental management (e.g., heat, air conditioning, water, custodial services), and depreciation on equipment. Indirect costs are usually calculated as a percentage of direct costs. Institutions that have worked with the U.S. government, including many universities, have an approved overhead rate. You might be shocked to learn that it can run as high as 60% or more of the direct costs. Thus, if you are developing a grant proposal budget, for example, and you know that the total amount of the award is fixed, you must be mindful of your indirect rate to know how much money you actually have to work with. Some donors will pay only a small percentage of indirect costs. Others, such as the National Institutes of Health, provide indirect costs on top of direct costs for research projects.

In-Kind Contributions

In the nonprofit world in which public health often operates, organizations frequently consider their time (e.g., time spent on activities by volunteers), their space, use of equipment, and other in-house resources as **in-kind contributions** to a project budget. These resources are used to produce program outputs but may not be factored into direct or indirect budget costs. Some donors expect to see a match made for their investment through direct financial resources, in-kind resources, or additional donations.

Total Budget

The **total budget** is the sum of direct and indirect costs, including in-kind contributions and additional donations. If the project will run for more than one year, an annual budget needs to be prepared as well as a budget for the total time period. Sometimes you will need to separate and track different funding streams for your overall budget. For example, if a charitable organization wants to know how you spent its contribution, you want to be able to tell this donor with some precision (e.g., not just "for 30% of the project"). In addition to a spreadsheet, you often need to provide a budget narrative that describes each expenditure and its purpose. **BOX 11-12** provides a

BOX 11-12   Budget Sample and Narrative

Kididdelnhopper Community Health Center (KHCHC)
"Kididdel Hopping Kids Health Improvement Project"
BUDGET NARRATIVE
January 1–December 30, 2017

Summary

The total amount budgeted for the January 1 to December 30, 2017, period is $109,062, which includes an indirect cost rate of 25%, or $21,812 and direct costs of $87,250.

Personnel Expenses

The total budget for salary expenses is $59,000. All salaries are based on a 12-month project period.

Project Director

This position is filled by the Director of Health Promotion at a 0.2 FTE level of effort. The Director of Health Promotion position is currently filled by Sarah Varpanta, MPH. The allocated budget for this salary expense is $13,000, based on a $65,000 annual salary and a 20% level of effort. This position is supervised by KHCHC's CEO, Dr. Claudia Kididdelhopper. The Director of Health Promotion supervises the Registered Dietitian, Youth Activity Specialist, and the Fitness Coordinator for the Center and this project.

Registered Dietitian

KHCHC's Registered Dietitian will provide individualized goal setting, nutrition education, diet planning, and weight monitoring for participants. The dietitian position is currently held by Maxine Threelegs. The allocated budget for this salary expense is $9,000, based on a $60,000 annual salary and a 15% level of effort.

Fitness Coordinator

The Fitness Coordinator has the responsibility of providing physical activity and additional recreational programs for the participants. The position will also maintain the project website, which includes an interactive database for participants to track their fitness challenge goals and accomplishments. The Fitness Coordinator position is currently held by Hayley Nelson, MPA, AT. The allocated budget for this salary expense is $25,000, based on a $50,000 annual salary and a 50% level of effort.

Youth Activity Specialist

The Youth Activity Specialist has the responsibility of coordinating and leading the daily afterschool and monthly weekend programs. This position is currently held by Lola Catt, BA. The allocated budget for this salary expense is $6,400, based on a $32,000 annual salary and a 20% level of effort.

Graduate Student Assistants

Two graduate students from the Exercise Physiology and Wellness Program at the University of the Sciences will provide formative and evaluation research assistance, as well as general assistance, to the project. Each student will provide approximately 10 hours per week for 14 weeks per semester, for a total of 560 hours provided to the project and a total cost of $5,600. Students are TBN (to be named).

Fringe Benefits

A total amount of $18,290 is budgeted to pay for fringe benefits for the project director, dietitian, fitness coordinator, and youth activity specialist for the specified employment periods. (Student workers do not receive fringe benefits.) Fringe benefits include FICA, unemployment insurance, worker's compensation, and health and disability insurance. Full-time employees (must work at least 32 hours a week) receive KHCHC's standard health, dental, life and disability insurance benefit package. Fringe benefits for current employees on staff are calculated at 31.1% of gross salary.

Non-Personnel Expenses

Travel

Local travel expenses include the costs of using public transportation ($1.75 per trip) as well as private automobiles to conduct project activities. Local travel will include sending project staff out to community centers, churches, and other after-school programs within our catchment area for special events. It also supports travel to attend off-site meetings, training, and regional conference sessions. Private automobile mileage will be reimbursed at the federally approved rate of $0.54/mile (2016), by means of a mileage log. The local travel budget for staff is budgeted at $1200 for the 12-month project period.

A travel budget of $600 is included for air and ground travel for two project staff to attend a 2-day professional conference related to youth obesity prevention.

The total budget for per diem and lodging for this conference is $600. This is the estimated cost for two project staff to attend a professional conference related to youth obesity prevention for 2 days and nights.

Other Non-Personnel Expenses

The total budget for out-of-pocket expenses is $7560. The largest amount will be spent on activity and educational supplies. Supplies include staff curriculum materials, participant materials, and parent materials, as well as outreach to promote the activity in the community. We have budgeted for the cost of two new laser printers with a year's worth of toner, as we intend to produce most of the materials in-house. We anticipate using very limited services of a graphic designer to provide a coherent look to our materials. We also intend to develop audiovisual materials to be used on site as well as sent home with children. For this, we intend using a recording device (mobile phone), and transferring videos onto flash drives or digital downloads. Finally, we will purchase sports equipment, games, light refreshments, and incentive items ($5.00 or less) for the after-school and weekend programs. We have set aside $1000 for all office supplies, postage, and telephone services related to the project.

Kiddidelhopper "Kiddidel Hopping Kids" Project Budget Spreadsheet		
Object	**% Time**	**Year 1**
A. DIRECT EXPENSES		
Personnel Expenses		
Project Director	0.20	$13,000.00
Registered Dietitian	0.15	$9,000.00
Fitness Coordinator	0.50	$25,000.00
Youth Activity Specialist	0.20	$6,400.00
Graduate Student Assistants		
2 (10 hours/week) × 28 weeks × $10/hour		$5,600.00
Total, Salaries		$59,000.00
Fringe Benefits (31.1%)		$18,290.00
Total, Personnel Expenses		**$77,290.00**
Non-Personnel Expenses		
Travel		$2,400.00
Laser printers 2 @ $250		$500.00
Paper		$2,000.00
Toner cartridges		$1,500.00
Recording software		$200.00

(continues)

BOX 11-12 Budget Sample and Narrative *(continued)*

Object	% Time	Year 1
A. DIRECT EXPENSES		
Recording devices		$300.00
DVDs		$200.00
Sporting equipment		$500.00
Incentives and refreshments		$1,000.00
Other office supplies		$400.00
Postage		$240.00
Telephone		$360.00
Professional services: graphics		$360.00
Total, Non-Personnel Expenses		**$7,560.00**
	Total Direct Expenses	$87,250.00
B. Indirect Expenses (25% of Base)		$21,812.50
Total Expenses		**$109,062.50**

sample budget and narrative for a community-based intervention.

Media costs are so variable by geographic location and other factors that it is impossible to provide generic guidance. However, **BOX 11-13** features a planning tool from California's First 5 Program which promotes early childhood education. The advertising budget tool is based on promoting a local town hall.

Finally, **BOX 11-14** provides CDC's minimum and recommended funding for overall campaigns as well as the mass media components for state tobacco control programs. As a rule, mass communication outreach efforts should amount to 10%-20% (25% or higher if mass media is the primary intervention) of total state tobacco control program funding—enough to support three such health communication efforts year-round. Although funding levels for mass communication may seem high, they amount to about $2-$3 per person.

Timeline

Larger-scale communication programs utilizing print or audiovisual media may take one year to plan and produce, including time spent on conducting formative research, developing and testing materials, and readying everything for dissemination to partners or media outlets. Those relying more on informal social media may go more quickly, but the formative research phase should not be skipped. Planning for evaluation begins as you develop your strategy. **BOX 11-15** shows a timeline for a fairly complex campaign with activities spread over three years.

Measurement and Evaluation

It is useful to include a set of metrics and the method by which they will be collected as part of your final plan. These metrics are used to ensure that program components are performing as planned. If something

BOX 11-13 Advertising Budget Planning Tool: CA First 5 Town Hall

Expense Items	Minimal Price	Moderate Price	Maximum Price	More Max Price	F5 Tips and Notes
Online advertising on Facebook and the Google Display Network	$0 — this is a "nice to have." There are plenty of opportunities to promote through media outreach and other avenues.	$200 direct costs (design in house) to run ads on Facebook for two weeks	$400 direct costs plus $200 for graphic design to run ads on Facebook and the Google Display Network for four weeks	$1,000 direct costs plus $200 for graphic design for a month-long buy on Facebook and the Google Display Network, as well as local media websites	Set per-day limits for your buy to ensure online advertising stays within budget.
Print advertising in local newspapers	$0 — this is a "nice to have." There are plenty of opportunities to promote through media outreach and other avenues.	$250 direct costs (design in house) to run a quarter-page ad in a small community paper	$500 direct costs plus $200 for graphic design to run a half-page ad in local paper	$1,500 direct costs plus $600 for design to run three ads in local papers for two weeks	Ads could be both in print and online. Focus on community papers, daily and weekly.
Radio advertising	$0 — this is a "nice to have." There are plenty of opportunities to promote through media outreach and other avenues.	$750 in direct costs to run ads for one week on one to two stations	$1,250 in direct costs plus $200 for graphic design to run ads for one week (with higher frequency and adding online ads on station websites)	$2,000 in direct costs to run ads for two weeks on multiple stations	Run 15- and 30-second ads for two to three weeks leading up to the town hall.
Local blogs	$0 — this is a "nice to have." There are plenty of opportunities to promote through media outreach and other avenues.	$0—outreach only, assuming internal staff do outreach	$100 to run ads on one to two blogs	$250 for ads/ messaging on five blogs	Outreach to local blogs geared toward families, policy, First 5 issue areas and community events.
Local retail/ community center outreach	$0 — this is a "nice to have." There are plenty of opportunities to promote through media outreach and other avenues.	$300 direct costs to print 10 posters (full-color, 18 × 24") (design in house)	$600 direct costs plus $200 for graphic design for 20 posters (full-color, 18 × 24")	$1,000 direct costs plus $200 for graphic design for 35 posters (full-color, 18 × 24")	Produce and place posters in windows of grocery stores, libraries, family activity centers (YMCA, kids gyms), and other community gathering places.
TOTAL	**$0**	**$1,500**	**$3,650**	**$6,750**	

BOX 11-14 Recommended Total and Mass-Reach Health Communication Funding Levels for Tobacco Control Programs, Selected States, 2014

| State | Total Funding—State Tobacco Control Programs | | Mass-Reach Health Communication Interventions Funding Only | |
	Minimum	Recommended	Minimum*	Recommended*
California	$248.6 million	$347.9 million	$52.8 million (15.9%)	$76.0 million (16.0%)
New York	$142.8 million	$203.0 million	$31.8 million (21.2%)	$45.7 million (21.8%)
Vermont	$6.1 million	$8.4 million	$1.1 million (18.0%)	$1.6 million (19.0%)
Wyoming	$6.2 million	$8.5 million	$0.6 million (9.6%)	$0.9 million (10.6%)

*Percentages represent the proportion of overall state tobacco control program funding

Data from https://www.cdc.gov/tobacco/stateandcommunity/best_practices/pdfs/2014/comprehensive.pdf.

is not working, adjust it to make it work. These metrics also set up the logic model for your outcome evaluation.

BOX 11-16 shows an application of an Association for Measurement and Evaluation of Communication (AMEC) framework from the U.K. government for its "Chip My Dog" campaign (a campaign to increase microchipping of dogs). This campaign was conducted primarily through social media.

▶ Summary Implementation Plan

The summary implementation plan is likely the one that will guide your program and be shown to potential collaborators or donors. For this reason, you do not want to go into all of the details included elsewhere in this text.

Your plan should include these key points:

- Background and justification, including your SWOT (strengths, weaknesses, opportunities, threats) analyses
- Intended audiences
- Communication objectives by audience
- Messages
- Settings and channels for conveying your messages

- Activities (including media, materials, and other methods)
- Available partners and resources
- Tasks and timeline (including persons responsible for each task, dates for completion of each task, resources required to deliver each task, and points at which progress will be checked)
- Budget

You can add more if you want. Realize that you will also have more detailed planning documents for working with your media productions partners (if any), the news media (if involved), and program implementers.

▶ Conclusion

Implementation is the distillation of what you want to happen, who you plan to reach, and how you are going to proceed. Implementation is limited by how much support you have and what you can afford, by external barriers, by the distraction of competing influences, and by imposed time limits. Implementation is the tip of the iceberg, supported completely by below-the-surface planning. It is an extended moment of truth—the time when your planning and expectations are embodied into action. How do you know if you did well? Evaluation is the next step.

BOX 11-15 Campaign Timeline

PHASE	Year 1												Year 2												Year 3											
	Jan	Feb	Mar	Apr	May	Jun	Jul	Aug	Sep	Oct	Nov	Dec	Jan	Feb	Mar	Apr	May	Jun	Jul	Aug	Sep	Oct	Nov	Dec	Jan	Feb	Mar	Apr	May	Jun	Jul	Aug	Sep	Oct	Nov	Dec
Management decisions and team building	■	■																																		
Formative research			■																																	
Analysis and creative briefs			■	■																																
Creative agency selection					■	■																														
Design team meetings						■	■																													
Materials development and review							■	■																												
Pre-testing completed									■																											
Produced TV, radio and print executions										■	■																									
Revisions to materials												■	■																							
Approvals														■																						
SMS content development and testing										■	■	■	■																							
Final approval														■																						

BOX 11-15 Campaign Timeline *(continued)*

Task	Y1 Jan	Feb	Mar	Apr	May	Jun	Jul	Aug	Sep	Oct	Nov	Dec	Y2 Jan	Feb	Mar	Apr	May	Jun	Jul	Aug	Sep	Oct	Nov	Dec	Y3 Jan	Feb	Mar	Apr	May	Jun	Jul	Aug	Sep	Oct	Nov	Dec
Finalization of materials															X	X																				
Partner collaboration finalized																	X	X																		
Launch planning																		X	X																	
Delivery of materials to partners																			X	X																
Radio spots on air																					X	X	X	X												
TV spots on air																								X	X	X										
SMS service implementation																								X	X	X	X	X	X	X						
Omnibus monitoring surveys																								X			X			X						
Evaluation planning														X					X	X																
Selection of research firm																		X	X																	
Evaluation fieldwork																					X	X	X													
Analysis and report writing																															X	X	X	X	X	
Planning for the future																																	X	X	X	X

Inspired by Wazazi Nipendeni (Parents, Love me) project conducted by the Ministry of Health, Tanzania with support from USAID and CDC, implemented by Johns Hopkins Center for Communication Programs.

BOX 11-16 Chip My Dog Example of Process Evaluation Metrics

Program Objective

Increase microchipping of dogs this year (target 100% increase) and move the public toward compulsory microchipping by April 2016. (Microchipping involves inserting a microchip under the dog's skin to aid identification of the animal in case of loss.)

Communications Subobjectives

- Encourages dog owners to chip their dogs
- Create online engagement level
- Achieve a joint credible voice with partner organizations
- Start to signpost that microchipping will become law

Audiences

- *Intermediary audiences:* Press, social media users, and animal welfare charities
- *End audience:* Dog owners and their friends and family

Sample Communications Activity

- Traditional media using ministerial quotes and partners/stakeholders
- Social media using #ChipMyDog, encouraging people to share photos of their dogs
- Facebook page "Chip My Dog"
- Google map of free microchipping locations
- Make a video of a dog being microchipped
- Ministerial visits to Dog centers
- Case studies on digital media
- Brief stakeholders and sought support
- Work with Dogs Trust
- Carry out #AskDefra Twitter Q&A sessions on the topic with the Chief Veterinarian
- Sell in Q&A to *Dogs Today* from Animal Welfare Minister

Use of AMEC[1] Criteria to Measure Efficacy of the Program

Department for Environment Food & Rural Affairs

 # ChipMyDog campaign

MENU	EXPOSURE	ENGAGEMENT	PREFERENCE	IMPACT	ADVOCACY	
PROGRAMME METRICS	• Opportunities to see from both DEFRA and dedicated Chip My Dog accounts • % increase in campaignrelated mentions	• Interaction rate on dedicated FB page and Google map • % comment or shares inc. questions at live Twitter Q&A • #ChipMyDog usage	• Increase in recognition of compulsory microchipping legal requirement	• New Influencers • Key message penetration rates • New enquires received	• Total Mentions % increase	This was the ultimate outcome of the campaign
BUSINESS METRICS	• Awareness level measure • Cost per assitional dog chipped	• Campaign mentions • Share of voice of partner and Defra • % increase in click throughs to the 'how to' pages	• % increase in map searches • % increase in map commentary relating to intention to chip their dog	• Actual increase in volume of dogs chipped compared with previous year • % increase in inbound requests for information	• Recommen dations via YouTube and FB shares % • % increase in number of likes of FB page	This was a stretch target in that it demonstrates organic promotion at no cost the tax payer.
CHANNEL METRICS	• Number of items (tweets, posts) • Mentions • Opportunities to see • Media tweets	• Post likes • Comments • Shares • Views • RTs/1000 • Followers % increase	• Tone and sentiment of user generated content • Favourable questions asked via Twitter Q&A • Stakeholder supporting comments/sign posts	• Unique visitors to website referred from each channel	• Organic posts by advocates • Comments supporting links to YouTube / ChipMyDog pages	

Social Media Measurement Solved
Your Question Answered.

 amec Measurement Week
15-19 September. 2014
a part of the Global Education Program

PRIME ☐ RESEARCH
presented by Excellennce in communication research

FIGURE 11-5 ChipMyDog campaign

---

1. Association for Measurement and Evaluation of Communication.

BOX 11-16 Chip My Dog Example of Process Evaluation Metrics *(continued)*

Result

- Approximately 130,000 dogs were microchipped in 2013–2014 compared with just 25,000 in 2012–2013, an increase of more than 500%.
- The campaign has provided benchmark metrics for the next phase of the campaign around compulsory microchipping of dogs in April 2016.
- DEFRA (Department for Environment, Food and Rural Affairs, Government of UK) and its partners are influencers in this topic and credible voices in the conversations about dog chipping.
- The advocacy level is high, which is also helpful for the next phase of activity.

Wrap-Up

Chapter Questions

1. Identify and define each SMART term.
2. Briefly describe the process of transforming a creative brief into a concept.
3. What is the importance of pre-testing concepts with audiences and gatekeepers?
4. Describe the content-focused and people-focused components in Rach's "quad" model of content management.
5. Why would you ever want something to have a home-made appearance?
6. What is the purpose of some redundancy in pre-test questions?
7. Describe at least two physiological and neuromarketing techniques used in high-tech testing and explain their purpose in pre-testing.
8. What are the key elements of a budget?

References

1. Gaglio B, Shoup JA, Glasgow RE. The RE-AIM framework: a systematic review of use over time. *Am J Public Health*; 2013;103(6):e38-e46.
2. What is RE-AIM. Virginia Tech College of Agriculture and Life Sciences. http://www.re-aim.hnfe.vt.edu/about_re-aim/what_is_re-aim/index.html. Accessed January 15, 2016.
3. Measures and checklists: RE-AIM planning tool and adaptation. Virginia Tech College of Agriculture and Life Sciences. http://www.re-aim.hnfe.vt.edu/resources_and_tools/measures/planningtool.pdf. Accessed January 15, 2016.
4. Noar, SM, Benac CN, Melissa SH. Does tailoring matter? Meta-analytic review of tailored print health behavior change interventions. *Psychol Bull.* 2007;133(4):673-693. http://dx.doi.org/10.1037/0033-2909.133.4.673.
5. Snyder LB, Hamilton MA, Mitchell EW, Kiwanuka-Tondo J, Fleming-Milici F, Proctor D. A meta-analysis of the effect of mediated health communication campaigns on behavior change in the United States. *J Health Commun.* 2004; 9(suppl1):71-96. http://doi.org/10.1080/10810730490271548.
6. Content strategy basics. Usability.gov. March 14, 2012. www.usability.gov/what-and-why/content-strategy.html. Accessed January 15, 2016.
7. Rach M. Brain Traffic blog [Internet]. From the archive: Brain Traffic lands the quad. July 5, 2012. http://blog.braintraffic.com/2012/07/from-the-archive-brain-traffic-lands-the-quad/. Accessed February 7, 2016.
8. Wilson R, Gaines J, Hill R. Neuromarketing and consumer free will. *J Consumer Affairs.* 2008;42(3):389-410.

Appendix 11

Campaign to Sustain Hand-Washing Behaviors in an Urban Informal Settlement in Kenya

Renée A. Botta, PhD; Kelly Fenson-Hood, MAD; Leah Scandurra, MA; and **Rina Muasya, MA candidate**

▶ Introduction and Problem Definition

Diarrhea kills an estimated 1.5 million young children globally every year,[1] and it is the leading cause of child mortality in Africa, resulting in an estimated 19% of child deaths.[2] In systematic reviews of hand washing studies conducted from 1990 to 2013, Freeman and colleagues concluded that hand washing with soap reduces diarrhea by 40%.[3] Cairncross et al. concluded that hand washing with soap reduces severe diarrheal outcomes by 48%.[4] Greenland, Cairncross, Cumming, and Curtis estimated that proper hand washing could prevent 607,000 deaths annually from diarrhea and pneumonia among children aged 1 to 5 years.[5] Although hand-washing campaigns have been successful at improving hand-washing behaviors, sustaining those changes over time has proved difficult.[6]

Hand washing with soap is a cost-effective method to prevent diarrhea; thus, it is appropriate to focus a prevention intervention on sustaining proper hand washing behaviors. Among Kenyan children younger than age 5 years, 2008 data indicate that death from diarrheal disease was the leading cause of mortality, accounting for 21% of deaths among children ≤5 years.[7] Informal settlements in the urban areas of Kenya are rife with poor sanitation and hygiene, causing urban children to die at a rate more than twice that for rural children.[7] The packed living circumstances of an estimated 500,000 or more people living within one square mile in what is colloquially known as a "slum" makes proper hygiene challenging.

We chose a community deep inside one of these settlements to implement a hygiene campaign as part of a larger Water, Sanitation, and Hygiene (WASH) program designed to reduce diarrheal disease. This case study focuses on the campaign to increase, improve, and sustain hand hygiene. A participatory communication framework in which key stakeholders were involved in the development, implementation, and evaluation of the campaign was used to improve the sustainability of the campaign.

Given the high incidence of diarrhea and preventable deaths due to diarrhea, and the well-established connection between proper hand hygiene and reduction in diarrhea-related deaths, this campaign sought to increase knowledge about and proper use of hand hygiene guidelines. To improve outcomes, the campaign focused on more than just the benefits of hand washing. Specifically, hand hygiene guidelines were introduced that included proper technique, amount of time needed to wash with soap, and key times to wash with soap.

▶ Campaign Goals

The goals for this campaign focused on the following:

- Collaborate with the community on hand hygiene solutions
- Develop community collaboration for hygiene training

This campaign was funded by grants from the University of Denver and the Rotary Club of Denver Southeast.

- Increase knowledge of hand hygiene guidelines within the community
- Increase frequency of proper hand hygiene practices within the community
- Increase the sustainability of hand-washing behavior change within the community

▶ Behavior Change Theories Used in the Development of the Campaign

The development of the campaign was based on the Theory of Planned Behavior (TPB),[8] which seeks to explain how and why behavior change occurs by focusing on a set of key beliefs related to the desired behavior that, as a set, predict intentions to perform the behavior. By increasing positive attitudes, subjective norms and perceived control about a particular behavior, TPB predicts there will be a subsequent increase in the intention to perform that behavior, which will lead to the adoption of the behavior.[8,9] Attitudes about the behavior follow from beliefs about the behavior's likely consequences. Subjective norms follow from normative expectations from important others about performing the behavior. Perceived behavioral control follows from the presence of factors that control behavioral performance.

How important others see the behavior constitutes normative beliefs. For example, do those important to the target audience believe hand washing is a good idea? Do they use proper hand-washing techniques? How motivated is the target audience to comply with these important other's beliefs about proper hand washing?

Control beliefs are the extent to which the target audience believes the issue is within their control, that they can properly wash their hands in spite of whatever barriers to hand washing they may encounter. Other theorists and behavior change specialists use a similar concept called self-efficacy, which has been defined as the confidence in one's own ability to carry out a behavior.

Behavioral beliefs are target audience attitudes about the behavior and its outcomes. For example, what do they get in return for the desired behavior? These can be positive or negative attitudes. For example, they could believe proper hand washing reduces diarrhea, which is positive, or they could believe proper hand washing wastes precious water, which is negative.

TPB suggests that if control beliefs, behavioral beliefs, and normative beliefs are all positive, the target audience should have a positive intention to perform the behavior—in this case, proper hand washing. In turn, these increased intentions are expected to lead to increased performance of the behavior. Thus, if we can establish positive normative expectations, obtain positive outcome evaluations, and reduce barriers to practicing hand hygiene, then we should be able to increase hand hygiene practices within the community.

▶ Formative Research

Focus groups and household surveys were conducted to better understand individual knowledge, normative beliefs, behavioral beliefs, control beliefs, barriers to hand washing with soap, and common practices within the community. A random sample of community households was chosen for baseline surveys to learn where the target audience stood relative to the theoretical underpinnings of the campaign and to more generally understand what they knew about proper hand washing techniques and what were their existing attitudes and practices toward them. We also gathered information on perceived health of family members, as well as diarrhea symptoms and frequency. We completed 210 surveys and conducted 15 focus groups, with 4 to 8 people participating in each focus group.

The formative research indicated that some knowledge of hand washing existed in the community, although knowledge of proper hand-washing guidelines (techniques, frequency, key times to wash) was scant. The frequency of hand washing varied, with the frequency of proper hand washing at most of the key times being least frequent.

Of the families surveyed, 58% had children younger than the age of 5 years. Of these, 86% reported their children experienced diarrhea at least some of the time. Of the 35% of families that had children aged 5 to 18 years, 70% reported their children experienced diarrhea at least some of the time. Only 28% of households with children reported that it was easy to keep their children free from diarrhea. Diarrhea was indeed a problem in this community.

We then sought to learn what community members knew about proper hand hygiene and its role in the reduction of diarrhea. Knowledge of the connection between poor hygiene and diarrhea was scant, as was knowledge of the ways that proper hygiene can prevent diarrhea. Knowledge of the proper times to wash hands with soap was also mostly limited to two key times: after toileting and before eating.

Of those surveyed, when asked when are the proper times to wash hands with soap:

- 97% said after using the toilet.
- 62% said before eating.
- 35% said before cooking.
- 14% said after changing a baby's diaper.
- 12% said after shaking hands with someone.
- 10% said after eating.

No one mentioned all six of these times, 4% mentioned five of the six times, 6% mentioned four of these times, 32% mentioned three of these times, 35% mentioned two of these times, and 22% mentioned only one of these times.

As for knowing the amount of time to wash with soap (20 seconds), only 25% were correct.

When survey respondents were asked to demonstrate proper hand washing, 33% demonstrated the appropriate technique for doing so.

Although 30% reported using soap most of the time to wash their hands, when asked more specifically about the better-known key times for using soap, the percentages increased. For example, 44% reported using soap most of the time when washing hands after using the toilet in the past week, and 42% reported using soap most of the time when washing hands before cooking in the past week.

Self-reported data for hand washing, however, are known to be overestimated;[10] thus people's estimates of others' washing habits may be more reliable. Also, because normative beliefs and expectations are an important factor in behavior change in the TPB, norms perceptions were queried.

Only 21% said that it was a norm in the community to wash hands with soap after using the toilet. Only 15% thought that it was a norm in the community to wash hands with soap before cooking.

TPB also suggests that intentions are a good predictor of behavior. When asked about intentions, 36% reported intending to wash their hands with soap before they ate in the next week, and 31% reported intending to wash their hands with soap after using the toilet in the next week.

Focus group discussions also revealed that as a collectivistic culture, the community would respond better to hand hygiene communications using "we" rather than "I" terminology. Relatedly, a sense of collective efficacy (in addition to self-efficacy) was found to be important, indicating the campaign needed to recognize community barriers to action as much as individual barriers to practicing proper hygiene.

Importantly, the formative research also revealed that people were at ease with talking about these issues.

To sum up, focus group and household survey research revealed that diarrhea was a problem in the community that community members thought was important to solve. Community members wanted solutions to barriers and believed improved behavioral control through the reduction of barriers would result in increased hand hygiene in the community. Before the campaign began, it appeared that community members were (1) low on normative expectations, (2) low on efficacy due to the cost barriers for soap and a lack of hand washing stations, (3) low on knowledge about the connection between hand hygiene and diarrhea reduction and (4) low on key knowledge about hand hygiene generally. Thus, many did not have the necessary knowledge or the belief system suggested by TPB (normative, control, and behavioral beliefs) to practice proper hand hygiene.

▶ Campaign Objectives

The formative research informed the development of campaign objectives. We learned that: people in the community were not well enough aware of the proper hand-washing guidelines, they were not educated about the proper hand-washing guidelines, not enough people in the community were practicing the proper hand-washing guidelines, and community members had a number of barriers for doing so. We also learned that people in the community were very interested to learn more about hand washing and to work as a community to decrease diarrhea by increasing proper hand washing.

Soon it became apparent that the norms in the community were not supportive of proper hand washing due to a lack of knowledge about the guidelines and because of barriers to obtaining affordable soap. The soap barrier, of course, also meant that people's control beliefs were not in support of the proper hand washing guidelines. Community members said they could not always wash their hands with soap because they could not afford to do so and because they did not always have access to a place to do so. In addition to being low on normative beliefs and control beliefs, community members demonstrated a combination of positive and negative attitudes toward the behavior, meaning mixed results for the behavioral beliefs. It was not surprising that people in the community were not practicing the hand-washing guidelines. It was also apparent that the lack of affordable soap was a barrier we would have to overcome if we wanted to have a successful campaign.

Ultimately, the campaign objectives for this community in the first six months were as follows:

- Increase awareness of, and knowledge about, hand hygiene guidelines by 50%
- Increase proper hand hygiene intentions by 25%
- Increase frequency of hand washing with soap by 15%
- Increase frequency of hand washing with soap at five key times by 10%
- Increase application of hand hygiene guidelines to hand-washing behaviors by 25%
- Increase efficacy for keeping children free from diarrhea by 25%
- Mobilize all 100 community health workers to conduct 100 community trainings

If we can help the community to sustain this campaign on its own, then the percentages will increase over time, rather than decrease as has been the case in previous interventions.

▶ Campaign Description and Methodology

Train-the-trainer sessions were conducted with community health workers and focused on hygiene KAP (knowledge, attitudes, practices) and health behavior change activities. Health messages and communications reinforced this training.

We worked with Kenya's Ministry of Health (MOH) to develop the training. MOH chose 10 of its community health education workers to participate in a week-long workshop in which we developed the training, which was designed to operate in an interactive and small-group format. A key tool involved in completing the training was a set of picture cards created by a local artist utilizing local visual cues about situations and behaviors within the community. Each set contained 50 cards to allow for a variety of responses to the various training cues. Activities were structured using the drawings, creating stories, and group discussions. We also created hygiene manuals for the trainers, which were written in English and in Kiswahili. Our head trainer was Kenyan and, therefore, fluent in Kiswahili; this individual was helpful not just in translating the manual, but also in making sure it was culturally appropriate.

According to Tufte and Mefalopulos, "Public participation is based on the belief that those who are affected by a decision have a right to be involved in the decision-making process. Public participation is the process by which an organization consults with interested or affected individuals, organizations, and government entities before making a decision. Public participation is two-way communication and collaborative problem solving with the goal of achieving better and more acceptable decisions."[11] They argue that participatory communication strategies are more likely to result in (1) increased feelings of ownership of a problem and a commitment to do something about it; (2) improvement of competencies and capacities required to engage with the defined development problem; and (3) actual influence on institutions that can affect an individual or community. Participatory communication emphasizes involving the stakeholders in the development process and the process of determining outcomes, rather than imposing pre-established (i.e., already decided by external actors) outcomes and processes.[11] "It requires academic members to become part of the community and community members to become part of the research team, thereby creating a unique working and learning environment before, during, and after the research."[11]

An advantage of participatory communication is that it benefits from four (rather than one) quadrants of knowledge in building communication campaigns. The Johari Window, proposed by Joseph Luft and Harry Ingham, and described by Tufte and Mefalopulos,[11] suggests the first quadrant involves dialogue based on the common knowledge shared by all parties; the second quadrant represents knowledge of the local players who have a stake in the campaign, and which is not known by the outside experts; and the third quadrant is knowledge from the outside experts that is shared with local stakeholders. The final quadrant represents that which is unknown to both groups. At this point, the knowledge, experiences, and skills of key stakeholders and campaign developers come together to develop the most appropriate options and solutions that will lead to the desired change.

When the team of outside academic experts and local MOH experts had completed the development of the hygiene training, a manual was written in both English and Kiswahili to facilitate a simpler process in conducting the trainings. The hygiene training consisted of five steps, each of which included two or more group activities.

The first step was problem identification, in which groups talked about diarrhea-related health problems in the community and discuss potential solutions to those health problems. The purpose of the first activity was to enable the community health workers to identify important diarrhea-related issues and problems in their community. The purpose of the second activity was to enable the community health worker participants to identify methods for solving diarrhea-related issues and problems facing their community.

The second step in the training, problem analysis, consisted of two hand hygiene activities. This step also included a safe water activity and sanitation practices activity, which were part of the larger project rather than the focus of this case study about hand hygiene. These activities were designed to enable the community health worker participants to closely examine common hygiene practices. Through this examination, participants identified normative practices in the community, discussed how practices might be good or bad for health, and enumerated the advantages and disadvantages of each practice.

In the first activity of this step, the community health workers discussed what they believed constituted all kinds of good and bad hygiene behaviors. In the second activity, they discussed hand hygiene more specifically; in the third activity, they discussed safe water use; and in the fourth activity, they discussed community sanitation practices.

The third step, planning for solutions, included an activity focused on identifying the spread of disease, an activity in which the community health worker participants discussed blocking the spread of disease, an activity focused on barriers to blocking the spread of disease, and an activity in which they discussed ways to overcome those barriers. These activities were focused on their community, how they saw disease being spread within their community, potential ways to block the spread of disease within their community, and recognizing and finding solutions for the barriers people in their community faced for stopping the spread of diarrheal disease. Participants analyzed the effectiveness of behaviors that block disease transmission and discussed how easy or difficult the behaviors were to practice in their daily lives in their community.

The final activity in this step was making hygiene messages. It was meant to help participants identify how to introduce, encourage, and reinforce positive hygiene behaviors in the community. Groups developed songs that incorporated hand hygiene guidelines, and they created posters using local artist renditions to spread the word about hand hygiene, safe water practices, and hygienic sanitation practices. For this case study, we have included examples of the posters created for hand hygiene. The community health worker participants created hygiene posters by thinking through what they would say to others to help motivate and remind them to practice good hygiene behaviors. They were given a set of large posters with locally drawn pictures that corresponded to hygiene in the community. Groups chose the pictures they thought would work best for posters and they requested additional pictures they would like to see drawn. Finally, they wrote their messages on them. The messages were then placed on the pictures via computer program and returned to the community health workers to serve as hygiene promotion posters displayed in the community for the remainder of the campaign.

Step four involved demonstrating hygiene guidelines and practices. There were four main purposes of this step. The first was hand and water hygiene education. The second was to work with participants in making their own portable hand washing station, known as a leaky tin. The third was to work with participants to make their own safe water storage containers and demonstrate water purification techniques. The last was to reduce the cost barrier for hand washing with soap by teaching participants how to make liquid soap at a cost significantly cheaper than bar soap.

Step five involved planning for change, as the community health worker participants developed their own single-day trainings and discussed and practiced peer education, motivational interviewing, and role playing. They were encouraged to use these communication techniques during their own training.

▶ Materials Used in the Campaign

Posters
Hand washing songs
Key messages
Training manuals

Communication Strategies

A participatory communication framework was used to create and conduct train-the-trainer sessions with community health workers.

Use of locally designed and context specific hygiene images in:

- Hygiene training workshops
- Posters

Use of key messages in:

- Hygiene training workshops
- Posters
- Hand washing songs

Examples of Some Key Messages

- We wash with soap every time. (*Sisi uosha mikono kwa sabuni kila mara.*)
- We protect our families from diarrhea. *(Sisi hulinda familia zetu lutokana na ugonjwa wa kuhara.)*
- Washing hands with soap prevents diarrhea. (*Kuosha mikono kwa sabuni huzuia ugojwa wa kuhara.*)
- Washing hands with soap is easy; use liquid soap. (*Kuosha mikono kwa sabuni ni rahisi; tumia sabuni ya maji.*)
- Ready to eat? Don't forget to wash your hands with soap. (*Uko tayari kula chakula? Usisahau kuosha mikono kwa sabuni.*)
- Don't forget to use soap after the toilet. (*Usisahau kutumia sabuni baada ya kutumia choo.*)

▶ Campaign Implementation

Next, the campaign was implemented. The training took place in three phases. In the first phase, we worked with MOH officials to develop the training; in the second phase, we worked with the MOH officials to train community health workers in the community (who were also community members). In the third phase, community health workers trained lay community members.

With the cooperation of the community and the Ministry of Health, 100 community health workers were brought together to be trained over 5 days in a church in the community. The lead facilitator, a Kenyan with a bachelor's degree in public health from a Kenyan university, worked as a part of the campaign development team. Her role was to lead the larger group and answer questions for the co-facilitators. She began each step of the training with a group discussion among the 100 community health workers and the 10 health education experts from the Ministry of Health. The 10 smaller groups, led by the MOH workers, would then complete an activity, after which the group as a whole would come back together.

After completing their own training, the community health workers led trainings in the community. They gathered groups of four to eight people and trained them in one day. They also sold the less expensive homemade liquid soap in the community as they went around doing their normal community health worker duties, reducing the soap cost barrier.

One weakness that was revealed during the implementation of the campaign was that it soon became apparent that some of the community health workers were more motivated and conducted more trainings than others. This also meant that some areas of the community had more frequent access to trainings. This limitation will be discussed more in the conclusions and lessons learned sections.

▶ Evaluation

We evaluated the effectiveness of the campaign through 211 random household post-test surveys collected in the community, which were compared with the results of the household surveys conducted before the start of the campaign. Survey interviews were conducted orally in the local language.

Evaluation for each objective:

1. *Increase awareness of and knowledge about hand hygiene guidelines by 50% in the community within 6 months of starting the campaign.* Community members increased knowledge of the key times to wash hands during the campaign. The four that were least known before the campaign increased by at least 50% and in some cases by as much as 100%. Of the two that were best known prior to the campaign, washing hands after using the toilet was already at 97% and stayed there. Knowledge of washing hands before eating jumped from 62% before the campaign to 80% after the campaign. The percentage of those who knew the correct amount of time to wash hands with soap (20 seconds) increased by 48%. Thus, the objective was successfully achieved.

2. *Increase proper hand hygiene intentions by 25% in the community within 6 months of starting the campaign.* Community members' intentions to wash their hands with soap at key times in the next week increased by 50% to 81%. Thus, the objective was successfully achieved.

3. *Increase frequency of hand washing with soap by 15% in the community within 6 months of starting the campaign.* Self-reported hand washing with soap increased by 8% during the campaign. Although this is a significant increase, it was not the amount we thought we could achieve; thus we did not accomplish this objective.

4. *Increase frequency of hand washing with soap at 5 key times by 10% in the community within 6 months of starting the campaign.* We thought that getting people to wash their hands with soap at the key times would be trickier than getting them to increase hand washing with soap in general, so we estimated a 10% increase. However, the increase of self-reported hand washing at key times actually ranged from 12% to 31%. Thus, community members reported behaviors that indicated greater increases in specific types of hand washing with soap, than with hand washing with soap in general. Future research should attempt to tease out why this disparity might occur. This objective was successfully achieved.

5. *Increase application of hand hygiene guidelines to hand washing behaviors by 25% in the community within 6 months of starting the campaign.* The number of community members who demonstrated the proper hand washing technique increased by 55%. Thus, this objective was successfully achieved.

6. *Increase efficacy for keeping children free from diarrhea by 25% in the community within 6 months of starting the campaign.* Before the campaign, 28% of people expressed positive efficacy for keeping children free from diarrhea. After the campaign, 51% of the community members surveyed expressed positive efficacy for keeping children free from diarrhea, which was an 82% relative increase. Thus, this objective was successfully achieved.

7. *Mobilize 100 community health workers in hygiene training to conduct 100 small-group community trainings within 6 months of starting the campaign.* In total, 100 community health workers were trained. They trained 145 people within the first 3 months following their own training. About half of the community health workers conducted the trainings, which fell short of the 100% objective. Also, they chose to conduct the trainings in teams of 2. The teams conducted a total of 106 community trainings within 6 months. Thus, we met the objective for number of community trainings, but with a smaller number of trainers.

▶ Conclusions

Given that we met or exceeded six of the seven objectives for the campaign, we feel that the campaign was very successful. Knowledge, efficacy, and intentions improved the most, all of which, according to TPB, should be precursors of increased behavior change. Normative beliefs did not shift during the campaign, and indeed remained quite low (15% to 21% pre-intervention and 16% to 23% post-intervention); if norms can be improved as the health workers continue conducting more trainings, then increased behavior change is likely to follow, given that the other TPB factors were in place by the completion of the campaign.

A community-based organization (CBO) has taken over and continues with the trainings, soap production and sales, and one-on-one hygiene education. This type of community buy-in should help to increase normative expectations. We will conduct further research to establish if that is the case and to see whether this type of community buy-in also increases the sustainability of the outcomes. The CBO indicated that the participatory nature of the campaign was the reason it became interested in continuing the campaign efforts.

Another indicator of the success of the campaign was evaluated outside of the list of objectives. As part of the post-test surveys, we asked whether respondents had attended a community training conducted by the health workers whom we had trained, and 15% indicated they had. Of those, 65% could recite key messages from the campaign without prompting. Another 32% correctly recalled key messages. Only one person who had attended a training could neither recall nor recite key campaign messages. Additionally, 94% said the trainings were helpful; 90% said they learned a lot; 74% said it was helpful for the community; and 79% of those with children said it was helpful to their family.

▶ Lessons Learned

■ Collaborating with multiple stakeholders is an excellent way to create buy-in and thus provides a better opportunity to sustain outcomes.

■ This campaign indicates that training based on participatory communication can create the kind of sustainable behavior change health promotion that scholars and practitioners have been trying to achieve.

■ TPB can help identify where to focus intervention efforts and may indicate areas where we fell short. A key to the next set of household surveys in the community will be looking at levels of normative expectations. Also, since the completion of the campaign, we have collaborated with the community on a hygiene festival that had broad participation and is another strategy to increase normative perceptions for hygiene behaviors.

■ Locally produced messages are memorable and relatable.

■ Not all community health workers will automatically feel motivated to conduct trainings on their own. Those interested in the income-generating activity of making and selling soap were much more motivated; they realized that increasing interest and motivation to wash hands with soap would increase soap sales and, therefore, generate more income.

■ Community members' self-reported behaviors indicated greater increases in specific types of hand washing with soap than hand washing with soap in general (12% to 31% increase versus 8% increase). Future research should attempt to tease out why this disparity might occur. Scholars have been seeking better ways to measure hand hygiene behaviors. Future campaigns should explore other methods.

References

1. World Health Organization (WHO), United Nations Children's Fund (UNICEF). *Diarrhoea: Why Children Are Still Dying and What Can Be Done*. New York, NY: UNICEF/ Geneva, Swizarland: WHO; 2009.

2. Black RE, Cousens S, Johnson HL, et al. Global, regional, and national causes of child mortality in 2008: a systematic analysis. *Lancet*. 2010;375:1969-1987.

3. Freeman MC, Stocks ME, Cumming O, et al. Systematic review: hygiene and health: systematic review of handwashing practices worldwide and update of health effects. *Trop Med Int Health*. 2014;19(8):906-916.

4. Cairncross S, Hunt C, Boisson S, et al. Water, sanitation and hygiene for the prevention of diarrhoea. *Int J Epidemiol*. 2010;39(suppl 1):i193-i205.

5. Greenland K, Cairncross S, Cumming O, Curtis V. Can we afford to overlook hand hygiene again? *Trop Med Int Health*. 2013;18:246-249.

6. Davis J, Pickering AJ, Rogers K, Mamuya S, Boehm AB. The effects of informational interventions on household water management, hygiene behaviors, stored drinking water quality, and hand contamination in peri-urban Tanzania. *Am J Trop Med Hygiene*. 2011;84(2):184-191.

7. World Health Organization. World health statistics 2010. 2010. http://www.who.int/whosis/whostat/2010/en/index.html. Accessed November 10, 2010.

8. Ajzen I. The theory of planned behavior. *Org Behav Hum Decision Proc*. 1991;50(2):179-211.

9. Ajzen I. The theory of planned behavior. In: Lange PAM, Kruglanski AW, Higgins ET, eds. *Handbook of Theories of Social Psychology*, Vol. 1. London, UK: Sage; 2012:438-459.

10. Ram P. *Practical Guidance for Measuring Handwashing Behavior: 2013 Update. Water and Sanitation Program*. Washington, DC: World Bank Publications; 2013.

11. Tufte T, Mefalopulos P. *Participatory Communication: A Practical Guide*. Washington, DC: World Bank Publications; 2009.

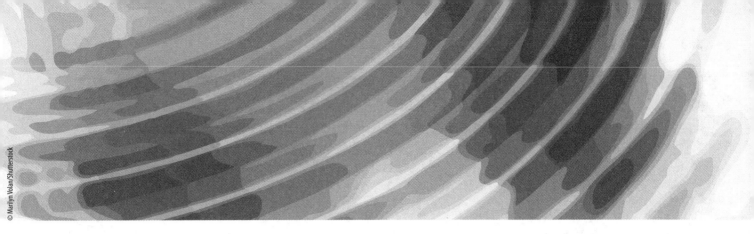

CHAPTER 12

Evaluating a Health Communication Program

May Grabbe Kennedy and **Jonathan DeShazo**

LEARNING OBJECTIVES

By the end of this chapter, the reader will be able to:

- Ask the central evaluation questions.
- Understand the role of evaluation frameworks.
- Identify the major communication program evaluation designs.
- List some issues to consider in evaluating interventions that use e-channels.
- Find e-health and other evaluation resources.

▶ Introduction

"Efficiency is concerned with doing things right. Effectiveness is doing the right things."

—Peter F. Drucker, 1973[1]

Program evaluation is too often a dreaded, funder-required procedure with a fixed deadline for an up-or-down verdict on the value or merit of a program. Such an assessment is essential when a program represents a heavy financial investment and has the potential to be a model for future projects. In other circumstances, evaluation is an iterative process designed to improve a particular program over time. Either way, evaluation is a balancing act. Typically, there are more questions about a program than can be answered convincingly with available resources. On top of that, various stakeholders have very different evaluation priorities. This chapter discusses some of the key tasks and trade-offs (**BOX 12-1**) in an evaluation study in a communication context.

The very use of the term "program evaluation" can be problematic, because a distinction has been drawn between program evaluation and research (e.g., in federal law, CFR 45, Part 46, on institutional review board [IRB] requirements). **BOX 12-2** lists some differences between research and evaluation. In practice, the methods of rigorously conducted program evaluation overlap with those of program operations research and intervention research. Be flexible about terminology, strive for the greatest rigor possible in a given set of circumstances, and

BOX 12-1 Competing Evaluation Considerations

To achieve this…	You might have to sacrifice this (and vice versa)…
The outcomes measured are the ones that program decision makers and other stakeholders believe and care most about.	Findings can be compared directly to those of studies of other programs that addressed the same health issue.
Evaluation questions and measures are informed by the detailed knowledge that program insiders have.	The evaluation is designed by an objective, external entity and satisfies accountability standards for large, high-profile programs.
Measures of knowledge, attitudes, and other psychological determinants of health behavior use valid and reliable (often multi-item) scales.	Measures of determinants are kept short to preserve respondents' goodwill.
Adequate time is taken to refine a study design, get it approved, implement procedures with care, analyze results methodically, and get peer review of reports.	Evaluation results are available in time to inform key program decisions.
Effects of each program component are assessed for each target audience of interest.	Evaluation stays within the limits of its finite resources.
The study design is strong, with minimal threats to validity and causal inference.	Evaluation is feasible practically, politically, and ethically.

For a more extended discussion of trade-offs, see Shadish WR, Cook TD, Leviton LC. *Foundations of Program Evaluation: Theories of Practice.* Newbury Park, CA: Sage; 1991.

BOX 12-2 Differences Between Program Evaluation and Research

Program Evaluation	Research
Intended to inform program decision makers	Intended to produce generalizable knowledge
Uses theory to test programs	Sometimes just tests theory
Emphasizes usefulness of findings	Emphasizes study design rigor
Sometimes exempt from institutional review board (IRB) review for ethical treatment of human subjects	Always subject to at least expedited IRB review when data are collected from program participants
Usually allocates a larger share of available resources to the program	Usually allocates a larger share of available resources to the study
Program activities are more likely to continue after the study	Program activities (e.g., research project) are less likely to continue after the study
Is conducted in a natural field setting	May be conducted in either a controlled, laboratory setting or a field setting
May put heavy weight on participant satisfaction with the program and unintended consequences of the program	Often ignores participant satisfaction or unintended consequences

Levin-Ronzalis, M. Evaluation and research: Differences and similarities. *Can J Program* Eval. 2003; 18(2):1-31.

build ethical review into your timeline if your study involves human subjects.

The process of understanding how and how well a health communication program works often is divided into **formative** (or pre-testing), **process** (or implementation monitoring), and **outcome** (or summative) evaluation phases. The first two phases are examined in depth elsewhere in this text. This chapter emphasizes outcome evaluation.

The *main task* of outcome evaluation in a health communication context is to *test for a connection between exposure* to messages that a program disseminates *and desired outcomes* of such exposure. That sounds straightforward enough, but understanding and measuring message exposure and its outcomes can be challenging, especially in today's rapidly evolving media environment. Moreover, the typical design of a health communication evaluation study is correlational, and does not warrant strong statements made about cause and effect.

▶ Three Central Evaluation Questions

Evaluating a health communication program can get very technical, but it boils down to answering three questions:[2]

- Outcome: *Are you doing the right things?*
- Implementation: *Are you doing them right?*
- Impact: *Are you doing enough of them make a difference?*

Doing the Right Things?

Long before a program or campaign is launched, you can take several steps to increase the likelihood that the effort heads in the right direction. One step is to conduct audience and other formative research, as described in other chapters. In addition, three forms of the "right things" question should be asked:

Is there empirical "proof of concept" from a well-conducted prior study?

While it is exciting to do something brand new, when planning a new intervention it is usually best to adopt or adapt existing intervention strategies that have established **efficacy**. Program procedures are considered efficacious if there is convincing evidence that they brought about a desired change under tightly controlled conditions.[3] **BOX 12-3** provides links to some databases of such evidence-based interventions. Even if an efficacious model is used, however, it is likely that some local evaluation will still be needed. It is important to establish that the **effectiveness** of a model program was retained when it was replicated under real-world conditions.[3]

Unfortunately, the results of most health communication program evaluations are never published, much less find their way into databases of effective programs.[4] To select the "right things" for your intervention, it may be necessary to contact staff from respected programs that are similar to yours and find out what worked for them.

BOX 12-3   Examples of Evidence-Based Strategy Databases

All Health Topics

- The Guide to Community Preventive Services: http://www.thecommunityguide.org/index.html
- The Cochran Collaboration systematic reviews of health research: http://www.cochrane.org
- The Campbell Collaboration systematic reviews of research on social and educational programs that can be relevant to social determinants of disease: http://www.campbellcollaboration.org

Specific Health Topics

- Substance Abuse and Mental Health Services Administration's National Registry of Evidence-Based Programs and Practices in mental health and substance abuse: http://nrepp.samhsa.gov
- National Cancer Institute's Research-Tested Intervention Programs: http://rtips.cancer.gov/rtips/index.do
- Centers for Disease Control and Prevention's Compendium of Evidence-Based Interventions and Best Practices for HIV Prevention: http://www.cdc.gov/hiv/prevention/research/compendium/index.html
- World Health Organization's e-library of evidence for Nutrition Actions: http://www.who.int/elena/en

See *The Community Tool Box Database of Best Practices* (http://ctb.ku.edu/en/databases-best-practices) for other databases.

Does the program plan specify how its objectives will be met in a theoretically plausible manner?

Before an evaluation study begins, the evaluator and program decision makers should review a draft of the program logic model to clarify inputs, outputs, and outcomes. Revisions should be made until all components of the logic model and their respective measures are acceptable from both perspectives. Often, good program logic models incorporate theoretical determinants of behavior change (e.g., knowledge, self-efficacy, or perceived social support) as short-term outcomes. In fact, many efficacious model programs consider a focus on theoretical determinants to be a **core element**—an essential driver of behavior change that must be preserved when a model program is adapted to fit local needs.[5] When an evaluator is the only health scientist on a program team, part of his or her role is to ensure that the logic model is theoretically sound. This input is required early in the planning process.

Are program procedures acceptable to the local community?

A local community review or advisory board may already exist. If so, explore proposed program concepts, procedures, and materials with its members. If no such body exists, look for a local program that set a procedural precedent, and for an alternative source of community feedback.

In part, community acceptance may rest upon whether the proposed communication channels reach *only* the intended audience. For example, an edgy sexually transmitted disease (STD) prevention campaign that posted messages in gay chat rooms could be acceptable, while the same attention-grabbing treatment could be offensive in radio ads broadcast to general audiences. A word to the wise: Consult the community *before* program funds are spent to produce campaign materials.

Doing the Right Things Right?

This question is really about careful program implementation, and it is never answered once and for all. Periodic collection of implementation data to verify that activities remain true to the initial program plan is called **fidelity monitoring**, and this kind of process evaluation is a necessary aspect of ongoing quality control (see phases 5 and 6 of

the *Social Marketing Edition of CDCynergy*).[2] In contrast, outcome evaluation (1) requires definite beginning and ending points so that data sets can be assembled for analysis and (2) may be optional if an evidence-based model is replicated and resources are scarce.

Evaluators and program planners need to work together to find ways to build fidelity into the structure of a health communication program; **BOX 12-4** offers some ideas on "fidelity by design." Then evaluators and program staff can work jointly to select the fidelity monitoring processes that will become standard operating procedure.

For a media-based program, fidelity data should be available from the media outlets themselves, or from website analytics reports[6] or third-party tracking services.[7] These data normally consist of lists of media placements and estimates of the number of impressions the placed messages created. In contrast, when you use interpersonal channels to get your health message across, you really must observe the program in action from time to time. One way is to drop by unannounced with a checklist to rate program conformity with a standard protocol.[3] Of course, you should explain the reason for the drop-by observations to program delivery staff in advance.

When fidelity monitoring detects drift from the original program plan, the reasons for the drift can be identified and appropriate corrective action can be taken. Fidelity data also can be helpful in interpreting outcome evaluation findings. Negative outcome evaluation results could mean that a program was based on a bad plan. An alternative explanation is that

---

BOX 12-4 Building Fidelity into a Program

- Automate, script, or otherwise "hard-code" core procedures where possible.
- Ensure that successive generations of creative ideas for a campaign are essentially consistent with the original creative brief.
- Offer both initial staff training and periodic "booster" training.
- Solicit staff concerns about program procedures so that they can be addressed in a uniform fashion that avoids undercutting the core elements of the program.

Adapted from: DHHS, Fidelity Monitoring Tip Sheet, Family and Youth Services Bureau, online at www.acf.hhs.gov/sites/default/files/fysb/prep-fidelity-monitoring-ts.pdf.

the negative results reflected a failure to implement a program as planned. The only way to know which explanation fits best is to monitor procedural fidelity during the study period.

Doing Enough of the Right Things to Make a Difference?

The last central evaluation question has two levels. On a practical level, the "difference" in question should be a behavior change that is explicit in an *a priori* program objective (see the section on SMART[ER] objectives later in this chapter). At a broader level, the "enough right things to make a difference" question asks whether a program changed enough risk behavior in enough people to have had an actual impact on overall rates of a disease or health problem.

Making Enough Noise, and Capturing Any Difference It Made

Doing "enough of the right things" means *exposing enough audience members* to a message to be able to detect a prespecified difference by using a planned evaluation procedure. In a review of the health campaign evaluation literature, Robert Hornik found that most campaigns that fail were not ill conceived, but rather were mounted on too small a scale.[8] In other words, those unsuccessful campaigns made insufficient "program noise" to break through the "background noise" from other health messages (often from less than credible sources) and the other distractions of everyday life.

Sample size is the other side of the effect detection "coin." Sample size is a major factor in statistical power—the ability to detect a program effect when it is actually present. An adequately powered study obtains data from enough audience members to detect program outcomes of at least a prespecified size using a particular statistical test, while taking other factors into account. The other major factors that feed into the power equation are audience diversity on the key outcome measure prior to the campaign, and the expected intensity of audience reactions to the campaign message. Note that the power calculation can be quite complicated. Although "fill-in-the-blanks" power calculators are available online, consulting with a statistician to set program and evaluation study participation targets in advance can be a sensible investment of program funds. No study should miss an opportunity to detect a real effect because of inadequate statistical power.

A common mistake is to "power" a study (i.e., estimate the number of participants needed) without considering (1) the likely loss of effect size at each stage in a chain of outcomes or (2) the inevitable participant attrition at each of a series of repeated measures. The latter oversight is well illustrated by an evaluation of *Change4Life*, a national mass-media campaign in England that attempted to prevent childhood obesity by changing parenting practices. At baseline, 3774 families with 5- to 11-year-old children were recruited into a study of the effects of supplementary print campaign materials. The 1829 families assigned to the intervention group received either a personalized mailing about their child's eating and activity (if they had returned an initial questionnaire) or a generic mailing (if they had not returned the questionnaire). Only 98 families returned the questionnaire and only 3 families remained in the no-mailing control group until the end of the study, so the study had insufficient power to detect differences in parenting practices related to personalized mailings.[9]

Differences That Make a Difference

Be prepared for program planners and stakeholders to have unrealistically high expectations about the ability of a single program to bring about a detectable, positive change in health risk behavior prevalence, community disease rates, or other health outcome measures. Arguments that even very large and unusually well-funded programs had a measurable disease impact often rest on complex mathematical models. State-of-the-art models are well beyond the scope of most program evaluations, and even the most sophisticated ones are often based on debatable assumptions. **BOX 12-5** identifies program impact modeling challenges, and the *VERB* campaign[10] and Box 12-12 later in this chapter offer examples of modeling efforts.

Negotiate a "success bar" of measured health behavior change in enough target audience members to matter to local program stakeholders. Ideally, the cumulative effects of sound behavior-change programs and other factors (e.g., institutional and governmental policy changes) will lower rates of the health problem of interest. For example, efforts directed against tobacco use have collectively lowered the incidence of smoking-related diseases in the United States.[11]

BOX 12-5 A First Look at Program Impact Modeling Challenges

- Models simplify reality. Meanwhile, an individual's health behavior can have a variety of influences, and disease trends are affected by a host of factors beyond just individual health behaviors.[1]
- Behavior change prompted by a program can be real and widespread, but short-lived.[2]
- Permanent behavior change can take years to be reflected in disease statistics.[3]

References

1. Garnett GP. An introduction to mathematical models in sexually transmitted disease epidemiology. *Sex Trans Infect*. 2002;78:7-12.
2. Marcus BH, Forsyth LH, Stone EJ, et al. Physical activity behavior change: issues in adoption and maintenance. *Health Psychol*. 2000;19(1 suppl):32-41.
3. Kaplan RM. Behavioral epidemiology. In: Suls JM, Davidson KW, Kaplan RM, eds. *Handbook of Health Psychology and Behavioral Medicine*. New York, NY: Guilford Press; 2011:203-216.

▶ Capturing the Basics

Program Exposure

Assessing exposure to a health message turns out to be more complicated than just asking audience members whether they heard the message. Moreover, when the communication program or campaign uses multiple channels to get a message across, the evaluator is faced with some major decisions, which are discussed next.

Exposure Complexities

Exposure to a communication program's message can be conceptualized as a process, rather than as an event. This process can include being in the physical presence of a communication product, noticing it, understanding and believing the message the product is intended to convey, and remembering the product and message over time.

Exposure is also influenced by audience expectations about channel-specific content and features, such as interactivity. For example, a single e-health game play on a mobile device is expected to take two minutes or less, whereas desktop game plays (although likely to be less frequent) are tolerated for longer periods. Unlike skill games that players expect to enjoy repeatedly, a narrative e-health game wears out quickly, suggesting a trade-off between message

repetition and message "stickiness." In addition, many recipients now expect to be able to add their own comments to the e-messages originally sent by health agencies, and then to be able to forward the expanded content to their network members, introducing peer influences on exposure that are not fully understood.

Measures of exposure should attempt to capture this complexity; **BOX 12-6** provides some suggestions on how to measure exposure most effectively. At a minimum, both what was *sent* and (at least something about) what audience members *took away* should be assessed. To document what was sent, use multiple process measures (e.g., website clicks, time spent viewing, proportions of "click-throughs" to deeper content),[6] and then address the question about what got across by collecting audience member self-report data.

Remember that program outputs estimate exposure more accurately for some communication channels than for others. For example, physicians who deliver

---

BOX 12-6 Tips for Measuring Exposure

1. Map the pathway by which message exposure will be achieved in your program, and collect the information necessary to raise or lower exposure estimates along the message's route. For example, multiply the number of posters inside buses by the average ridership per bus during the study period, and multiply that result by the percentage of riders in a convenience sample who say they saw the ads.
2. Measure both recognition and recall of messages, slogans, and other content. Recognition will yield higher estimates because it is easier to pick an option from a list than to fill in a blank, but recognition is more vulnerable to false-positive responses.
3. Ask about exposure to any other local or national programs or campaigns that addressed your health topic during the evaluation period. Start with the health topic, and then use the campaign name.
4. Add "ringer" messages (i.e., those that were never sent) to recognition items to derive correction factors for false reporting.
5. When using web-based channels (e.g., Facebook, Twitter), include a comment box for open-ended input, and provide a link to an online questionnaire (e.g., via *Survey Monkey* or *RedCap*) to get structured/closed-ended information from audience members.

The Communication Evaluation Expert Panel, Abbatangelo J, Cole G, Kennedy MG. Guidance for evaluating mass communication health initiatives: Summary of an expert panel discussion sponsored by CDC. *Eval Health Prof*. 2007;30(3):229–253.

health messages face-to-face usually have the attention of their patients, and the "teach back" method can verify that the messages were heard and understood.[12] By contrast, the number of views of Facebook pages *containing* ads may overestimate the number of ads *noticed* by a large margin. Measures such as billboard impressions (i.e., the number of people driving by a billboard) and tweets sent should be interpreted as upper boundaries of exposure estimate ranges.

Measuring Exposure by Channel

Controversy surrounds the process of evaluating channel-specific effects in multichannel programs, especially when exposure information is self-reported. Sending *new* information through *multiple* channels has been associated with positive health program outcomes,[13] but memories of message exposure through particular channels are not very reliable. Some call this the "saw it on the radio" problem. Because individual channel effects often are synergistic by design, some have argued that it is inappropriate to evaluate their separate effects on outcomes.[7] In any event, few analyses have shown differential outcomes by broad communication approach utilized (e.g., ad campaigns versus entertainment education),[14] much less by message channel.

Nevertheless, media channels may have characteristic effects, and more information about channel-specific outcomes can help program planners make the best use of their resources.[15] Importantly, collecting self-reported channel-specific exposure information, at least by means of a checklist (e.g., heard radio ad [yes/no], saw billboard [yes/no]), allows an evaluator to construct a campaign *exposure dosage* variable. The evaluation of the Prevention Marketing Campaign demonstration site in Sacramento, California, provides a good example.[16] Dosage variables have a range of values, so they can be more sensitive than a dichotomous variable (i.e., exposed versus unexposed) to program outcomes. An evaluator could include questions about within-channel exposure (e.g., how many times a certain ad was seen) if a survey were not too long already, and if the resulting frequency estimates were taken with a big grain of salt. If the reported exposure pattern closely mirrored actual media buys and other program outputs, channel frequency weights could be incorporated into a dosage variable. However, such a weighted variable might be misleading in terms of its implied precision.

Before moving on to program outcomes, we note that the line between exposure and outcome is blurring as media become more interactive. Clicking on a hyperlink in a text message may be required for full message exposure, but it also constitutes an information-seeking activity. In turn, information-seeking can be viewed as a behavioral outcome, especially for campaigns that aim to inform instead of persuade. Additional gray areas emerge when audiences can make choices about when broadcasts are consumed, how often, and which parts are skipped and repeated.[17]

Program Outcomes
Goals and Smart(er) Objectives

An evaluation gets off on the right foot when worthwhile, sensible goals inform the program's logic model (or "theory of action"), and its products and outcomes are then translated into objectives that are SMART(ER)—that is, **S**pecific, **M**easurable, **A**chievable (in principle), **R**ealistic (for this program), **T**ime bound, **E**xtending/challenging, and **R**eviewed. "Extending" means that the program will stretch to achieve a public health impact. "Reviewed" means that draft objectives have been shared with stakeholders, and that those stakeholders' input has been incorporated. The purpose of outcome measures is to show how well the carefully crafted and vetted objectives of the program were met.

Short-Term and Longer-Term Objectives

Typically, a good evaluation plan includes both shorter-term and longer-term objectives,[18] with good (and preferably multiple) measures of the most critical ones. Measures of long-term health conditions, if possible to include at all, should be accompanied by measures of behavior that can change in the relatively near future, and well as measures of theoretical outcomes (e.g., recall, attitudes, or intentions) that can change even more quickly. **BOX 12-7** identifies some advantages of including short-term outcomes in the program plan.

Measures of Outcomes

The wording of questions about theoretical determinants of behavior matters a great deal. One good source of standard wording for questions about constructs from behavior change theories is the National Institutes of Health's (NIH) online Grid-Enabled Measures (GEM) database.[19] You should also search the scientific literature for scales and items that have been used in previous research to measure determinants of your focal health behavior, and of the behavior itself.

Some theory-based measures *progress* from questions about determinants of behavior to questions about behavior performed.[15] Such hybrid "stages of change" or behavioral readiness measures (e.g., those based on the Transtheoretical Model or the levels of McGuire's

---

BOX 12-7 Advantages of Including Short-Term Outcomes

- Program exposure and determinant change sometimes can be documented in the same data collection session, eliminating the need for the audience member to have an opportunity to perform a health behavior. This saves time and money and may help tie exposure directly to outcomes.
- Short-term determinant changes may be all you need to show if you are replicating a model program that changed those determinants and your behavioral objective.
- Reliance on short-term outcomes minimizes participant attrition.
- Short-term change in theoretical determinants helps validate correlational evidence of behavior change by showing that you understand how the behavior change came about.
- Measuring determinants can increase the number of outcomes measured, thereby increasing the odds that some measure will be sensitive to program effects.

The Communication Evaluation Expert Panel, Abbatangelo J, Cole G, Kennedy MG. Guidance for evaluating mass communication health initiatives: Summary of an expert panel discussion sponsored by CDC. *Eval Health Prof*. 2007;30(3):229–253.

---

hierarchy) can be quite sensitive to changes compelled by health communication campaigns. **BOX 12-8** suggests some advantages of using these kinds of behavioral readiness measures in program evaluation.

Cost-Effectiveness

Cost-effectiveness is not a basic evaluation topic, but discussion of it is included here because program planners and stakeholders often *request* evidence of a program's cost-effectiveness. Generating a credible cost–benefit estimate is a major undertaking that requires specialized economic expertise (e.g., see the cost analysis of the national Truth anti-tobacco campaign by Holtgrave and colleagues[20]). Furthermore, such estimates (1) are biased when start-up costs are mixed with fixed costs in new programs and (2) require data on costs and outcomes from other types of programs for purposes of comparison.

Even though a technically sound cost-effectiveness analysis would go beyond the resources of most evaluations, we still advise evaluators to collect a limited

---

BOX 12-8 Advantages of Hybrid Measures of Behavioral Readiness

- They acknowledge that behavior change does not happen all at once.
- They can capture an individual's stage in the behavior change process at which program exposure occurs.
- They give a program credit for spurring movement along the path to the ultimately desired behavior.
- They make intuitive sense to program staff and other stakeholders and are fairly easy to administer.

Glanz K. Health behavior and health education: Theory, research and practice. Ed. 4, Wiley, 2008.

---

amount of data on program expenditures. With the disclaimer that cost-effectiveness has not been estimated formally, you can present this information alongside data on the program's reach and outcomes to help improve the program now, and to contribute later to more sophisticated studies.

▶ E-Media Considerations

New E-Health Sources of Information

E-media have created a wealth of new sources of health data, ranging from physicians' notes in electronic medical records to posts in health chat rooms. From both program development and evaluation perspectives, e-media represent rich new sources of information about the characteristics and health-relevant behaviors of audience members. For example, participants in a nutrition study can now take smartphone pictures of what they eat instead of entering partial and somewhat unreliable reports of their food choices in a diary. Also, after major health events, "social listening" can reveal changes in the content of online conversations.[21] Finally, although slow to come online,[22] electronic medical records in primary care practices should add immeasurably to what we will be able to find out about health message dissemination and utilization in the future.

E-Health as a Source of New Research Questions

E-health is also a treasure trove of research topics, and real-world program evaluation findings that are relevant to e-health can validate, qualify, and extend evidence from more controlled investigations of e-health questions. One key research question is whether the effectiveness of a medium is positively associated with its degree of interactivity, as many believe. To answer this question, interactivity must be operationalized in a variety of ways and its effects tested in multiple health domains. A related—and still unresolved—question is whether interaction metrics (e.g., number of click-throughs), which are widely used by ad agencies and others as short-term outcomes, actually do predict health behavior.

E-Media Advantages and Disadvantages for Research

E-media such as social network channels and mobile apps have a number of research-specific advantages, such as their ability to reduce experimenter effects, but they also have some disadvantages for research.[23] Usability issues, for example, may interact with intervention effects. Some applications restrain user comments to 140 characters in length, or content to a subset of website information that fits on a mobile phone screen. Conversely, the extent of the qualitative content sent through e-media can be overwhelming. "Lurking" unobtrusively in the background of a message board (where there may be an expectation of privacy) can present IRB issues.[24] Invitations to participate in an online study can be seen as spam, and online survey response rates tend to be low (**BOX 12-9** identifies some ways to increase response rates for online studies). Finally, social and mobile media fail to reach a sizable proportion of many audiences,[25] and that inability can compromise sample representativeness.

BOX 12-9 Ways to Boost Response Rates in Online Studies

1. Keep the URL short and the layout sober, and emphasize the goal and importance of the study.
2. Include the name of the research organization, mention IRB approval, and state that the site is not commercial.
3. Indicate in advance how long the test takes, and provide an opportunity to comment or ask questions.
4. Offer a financial incentive.
5. If project funds allow, use large, nationally representative panels of people who have already agreed to participate in periodic web surveys.[a]

---

a Baker LC, Bundorf MK, Singer S, Wagner TH. *Validity of the Survey of Health and Internet and Knowledge Network's Panel and Sampling.* Stanford, CA: Stanford University; 2003.

Fan W, Yan Z. (2010). Factors affecting response rates of the web survey: A systematic review. Computers in human behavior, 26(2), 132-139.

▶ Study Designs

Study design is of central importance to program evaluation and any other kind of empirical inquiry. The design of a study sets limits on the conclusions that can be drawn from its results. Basic study designs are summarized here, but many variations and combinations exist. You should choose a study design for its ability to capture the types of program effects that you expect.[26,27]

Randomized Controlled Trials

Randomized controlled trials (RCTs) are defined by *random assignment* of study participants to either the treatment/intervention or the control condition. This design provides the soundest logical basis for concluding that a specific intervention caused certain effects. Unfortunately, RCTs are ill suited to detecting mass-media campaign effects that develop slowly, lag behind the campaign by an unknown period, are small in size, diffuse through social networks, result from saturating the environment with media messages, or occur primarily at an institutional policy level.[26]

BOX 12-10 lists some other challenges for performing RCTs at a community scale. Note that it may be possible to achieve sufficient exposure control to conduct an RCT if messages are disseminated for a relatively short period of time and sent to individual audience members directly. In fact, a meta-analysis found that RCTs of text-message interventions have been conducted in 13 countries, and that this type of intervention can be effective.[28]

BOX 12-10 Challenges in Performing Randomized Controlled Trials for Full-Coverage Programs with Media

- Lack of initially comparable control areas for national or other very large programs
- Prohibitive cost and analysis challenges (e.g., clustering on an unknown set of variables) when randomizing at the community level of analysis
- "Contamination" of control communities or target audiences by unintended exposure to campaign messages
- Community resistance to no-treatment control status when an intervention has face validity and the health issue is urgent
- Unpredictable activities in the control community that parallel or exceed intervention activities

---

The Communication Evaluation Expert Panel, Abbatangelo J, Cole G, Kennedy MG. Guidance for evaluating mass communication health initiatives: Summary of an expert panel discussion sponsored by CDC. *Eval Health Prof.* 2007;30(3):229–253.

Quasi-experiments

Quasi-experiments are similar to RCTs: They have both intervention conditions and comparison (not control) conditions or groups. Because assignment of participants to the conditions is not random in a quasi-experiment, preexisting groups can participate, making quasi-experiments less disruptive than RCTs to host settings such as schools and churches. Even so, when quasi-experiments are very large, they face many of the same challenges as full-coverage RCTs. The classic books by Donald Campbell and his colleagues describe the various types of quasi-experiments and the threats to the validity of causal inferences associated with these designs.[29]

In one type of quasi-experiment called an **interrupted time-series study**, the comparison condition is a period of time rather than a group of people. The outcomes of interest are measured multiple times before and after the "interruption" constituted by the program. If a significant change in the slope of an outcome trend line occurs in concert with the introduction of the program, one can infer that the program was likely to have been responsible for the change. This inference is strengthened if an analogous set of observations made in a comparison community over the same period of time show no slope discontinuity.

For evaluating national campaigns, the interrupted time-series design may be more suitable than other quasi-experimental designs, given that there is no appropriate control group or area. This design also has been used to evaluate news media outreach efforts. For example, a time-series approach was used to show that news stories mentioning breast cancer screening coincided with increases in online searches for information, but only when the stories covered the controversy surrounding the changes in the mammography guidelines in 2009.[30]

Correlational Studies

Correlational studies are the rule, rather than the exception, when evaluating programs that employ broadcast channels to reach large audiences ("full coverage" programs). This design often employs surveys to collect information on (1) program exposure as it is experienced, (2) the outcome of interest, and (3) other variables that could affect the relationship between exposure and outcomes (e.g., demographics). Regression and other multivariate analysis methods are used to control statistically for major potential confounding factors. Measures of association, such as odds ratios, are calculated to assess the statistical connection between exposure and outcomes. This kind of study is referred to as "observational" because, lacking control over program exposure, the evaluator is relegated to observing changes in outcomes that may or may not be program effects.

Some observational studies collect respondent outcome data at multiple points in time. The studies can be cross-sectional (i.e., sampling different participants at each time point), longitudinal/cohort (i.e., taking repeated measures of the same people over time), or both (e.g., when a small cohort is embedded within a larger cross-sectional study). More commonly, researchers seek to save money and preserve the anonymity of respondents by using a single-wave, cross-sectional, post-program design in which outcomes among exposed respondents are compared with those of unexposed respondents.

There may be serious threats to the validity of causal conclusions based on data drawn from single-wave, cross-sectional studies. The major threat is self-selection; in other words, there may be a preexisting propensity for participants to be exposed to a message, which in turn creates a spurious correlation between exposure and outcome. For example, a teenager already planning to start using contraception might be unusually likely to notice an ad for a family planning clinic, but she also would have been relatively likely to find the clinic without the ad. If a survey contains enough information about respondents, it is possible to control for self-selection bias (at least partially) by creating **propensity scores**. These scores can be held statistically constant in analyses, helping to rule out the possibility that people who changed were both more likely to notice a health message and already primed to change a relevant behavior.[31]

Self-selection is only one of several rival explanations for apparent associations between exposure to a program and a desired outcome. **BOX 12-11** highlights

---

BOX 12-11 Countering Threats to the Validity of Nonexperimental Study Conclusions

- Collect data from a comparison community to show that positive outcomes in the program community were not just a function of historical or "secular" trends that would have unfolded anyway, without the program.
- Include measures of exposure dosage in surveys; increases in outcomes that are significantly associated with exposure dosage help legitimize causal inferences.
- Time survey waves to be able to show that outcomes rise and fall in synchrony with campaign waves.

The Communication Evaluation Expert Panel, Abbatangelo J, Cole G, Kennedy MG. Guidance for evaluating mass communication health initiatives: Summary of an expert panel discussion sponsored by CDC. *Eval Health Prof*. 2007;30(3):229–253.

some other threats to validity that are common when correlational data are employed, and offers some suggestions for ruling out validity threats.

Sampling

Evaluations typically do not collect data from every member of a target population. Instead, the population is sampled. A sample's characteristics determine the external validity of the findings—that is, the degree to which they can be generalized to the rest of the population.

Random samples, which yield the most generalizable results, are possible only when the population has known boundaries and has been counted. Random samples may be multistage (e.g., sampling schools within districts, and then classrooms within schools), and they sometimes include quota sampling or oversampling of groups that are small but important from a public health perspective.[32] Boosting the representation of minority groups helps to detect disparate campaign effects across audience segments.

Random samples of phone numbers or addresses within specified geographic areas can be purchased from commercial vendors. Increasingly, low survey response rates are threatening the reliability of survey information collected today, but prompt/reminder procedures can boost response rates substantially, especially when used in combination with incentives.[33]

Many important public health issues affect populations that are somewhat hidden (e.g., those engaging in stigmatized or illegal behavior) and, therefore, lack the fully specified sampling frame necessary for random sampling. If there are networks of ties between members of these populations, respondent-driven sampling[34] or some other variant of snowball sampling (i.e., asking known target audience members to identify similar others) can map an "underground" population effectively. Even if there are few network ties in the population of interest, convenience samples at venues frequented by the population may provide some guidance for program managers.

Finally, note that samples are not always composed of people. A sample of news stories, for example, can also be very revealing. One purpose for performing this kind of retrospective media monitoring would be to evaluate an attempt to "earn" health message dissemination by holding press events. Sampling news coverage entails searching a news archive such as Google News or Nexis/Lexis. Purposive sampling choices are made about including certain geographic areas, time periods, types of media, types of coverage (e.g., news and editorials, but not letters to the editor), and content placement (e.g., title or first paragraph). The sample may be further restricted to specific stations or newspapers or websites (e.g., elite and local). Within this narrowly defined sample, keyword searches are performed to generate a large initial number of stories for quantitative analysis. A random subsample then may be read in full for qualitative analysis.[35]

Evaluation via Indicators

In most low-income countries, the government supports periodic surveillance of population health status using a small number of variables called indicators. Indicator data (e.g., infant deaths in the first three months of life) reflect the *cumulative* effects of all prior programs and other influences. If an indicator spikes or plummets, a formal evaluation study can be commissioned to investigate the cause.

Routine health behavior surveillance is conducted in the United States as well, by means of state-wide surveys such as Centers for Disease Control and Prevention's (CDC) Behavioral Risk Factor Surveillance System,[36] and national surveys such as the National Cancer Institute's HINTS.[37] If relevant indicator data can be disaggregated down to a campaign's jurisdiction, it may be possible—and worthwhile—to add a campaign exposure item to a standard survey that is scheduled to go into the field at an opportune time. If the campaign did *enough of the right things* to make a difference, and indicator trend discontinuities co-occur with the campaign, you can make a case that your program contributed to the change in the surveillance data pattern. Ordinarily, such a claim is likely to require backup by data from other sources.

▶ Using Qualitative and Quantitative Data

Outcome evaluations can include *qualitative* data (i.e., themes based on rich, in-depth information about a few people or a few cases), *quantitative* data (i.e., numerical information about a large number of people or cases), or both. There are several methods for collecting each of these types of data, and many ways to mix qualitative and quantitative methods.[38] A choice of a particular **mixed method** should be driven by the study question, rather than the other way around.[39]

Randomized quantitative studies are the gold standard when it comes to internal validity. Nevertheless, even in the absence of an RCT design, quantitative data from several sources that "triangulate" to validate each other can be combined to form a very convincing argument that your campaign was, in fact, responsible for certain observed effects; see **BOX 12-12** for an example.

BOX 12-12   Evaluation of the 2012 *Tips From Former Smokers* Campaign

The CDC's *Tips from Former Smokers* (*Tips*) campaign aired nationwide for 3 months during the spring of 2012. Through television, radio, outdoor, magazine, newspaper, and online advertisements, the *Tips* campaign shared true stories of former smokers who described in personal and emotional terms the toll that smoking has taken on their health, their lives, and the lives of their loved ones.[1] The evaluation of the 2012 *Tips* campaign consisted of three main components:

1. Pre- and post-longitudinal surveys were conducted online using the nationally representative Knowledge Panel. The surveys gathered information on smokers' and nonsmokers' exposure to *Tips* ads and relevant outcomes, including measures of recent quit attempts; knowledge, attitudes, and beliefs related to smoking; and nonsmokers' referrals of family and friends who smoke to cessation services.[1]
2. Traffic to campaign-related cessation resources (e.g., quitline and campaign website) was examined. Particularly, data on weekly call volume to 1-800-QUIT-NOW were analyzed to evaluate more directly the campaign's impact on calls to the national quitline portal. These data were combined with measures of the intensity of *Tips* campaign media placements to identify the relationship between weekly variations in advertising and weekly fluctuations in calls to 1-800-QUIT-NOW.[2]
3. A cost-effectiveness analysis was conducted to quantify reduced smoking-attributable morbidity and mortality among the national population of smokers and to determine the return on investment for campaign expenditures.[3]

The prevalence of smokers reporting a quit attempt for 1 day or longer in the past 3 months increased from 31.1% before the campaign to 34.8% after the campaign ($p < 0.05$), a 12% relative increase. There was also a strong relationship between self-reported frequency of exposure to campaign ads and an increased likelihood of making a quit attempt. This relationship was strongest among smokers who had not previously made a quit attempt during the 3 months prior to the *Tips* campaign, suggesting that the campaign motivated new quit attempts among smokers who had not previously tried quitting. These relationships also persisted after controlling for potential confounding factors at the individual, state, and market levels.[1]

Applying the pre-post rate of change in quit attempts to U.S. Census data suggests the *Tips* campaign was responsible for approximately 1.64 million smokers attempting to quit. In addition, an estimated 13.4% of smokers who attempted to quit during the *Tips* campaign remained smoke-free at the post-campaign follow-up point, translating into approximately 220,000 total smokers. Based on these projections, and other literature that has estimated longer-term quit rates, we conservatively estimate that approximately 100,000 of those smokers who were cigarette abstinent at follow-up would not relapse in the future (i.e., would remain quit).[1]

Total call volume during the 2012 campaign was 365,194 calls, compared with 157,675 calls (a 132% increase) during the corresponding 12 weeks in 2011. Compared to the corresponding weeks in 2011, weekly increases in calls during the campaign ranged from 86% to 160%. The website received a 428% increase in unique visitors during the campaign, compared to the same period in 2011. Weekly increases in visitors compared to the corresponding weeks in 2011 ranged from 355% to 484%.[2]

Cost-effectiveness analysis was conducted to evaluate the campaign from the perspective of the funding agency and to provide estimates of sustained cessations, premature deaths averted, raw life-years saved, and quality-adjusted life-years gained as a result of the campaign. Findings from this analysis suggest that the *Tips* campaign prevented more than 17,000 premature deaths in the United States. Based on a total campaign cost of roughly $48 million, the *Tips* campaign spent approximately $480 per quitter and $2820 per premature death averted.[3] These estimates easily surpass accepted minimum standards of cost-effectiveness for public health interventions.[3]

The *Tips* campaign was the first national, mass-media antismoking initiative to be funded by the U.S. government. It reached nearly 80% of U.S. smokers and was associated with a 12% relative increase in quit attempts within a nationally representative cohort. Based on the absolute increase in quit attempts (i.e., 3.7%), the public health effect of *Tips* was substantial, with an estimated 1.64 million campaign-attributable quit attempts made and 220,000 smokers remaining abstinent at the campaign's culmination.[1] The campaign was also successful at reducing smoking-attributable morbidity and mortality while achieving these reductions in a cost-efficient way.[3] The evaluation results show the effectiveness of a national-level antismoking campaign using hard-hitting messages delivered in emotional, graphic personal stories.

References

1. McAfee T, Davis KC, Alexander R Jr, Pechacek TF, Bunnell R. Effect of the first federally funded US antismoking national media campaign. *Lancet.* 2013;382(9909):2003-2011.

2. Centers for Disease Control and Prevention. Increases in quitline calls and smoking cessation website visitors during a national tobacco education campaign—March 19–June 10, 2012. *MMWR.* 2012;61(34):667-670.

3. Xu X, Alexander R Jr, Simpson S, Goates S, Nonnemaker J, Davis KC, McAfee T. A cost-effectiveness analysis of the first federally funded antismoking campaign. *Am J Prev Med.* Mar 2015; 48(3):318-325.

Insights based on qualitative data (e.g., archival records, key informant interviews or video tapes) can make numeric findings more interpretable. In an evaluation context, quotes from target audience members can bring numeric findings to life. Qualitative data can be especially useful when little is known about a health problem; for example, a qualitative case study of a newly discovered health threat can be an excellent source of hypotheses that can be tested quantitatively at a later time. Also, when a quantitative study shows that a program has failed, post hoc qualitative interviews with program participants, staff, and stakeholders may help explain why the failure occurred.

To see how important qualitative data can be in interpreting quantitative data, consider the evaluation of One Tiny Reason to Quit (OTRTQ).[40] This social marketing campaign promoted 1-800-QUITNOW, an evidence-based smoking "quitline," to pregnant African American smokers. The coalition-based intervention was launched in Richmond, Virginia, and replicated there 2 years later. For each campaign wave, the number of calls to the quitline from pregnant women during the 3-month campaign was contrasted with the number of calls from pregnant women in the 3 months before the campaign. Also, to help rule out seasonal effects (e.g., calls prompted by New Year's resolutions to quit smoking), calls made during the campaign were contrasted with same-season calls from the previous year. Compared with any of these other periods, there were striking and highly statistically significant spikes in calls from pregnant women in the Richmond area during the OTRTQ campaign waves. Nonetheless, because the quitline is promoted in various ways by the Virginia Department of Health (VDH), it was essential to conduct qualitative interviews with VDH staff to rule out possible non-campaign-related causes of the quantitative call spikes observed during the OTRTQ waves. According to the key informants, there were no special quitline promotions in Richmond during the evaluation periods. Thus, evaluators attributed the increased number of calls from pregnant women to the OTRTQ campaign, and it was subsequently accepted into two EBI databases.[41]

Initially unstructured records become useful qualitative data when structured into discrete categories or themes,[42] which is a laborious process. To cope with a flood of unstructured data, "text mining" tools may be used that perform natural language processing; they miss a lot of instances of themes, but their capabilities are improving.[43] Several commercial programs offer "sandbox" versions at no charge, and there is also freeware for generic text, medical records, and press content (e.g., at http://nlp.stanford.edu/software/, https://www.i2b2.org/software/index.html, and https://gate.ac.uk/).

▶ Evaluation Frameworks

Before putting the final touches on an evaluation plan and submitting it for approval by program stakeholders, it is helpful to step back and consider the program in the larger scheme of things. Several conceptual frameworks are available to help put program activities into a broader perspective. Viewing a program through such a "big picture" lens may well prompt you to revise your evaluation plan.

Some frameworks focus on evaluation itself, others treat evaluation as one aspect of the larger program planning process, and others highlight features of a communication approach or class of channels. Examples of both well-known and newer frameworks are described in this section.

CDC Evaluation Framework

The CDC framework begins with engaging stakeholders in the process of choosing evaluation outcomes and outcome measures (**FIGURE 12-1**).[44] That starting point acknowledges the fact that, regardless of the quality of the evaluation, its findings will not be applied to improve the program if stakeholder concerns were not addressed. In other words, evaluations should be *use-focused*.[45] Correspondingly, most of the website links, evaluation handbooks, and other resources available on CDC's Program Performance and Evaluation Office website (http://www.cdc.gov/eval) emphasize stakeholder collaboration.

Another key feature of the CDC framework is that it is a circle—a form with no endpoint—signifying that evaluation is an ongoing process. Of course, evaluating a program on an ongoing basis does not necessarily mean that the same study is conducted repeatedly. A better use of resources might be conducting a series of studies, each of which adds a different kind of information about how or how well the program works. An example of a multiyear campaign consistent with this

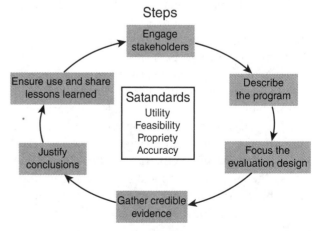

FIGURE 12-1 CDC Evaluation Framework.

Available at http://www.cdc.gov/eval/framework/. Accessed December 15, 2015.

framework is "Get Yourself Tested" (GYT). The GYD program, which focuses on STD testing, diagnosis, and treatment, is a collaboration among the American College Health Association (ACHA), Kaiser Family Foundation (KFF), the National Coalition of STD Directors (NCSD), MTV, and the Planned Parenthood Federation of America, with technical assistance from CDC.[46] **Appendix 12A** describes the evaluation of the GYT program.

RE-AIM, PRECEDE–PROCEED, and Inform-Persuade

A popular sequence of research foci in ongoing, multi-study evaluation efforts is the one spelled out in the RE-AIM framework developed by Russ Glasgow and colleagues. The letters in this acronym stand for *reach, effectiveness, adoption, implementation,* and *maintenance.* For each of these aspects of program functioning, there are sample research questions, measures, and suggestions for using findings to enhance program impact on a website dedicated to RE-AIM.[47]

The PRECEDE-PROCEED framework is a systematic program planning model that guides communities in setting and addressing public health priorities.[48] There are five phases analogous to formative evaluation in PRECEDE; they culminate in a plan that is pertinent to the first "right things" question. The second and third central evaluation questions are raised during the PROCEED phase.

The **inform/persuade paradigm** (following initial engagement) divides health communication programs into those that set out to deliver new information to audiences and those that attempt to motivate audience members to put knowledge into practice. Because the intended objective of a program should be measured well and thoroughly, programs designed to inform should assess the degree to which new, accurate information was actually imparted to the target audience, how long audience members retained the new information, and the degree to which they disseminated it. Programs designed to persuade, in contrast, should be evaluated in terms of message credibility and attitude change at a minimum. For an example of a more thorough evaluation in the "persuade" category, think about persuasive communication as one part of a multipronged strategy to change behavior by altering its actual or perceived costs and benefits. In such a case, the entire effort should be evaluated in terms of the behavior change, its perceived costs and benefits, and other major theoretical determinants such as intentions.[15]

E-Health Frameworks

Several attempts to articulate a framework for e-health activities have been made. Early on, Eysenbach listed **"10 E's"** (e.g., efficiency, empowerment, extending) that were dimensions along which e-health held promise.[49] If the opportunity arises (perhaps as systems are running in parallel, in preparation for a switch to automation), evaluators could choose to allocate some of their resources to determining whether the newer strategies are, indeed, superior in terms of one or more E's.

The **Community of Inquiry (CoI) framework** assumes that online learning is a function of the interaction of three presences: (1) social presence, (2) cognitive presence, and (3) teaching presence.[50] It reflects John Dewey's insight that inquiry is an essentially social process of practical problem solving[51]—an apt description of crowd-sourced online information.

Recently, the **Comprehensive E-Health Research Framework** was synthesized from 16 others; this composite is intended to provide a conceptual map of the fit and recursive dynamics among technological, human, and contextual systems.[52] This framework's notable additions to traditional frameworks used in public health include (1) an emphasis on the business model that undergirds an e-health strategy and (2) e-application design and testing phases, which are separate from, but iteratively connected to, outcome evaluation.

▶ Conclusion

Evaluation of health communication programs is part science and part art. Experienced practitioners follow some conventions, but also utilize some "tricks of the trade." Our discussion of program evaluation closes with practice recommendations from national experts in health communication evaluation who were convened by the CDC:[15]

- Be on the lookout for new, low-cost, qualitative and quantitative data collection strategies, many of which will be new media-tracking resources.[53]
- Perform cognitive testing of your interview or questionnaire. Words and questions may not mean the same thing to you as they do to the target audience. Find out if your questions are clear by asking a small sample of audience members to think out loud as they read a questionnaire and translate the questions into their own words. If you are collecting data electronically, you should also test usability. Online resources such as *Mechanical Turk Sandbox* may help you perform such tests affordably.

- If there is no efficacious model program, it is best to test the efficacy of proposed procedures with a small group *before* trying to expose a large target audience to the procedures. If a program is replicating one that worked, a less rigorous evaluation design may provide "good enough" evidence of effectiveness.
- Quantify program outputs and evaluate only those programs that have exposed expose enough members of the target audience to a message enough times for the message to register.
- Nothing works forever in health communication. Determine when it is time to refresh a campaign.

Examine data from periodic tracking "pulse checks" (e.g., media ratings, low-cost surveys of convenience samples) to detect a fall-off in campaign response.
- Track both intended and unintended campaign effects. This step is both an ethical issue and a political consideration. It helps to have evidence that potentially controversial health messages (especially those targeted to groups who already suffer negative health disparities) did no harm. Paradoxically, unintended consequences can be positive, or suggestive of additional avenues of study.

Wrap-Up

Chapter Questions

1. What is the basic purpose of a health communication program evaluation?
2. What are the central research questions that a health communication program evaluation asks?
3. At which points and how should stakeholders be involved in evaluation?
4. Which major study designs are used to evaluate health communication programs, and how can qualitative data complement quantitative data in evaluation studies?
5. What are some commonly used e-health metrics, and how predictive are they of change in health risk behavior?

References

1. Drucker PF. *Management: Tasks, Responsibilities, Practices.* New York, NY: Harper & Row; 1973: 45.
2. CDCynergy. Social marketing edition, version 2. http://www.orau.gov/cdcynergy/soc2web/. Accessed March 22, 2016.
3. Flay BR. Efficacy and effectiveness trials (and other phases of research) in the development of health promotion programs. *Prev Med.* 1986;15(5):451-474.
4. Evans WD, Uhrig J, Davis K, McCormack L. Efficacy methods to evaluate health communication and marketing campaigns. *J Health Commun.* 2009;14:315-330.
5. Carvalho ML, Honeycutt S, Escoffery C, Glanz K, Sabbs D, Kegler MC. Balancing fidelity and adaptation: implementing evidence-based chronic disease prevention programs. *J Public Health Manag* Pract. 2013;19(4):348-356.
6. Centers for Disease Control and Prevention. The health communicator's social media toolkit. July 2011. http://www.cdc.gov/SocialMedia/Tools/guidelines/index.html. Accessed March 22, 2016.
7. Freimuth V, Cole G, Kirby S. Issues in evaluating mass media-based health communication campaigns. In: Detrani JR, ed. *Mass Communication: Issues, Perspectives and Techniques.* Oakville, ON: Apple Academic Press; 2011:77-98.
8. Hornik RC. *Public Health Communication: Evidence for Behavior Change.* Mahwah, NJ: Lawrence Erlbaum Associates; 2008.
9. Croker HF, Lucas R, Wardle J. Cluster-randomised trial to evaluate the "Change for Life" mass media/social marketing campaign in the UK. *BMC Public Health.* 2012 6;12:404.
10. Bauman A, Bowles HR, Huhman M, et al. Testing a hierarchy-of-effects model: pathways from awareness to outcomes in the VERB campaign 2002-2003. *Am J Prev Med.* 2008;34(6suppl): S249-S256.
11. Jamal A, Agaku IT, O'Connor E, King BA, Kenemer JB, Neff L. Current cigarette smoking among adults—United States, 2005-2013. *MMWR.* 2014;63(47):1108-1102.
12. Osborne H. In other words...confirming understanding with the teach-back technique. American Medical Foundation. http://www.healthliteracy.com/article.asp?PageID=6714. Accessed March 22, 2016.
13. Snyder LB, Hamilton, MA, Mitchell EW, Kiwanuka-Tondo J, Fleming-Milici F, Proctor D. A meta-analysis of the effect of mediated health communication campaigns on behavior change in the United States. *J Health Commun.* 2004;9(6 suppl 1):74-96.
14. Randolf KA, Whitaker P, Arellano A. The unique effects of environmental strategies health promotion in campaigns: a review. *Eval Prog Plan.* 2012;35:344-353.
15. Communication Evaluation Expert Panel, Abbatangelo J, Cole G, Kennedy MG. Guidance for evaluating mass communication health initiatives: summary of an expert panel discussion sponsored by CDC. *Eval Health Prof.* 2007;30(3):229-253.

16. Kennedy MG, Mizuno Y, Seals BF, Myllyluoma J, Weeks-Norton K. Increasing condom use among adolescents with coalition-based social marketing. *AIDS.* 2000;14(12):1809-1818.

17. Heeter C. Interactivity in the context of designed experiences. *J Interactive Advert.* 2000;1(1). http://s3.amazonaws.com/academia.edu.documents/27070245/Interactivity_in_the_Context_of_Designed_Experiences.pdf?AWSAccessKeyId=AKIAJ56TQJRTWSMTNPEA&Expires=1482446233&Signature=t1uxkFnadmkIa9cQOdU%2Fb7YIMSE%3D&response-content-disposition=inline%3B%20filename%3DInteractivity_in_the_context_of_designed.pdf. Accessed March 23, 2016.

18. National Center for Chronic Disease Prevention and Health Promotion. Developing an effective evaluation plan. http://www.cdc.gov/obesity/downloads/CDC-Evaluation-Workbook-508.pdf. Accessed March 23, 2016.

19. National Cancer Institute. Grid-enabled measures database. http://www.gem-measures.org/Public/Home.aspx. Accessed March 23, 2016.

20. Holtgrave DR, Wunderink KA, Vallone DN, Healton CG. Cost-utility analysis of the national truth campaign to prevent youth smoking. *Am J Prev Med.* 2009;36(5):385-388.

21. Jones SC, Adams S, Takata Schneider Y. Using social listening and web traffic analysis following major media health events to inform public health campaigns. Presented at the NCHCMM Conference; August 2014.

22. Goetz Goldberg D, Kuzel AJ, Feng LB, DeShazo JP, Love LE. EHRs in primary care practices: benefits, challenges, and successful strategies. *Am J Manag Care.* 2012;018(2):e48-354.

23. Wright KB. Researching Internet-based populations: advantages and disadvantages of online survey research, online questionnaire authoring packages, and web survey services. *J Computer-Mediated Commun.* 2006;10(3). doi: 10.1111/j.1083-6101.2005.tb00259.x.

24. Allison S, Bauermeister JA, Bull S, et al. The intersection of youth, technology and new media with sexual health: moving the research agenda forward. *J Adolesc Health.* 2012;51(3);207-212.

25. Pew Research Center. Social media usage: 2005-2015. http://www.pewinternet.org/2015/10/08/social-networking-usage-2005-2015. Accessed March 23, 2016.

26. Robert Wood Johnson Foundation. Evaluating communication campaigns. https://folio.iupui.edu/bitstream/handle/10244/617/evaluatingcommcampaigns2008.pdf. Accessed March 23, 2016.

27. Valente TW. *Evaluating Health Communication Programs.* New York, NY: Oxford University Press; 2002.

28. Head KJ, Noar SM, Iannarino NT, Grant Harrington N. Efficacy of text messaging-based interventions for health promotion: a meta-analysis. *Soc Sci Med.* 2013;97:41-48.

29. Cook TD, Campbell DT. *Quasi-Experimentation: Design and Analysis Issues for Field Settings.* Boston, MA: Houghton Mifflin; 1979.

30. Weeks BE, Friedenberg LM, Southwell BG, Slater JS. Behavioral consequences of conflict-oriented health news coverage: the 2009 mammography guideline controversy and online information seeking. *Health Commun.* 2012;27(2):158-166.

31. Yanovitsky I, Zannuto E, Hornik R. Estimating causal effects of public health education campaigns using propensity score methodology. *Eval Prog Plan.* 2005;28:209-220.

32. Noar SM, Palmgreen P, Zimmerman R. Reflections on evaluating health communication campaigns. *Commun Meth Meas.* 2009;31(1-2):29-46.

33. Messer BL, Dillman DA. Surveying the general public over the Internet using address-based sampling and mail contact procedures. *Public Opin Q.* 2011; 75(3):429-457.

34. Lansky A, Drake A, Wejnert C, Pham H, Cribbin M, Heckathorn DD. Assessing the assumptions of respondent-driven sampling in the national HIV Behavioral Surveillance System among injecting drug users. *Open AIDS J.* 2012;6:77-82.

35. Casciotti DM, Smith KC, Andon L, Vernick J, Tsui A, Klassen AC. Print news coverage of school-based human papillomavirus vaccine mandates. *J Sch Health.* 2014;84(2):71-81.

36. Centers for Disease Control and Prevention. Behavioral Risk Factor System. http://www.cdc.gov/brfss/. Accessed March 23, 2016.

37. National Institutes of Health, National Cancer Institute. Health Information National Trends Survey. http://hints.cancer.gov/. Accessed March 23, 2016.

38. Leech NL, Onwuegbuzie AJ. A typology of mixed methods research designs. *Qual Quant.* 2009;43:265-275.

39. Creswell JW. *Research Design: Qualitative, Quantitative, and Mixed Methods Approaches* (4th ed.). Thousand Oaks, CA: Sage; 2014.

40. Kennedy MG, Wilson-Genderson M, Sepulveda AL, et al. Spikes in calls to a smoking quitline: results of the One Tiny Reason to Quit campaign for pregnant African-American women in urban and rural settings. *J Women's Health.* 2013;22(5):432-438.

41. Association of Maternal and Child Health Programs. Innovation Station: a best practices database. http://www.amchp.org/programsandtopics/BestPractices/InnovationStation/Pages/default.aspx. Accessed March 23, 2016.

42. Parvanta S, Gibson L, Forquer H, et al. Applying quantitative approaches to the formative evaluation of antismoking campaign messages. *Soc Mar Q.* 2013;19(4):242-264.

43. Patton MQ. *Utilization-Focused Evaluation: The New Century Text* (3rd ed.). Thousand Oaks, CA: Sage; 1997.

44. Beitzel SM. *On Understanding and Classifying Web Queries.* PhD thesis, Illinois Institute of Technology; 2006. http://citeseerx.ist.psu.edu/index;jsessionid=5D2C6073F8EF38AB18D0EA11C0AA3978. Accessed March 23, 2016.

45. Centers for Disease Control and Prevention. Framework for program evaluation in public health. *MMWR.* 1999;RR-11:48.

46. Friedman AL, Brookmeyer KA, Kachur RE, et al. An assessment of the GYT: Get Yourself Tested campaign: an integrated approach to sexually transmitted disease prevention communication. *Sex Trans Dis.* 2014; 41(3):151-157\.

47. Glascow R. RE-AIM. http://www.re-aim.hnfe.vt.edu/. Accessed March 23, 2016.

48. Green LW, Kreuter MW. *Health Promotion Planning: An Educational and Ecological Approach* (3rd ed.). New York, NY: McGraw-Hill; 1999.

49. Eysenbach G. What is e-health? *J Med Internet* Res, 2001;3(2):e20. doi: 10.2196/jmir.3.2.e20.

50. Swan K, Garrison DR, Richardson JC. A constructivist approach to online learning: the Community of Inquiry framework. In: Payne CR, ed. *Information Technology and Constructivism in Higher Education: Progressive Learning Frameworks*. Hershey, PA: IGI Global; 2009:43-57.

51. Dewey J. My pedagogic creed. In: Dewey J. *Dewey on Education*. New York, NY: Teachers College, Columbia University; 1959:19-32. (Original work published 1897).

52. van Gemert-Pijnen JE, Nijland N, van Limburg M, et al. A holistic framework to improve the uptake and impact of eHealth technologies. *J Med Internet Res*. 2011;13(4):e111. doi: 10.2196/jmir.1672.

53. Fitzpatrick JL, Sanders JR, Worthen BR. *Program Evaluation: Alternative Approaches and Practical Guidelines* (3rd ed.). Boston, MA: Allyn & Bacon; 2003.

Appendix 12

Evaluation of the National GYT (Get Yourself Tested) Campaign

Allison Friedman, Sarah Levine, Melissa Habel, Elizabeth Clark, Rachel Kachur, Kathryn Brookmeyer, Mary McFarlane, and **Tina Hoff**

▶ Problem Description

Youth (ages 15–24) in the United States are disproportionately affected by sexually transmitted diseases (STDs). Although they make up only a quarter of the sexually active population, youth account for half of the estimated 20 million STDs each year. Chlamydia, the most commonly reported infection in the United States, is often asymptomatic and can lead to infertility in women, if left untreated. Yet challenges to access (such as cost and location), a lack of information, fear, misconceptions, and stigma keep many youth from seeking needed testing or treatment. In March 2008, new information was released by the Centers for Disease Control and Prevention (CDC) indicating that as many as one in four teen girls has an STD, which prompted national provider, public health, media, and nonprofit agencies to mobilize for action.

GYT: Get Yourself Tested was launched in April 2009 as an ongoing promotion under "It's Your (Sex) Life," MTV's Emmy and Peabody Award–winning public information campaign to support young people in making responsible decisions about their sexual health. Supporting partners of GYT include American College Health Association (ACHA), Kaiser Family Foundation (KFF), National Coalition of STD Directors (NCSD), MTV, and Planned Parenthood Federation of America. Technical consultation is provided by CDC.

▶ Market Research

CDC and KFF conducted consumer surveys, focus groups, and interviews to better understand youth knowledge, attitudes, and beliefs about STDs and testing. Formative research revealed that many youth are unaware of the potentially asymptomatic nature and prevalence of STDs; that routine STD screening is recommended; that providers do not automatically test for STDs during routine clinical visits; and that confidential, noninvasive, and youth-friendly services are available. Research indicated that youth did not perceive themselves to be at risk for STDs (particularly those in relationships) and feared various aspects of STD testing (e.g., uncomfortable procedures and what parents and peers might think and say). Other key barriers included concerns about confidentiality and cost, embarrassment, and sex partner concerns related to testing, including implied distrust or cheating. Key benefits that emerged were knowing one's status, confirming one's negative status, and being able to take action in the case of testing positive.

▶ Market Strategy

The GYT campaign seeks to promote STD testing (and treatment, as appropriate) among sexually active youth, ages 25 and younger, through a youthful, empowering social movement. It aims to:

- Increase STD awareness and perceived risk—by emphasizing the high prevalence and asymptomatic nature of STDs.
- Reduce STD testing fears and stigma—by normalizing testing as something that all sexually active youth do.
- Connect youth to STD testing services through a national testing locator tool (https://www.findSTD test.org or https://www.gettested.cdc.gov) as well as linking them to testing events and promotions.

- Promote open communication with sex partners and healthcare providers (as intermediaries for behavior change)—by normalizing conversations around sexual health and offering talking tips and other support tools. The "GYT" acronym offers an easy way to talk about STD testing in a short-hand that is familiar to young people.

Campaign messaging (informed by consumer research and key constructs of the Health Belief Model and theory of planned behavior) avoids targeting "high-risk" subgroups, instead aiming to normalize testing for *all* sexually active youth. GYT campaign messaging uses a humorous, light-hearted approach to reach youth. In 2009, its first year, messaging was designed to promote brand exposure by piquing interest in the campaign (e.g., with messages such as "WTF is GYT?") and driving traffic to informational and testing resources. In year 2, the campaign focused on talking about STDs/testing with one's partner and provider, emphasizing the ease of testing with the "Get yourself talking. Get yourself tested." tagline. In its third year, GYT introduced a new look and feel to appeal to Millennials (Generation Y) and shifted to a "lifestyle brand," supported by diverse youth leaders ("Team GYT") who served as campaign ambassadors, promoting the campaign through their own social networks and social media channels. With a youth empowerment theme, the tagline evolved to "Know yourself. Know your status." Campaign themes and strategies continue to evolve to stay relevant to youth audiences.

▶ Intervention

GYT is a year-round initiative that refreshes each April (National STD Awareness Month), with special promotions during other key periods of the year, including Valentine's Day, spring break, National HIV Testing Day, back-to-school period, and World AIDS Day. The campaign has used multimedia platforms, including television (advertising and original programming), web, print, short message service (SMS) and on-the-ground outreach efforts. Targeted messaging is integrated across partner platforms, including MTV's on-air and online programming and communications. The campaign runs special promotions (e.g., sweepstakes, contests), events, and audience engagement activities (e.g., concert series, testing events) to incentivize STD testing among youth. In addition, musical artists and celebrities speak out on behalf of the campaign. Finally, the national GYT campaign is supported by state and local partners through their own media, marketing, advocacy, events, promotions, and outreach efforts. GYT toolkits containing promotional materials are provided at no cost (as available) to facilitate local efforts. Examples of campaign platforms including the following:

- GYT offers information and testing resources, including an interactive website (GYTNOW.org) with basic information about common STDs, talking tips and tools, and a testing locator to find nearby free or low-cost and youth-friendly STD testing services.
- Original GYT on-air promotions and programming, including digital and social elements, are featured on MTV, mtvU (broadcasting to more than 750 college campuses nationwide), MTV2 (the number one network among males ages 12–34), and Tr3s (reaching bicultural U.S. Latinos ages 18–34). Innovative programming has included the *Top 10 Most Outrageous Sex Myths*, a countdown show featuring popular artists debunking misconceptions about sexual health issues, and *I'm Positive*, a documentary following three young people living with HIV.
- GYT works with MTV's producers to integrate sexual health messaging into existing television programming (e.g., *Girl Code, The How-To Show, MTV News, Dean's List*) and social media properties, driving audiences to online resources for more information.
- GYT is on Facebook and Twitter, serving as a digital meeting place connecting health centers and clinics, community organizations, and student groups promoting STD testing. It has partnered with businesses and organizations in the social media space, including Foursquare, through which consumers who got tested could "check in" to clinics and receive a GYT badge, and now works in partnership with *It's Your Sex Life* social media.
- GYT cross-promotions and activities take place on the ground through Planned Parenthood's more than 700 health centers across the country, ACHA's network of college health clinics, and private-sector and community-based partnerships. For example, GYT has been promoted through concert series in select cities nationwide to promote testing for STDs and HIV.

▶ Evaluation

Efforts to evaluate GYT's reach and impact have included media and materials tracking; monitoring of STD testing and positivity rates at participating Planned Parenthood health centers, college health, and other partner clinics; and college, clinic, and online national surveys of youth.

Select Process Evaluation Results

In its first year of implementation alone, GYT produced more than 20 public service ads and original programs, airing more than 2000 times on MTV stations, and received more than 100,000 clinic referrals from web and SMS clinic locator tools.

In the five-year period from launch through March 31, 2014, more than 4.1 million people accessed information through the website.* The campaign remained among the top-10 referring sites to CDC's STD testing locator as of August 2014. GYT has been nominated for and has received multiple awards, including several Beacon Awards.

Selected Outcome Evaluation Results

Key outcome measures assessed were campaign awareness, STD testing behavior, HIV testing behavior, and communication with partners and providers.

Reported Youth Behaviors

National Survey of Youth A 2013 nationally representative survey of youth ages 15–25 ($n = 4017$) found that GYT reached about one-fifth of youth in the United States. Those who reported hearing about the campaign (i.e., with or without a visual prompt) were significantly more likely to report STD and HIV testing and communication with a provider or partner compared to those who were unaware ($p < 0.05$). Testing and communication behaviors increased with the number of channels/settings in which youth reported seeing GYT materials, indicating a possible dose–response relationship. Among those aware of the campaign, 47.6% of those who reported seeing/hearing GYT messages through one channel had ever been STD tested, compared to 50.5% among those exposed through two to four channels, and 70.7% among those reporting exposure through five or more channels. HIV testing also increased linearly with the number of reported exposures/channels, from 31.1% (zero channels) to 75.6% (five or more channels).[1]

STD Testing Data

Planned Parenthood Affiliate Data In the first six years of GYT (2009–2014), 798,537 people were tested for selected STDs (chlamydia, gonorrhea, and HIV) during the month of April (peak promotion period)

at Planned Parenthood health centers nationwide. Increases in STD testing during the month of April were strongest in the first years of the campaign, but have been sustained over time.[2]

From April 2008 (pre-campaign) to April 2010 (year 2 of campaign), there was a 71% increase in STD testing at nine reporting Planned Parenthood affiliates, representing approximately 118 health centers nationwide. This was supported by national trend data, which indicated that testing was higher in spring 2009–2010 compared to other periods during those years.[3]

From April 2009 to April 2014, there was a 12% increase in STD testing at 35 reporting Planned Parenthood affiliates. Notably, the percentage of patients testing positive for chlamydia and gonorrhea reflect national positivity rates, indicating that those seeking testing represent at-risk populations. More than 50% of those seeking STD testing at last report (April 2014) were younger than the age of 25, the target of GYT.[2]

Local Evaluations from School, Community, and Health Partners GYT worked with ACHA-member institutions to conduct a brief survey assessing the impact on 12 college campuses of varying sizes, locations, and demographics in April 2012 ($n = 1986$) and 2013 ($n = 1733$). Of the total sample ($N = 3719$), 55.4% had seen or heard of the GYT campaign. Of those who had seen or heard about the campaign, 57% reported coming to the clinic for STD testing, with 42.6% indicating that this visit was due in part to the GYT campaign. Students aware of GYT were also more likely to have discussed sexual health issues with a doctor, nurse, or healthcare provider (62.6% versus 37.4%, $p < 0.001$) as well as a boyfriend, girlfriend, or partner (63.1% versus 36.9%, $p < 0.001$) within the past 12 months, compared to those who had not seen/heard of GYT.[4]

GYT supported nine geographically diverse community, health, and school agencies to implement and evaluate their own local GYT campaigns in 2011. Programs collected STD testing data at participating sites during campaign implementation and compared it to comparable periods in the previous year (baseline data). Among the nine sites, nearly 7000 individuals got tested for chlamydia during the campaign promotion period (which varied by site), representing a 14.8% increase at these sites compared to baseline.

---

* This includes visitors to itsyoursexlife.org (GYTNOW.org is hosted on MTV.com, as part of itsyoursexlife.org). Not all web visitors are connected to GYT-specific promotions; likewise, visitors entering through *It's Your (Sex) Life*-related promotions may visit GYT content.

Despite staffing and organizational challenges at some sites, all but one site reported increases in the number of people tested (increases were significant for seven sites; $p < 0.01$), with increases ranging from 0.5% to 128%. Positivity rates for chlamydia remained high during campaign implementation periods, ranging from 6.3% to 15.5%, suggesting that the campaign was reaching those at risk.[5]

References

1. Friedman A, McFarlane M, Habel M, Hogben M, Kachur R, Brookmeyer K. GYT exposure among youth and effects by dose. Presented at the National Conference on Health Communication, Marketing and Media; Atlanta, GA; August 19-21, 2014.

2. Planned Parenthood Federation of America. *GYT '14 Campaign: National STI Testing Month Survey.* July 15, 2014.

3. Friedman AL, Brookmeyer KA, Kachur RE, Ford J, et al. An assessment of the *GYT: Get Yourself Tested* campaign: an integrated approach to sexually transmitted disease prevention communication. *STD.* 2014;41(3):151-157.

4. Habel MA, Eastman-Mueller H. The evolution of a public health social marketing approach to STI prevention: what is your role? Presented at the Annual Meeting of the American College Health Association; Orlando, FL; May 26-30, 2015.

5. Friedman AL, Bozniak A, Ford J, et al. Reaching youth with sexually transmitted disease testing: building on successes, challenges, and lessons learned from local *Get Yourself Tested* campaigns. *Soc Market Qtly.* 2014;20(2):116-138.

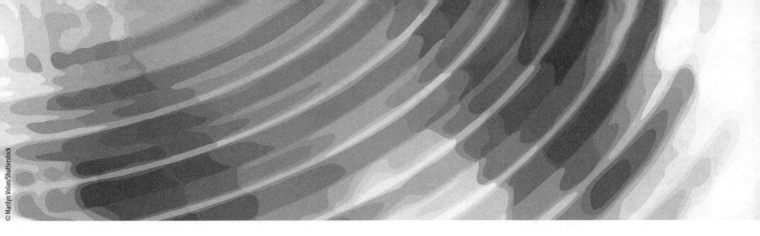

CHAPTER 13

Clinician–Patient Communication

Richard N. Harner

LEARNING OBJECTIVES

By the end of this chapter, the reader will be able to:

- Describe the relationship between patients and clinicians in terms of multiple goals, barriers, and levels of communication.
- Identify key tools the clinician may use to communicate effectively with the patient.
- Practice empathetic and effective listening and speaking with a study partner or model patient.

▶ Introduction

This chapter focuses on **clinician–patient communication (CPC)**, meaning the face-to-face communication between healthcare providers and their patients. Fifty years ago, this would have been mostly about the doctor–patient relationship.[1–5] Since then, the nature of healthcare communication has changed. New technologies and new demands on time—in particular, the need to maintain the electronic health record (EHR; see **BOX 13-1**) have changed the way physicians and other clinicians interact during a patient encounter.[6,7] In parallel, and in part as a consequence, new health professions have arisen (e.g., scribes for EHR-challenged clinicians); more nurses are becoming nurse practitioners, assistants are becoming physician assistants, and pharmacists, physical therapists, emergency medical technologists, and other specialists increasingly function as independent practitioners. When we add on growing interest in improving public health through pharmacy, hospital, and community sites, we find that the spectrum of clinicians communicating with individual patients is greatly broadened.

Physicians, other clinicians, and healthcare workers in general all must communicate effectively with individual patients (sometimes referred to as clients—see **BOX 13-2**) to diagnose, treat, care for, and assist those in need. In this chapter we develop a conceptual framework for CPC; emphasize the multifaceted, bidirectional nature of this communication process; and outline the steps toward more effective interaction. While this framework can be used to facilitate communication with patients at a distance through electronic, postal, or other means, in this chapter we focus on the face-to-face clinician–patient encounter with its rich mix of verbal and nonverbal elements.

BOX 13-1 Barriers to Communication

Just as the number and types of providers are increasing, so are the number and types of communication needs and communication channels. You cannot just drop by your doctor's office if you have a severe headache and a fever of 103°F. Telephone calls, emails, and text messages to the receptionist, nurse, and/or physician may lead to a squeezed-in appointment with a busy primary care physician or, more likely, a referral to an equally busy emergency department that may or may not have access to your EHR and health insurance information, and that will initiate a *de novo* inquiry into your health and payment options. Meanwhile, you are texting your friends or family to allay their concerns or get their advice. It may be hours before you get to someone who knows that severe headache and high fever in a student need to be addressed quickly because of the rare, but serious possibility of meningitis that requires urgent treatment. See, for example, Køster-Rasmussen RA, Korshin A, Meyer CN. Antibiotic treatment delay and outcome in acute bacterial meningitis. *J Infect.* 2008;57(6):449-454.

BOX 13-2 Client or Patient?

What distinguishes a patient from a client? Wing noted that the question of patient autonomy versus medical paternalism is occasionally raised as a possible reason to justify the use of the term "client" rather than "patient."* He concluded that patients sought out the protection and care of a physician, and did want to think of themselves as clients or as "consumers" of medical services.

* Wing PC. Patient or client: if in doubt, ask. *Can Med Assoc J.* 1997:157287-157289.

▸ Conceptual Framework for Effective Clinician–Patient Communication

We begin by recognizing five dichotomies that help frame the interaction between patients and clinicians. These dichotomies, along with goals, barriers, levels, modes, tools, and external issues, to be discussed later, form the conceptual framework for effective CPC (**FIGURE 13-1**).

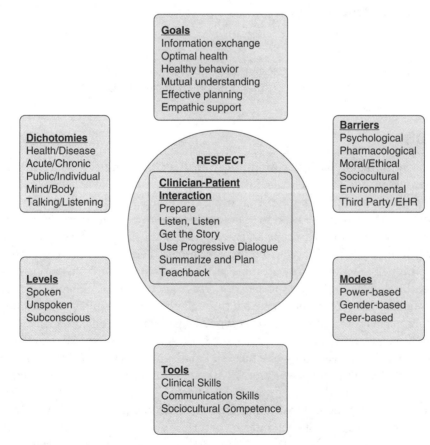

FIGURE 13-1 Conceptual Framework for Clinician–Patient Communication.

Dichotomies

- *Health versus disease:* Are we approaching our interaction from a predominately health-oriented or a predominately disease-oriented perspective—a routine checkup (e.g., physical examination) or an evaluation of recent weight loss and abdominal pain?

- *Acute versus chronic:* Acute medical problems can often be addressed and resolved by a single health-care clinician. Chronic disorders such as cancer, heart disease, diabetes, and dementia often require the participation and coordination of healthcare professionals from multiple disciplines. This leads to new communication issues and the need for well-developed team communication skills, both face-to-face and electronic. Because of the huge and increasing impact of chronic disease, team approaches such as the patient-centered medical home (PCMH; discussed later and in Box 13-10) are being developed.

- *Public versus private:* Is our intervention at the public level or predominately at the individual/private level? In this chapter, we focus on the individual level.

- *Mind versus body:* While mind cannot easily be separated from body, it is essential to ensure that both are considered fully, even though the initiating complaint/event may seem wholly physical or mental. **BOX 13-3** addresses the "soul of communication."

- *Talking versus listening:* We cannot overemphasize the essential bidirectional nature of effective CPC. We want to talk, but we must also listen. As we will see later, most often listening should form the larger part of the clinician's intervention to achieve the goals of patient-centered communication.[8]

BOX 13-3 The Soul of Communication

Sue Checchio

Archetypal psychologist and bestselling author Thomas Moore maintains that the single most important aspect of a physician's job is to listen and to create an environment where good communication can take place. The good doctor must also carefully listen not only to what is being said, but for what is not being said. Moore speaks of the "soul in medicine and illness rather than the mind" and of the "deep history, the profound emotions, the many thoughts and fantasies" that are especially intense and extensive during illness.

The enlightened provider will "grasp the deep poetry in the body and in illness: A heart problem is not just that of an organ or a pump but also of the heart as the seat of emotions and relationships." He or she "knows the wide world and therefore can practice medical skills with wisdom and humanity [and] doesn't reduce human experience, including illness, to the physical body, but understands that issues of soul and spirit play themselves out in our illness and therefore have an important role in healing."

Moore stresses, "Here we see the soul in medicine: a deep feeling for humanity showing itself in many compassionate and creative modes of service."

On the soul, Moore says: "The soul is the invisible factor that draws people together, brings out their humanity, and gives depth and meaning to whatever they do. When you treat people as objects, as cases and syndromes and machines in need of repair, you will not be a healer, you will be a technician, a human repair person, a functionary in a world of objects. Soul will not enter into your work, not into your skillful use of techniques, and not into your relationship with your patients. Your work will not satisfy you, not because it isn't worthy work, but because there is no soul to give it a deep human pulse.

"On the other hand, when soul is present, when you are capable of being present as a human being and making a connection to a patient, even simple applications of your skills will make your work fulfilling and bring you close in touch with the people who come to you for help. A hospital with soul is a place of healing. A hospital without soul is a body repair shop. The depth of human feeling and care will show itself in the people, in the building, and in the atmosphere. In a sense, it is the atmosphere that heals!"

References

1. Groopman JE. *How Doctors Think*. Boston, MA: Houghton Mifflin; 2007.
2. Moore T. *Care of the Soul in Medicine: Healing Guidance for Patients, Families, and the People Who Care for Them*. Carlsbad, CA: Hay House; 2010.
3. Moore T. Telephone interview with Thomas Moore. January 15, 2015.
4. Moore T. Email interview with Thomas Moore. December 7, 2014.

Goals

We may also view a clinician–patient encounter as in an exercise in goal setting. What do patients and clinicians want? Consider the following goals, all or most of which are relevant to every clinician–patient encounter:

- Information exchange
- Optimal health
- Healthy behavior
- Mutual understanding
- Effective planning
- Empathic support

When the patient comes to a physician for diagnosis and treatment of a heart attack, a different set of priorities is involved than, say, when obesity control is the goal. In the first case, accurate diagnosis and institution of urgent care are paramount. In the second case, the health behavior issues of adherence to dietary programs, lifestyle changes, and medical treatment are crucial and require empathic support and shared planning.

Finally, the goals of promoting mutual understanding and providing empathetic support in and of themselves need to be emphasized. Many studies now document that attention to these "soft" goals is essential to build patient trust, satisfaction, and participation in achieving the "hard" goals of direct patient care.[9–12]

Barriers

Clinicians and patients alike approach the communication process with a set of barriers:

- Psychological
- Pharmacological
- Ethical/moral
- Sociocultural
- Environmental
- Third party

Barriers at the psychological level include disinterest, fear, anxiety, depression, and reality distortion by underlying psychosis. Pharmacologic interventions such as overmedication may reduce alertness and interaction. Overriding ethical and moral standards may reduce the ability of clinicians to take certain actions, or for patients to respond in ways that may be considered healthy. Sociocultural barriers accompany sociocultural diversity and include issues with language, gender, income, health literacy, education, intellect, and ethnicity. Environmental distractions are relevant: Excessive noise, inadequate time, telephone and texting interruptions, and inappropriate settings or dress may all interfere with communication.

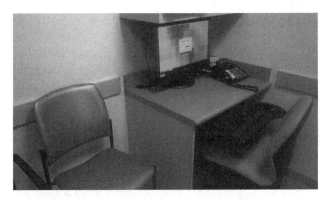

FIGURE 13-2 Optimal Locations for EHR and Patient Interaction.

The EHR and data entry are now a part of most clinician–patient encounters in the form of a computer screen and keyboard. Ideally, these are placed near but outside the direct line of visual interaction (**FIGURE 13-2**). While the need to enter data into the EHR and its review in a timely manner are not questioned, each clinician must find ways to reduce the negative impact of EHR interaction on clinician–patient communication (**BOX 13-4**).

Third-party interference with CPC is common with children and not rare with adults. Parents, family, significant others, and friends—all have their own agenda that is not identical to, and may even be at

---

BOX 13-4 Approaches to Data Entry During the Patient Encounter

- Enter data after the patient visit is concluded (time consuming, error prone for longer communications).
- Pause the clinician–patient encounter and perform data entry/review before returning to full-time interaction (time consuming).
- Enter data interactively as the patient responds to questions (challenging for nonverbal communication).
- Position the patient within your range of vision, if not straight ahead. Never turn your back.
- Try sharing the EHR with both you and the patient viewing the screen side by side (no secrets).
- Give the patient a printout of your completed patient encounter data as a take-away (added value).
- Use a scribe assistant to complete the EHR during and after the encounter (becoming more common—increases clinician time with patients and/or allows more patients to be seen).

Hafner K. January 12, 2014. http://www.nytimes.com/2014/01/14/health/a-busy-doctors-right-hand-ever-ready-to-type.html.

odds with, that of the patient. When the third party is present during the encounter, that person's interaction with the patient can be considered and interpreted. For the clinician, it is still important to get some time alone with the patient to gain a sense of his or her independent goals and needs. Even when no one else is present and communication is failing, it may be worthwhile to ask yourself, "How many people are in the room?" Sometimes the words of a dominant family member, colleague, or friend may drone in the patient's (or clinician's!) head and interfere with what otherwise would have been effective communication.

With the advent of team medicine, patients may find themselves literally surrounded by clinicians (physicians, residents, nurses, physician assistants, pharmacists, physical therapists, students, and on and on), each with a different message and approach (often uncoordinated) that can severely tax the comprehension of even the most attentive patient. While health professions students are learning to work together through "integrated professional education," this should not be construed as a license for "ganging up" on the patient all at one time.

As clinicians, we do want to communicate, and we know that good communication is essential to the achievement of patient-centered health goals. But how much communication is enough, how much is too much, and which channels are most effective, singly or in combination, can be challenges to this process.

While there are many barriers to successful CPC, all is not lost!

▶ Getting Started

If two natural communicators with similar social, cultural, language, and educational backgrounds were to meet as patient and clinician with a shared healthcare goal, their interaction might be simple, brief, and effective. For the rest of us, we need to keep in mind the multiple levels at which communication takes place and the multiple goals that may be present within the minds of both the sender and the receiver in the communicative process.

When entering into a healthcare encounter, both clinician and patient must be prepared to shift between providing information and giving feedback in a flexible and progressive fashion. The clinician may juggle goals and approaches to achieve the overall communication goal.

Much has been written about interpersonal communication.[13–22] While communication in relation to health shares some features—such as effective give-and-take, agenda setting, and the like—the context

of the health encounter often sets a difficult tone. Often, emotional issues are overriding, bringing relief, despair, or euphoria into an encounter. Life-and-death issues may charge seemingly harmless words with great intensity and unexpected meaning. The following subsections make explicit some of the features of successful CPC. Threads running throughout this discussion—and key to CPC effectiveness—relate to respect, motivation, momentum, story, and soft-focus approaches to communication.

Levels

It can be very difficult to keep in mind the multiple goals brought to an encounter by both patient and clinician, particularly when time is short and emotions are running high. The successful communicator will engage on three distinct levels of goal/need communication:

- Unspoken (what is left unsaid)
- Spoken (what is said)
- Subconscious (what is below awareness)

We all tend to focus on spoken communication, but even well-chosen, well-spoken words are best interpreted in context. As we become more aware of context, our understanding of a patient's needs and goals can expand to a degree "that words cannot express." We begin listening to the unspoken communication—to what is not said. The patient who faces a diagnosis of cancer and never asks about his or her short-term and long-term prospects is expressing a major fear—and perhaps signaling a desire to not know more at that particular time. What remains unspoken also provides information about a patient's background, fears, upbringing, political concerns, and religious convictions and beyond. It is a wealth of information.

Subconscious goals and needs are expressed in the posture, movements, and expressions that make up our body language. In addition to body language, dress, punctuality, and the choice of accompanying persons provide information about unconscious needs and goals. The mythical perfect communicator knows and uses all of this information. For the rest of us, it helps to begin by consciously searching for communication opportunities at all levels until the search becomes implicit in our own communication behavior.

Modes

There are three modes of CPC in common use:

- Power-based
- Gender-based
- Peer-based

Authoritarian, power-based doctor–patient interaction has a long history. We now know that physicians are not infallible and that diagnoses, treatments, opinions, and technical skills can vary widely. Even so, according to surveys of public opinion, the respect given to physicians and other clinicians infuses their direct communication with the power to produce change beyond that of any other healthcare channel.

A second factor in CPC relates to gender roles.[23-32] Gender differences and similarities influence the encounter at spoken, unspoken, and unconscious levels, offering both opportunities and risks for the participants. Historically, a paternalistic role for physicians has been assumed and expected by patients seeking care for their illness. When the clinician is a woman, a maternalistic relationship may result. Patients do assign roles that empower clinicians, but these roles also complicate CPC and the clinician-patient relationship. Hall and colleagues have shown that gender-based communication is a factor in patient satisfaction and adherence to treatment programs.[19-22] Women as clinicians are often more effective in this regard; indeed, women now account for more than half of medical school applicants and one-third of practicing physicians.

A look back at the television program *Private Practice* (2007–2012, American Broadcasting Company) gives an example of peer-based CPC. Ties and white shirts are avoided, as are long white coats. Doctors become friends and advisers, and the less formal peer–peer communication is used to effect change.

Shorn of the power and respect inherent in the classic doctor–patient model, the clinician must earn respect and empowerment through effective communication and actions. Reaching this level in the clinician-patient relationship can take a while.

Power-based, gender-based, and peer-based communications all have the potential to enhance communication, yet also have associated risks.[32] Their use depends on the background and spirit of the communicators—patient and clinician alike. The best approach is a flexible one, in which the clinician chooses or changes modes to best fit the needs of the patient and the skills of the clinician.

Tools

Each clinician can use a variety of tools to deal with the many barriers to effective communication just described. These can be grouped under three headings:

- Clinical skills
- Communication skills
- Sociocultural competence

In the classical clinician–patient relationship, the healthcare provider brings a broad spectrum of knowledge and clinical skills to bear on the patient's problems, providing answers and therapeutic plans and addressing questions of concern on behalf of the patient. Relevant clinical skills remain the cornerstone of patient care.

In recent decades, faced with increasing demands on their professional time and a startling expansion of the medical knowledge base, generalists and specialists alike have begun to find their medical knowledge increasingly incomplete.[33-36] At the same time, patients have become more knowledgeable about their own diseases, diagnoses, and treatments—especially through widespread availability of information on the Internet. As the knowledge differential between patient and clinician diminishes, the clinician–patient interaction is altered. To put it another way, because information can now be easily obtained from a variety of sources, the clinician has become less of a source of information and more of an adviser, organizer, and facilitator. Thus, any clinician, whether medically trained or not, will need to have full array of communication skills in addition to clinical competence in his or her chosen area.

The third element in the toolset for CPC is that of **sociocultural competence**—that is, the ability to understand and relate to behavioral patterns that are determined in part by membership in racial, ethnic, and social groups. This term is used here in preference to the more widely used "cultural competence" to emphasize the major role of social factors (e.g., age, income, gender, living circumstance) in successful CPC.[37] ("Cultural competence" *should* have the same meaning, but too often is limited to racial and ethnic issues by common usage.)

It is the rare healthcare encounter in which social and cultural factors are not significant elements in determining the ultimate outcome. This reality requires preparation to overcome the barriers, especially on the part of the clinician:

- Awareness and acceptance of the need for social and cultural competence
- Language and social skills that allow cultural barriers to be franchised
- Cross-cultural training and/or experience whenever possible

Numerous sociocultural factors affect communication, including community, customs, morals, ethics, income, language, style, and body language. For example, norms for body language, eye contact, and choice of interpersonal distance for communication are culturally determined.[38–41] To be unaware of the potential for a mismatch in such cultural norms risks being misunderstood or even giving offense with a simple gesture or movement.

External Issues

While external issues in the encounter environment are usually less important than the interpersonal considerations described earlier, location, time of day, and environmental factors such as noise, distraction, furnishings, dress, lighting, and more can either facilitate or impair communication. Emergency care in the middle of a busy street is a setting in which CPC is vital but difficult. In a controlled setting such as a doctor's office, CPC can be facilitated by supportive personnel and environments for reception, waiting, examining, and consultation.

To this point, we have outlined dichotomies, goals, barriers, levels, modes, tools, and external issues that relate to CPC. While this approach may seem overly deconstructed, the purpose is to underline the multiple factors[42] that contribute to effective CPC. As we learn how to apply this framework, the details will be replaced as CPC skills become second nature.

▶ Clinician–Patient Encounter

Each of the following aspects or actions is an important consideration in the clinician–patient encounter:

- Respect
- Preparation
- Listen first
- The "story"
- Progressive dialogue
- Review and summation
- Teach-back technique

We will use a new-patient visit to a doctor's office to illuminate the process. The "doctor" may be another type of clinician such as a nurse practitioner or a physician assistant. The patient is a stranger, unknown to the doctor.

Respect

As Purtilo, Haddad, and Doherty state in their preface and emphasize throughout their book, "Respect is the thread that weaves together discussions regarding professional and patient encounter in the healthcare environment."[6] Throughout the health encounter, the need and search for respect on the part of clinician and patient alike are never absent. Respect sets

the tone of CPC before the first word is spoken and then allows one to listen, think, move, speak, disagree, cajole, encourage, plan, share, and more—respectfully. Respect for values, customs, language, education, economic, age, and gender diversity is essential to the application of sociocultural competence to CPC.

To get respect, however, you must give it. That exchange is the essence of effective CPC.

Preparation in Environment, Body, and Mind

If the patient feels valued from the moment of entry into the encounter environment, that feeling will enhance the subsequent face-to-face communication. If the wait is long, the staff abrupt, or the waiting area less than serene, the effect on CPC may be negative. Even the face-to-face communication process begins before any words are spoken.[43] Do you place a big desk (or a big computer screen) between you and your patient, or talk across the corner of a table, or sit on the floor with a child?

Nonverbal cues such as dress, demeanor, grooming, and touch are extremely important. The first impressions of doctor and patient alike will influence the rest of the discussion in a more powerful way than might ordinarily be appreciated.[44]

The prime factor in selection of dress should be meeting the patient's needs. In support of earlier (and continuing) patients' need to place the doctor at a higher level, long white coats, white shirts, ties, and the like can be useful. Open shirts and casual attire help to establish a peer-based CPC. An active, patient-oriented choice on the part of the clinician is required for best CPC. When it comes to grooming and cleanliness, there is no choice: Bad grooming and lack of cleanliness are always perceived in a negative manner.

On the heels of the nonverbal cues comes the verbal greeting, which will cement the patient's first impression and set a tone for the rest of the encounter. I recently accompanied my daughter to an appointment with a physician whom I had never met. When he entered the examination room, he did not acknowledge my presence or even greet my daughter, but instead began with a command: "Rate your pain on a scale of 1 to 10." You can imagine the impression he made.

Even though your greeting is brief, it can also be welcoming, informative, reassuring, and empathetic. A good start might begin with a friendly expression, followed by "Good morning, I'm Dr. Johnson" or "Robert Johnson," or "Robert Johnson, nurse-clinician," or

"Hi, I'm Bob, I'll be checking your blood pressure and weight." Opening with "Sit down; I'll be with you in a moment" or "I'm a little behind schedule—what's your main problem?" does not work, either. Instead, finish up whatever else you were doing, and clear your head before any patient contact. Make each patient feel as if he or she were your first or most important patient of the day.

When possible and appropriate, some type of tactile contact can be useful in setting the tone for a clinical encounter (**BOX 13-5**). First, however, based on a sociocultural awareness and nonverbal cues, the clinician must quickly establish which limits should be set on physical contact before any touch is extended to the patient.

In Western cultures, an offered handshake is often worth a try, even with children. If nonverbal cues of fear or distance are perceived or suspected, the touch communication will have to wait or be avoided altogether.

Listening

From the physician's standpoint, listening is the next step.[45] For the clinician to listen, the patient must be talking; for the patient to talk, the patient has to be motivated. Both doctor and patient will need to listen carefully to what the other person is saying to find out which communication channels will be open. The best approach is to establish some simple communication at the level of "How are things?" or "How is your day going?" The time-honored "What brings you to see me today?" too often leads to responses like "My wife" or "The subway"—and should probably be avoided. Sometimes, a clinician can initiate patient verbalization by simply waiting or making a welcoming gesture that seems to say, "What can you tell me?" Much is to be gained by not forcing a particular direction or focus on the conversation. Sometimes a nonmedical question is needed to break the ice, as described in **BOX 13-6**.

To learn more about the origins of a patient's concern, it is often useful to ask, "What was going on when or before all of this started?" That query focuses on the possibly related events leading up to the onset of symptoms. The beginning of the symptom story often contains useful diagnostic information that can guide the subsequent medical inquiry. Sometimes medical history taking is called *anamnesis*, indicating it is a kind of anti-amnesia process. The clinician can use subtle, nondirective probes to avoid biasing recall and to enhance the patient's memory of important but seemingly insignificant events that were not actively committed to memory.

BOX 13-5 Touch and More

A patient's report:

> When my doctor comes into the room, he always breaks the ice by greeting me and giving me a light touch. He asks how I am doing and is interested in who I am as a person. He'll take my hand and say, "We're going to take care of this."… Why can't all doctors have that level of compassion for their patients? Don't they learn that in medical school?

BOX 13-6   "How 'Bout Them Red Sox!"

In his book *Better*, Atul Gawande, a Boston surgeon, focuses on the need to make human connection with each patient. Even one nonmedical question will underline that a patient is more than a disease or a problem to be solved.

> But consider, at an appropriate point, taking a moment with your patient. Make yourself ask an unscripted question: "Where did you grow up?" Or: "What made you move to Boston?" Even: "Did you watch last night's Red Sox game?" You don't have to come up with a deep or important question, just one that lets you make a human connection.*

Even when the patient comes with a specific lump or question, after responding to the expressed need, Gawande counsels asking, "How are things otherwise?" That inquiry opens the door for other concerns that may be hard to express without a little encouragement.

*Gawande A. *Better*. New York, NY: Henry Holt; 2007:151.

Story

Once a health encounter is initiated, and one has obtained some sense of the levels (spoken, unspoken, unconscious) on which the patient is communicating, the next step is to obtain the story. The value of the narrative in health communication has been the subject of considerable interest.[46,47] Indeed, the illumination of narrative is what we seek. How did it all start? What was the context? What happened next? Then what? After that? Now? Feelings? Fears? In actual practice, the narrative is usually disjointed, delayed, confused, and difficult to obtain. Typically, the patient cannot tell you the story of his or her problem in one pass with any of the clarity that you would like. Instead, you have to work with various bits and pieces through the entire encounter, letting the details drift in before a coherent narrative can be formulated.

It may be difficult for a patient to stay in focus. Patients arrive with a bewildering array of symptoms and complaints, supplemented with a list of doctor's visits and medications. While all of these things are important, it is sometimes (that is to say, almost always) useful to focus on the narrative or story of the illness, if indeed diagnosis and empathy are goals of the encounter.

A useful approach, developed in the 1950s by Carl Rogers,[48] involves the use of nondirective statements whenever possible, rather than asking questions. How does one get information if no questions are asked? One strategy to get the patient talking is through a simple statement such as "Tell me about it" or "Tell me more." As the patient begins to talk, brief, affirmative, repetitive, conjunctive statements ("OK…," "You say you felt weak…," "and…") can be used to maintain the flow. When a patient says something dramatic, a silent response and a supportive body language may allow the patient to develop the drama in terms that he or she understands better than you.

The patient's idea of narrative may be less useful than desired. For example, the patient may see the story of his or her illness as a series of doctor's visits, tests, test results, and treatments prescribed. From a medical standpoint—and a sociocultural standpoint—we look for something else—we look for what is going on within the patient more than what has been done to the patient. It is often useful to say to the patient, "It would help to hear more about you and your symptoms first and leave your previous medical care for later." This is often a difficult point to get across but an important one if the underlying story of the disease and the person is to be developed coherently.

With a focus on the patient symptoms and feelings (rather than diagnoses and treatments), the details of the patient's personal life are presented along with disease symptoms and provide a broader understanding of the illness (the individual's response to disease) to be diagnosed and treated. The result is **patient-centered health communication**.[49–52]

During this time and during subsequent encounters, emphasis should be placed on patient verbalization. Conversation analysis[53] of recorded or transcribed clinician–patient interactions probes the many factors that may influence impact and outcome. Quantitative studies of doctor–patient communication indicate that some doctors talk 70% of the time, while patients speak 30% of the time or less. Patients ordinarily view these interactions as unrewarding.[54–56] It is first goal of the clinician to encourage patient verbalization before turning to a list of need-to-know questions.

This next step may be called the "interrogative step"; it is the point at which the clinician begins to ask specific details about symptoms, treatments, circumstances, medications, and responses, and beyond. At the same time, the patient's background needs to be filled in. The clinician needs to know about the patient's local and extended family. The clinician also needs to know about the individual's work circumstance, which may be directly related to the disorder for which the patient is seeking help.

Physicians are taught that the **past medical history (PMH)** and the review of symptoms (ROS) are crucial features of the medical history. In truth, specific questions about PMH and ROS need to be delayed until the most of the story has been told to avoid biasing or even obliterating the crucial story of the patient and the illness. The classic trap of "Have you ever had this before? Yes? Well, you've got it again" has to be avoided until all the information is obtained.

Toward the end of a successful health encounter, the patient and the physician are beginning to develop a mutual understanding of the patient's story and can start to formulate the next step in health care. But before that step can be taken, the clinician should widen his or her scope to look for important information that may have been left out or inappropriately included. It is at this point where the symptom checklist that has often been given in the waiting room may be usefully reviewed.

Expert communicators will develop a sense of timing and patience in obtaining information from a patient about his or her disease or life. Often, specific or sensitive questions about medical history and symptoms can be usefully delayed, even until the time of physical examination. In any case, simple questions are often of more value than complex questions, leading questions, or questions containing medical jargon.

Physical Examination

If this is a medical visit for a new patient, then a physical examination usually takes place. However, the history taking and the storytelling does not stop, but rather is stimulated by the examination itself. As one examines the eyes, ears, nose, throat, chest, abdomen, legs, and beyond, regional questions or comments can elicit information relevant to the "story."

To prevent the examination from interfering with interpersonal communication (and actually enhance it), it is important to begin an examination with non-threatening behavior. The inexperienced medical student who begins an examination by taking out an ophthalmoscope and shining its bright light directly in the eye of the patient knows that it is important to examine the eyes; he or she is not fully aware of the fear that can be induced from suddenly placing such a bright and sharp object an inch from an unsuspecting patient's eye.

Perhaps the best way to begin a physical examination is to take the patient's hands and gently raise both arms to a forward extended position and ask that the position be maintained. This allows an initial touch, which can be comforting and reassuring, and also enables the physician to gauge any weakness or instability or inability to follow directions on the part of the patient. This tactile contact can be used as part of the overall CPC as well as in the systematic physical examination.

Progressive Dialogue

During a doctor–patient visit, a progressive dialogue develops that is second in importance only to the story itself. As information is shared, symptoms, causes, and needs are clarified. A mutual momentum and motivation are established, leading to goals that are shared rather than imposed. An effective progressive dialogue makes the process of later planning, encouragement, or persuasion much easier.

Review and Summation

All the work (and fun!) of CPC culminates in the explicit summation of what has been learned, what is to be done, and how to go about it. Sometimes it helps to say, quite explicitly, "Let's sum up where we are and what we need to do." The summation process is facilitated by keeping the key steps of this exchange in mind:

- Inform
- Teach-back
- Support
- Comfort

The clinician provides information, opinions, and plans based on everything learned in the encounter, choosing words that are informed by what has been learned during the encounter about the language, sociocultural background, and goals of the patient. The patient is then asked to say what he or she understands to have been said. This is the crucial **teach-back** step (**FIGURE 13-3, BOX 13-7**). These steps are iterated as necessary to enhance mutual understanding at best; at worst, they lead to the recognition that communication is incomplete.

In either case, the clinician gives support for the patient and the patient's point of view, and avoids recrimination for any failures in communication or understanding. In every case, the patient must leave with the feeling that "The doctor understands me." When the clinician has gained some understanding and when this state is associated with unfeigned empathy (**BOX 13-8**), a patient begins to feel comforted. Patient comfort is always a goal in itself, but is also an aid in producing behavior change, adherence to treatment program, or acceptance of unachievable goals for the individual patient.

▶ Special Cases

Language Barriers

Of all the sociocultural barriers to CPC, language is the most obvious. Language barriers can be due to a patient's age, disease, emotional factors, education,

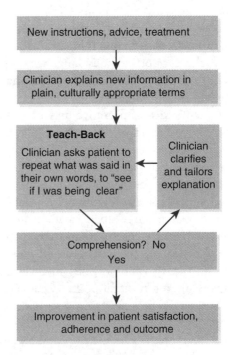

FIGURE 13-3 The Teach-Back Method.

BOX 13-7 Teach-Back Is a Special Case of Feedback

Since 1948, when Norbert Weiner's book *Cybernetics* (New York, NY: John Wiley & Sons) was published, feedback has been recognized as a crucial element of communication for both man and machine. Although the teach-back method is an example of a classic feedback loop, its importance for assessing and enhancing patient–provider communication has been fully appreciated only in the past decade or so.[*] Communication—verbal, electronic, or by some other means—is a fallible process, and error-checking routines are used in all serious communication systems. It is in some way a tribute to past physicians' sense of infallibility that error checking in clinician–patient communication (teach-back) took so long to be taken seriously.

* AHRQ Publication No. 10-0046-EF; April 2010.

BOX 13-8 A Patient's Cry for Empathy

Sue Checchio, MS Health Communication

Essayist and *New York Times* editor Anatole Broyard was diagnosed with prostate cancer in 1989 and lived with cancer for 14 months before he died in October 1990. Many of his writings center on the type of doctor he would have liked: "Just as he orders blood tests and bone scans of my body, I'd like my doctor to scan me, to grope for my spirit as well as my prostate. Without some such recognition, I am nothing but my illness." He elaborated: "I would like a doctor who is not only a talented physician, but a bit of a metaphysician, too. Someone who can treat body and soul."

When a patient is dealing with a terminal diagnosis often, few people know of their internal struggles, as they appear to "handle it well" with a false bravado. Broyard addresses this phenomenon: "My friends flatter me by calling my performance courageous or gallant, but my doctor should know better. He should be able to imagine the aloneness of the critically ill… To the typical physician, my illness is a routine incident in his rounds, while for me it's the crisis of my life. I would feel better if I had a doctor who at least perceived this incongruity."

Broyard understood that while not every patient could be saved, patients could *feel* better simply by being listened to and by being *seen* by the physician. He believed that this shift in interaction had the ability to profoundly change the doctor. The physician must to allow himself to be vulnerable; "to dissect the cadaver of his professional persona; he must see that his silence and neutrality are unnatural. It may be necessary to give up some of his authority in exchange for his humanity, but as the old family doctors knew, this is not a bad bargain. In learning to talk to his patients, the doctor may talk himself back into loving his work."

The world of a physician is filled with illness and death. The medical community "has little to lose and much to gain by letting the sick man into his heart. If he does, they can share, as few others can, the wonder, terror and exaltation of being on the edge of being, between the natural and the supernatural."

Reference

Broyard A. *Intoxicated by My Illness: And Other Writings on Life and Death.* New York, NY: C. Potter; 1992.

---

or simply not speaking the language of the clinician. It is the responsibility of the clinician to find the best means of communication, using patience, words, gestures, and/or an interpreter.[57,58] A few shared words of a common language can enhance trust and respect, and perhaps even communication.

The use of an interpreter deserves special mention because additional elements of uncertainty are added by the translation. Is the interpreter translating exactly? Can the words even be translated? Is the interpreter adding a personal bias to the translation? Most often, a

family member serves as an ad hoc interpreter. During this kind of translation process, lack of training and family biases can obscure or alter the patient's needs and symptoms as well as the clinician's intentions and opinions. In the case of recent immigrants, their children often end up as interpreters. Their assumption of this role may prevent parents from expressing feelings or problems that they consider inappropriate for their child's ears.

The best interpreters translate accurately without adding or removing words or phrases (**BOX 13-9**). Only

BOX 13-9 Using an Interpreter

Medical interpretation is a two-way process. The interpreter must understand not only the culture and language of the patient, but also that of the provider. This is why experts agree that asking family members to interpret should be avoided. "What if the relative does not know medical terminology and the doctor says appendicitis?" says Dharma E. Cortés, PhD, who trains medical interpreters at Cambridge College. "You don't know how the family member is translating that to the patient. If a child is interpreting for a parent, the child may be experiencing an undue emotional burden as he learns more about his parent's health in the process of translating the conversation between his parent and the doctor. Also, a parent may not disclose information relevant to his/her medical condition because he/she may not want his/her child to know about it."*

* Dharma E. Cortés, personal communication, January 22, 2010.

if they know the culture as well as the language being translating are supplementary comments on the cultural significance of words or body language appropriate.

Patient and clinician alike should be alert for signs of inappropriate translation. If several sentences of speech are translated as "She says 'no,'" then you have assuredly missed the flavor of that negative response and know to be alert for other mismatches.

A few words about automatic electronic translation are in order as well. Patil and Davies noted a poor success rate using the Google Translate service. In one study, they used Google to translate 10 phases into 26 languages with only 57% accuracy. Some of the translations were humorous but could have been misleading or even dangerous at worst.[59] A better option might be a new application for Android and Apple devices that provides a book of phrases commonly used in eight medical specialties and translates them verbally and visually into any of 15 languages. It also offers one-click access to a live translator as backup and medical language training for healthcare clinicians (http://www.canopyapps.com). For medications and devices, the Polyglot online application created with National Institutes of Health (NIH) funding, known as Meducation, allows practitioners to produce prescription-specific print and video instructions in mutiple languages (http://www.pgsi.com/products1.html). Given the vast cultural diversity in many parts of the United States, and the inability to have at least one staff member to speak each language, many healthcare facilities subscribe to a telephone or video-enhanced (e.g., "Skype") language line. These services can often accommodate any language on a 24-hour basis, depending on the subscription.

Informed Consent

An extensive literature has developed concerning **informed consent**—that is, obtaining the permission, or consent, of a patient or guardian before performing a medical procedure or service. How much information for informed consent is enough? How much information is too much? Often, the answers to these questions can be found in the early and progressive understanding of the patient's needs and goals. When this foundation is well established, tailoring of information to the patient's understanding, attention, and language can be most successful. In fact, consent forms are not tailored but prepared ahead of time to meet institutional approval. Such consent forms are often too long, covering all the possible medical and legal aspects of the decision being made. While these documents are necessary to protect the patient (and the physician), they require unhurried explanation to avoid serious misunderstanding or non-acceptance on the part of the patient.

If progressive dialogue is important in all clinician–patient encounters, it is of paramount in obtaining informed consent. In this situation, as in perhaps in no other, the presence of a third party—a patient advocate in the room—can be of value. Obtaining informed consent requires a high level of both clinical and communication skills to be successful. This is not a task to be delegated to the unaccompanied student, trainee, or intern. The clinician must be willing to evaluate the consent form paragraph by paragraph, providing excellent explanation where necessary and an explanation of options at all times. This is always easier if the clinician is known to the patient and has already established a working level of mutual communication.

The Dying Patient

The counseling of a dying patient causes concern to arise at the individual, family, social, cultural, religious, and political levels. Witness the intense political debate in the U.S. Congress in 2009 when a new health program was to contain provisions for financial support for counseling of the dying patient. The dispute is based on the potential for conflicting goals of the dying patient and those of other "interested" parties. How much should the government say about how we choose to die? How much influence should the doctor or family have on the patient's exit? In October 2015, Governor Jerry Brown, a former Jesuit seminary student, took the patient's side and signed the *End of Life Option Act*; This law made California the fifth state to allow physicians to prescribe lethal doses of drugs to terminally ill patients who want to hasten their deaths.

While it is easy to support the supremacy of the patient's own wishes, it is also impossible to ignore the societal pressures that bear on such decisions. No one prescription can be given to navigate this potentially treacherous path.[60-66] Perhaps the most useful path would be a return to the CPC encounter process. The patient's story remains central. The patient's needs and goals at spoken, unspoken, and unconscious levels are clarified. Third-party interests are addressed. Mutual understanding is sought. Then final decisions are made, based on the patient's interests, within the constraints of the existing local, legal, and sociocultural limits.

▶ Prospects

As discussed earlier, recent decades have seen a progressive increase in the role of nonphysician clinicians in CPC. Part of this trend reflects the reduction of CPC by physicians because of greater demands on their time and the increasing technical demands of the medical diagnostic and therapeutic process. But the external constraints are not the only factors involved in this evolution. In the past, physicians had little specific training in communication. They learned by observing their elders—some of whom were good communicators, and some of whom were not. The social climate in earlier eras allowed physicians to be less than good communicators if their medical skills were exemplary.

This milieu has now changed. We have high expectations for our physicians at all levels; expectations that cannot realistically be met. Doctors still do not have enough time to see and effectively interact with their patients. The amount of information that a doctor is required to know is beyond the capacity of most physicians and specialists unless their focus is in a very narrow field. Faced with the sobering impossibility, for generalists and specialists alike, to achieve and maintain an exhaustive knowledge of medical science, even specialist physicians are becoming more like general practitioners. In this setting, the importance of communication and cultural competency skills looms ever larger.[34]

As a by-product, other clinicians, especially nurse practitioners and physician assistants, are playing an increased role and gaining parity with physicians in promoting good health and health communication. The burdens and opportunities of interpersonal healthcare communication will be increasingly shared among health professionals from a variety of backgrounds. All are joined by the idea of developing of mutual, two-way CPC that facilitates diagnosis, treatment, and long-term health care for individuals and the community at large.

A concept that combines several aspects of health information and health communication into a potentially viable working model is the **patient-centered medical home (PCMH)**, as described in **BOX 13-10**. Whole-person, patient-centered CPC is essential to this concept.

BOX 13-10 Patient-Centered Medical Home

The primary care (or patient-centered) medical home (PCMH) model holds promise as a way to improve health care in the United States by transforming how primary care is organized and delivered. Building on the work of a large and growing community, the Agency for Healthcare Research and Quality (AHRQ) defines a medical home not simply as a place, but as a model of the organization of primary care that delivers the core functions of primary health care.

The medical home encompasses five functions and attributes.

Comprehensive Care

The PCMH is accountable for meeting the large majority of each patient's physical and mental healthcare needs, including prevention and wellness, acute care, and chronic care. Providing comprehensive care requires a team of care providers. This team might include physicians, advanced practice nurses, physician assistants, nurses, pharmacists, nutritionists, social workers, educators, and care coordinators. Although some medical home practices may bring

(continues)

BOX 13-10 Patient-Centered Medical Home *(continued)*

together large and diverse teams of care providers to meet the needs of their patients, many others, including smaller practices, will build virtual teams linking themselves and their patients to providers and services in their communities.

Patient-Centered Care

The PCMH provides health care that is relationship-based, with an orientation toward the whole person. Partnering with patients and their families requires understanding and respecting each patient's unique needs, culture, values, and preferences. The medical home practice actively supports patients in learning to manage and organize their own care at the level the patient chooses. Recognizing that patients and families are core members of the care team, medical home practices ensure that they are fully informed partners in establishing care plans.

Coordinated Care

The PCMH coordinates care across all elements of the broader healthcare system, including specialty care, hospitals, home health care, and community services and supports. Such coordination is particularly critical during transitions between sites of care, such as when patients are being discharged from the hospital. Medical home practices also excel at building clear and open communication among patients and families, the medical home, and members of the broader care team.

Accessible Services

The PCMH delivers accessible services with shorter waiting times for urgent needs, enhanced in-person hours, around-the-clock telephone or electronic access to a member of the care team, and alternative methods of communication such as email and telephone care. The medical home practice is responsive to patients' preferences regarding access.

Quality and Safety

The PCMH demonstrates a commitment to quality and quality improvement by ongoing engagement in activities such as using evidence-based medicine and clinical decision-support tools to guide shared decision making with patients and families, engaging in performance measurement and improvement, measuring and responding to patient experiences and patient satisfaction, and practicing population health management. Sharing robust quality and safety data and improvement activities publicly is also an important marker of a system-level commitment to quality.

Defining the PCMH. Available at: https://pcmh.ahrq.gov/page/defining-pcmh Accessed Dec 15, 2015.

Opportunities and challenges occur on the patient side as well. Given the increasing complexity of health care and healthcare communication, patients need to be active participants in CPC, not just passive receivers of information. **BOX 13-11** describes one example of an intervention designed to empower patients, the Ask Me 3 program, which encourages active self-advocacy for patients.

Many patients are now informed health seekers whose search of the Internet offers a panoply of options. The burden of too much information is real. One may read about a disease one week and as a result develop the symptoms the next week. As a species, humans are suggestible creatures. The need for restraint and judgment before jumping to medical conclusions is greatly needed. Restraint can be developed, but judgment can be realized only through broad clinical training in symptom analysis and the spectrum of underlying disease. Nevertheless, for all its problematic features, the Internet does provide a remarkable source of medical information that reduces the chance that important aspects of health and disease will go unconsidered.

Better understanding of nondominant cultures is also needed in health care across the board. The rapid influx of non-English-speaking groups into the United States provides a good example for a need of cross-cultural training at all levels of healthcare interaction. Patients and clinicians who misunderstand even the simplest of words and bring disparate cultural backgrounds to CPC present a challenge that is not easily met. The first step toward meeting this challenge is to recognize and address cultural differences before jumping to conclusions about understanding, diagnosis, or intervention.

▶ Conclusion

This chapter has developed a conceptual framework for clinician–patient communication; emphasized the multifaceted, bidirectional nature of CPC; and

BOX 13-11 Ask Me 3

Ask Me 3 (http://www.npsf.org/askme3) is a patient-education program designed to promote communication between healthcare providers and patients so as to improve health outcomes. The program encourages patients to understand the answers to three questions:

1. What is my main problem?
2. What do I need to do?
3. Why is it important for me to do this?

Patients should be encouraged to ask their providers (doctors, nurses, pharmacists, therapists) these three simple but essential questions in every healthcare interaction. Likewise, providers should always encourage their patients to understand the answers to these three questions.

Studies show that people who understand health instructions make fewer mistakes when they take their medicine or prepare for a medical procedure. They may also get well sooner or be able to better manage a chronic health condition.

Partnership for Clear Health Communication, National Patient Safety Foundation.

outlined the steps toward more effective CPC that are either now under way or still needed. For the clinician who is seeking to improve CPC, the most important concepts are as follows:

- The CPC framework
- The need to respect both the CPC process and its participants
- The need to find open communication channels

- The value of listening and silence in communication
- The power of story to inform
- The humility to put the patient first
- The satisfaction of making it all work

If you are motivated by these concepts, then you already have within your grasp the opportunity to dramatically improve health and the healthcare experience, one life at a time.

Wrap-Up

Chapter Questions

1. What are the three main levels of clinician–patient communication interaction?
2. Name three ways of facilitating verbal communication with the patient.
3. How would the approach to clinician–patient communication described in this chapter apply to a health communication trainee delivering door-to-door surveys on obesity in the inner city?
4. Could the suggestions to clinicians for improved communication given in the chapter also be used by patients? If so, how?

Additional Resources

1. Doctor–patient communication has a real impact on health. *Science Daily*. April 10, 2007. http://www.science daily.com/releases/2007/04/070409144754.htm.
2. Ha JF, Anat DS, Longnecker N. Doctor-Patient Communication: A Review. *Ochsner J.* 2010; 10(1): 38-43.
3. Houghton A, Allen J. Understanding personality type: doctor–patient communication. *BMJ Career Focus*. 2005;330:36-37. http://careers.bmj.com/careers/advice/view-article.html?id=629.
4. Mutha S, Allen C, Welch M. *Toward Culturally Competent Care: A Toolbox for Teaching Communication Strategies.* San Francisco, CA: Center for the Health Professions, University of California, San Francisco; 2002.
5. Teutsch C. Patient–doctor communication. *Med Clin North Am.* 2003;87(5):1115-1145.
6. Thompson TL, Parrott R, Nussbaum JF, eds. *The Routledge Handbook of Health Communication* (2nd ed.). New York, NY: Routledge; 2013.
7. Truog RD, Browning DM, Johnson JA, Gallagher TH. *Talking with Patients and Families about Medical Error: A Guide for Education and Practice.* Baltimore, MD: The Johns Hopkins University Press; 2011.
8. Wachter R. *The Digital Doctor: Hope, Hype, and Harm at the Dawn of Medicine's Computer Age.* New York, NY: McGraw Hill Education; 2015.

References

1. Raimbault G, Cachin O, Limal JM, Eliacheff C, Rappaport R. Aspects of communication between patients and doctors: an analysis of the discourse in medical interviews. *Pediatrics*. 1975;55(3):401-405.

2. Charney E. Patient–doctor communication. implications for the clinician. *Pediatr Clin North Am*. 1972;19(2):263-279.

3. Ziegler JL. *Ethical Dilemmas in the Doctor–Patient Relationship*. Lexington, VA: Washington and Lee University; 1976.

4. Hasler J, Pendleton D. *Doctor–Patient Communication*. London, UK/New York, NY: Academic Press; 1983.

5. Reiser DE, Rosen DH. *The Doctor–Patient Relationship*. Baltimore, MD: University Park Press; 1984.

6. Purtilo R, Haddad AM, Doherty RA. *Health Professional and Patient Interaction* (7th ed.). St. Louis, MO: Elsevier Saunders; 2014.

7. Wachter R. Unanticipated consequences. In: *The Digital Doctor: Hope, Hype, and Harm at the Dawn of Medicine's Computer Age*. New York, NY: McGraw-Hill Education; 2015:71-90.

8. Davis K, Schoenbaum SC, Audet A-M. A 2020 vision of patient-centered primary care. *J Gen Intern Med*. 2005;20(10):953-958.doi:10.1111/j.1525-1497.2005.0178.x.

9. Steinhausen S, Ommend O, Thümb S, et al. Physician empathy and subjective evaluation of medical treatment outcome in trauma surgery patients. *Pat Educ Counsel*. 2014;95:53-60

10. Kelley JM, Kraft-Todd G, Schapira L, Kossowsky J, Riess H. The influence of the patient-clinician relationship on healthcare outcomes: a systematic review and meta-analysis of randomized controlled trials. *PLoS One*. 2014;9:e94207.

11. Hojat M, Louis DZ, Markham FW, Wender R, Rabinowitz C, Gonnella JS. Physicians' empathy and clinical outcomes for diabetic patients. *Acad Med*. 2011;86:359-364.

12. Jean Decety J, Fotopoulou A. Why empathy has a beneficial impact on others in medicine: unifying theories. *Front Behav Neurosci*. January 14, 2015. doi: 10.3389/fnbeh.2014.00457.

13. O'Toole G. *Communication: Core Interpersonal Skills for Health Professionals*. Philadelphia, PA: Churchill Livingstone; 2009.

14. Adler RB, Rosenfeld LB, Proctor RF II. *Interplay: The Process of Interpersonal Communication*. New York, NY: Oxford University Press; 2009.

15. Beebe SA, Beebe SJ, Redmond MV. *Interpersonal Communication: Relating to Others* (6th ed.). Boston, MA: Allyn & Bacon; 2010.

16. DeVito JA. *Interpersonal Messages: Communication and Relationship* (2nd ed.). Boston, MA: Allyn & Bacon; 2010.

17. Baxter LA, Braithwaite DO, eds. *Engaging Theories in Interpersonal Communication*. Thousand Oaks, CA: Sage; 2008.

18. Monaghan L, Goodman JA. *Cultural Approach to Interpersonal Communication: Essential Readings*. Malden, MA: Wiley-Blackwell; 2007.

19. Lustig MW, Koester J. *Intercultural Competence: Interpersonal Communication Across Cultures* (6th ed.). Sudbury, MA: Allyn & Bacon; 2009.

20. Knapp ML, Daly JC. *Interpersonal Communication*. Thousand Oaks, CA: Sage; 2010.

21. Trenholm S, Jensen A. *Interpersonal Communication*. New York, NY: Oxford University Press; 2007.

22. Verderber KS, Verderber RF, Berryman-Fink C. *Inter-Act: Interpersonal Communication Concepts, Skills, and Contexts*. New York, NY: Oxford University Press; 2006.

23. Kalbfleisch PJ, Cody MJ. *Gender, Power, and Communication in Human Relationships*. Hillsdale, NJ: Erlbaum; 1995.

24. Blanch DC, Hall JA, Roter DL, Frankel RM. Medical student gender and issues of confidence. *Patient Educ Couns*. 2008;72(3):374-381.

25. Hall JA, Irish JT, Roter DL, Ehrlich CM, Miller LH. Satisfaction, gender, and communication in medical visits. *Med Care*. 1994;32(12):1216-1231.

26. Hall JA, Irish JT, Roter DL, Ehrlich CM, Miller LH. Gender in medical encounters: an analysis of physician and patient communication in a primary care setting. *Health Psychol*. 1994;13(5):384-392.

27. Hall JA, Roter DL. Do patients talk differently to male and female physicians? A meta-analytic review. *Patient Educ Couns*. 2002;48(3):217-224.

28. Hall JA, Roter DL, Katz NR. Meta-analysis of correlates of clinician behavior in medical encounters. *Med Care*. 1988;26(7):657-675.

29. Roter D, Lipkin M Jr, Korsgaard A. Sex differences in patients' and physicians' communication during primary care medical visits. *Med Care*. 1991;29(11):1083-1093.

30. Roter DL, Hall JA. Physician gender and patient-centered communication: a critical review of empirical research. *Ann Rev Public Health*. 2004;25:497-519.

31. Roter DL, Hall JA. How physician gender shapes the communication and evaluation of medical care. *Mayo Clin Proc*. 2001;76(7):673-676.

32. Power, Asymmetry and Decision-Making in Medical Encounters. In: Gwyn R. *Communicating Health and Illness*. London, UK: Sage; 2002:61-91.

33. Lloyd M, Bor R. *Communication Skills for Medicine* (3rd ed.). Edinburgh, UK/New York, NY: Churchill Livingstone/Elsevier; 2009.

34. Patak L, Wilson-Stronks A, Costello J, et al. Improving clinician-patient communication: a call to action. *J Nurs Admin*. 2009;39(9):372-376.

35. Wright KB, Sparks L, O'Hair D. *Health Communication in the 21st Century*. Malden, MA: Blackwell; 2008.

36. Bergmo TS, Kummervold PE, Gammon D, Dahl LB. Electronic clinician–patient communication: will it offset office visits and telephone consultations in primary care? *Int J Med Inform*. 2005;74(9):705-710.

37. Wissow L. Assessing socio-economic differences in clinician-patient communication. *Patient Educ Couns*. 2005;56(2):137-138.

38. Ngo-Metzger Q, Telfair J, Sorkin DH, et al. *Cultural Competency and Quality of Care*, Vol. 39. New York, NY: Commonwealth Fund; October 2006.

39. Stewart J, Zediker KE, Witteborn S. *Together: Communicating Interpersonally: A Social Construction Approach*. New York, NY: Oxford University Press; 2004.

40. Nápoles-Springer A, Pérez-Stable EJ. The role of culture and language in determining best practices. *J Gen Intern Med*. 2001;16(7):493-495.

41. Spencer-Oatey H. *Culturally Speaking: Managing Rapport Through Talk Across Cultures*. London, UK/New York, NY: Continuum; 2000.

42. Roter D, Hall JA. How medical interaction shapes and reflects the physician-patient relationship. In: Thompson TL, Parrott R, Nussbaum JF, eds. *The Routledge Handbook of Health Communication* (2nd ed.). New York, NY: Routledge; 2013:55-68.

43. Philippot P, Feldman RS, Coats EJ. *Nonverbal Behavior in Clinical Settings.* New York, NY: Oxford University Press; 2003.

44. Amer A, Fischer H. "Don't call me 'mom'": how parents want to be greeted by their pediatrician. *Clin Pediatr (Phila).* 2009;48(7):720-722.

45. Hart V. *Clinician-Patient Communications: Caring to Listen.* Sudbury, MA: Jones and Bartlett; 2010.

46. Gwyn R. *Narrative and the Voicing of Illness.* Thousand Oaks, CA: Sage; 2002:139.

47. Hinyard LJ, Kreuter MW. Using narrative communication as a tool for health behavior change: a conceptual, theoretical, and empirical overview. *Health Educ Behav.* 2007;34(5):777-792.

48. Rogers CR. *Client-Centered Counselling.* Boston, MA: Houghton-Mifflin; 1951.

49. Wilson EV. *Patient-Centered e-Health.* Hershey PA: Medical Information Science Reference; 2009.

50. Chapman BP, Duberstein PR, Epstein R, Fiscella K, Kravitz RL. Patient centered communication during primary care visits for depressive symptoms: what is the role of physician personality? *Med Care.* 2008;46(8):806-812.

51. Keselman A, Logan R, Smith CA, Leroy G, Zeng-Treitler Q. Developing informatics tools and strategies for consumer-centered health communication. *J Am Med Inform Assoc.* 2008;15(4):473-483.

52. Stewart A. *Patient-Centered Medicine: Transforming the Clinical Method* (7th ed.). Thousand Oaks, CA: Sage; 1995.

53. Robinson JD. Conversation analysis and health communication. In: Thompson TL, Parrott R, Nussbaum JF, eds. *The Routledge Handbook of Health Communication* (2nd ed.). New York, NY: Routledge; 2013:501-518.

54. Ellington L, Roter D, Dudley WN, et al. Communication analysis of *BRCA1* genetic counseling. *J Genet Couns.* 2005;14(5):377-386.

55. Roter D, Larson S. The Roter Interaction Analysis System (RIAS): utility and flexibility for analysis of medical interactions. *Patient Educ Couns.* 2002;46(4): 243-251.

56. Roter DL, Hall JA. Studies of doctor-patient interaction. *Ann Rev Public Health.* 1989;10:163-180.

57. Aranguri C, Davidson B, Ramirez R. Patterns of communication through interpreters: a detailed socio-linguistic analysis. *J Gen Intern Med.* 2006;21(6):623-629.

58. Hudelson P. Improving clinician-patient communication: insights from interpreters. *Fam Pract.* 2005;22(3):311-316.

59. Patil S, Davies P. Use of Google Translate in medical communication: evaluation of accuracy. *BMJ.* 2014. doi. org/10.1136/bmj.g7392.

60. Hunt LM, de Voogd KB. Are good intentions good enough? Informed consent without trained interpreters. *J Gen Intern Med.* 2007;22(5):598-605.

61. Mayer GG, Villaire M. *Health Literacy in Primary Care: A Clinician's Guide.* New York, NY: Springer; 2007.

62. Curtis JR, Patrick DL, Caldwell E, Greenlee H, Collier AC. The quality of patient–doctor communication about end-of-life care: a study of patients with advanced AIDS and their primary care clinicians. *AIDS.* 1999;13(9): 1123-1131.

63. Mack JW, Hilden JM, Watterson J, et al. Parent and physician perspectives on quality of care at the end of life in children with cancer. *J Clin Oncol.* 2005;23(36):9155-9161.

64. Yedidia MJ. Transforming doctor–patient relationships to promote patient-centered care: lessons from palliative care. *J Pain Symptom Manage.* 2007;33(1):40-57.

65. Formiga F, Chivite D, Ortega C, Casas S, Ramon JM, Pujol R. End-of-life preferences in elderly patients admitted for heart failure. *QJM.* 2004;97(12):803-808.

66. Barnard D, Quill T, Hafferty FW, et al. Preparing the ground: contributions of the preclinical years to medical education for care near the end of life. Working Group on the Pre-clinical Years of the National Consensus Conference on Medical Education for Care Near the End of Life. *Acad Med.* 1999;74(5):499-505.

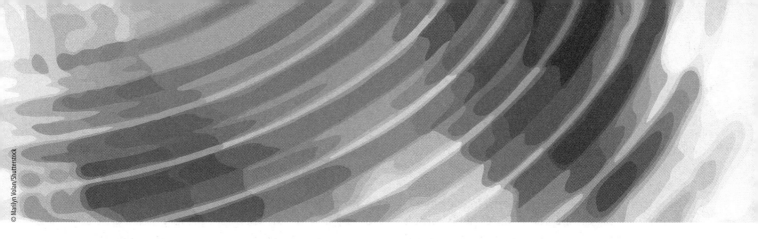

CHAPTER 14

The Role of Communication in Cancer Prevention and Care

Wen-ying Sylvia Chou, Danielle Blanch-Hartigan, and **Chan Le Thai**

LEARNING OBJECTIVES

By the end of this chapter, the reader will be able to:

- Discuss the origin and significance of the cancer control continuum.
- Describe "patient-centered communication" for cancer care.
- Discuss the difference between end-of-life and palliative care.
- List the main issues related to developing effective cancer communication campaigns and interventions.

▶ Introduction

Despite the tremendous advances in treatment and improvement in survivorship, cancer continues to affect and alter the lives of individuals, families, and communities significantly. In the words of one cancer survivor who went through the most debilitating treatments noted, "The day a diagnosis of cancer is given, everything profoundly changes." There are numerous delicate and crucial moments throughout a cancer journey, from prevention to the end of life, where communication plays a vital role and can fundamentally affect not only the patient's illness experience, but also the patient's health outcomes.

Background

Approximately 14 million people in the United States have been diagnosed with cancer, and more than 1.6 million new cases are diagnosed each year.[1] By 2022, it is projected that there will be 18 million cancer survivors in the United States.[2] This trend is shared across the global community, with more than 14 million new cancer cases being diagnosed on a worldwide basis each year, making cancer a leading cause of mortality and morbidity around the world.[3] Moreover, it is estimated that as many as 30% of cancers globally could be prevented through changes in modifiable risk factors including diet, physical activity, and tobacco and alcohol use. For example, tobacco use alone accounts for more than 70% of lung cancer deaths globally.[4] The financial burden of cancer is tremendous: In the United States, the cost of cancer care is projected to exceed $150 billion by 2020.[5] Globally, the economic cost from premature death and disability, not including direct medical care, is estimated at almost $900 billion—an amount larger than that for any other communicable or noncommunicable disease.[6]

These statistics suggest that cancer is not simply a disease that should be treated in oncology or medical settings, but rather one that requires public health attention to address its tremendous impact on world populations. In particular, communication efforts aimed at cancer prevention and control may present effective ways to address and alleviate the physical, psychosocial, and financial burdens of cancer, for both individuals and society as a whole.

Information and Communication

While communication efforts are important in public health and cancer prevention, the key role of communication has also been clearly demonstrated in the cancer clinical care setting. Not only are patients' and caregivers' needs for information and support great while coping with a cancer diagnosis, but their relationships with providers also affect their overall experience and disease outlook in myriad ways. Moreover, as cancer information penetrates the Internet and social media, communication about all aspects of cancer outside of the clinical care context increasingly shapes individuals' beliefs, attitudes, and knowledge about cancer. According to the most recent nationally representative estimates from the Health Information National Trends Survey (HINTS, tracks public use of cancer-related information in the United States) more than 55% of American adults have actively sought cancer information from a variety of sources.[7] The percentage is even greater for those with a personal or family history of cancer.[8] In addition, individuals are exposed to cancer-related information (credible or otherwise) through mass media and personal social networks even when they are not actively searching for it. How can public health practitioners leverage cancer information seeking, patient information needs, and the ubiquitous cancer information environment to alleviate the burden of cancer among individuals and in the larger population?

Chapter Goals

This chapter introduces the many issues related to cancer communication by providing a framework for considering priorities in cancer control and highlighting the contexts in which cancer communication may

occur. We begin with a summary of the cancer control continuum, a framework used by the U.S. National Cancer Institute (NCI) and NCI-designated Cancer Centers to delineate relevant points and actionable steps toward alleviating the burden of cancer. Key aspects of communication along this continuum will be discussed. Next, we survey the broader cancer communication landscape, focusing on the role of the media and the Internet in shaping cancer-related knowledge, attitudes, and beliefs. Turning back to clinical cancer care, we then define and illustrate "patient-centered communication" in cancer care and discuss the importance of care coordination and continuity of care. We close with some examples of cancer communication efforts aimed at alleviating the burden of cancer and by addressing key issues for cancer control communication and future directions for research and practice.

▶ The Cancer Control Continuum

The NCI and Cancer Centers across the United States have adopted the cancer control continuum as a framework to describe the trajectory of care and relevant areas of focus.[9] This model (**FIGURE 14-1**) includes prevention of cancer, disease detection, diagnosis, treatment and care, and end-of-life and cancer survivorship. In the following subsections, we highlight the key role of communication across this continuum.

Prevention

To promote cancer prevention, there have been increasing efforts to employ communication strategies aimed at addressing the modifiable risks and behaviors associated with cancer. Such activities include *primary prevention* efforts such as behavioral and lifestyle interventions for tobacco control, to increase physical activity, to promote consumption of a healthy diet, to reduce obesity, to increase human papillomavirus (HPV) vaccination uptake, and to promote sun safety.

Prevention also includes *secondary prevention* through early detection and cancer screening. The U.S. Preventive Services Task Force (USPTF) offers recommendations for mammography for breast cancer prevention, colonoscopy and blood testing, e.g., Fecal Occult Blood Testing (FOBT), for colorectal cancer prevention, prostate-specific antigen (PSA) testing for prostate cancer prevention, and low-dose computed tomography (LDCT) for individuals at increased risk for lung cancer. These cancer screening guidelines have been some of the most publicized and debated public health recommendations in recent years. Thus,

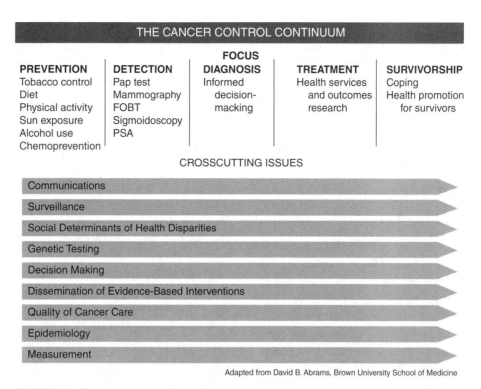

FIGURE 14-1 The cancer control continuum.

National Cancer Institute. The Cancer Control Continuum. Retrieved on December 8, 2015 from http://cancercontrol.cancer.gov/od/continuum.html.

when screening recommendations change, the task of developing communication campaigns becomes even more challenging and complicated. As an example, when the USPTF stopped recommending PSA testing due to emerging cancer epidemiologic evidence that this testing was associated with over-diagnosis and false-positive results, public attitudes and sentiment were rife with confusion and skepticism. Carefully planned and responsive public health communication campaigns may be needed to clarify recommendations and to improve public understanding of the state of the science about cancer screenings, including the associated risks and benefits.

Detection and Diagnosis

When cancer detection and diagnosis are the key concerns, the need for effective communication is salient. Information about the diagnosis needs to be presented in a manner that is understood by patients and their caregivers. Especially relevant at this point along the continuum is the need for shared decision making about treatment choices and goals of care by the patient, caregivers, and providers. Communication tools for patients, such as decision aids, may be developed to support patients and facilitate patient-provider communication. A cancer diagnosis does not necessarily follow the same treatment trajectory for all patients. For instance, with a diagnosis of prostate cancer, active

surveillance or "watchful waiting" may be appropriate for some patients, while a course of surgery, chemotherapy, or radiation may be recommended for others. Individuals may have different values and priorities that inform their decisions about care, and their goals need to be elicited and discussed. Arriving at the most appropriate treatment decision involves communicating complex risk concepts in a clinical setting. Thus, in addition to communication tools for patients and caregivers, providers need to be trained and mentored in communication skills with the goal of facilitating patient-centered cancer care—in other words, care that is focused on patient needs.

Treatment

After treatment decisions are made, effective communication continues to be required during treatment. Cancer patients are almost always cared for by a team of providers, which may include oncologists, nurses, primary care physicians, nutritionists, social workers, surgeons, radiologists, and other specialists. Each of these practitioners may have a specific task to perform with regard to his or her role in caring for the patient. Collectively, however, the patient's care plan comprises all of the tasks performed by each practitioner—hence effective communication among healthcare team members is key for quality, nonduplicative, and timely care.

In addition, patients as well as their caregivers often face increased psychosocial stress during the course of cancer treatment. Communication interventions at this stage of the continuum often focus on providing social and informational support, including offline and online support groups. Such support can improve treatment adherence, ensure patient-centered care, and provide instrumental support such as transportation and assistance with household responsibilities during a challenging time.

Palliative Care and End of Life

For individuals with advanced cancers, communication about palliative care and end of life is challenging but important. One distinction that often becomes lost in this conversation is the difference between palliative care and hospice/end-of-life care. Palliative care—which comprises a philosophy of care as well as a structured system for delivering it—aims to prevent and relieve suffering for patients with life-threatening or debilitating illness.[10] It can be delivered concurrently with other life-prolonging treatments, or it can be the main focus of care at any stage of terminal or life-threatening illness. In contrast, hospice care includes only supportive efforts aimed at ensuring good quality of life and is administered only when end of life is certain and curative treatment is no longer part of the care plan.[11]

One of the communication challenges at this stage of the continuum is knowing when and how to shift the focus from a discussion oriented toward cure while alleviating symptoms to a discussion that is purely focused on palliation and quality of life without curative treatment. Studies suggest that discussions about palliative care often come too far along in the care continuum and do not give patients and their families a chance to make informed, shared decisions that best address the patients' preferences and values. Many providers focus on communicating hope, and some avoid or delay end-of-life discussions. For example, a study of 1193 patients with advanced, terminal cancer being treated to slow progression or palliation demonstrated that 70% to 80% incorrectly believed their chemotherapy had curative potential.[12] It is important to help the public become aware of palliative care and end-of-life issues and to facilitate conversations about these topics so that patients and families are informed before they have to make a decision.

Survivorship

In discussing cancer communication, it is important to highlight the growing importance of cancer survivorship. Cancer-related communication needs do not necessarily end when a patient becomes cancer free. In fact, cancer survivors often have complex communication needs.[13] They may face late and long-term consequences from treatment. For example, removal or damage to the lymph nodes can cause lymphedema—swelling in the arms and legs—that must be monitored and treated. Aggressive radiation can lead to cardiovascular toxicity. In addition to the physical effects of treatment, survivors transitioning from active treatment to survivorship have psychosocial needs, including dealing with the fear of recurrence and adjusting to a "new normal" after cancer.

To effectively manage all of these consequences, *survivorship care planning* is a communication tool that can be used to meet survivors' needs: It facilitates communication with providers and outlines a plan for follow-up and surveillance, provides resources, and encourages communication about psychosocial needs. The Institute of Medicine (IOM) recommends that all cancer patients be provided with a comprehensive treatment summary and survivorship care plan to ensure effective communication at this stage of the cancer care continuum.[13]

Many have suggested the need to re-envision the Cancer Control Continuum to incorporate survivorship concerns. These critics would depict the continuum not as a linear framework, but rather as a cyclical continuum in which palliative care is a part of the process once a diagnosis is made, and survivorship does not signal an end to cancer care, but rather survivors' need to focus on prevention of recurrence.

For some survivors, cancer may be a "teachable moment," during which they are encouraged to make healthy lifestyle and behavioral changes, such as quitting smoking and engaging in regular physical activity. In addition, cancer survivors have unique screening guidelines that are distinct from the general population; for example, it is recommended that all cancer survivors be screened for fatigue upon completing active treatment.[14] In addition, there is an increased appreciation for viewing cancer as a chronic disease, as it can reoccur a second or even a third time.

Finally, the types of communication occurring during each phase vary across the cancer care continuum, moving from public health communication strategies (e.g., media campaigns) in prevention to increasingly individualized/interpersonal communication needs in the diagnosis, treatment, survivorship, and end-of-life phases. In addition to the shifting focus based on stage in the continuum, communication needs vary because cancer is a heterogeneous disease. Even within the continuum, communication approaches depend on the specific cancer type. Some cancer communities have a louder voice and more established advocacy networks than do others. The breast cancer community and associated campaigns, such as the Pink Ribbon campaign and the Susan G. Komen Race for the Cure, are highly recognized and organized efforts to generate awareness about and communicate information to those affected by breast cancer. By comparison, other types of cancer receive much less public attention and recognition. Moreover, communication needs extend beyond those of the patient. Most individuals have had either a personal or family experience with cancer. Caregivers, family members, friends, coworkers, and individuals in a patient's broader social network, including online social networks, may all seek and share cancer-related information.

Communication about cancer is complex and dynamic. In turn, thinking about how and where people communicate about cancer is important when developing public health campaigns to raise awareness and educate the public about this disease.

▶ The Cancer Information Landscape

Many people seek information about cancer before they personally encounter it; after a diagnosis, they are even more likely to seek information pertaining to treatment options, potential side effects, and prognosis. For most individuals (more than 70%), the Internet is the first place they go when looking for cancer information.[15] Approximately 80% of Americans report that they have searched for health-related information for themselves as least once in the past year,[16] and most individuals trust the Internet at least somewhat as a source of health information.[17]

The Internet

There are many websites and other online platforms where people can find basic information about the many different types of site-specific cancers, including etiology of disease, prevalence rates, diagnosis, and treatment options. There is also an abundance of unfiltered information online about research studies, doctors, cancer treatment centers, drugs, and complementary treatments. The scope and amount of this information can be overwhelming. Much of the information also needs to be carefully assessed: Is all of it accurate? Which sources can be trusted? The National Cancer Institute has developed a checklist of questions to help people determine whether they should trust

the information they find when searching for information on the Internet:

1. Who manages the information?
2. Who is paying for the project, and what is the funder's purpose?
3. What is the original source of the information that is posted?
4. How is information reviewed before it gets posted?
5. How current is the information?
6. If the site is asking for personal information, how will it use that information and how will it protect your privacy?

For public health practitioners, it is important to consider which types of information are available and how people determine which information is the most trustworthy. These issues of quality and accuracy of information also apply to other domains of information, including mass media such as television.

Television

Television may relay information about cancer in many different formats: news coverage, talk shows, narratives that include characters who are diagnosed with cancer, and advertisements.[18] News programs often feature stories about new research findings related to causes or prevention of cancer. However, the reporting of findings may oversimplify the studies' complexities and inadvertently promote inaccurate understanding or fatalistic beliefs about cancer.[19]

Opportunities exist to leverage media reporting to demystify certain beliefs and encourage healthy behaviors in alignment with the goals of cancer control. One possible strategy is to collaborate with television producers and writers. For example, talk shows, and particularly those with a health focus (e.g., *The Doctors*), often devote entire episodes to a specific topic, with cancer being a frequent subject of discussion. These shows may include information on the ways cancer can be prevented or feature a survivor describing his or her cancer journey. Unfortunately, it has been found that about half of the recommendations stated on these programs are either unsupported by research evidence or—even worse—contradicted by research evidence.[20] Many of these recommendations focus on cancer-related prevention or treatment.

The proliferation of reality television shows and celebrities sharing their cancer experiences (e.g., Angelina Jolie, Robin Roberts, Stewart Scott) provides yet another venue through which personal stories about cancer are shared. Entertainment programming such as soap operas or serial dramas may also portray occurrences of cancer through the characters in these shows. Sometimes, these cancer-related storylines are embedded at the behest of public health agencies to convey important health messages,[21] but more often they are unplanned communication platforms. An analysis of three seasons (2004-2006) of the top 10 shows found that nearly 6 out of 10 episodes had at least one health-related storyline.[22] This type of entertainment presents yet another channel through which people may receive information about cancer (regardless of whether the portrayals are accurate).

In addition, advertisements for drugs or certain treatment centers are readily encountered on television. These ads may also provide information about cancer and treatments.

Social Media

In addition to traditional types of media, the proliferation of online user-generated content and social networking sites has facilitated searching for and sharing of cancer information in various online groups, on discussion boards, and on blogs.[26] These online communities provide a space where information and emotional support can be offered and exchanged, transcending physical and geographical barriers. However, such user-generated content and networks lack traditional editorial filters. Because anyone can become a part of a group and share information, the accuracy and trustworthiness of the information may be called into question, with such forums sometimes causing confusion and leading to the spread of misinformation. It is imperative to ensure that the public understands how to determine the credibility of the information they encounter in social media.

Peer Groups

Cancer-related information available from a variety of sources—including peer support groups, many of which may not be focused on the accuracy of its content—can lead to conflicting or confusing messages about cancer prevention, etiology, treatment efficacy, and symptom management. This can then lead to uncertainty about individual choices and concerns about the validity of research.[23] Cancer survivors are a particularly active group in terms of seeking information. They seek cancer-related information from an average of five distinct sources, including peer support groups.[24] This abundance of information often leads to confusion about which information to pay attention to and trust. Two out of three Americans have been reported to agree with the statements

that "It seems like everything causes cancer" and "There are so many recommendations about preventing cancer that it is hard to know which ones to follow." Given the prevalence of cancer information in mass media and social media, it is no wonder that the public is often "frustrated and confused" by what they hear about what causes cancer and how to prevent it.[25]

Cancer information can be readily found in many different locations, whether through an Internet search at home or through talking to a healthcare practitioner. The key concern for patients and families is to ensure that the information on which they rely is credible and trustworthy. Opportunities for public health practitioners in this arena include developing accurate, useful educational campaigns and materials and in helping people develop media literacy skills to better interpret and assess information about cancer and other health topics.

▶ Cancer Communication in Clinical Settings

Although cancer information is increasingly available, patients still report that their top sources for cancer-related information and—by an overwhelming margin—their most trusted sources of information, are their oncologists and other providers. Therefore, communication in clinical settings continues to be of utmost importance for delivering patient-centered care.

Patient-Centered Care

The Institute of Medicine defines patient-centered care as "healthcare that establishes a partnership among practitioners, patients, and their families (when appropriate) to ensure that decisions respect patients' wants, needs, and preferences and that patients have the education and support they need to make decisions and participate in their own care."[27] The trend toward patient-centered care has gained momentum in research, medical education, and clinical practice. More than a buzzword or a "feel good" way to practice medicine, patient-centered care supports many positive outcomes, including improved patient perceptions of care, adherence to treatment recommendations, reduced medical costs and malpractice claims, and even better physiological outcomes. Thus, increasing patient-centered care is a fundamental goal of the current healthcare system and should be considered a public health issue.

Patient-centered care encompasses a host of communication-relevant functions that enable providers and healthcare systems to care for and engage the patient as a whole person. An NCI monograph identified six basic functions of patient-centered care:

- *Exchanging information:* Making sure the patient has all the information needed and the patient shares relevant information
- *Making decisions:* Involving the patient in a shared decision-making process
- *Fostering healing relationships:* Developing a trusting, positive, and productive relationship
- *Enabling patient self-management:* Helping patients take care of themselves when appropriate
- *Managing uncertainty:* helping patients understand and cope with the uncertainty in their care and outcomes
- *Responding to emotions:* Acknowledging and addressing patients' complex emotional needs

Connecting back to the cancer care continuum, patient-centered goals and specific communication tasks vary as patients move across the continuum.[28]

Complexity

As previously mentioned, cancer care is complex and involves a team of healthcare providers; consequently, improving care <u>coordination</u> is also central to patient-centered care. This means an increased focus not only on the communication between patients and providers, but also on the communication among providers and with family members. Given the many people involved (patients, caregivers, providers) and the many settings in which communication takes place, communication about cancer involves a complex system of stakeholders. To maximize message impact, an effective intervention or campaign design will identifying the stage at which the intervention is needed, tailor messages to the appropriate audiences, and understand how these audiences are embedded within the complex system. From prevention to diagnosis, and from treatment to survivorship, communication efforts are needed to build awareness, impart knowledge, shift attitudes, and impact behaviors related to cancer prevention and control.

Health Literacy

Central to any effective cancer communication is health literacy—that is, the ability of individuals to receive, understand, and use health information. **Appendix 14A** describes a detailed, 10-year, institution-wide evaluation of health literacy awareness, and implementation of a health literacy campaign including organizational support, printed materials, patient navigation, signage, and more within a major cancer facility. The scope and details of this study provide a great example of the importance that needs to be according to health literacy in cancer care.

▶ Examples

In this section, we share concrete examples of effective communication efforts across the cancer control continuum, all with the goal of reducing the burden of cancer.

Preventing Cervical Cancer

One current cancer *prevention* communication effort is focused on increasing uptake of the HPV vaccine among preteens and teenagers for cervical cancer prevention. Human papillomavirus is the most common sexually transmitted infection (STI). The primary concern over HPV vaccination for cancer control is that infection with high-risk HPV is the cause of almost all cervical cancer cases now being diagnosed. The two approved vaccines on the market are highly effective in preventing HPV infections and, therefore, a large proportion of cervical and anal cancers. Due to its public health impact, efforts are being made nationally and locally to increase the uptake of the vaccine, particularly among 11- to 12-year-olds (both boys and girls), the ages at which the vaccines are the most effective. In its initial communication campaign, the Centers for Disease Control and Prevention (CDC) presented the vaccine as an STI prevention measure; however, due to the associations of the vaccine with sexual activity, its acceptance remained low due to parental opposition. A revised national media campaign that began in 2013 reframed the vaccine as an "anticancer" vaccine and branded uptake of the vaccine as a public health concern. This example shows the importance of considering the social norms and values of both primary and secondary target audiences when designing a mass-media campaign.

Shared Treatment Decisions

Communication in the *treatment* phase involves a great deal of clinical or patient–provider communication as patients, families, and their healthcare team make important decisions about treatment options. Shared decision making is an essential component of patient-centered cancer communication. Decision aids are communication tools that can help patients and providers work together to make decisions. They are often used to communicate possible treatment options and convey complex concepts of potential risks and benefits associated with those options. For example, decision aids aiming to promote shared decision making about cancer treatment are implemented for patients newly diagnosed with prostate cancer.[29]

LIVESTRONG for Survivors

To address the needs of cancer survivors, the LIVESTRONG organization (www.livestrong.org) undertook a comprehensive effort to provide information across a broad range of topics, from diet and nutrition to managing finances and the cost of health care. The LIVESTRONG campaign and website are excellent resources for those seeking information about the unique needs and challenges of cancer patients and survivors. While originally developed to improve the quality of life of cancer survivors, the organization has since extended its scope to include anyone affected by cancer, including families and loved ones of cancer patients and survivors. The LIVESTRONG Foundation, which supports and manages the LIVESTRONG campaign, engages in a number of communication activities in support of those affected by cancer, including advocacy efforts, conducting and disseminating research, and free direct support services. For example, the website includes a tool for survivors to help them develop individualized survivorship care plans that they can share with providers and use to facilitate communication about follow-up care. Thus, LIVESTRONG is an illustration of a comprehensive cancer survivorship support organization that is addressing cancer as a public health issue through multiple communication strategies.

▶ Conclusion

Given the large number of people affected by cancer and its tremendous economic and social impact on the population, coupled with the growing body of evidence about the contribution of lifestyle choices to the etiology of cancer, it is important to address cancer control and prevention as a public health priority. Communication can play an integral role in reducing the burden of cancer on our population. In light of current research in cancer communication science, we offer some closing suggestions for best practices in developing cancer communication campaigns and interventions:

- Consider the target intervention in light of the stage of the cancer control continuum and determine the most important communication needs in regard to the goal of relieving the burden of cancer at that stage.
- Keep up with the changing communication landscape brought about by the Internet and social and mobile media. Leverage the promises of technology-mediated communication and innovations (e.g., e-health, wearable censors such as Fitbit, electronic patient portals).
- Identify and address cancer health disparities and particularly the community's need for culturally appropriate/sensitive communication, as there may be different information needs and health information–seeking behaviors in different groups, including underserved and minority communities.
- Leverage existing knowledge about program dissemination and implementation when planning and evaluating any broad-scale cancer communication campaigns or interventions.
- Understand the meaning and implications of "patient-centered communication" in the (messy) real world—given the demands on provider time, policy, and billing challenges in accounting for time spent with patients, providing patient-centered, tailored information in a complex healthcare system is a high priority.
- Consider the multilevel nature of cancer communication, from the policy level all the way to individual-oriented efforts affecting health decisions and behaviors. Communication efforts cut across multiple levels—from policy makers to the media (e.g., agenda setting in health journalism), to the community (e.g., geographic community, patient community), to communication within a family/workplace, and to individuals.

Wrap-Up

Chapter Questions

1. What are the main features of the cancer communication landscape?
2. How does patient-centered care affect cancer communication?
3. What are the most the important sources of cancer information for patients?
4. Why did the CDC reframe its communication for the HPV vaccine in 2013?
5. What are four ways to decide whether cancer information is trustworthy?

References

1. de Moor JS, Mariotto AB, Parry C, et al. Cancer survivors in the United States: prevalence across the survivorship trajectory and implications for care. *Cancer Epidemiol Biomarkers Prev*. 2013;22(4):561-570.

2. Institute of Medicine. *Delivering High-Quality Cancer Care: Charting a New Course for a System in Crisis*. Washington, DC: National Academies Press; 2013. http://nationalacademies.org/hmd/reports/2013/delivering-high-quality-cancer-care-charting-a-new-course-for-a-system-in-crisis.aspx. Accessed January 9, 2015.

3. Stewart BW, Wild CP. *World Cancer Report 2014*. Geneva, Switzerland: World Health Organization; 2014.

4. World Health Organization. WHO online cancer fact sheet. http://www.who.int/mediacentre/factsheets/fs297/en/. Accessed January 29, 2015.

5. Mariotto AB, Yabroff KR, Shao Y, Feuer EJ, Brown ML. Projections of the cost of cancer care in the United States: 2010-2020. *J Natl Cancer Inst*. 2011;103(2):117-128.

6. John RM, Ross H. The global economic cost of cancer. American Cancer Society; 2010. http://www.cancer.org/acs/groups/content/@internationalaffairs/documents/document/acspc-026203.pdf. Accessed January 29, 2015.

7. National Cancer Institute. Health Information National Trends Survey: Cycle 3 results. http://hints.cancer.gov/question-details.aspx?dataset=43&qid=401&qdid=5610. Accessed January 29, 2015.

8. Finney Rutten LJ, Agunwamba AA, Wilson P, et al. Cancer-related information seeking among cancer survivors: trends over a decade (2003-2013). Unpublished manuscript under review; 2014.

9. National Cancer Institute. The cancer control continuum. http://cancercontrol.cancer.gov/od/continuum.html. Accessed January 29, 2015.

10. National Consensus Project. *Clinical practice guidelines for quality for palliative care*, 2nd ed. Pittsburgh, PA: National Consensus Project; 2009.

11. Billings JA. What is palliative care? *J Palliat Med*. 1998;1:73-81.

12. Weeks JC, Catalano PJ, Cronin A, Finkelman MD, Mack JW, Keating NL, Schrag D. Patients' expectations about effects of chemotherapy for advanced cancer. *N Engl J Med*. 2012;367(17):1616-1625.

13. Hewitt M, Greenfield S, Stovall E, eds. *From Cancer Patient to Cancer Survivor: Lost in Transition*. Washington, DC: National Academies Press; 2005.

14. Bower JE, Bak K, Berger A, Breitbart W, Escalante CP, Ganz PA, ... & Ogaily MS. Screening, assessment, and management of fatigue in adult survivors of cancer: an American Society of Clinical Oncology clinical practice guideline adaptation. *J Clin Oncol*. 2014;32(17):1840-1850.

15. National Cancer Institute. Health Information National Trends Survey: results. http://hints.cancer.gov/question-details.aspx?qid=688. Accessed January 29, 2015.

16. National Cancer Institute. Health Information National Trends Survey: results. http://hints.cancer.gov/question-details.aspx?dataset=43&qid=757&qdid=5622. Accessed January 29, 2015.

17. National Cancer Institute. Health Information National Trends Survey: results. http://hints.cancer.gov/question-details.aspx?dataset=43&qid=677. Accessed January 29, 2015.

18. Wakefield MA, Loken B, Hornik RC. Use of mass media campaigns to change health behaviour. *Lancet*. 2010;376(9748):1261-1271.

19. Niederdeppe J, Fowler EF, Goldstein K, Pribble J. Does local television news coverage cultivate fatalistic beliefs about cancer prevention? *J Commun*. 2010;60(2):230-253.

20. Korownyk C, Kolber MR, McCormack J, ... & Banh HL. Televised medical talk shows: what they recommend and the evidence to support their recommendations: a prospective observational study. *BMJ*. 2014;349:g7346.

21. Hether HJ, Huang GC, Beck V, ... & Valente TW. Entertainment-education in a media-saturated environment: examining the impact of single and multiple exposures to breast cancer storylines on two popular medical dramas. *J Health Commun*. 2008;13(8):808-823.

22. Murphy S, Hether H, Rideout V. *How Healthy Is Prime Time? An Analysis of Health Content in Popular Prime Time Television Programs*. Menlo Park, CA: Henry J. Kaiser Family Foundation; September 16, 2008.

23. Nagler RH. Adverse outcomes associated with media exposure to contradictory nutrition messages. *J Health Commun*. 2014;19(1):24-40.

24. Blanch-Hartigan D, Blake KD, Viswanath K. Cancer survivors' use of numerous information sources for cancer-related information: does more matter? *J Cancer Educ*. 2014:1-9.

25. Arora NK, Hesse BW, Rimer BK, ... & Croyle RT. Frustrated and confused: the American public rates its cancer-related information-seeking experiences. *J Gen Intern Med*. 2008;23(3):223-228.

26. Chou WY, Lui B, Post S, Hesse B. Health-related Internet use among cancer survivors: data from the Health Information National Trends Survey, 2003–2008." *J Cancer Surviv*. 2011;5(3):263-270.

27. Institute of Medicine, Committee on Quality of Health Care in America. *Crossing the Quality Chasm: A New Health System for the 21st Century*. Washington, D.C. National Academies Press; 2001.

28. Epstein R, Street RL. *Patient-Centered Communication in Cancer Care: Promoting Healing and Reducing Suffering*. National Cancer Institute, NIH Publication No. 07-6225. Bethesda, MD, 2007.

29. Agency for Healthcare Research and Quality. Knowing your options: a decision aid for men with clinically localized prostate cancer. http://www.effectivehealthcare.ahrq.gov/ehc/decisionaids/prostate-cancer/. Accessed January 30, 2015.

Appendix 14

Health Literacy in the Context of Cancer Care: Fox Chase Cancer Center

Linda Fleisher, Stephanie Raivitch, and Rima Rudd

The concept of health literacy, which was first defined by Nutbeam in the 1998 World Health Organization (WHO) health promotion glossary, has been undergoing a transformation.[1,2] Early researchers focused on the skills of individuals to establish links between literacy and health outcomes. Over time, health literacy scholarship inquiries and policy initiatives have increasingly focused on the ability of health systems and health professionals to support the public's access to information as well as access to care and services.[3–5] Indeed, the initial report in 2004 from the Institute of Medicine (IOM) noted that health literacy was an "interaction between the skills of individuals and the requirements and assumptions of health and social systems.[6] However, a relatively recent paper from the IOM Roundtable on Health Literacy is spurring interest into the notion of a health-literate organization and encouraging research into those organizational attributes and professional skills that might either support or impede health literacy.[7]

This case study focuses on an early exploration of factors related to health literacy undertaken by a prestigious institution and offers insight into strategic developments for efficacious change.

▶ One Institution's Approach

Recognizing the significance of the problem of low health literacy, and the impact it could be having on our institution and its patient population, the first author and colleagues initiated a multistep, multiyear process ultimately resulting in institutionally supported changes in practice (**FIGURE 14A-1**). We began building momentum for health literacy work by creating a stakeholder committee and conducting awareness-raising activities throughout the Fox Chase

Cancer Center (FCCC), located in Philadelphia. These relatively simple activities included cafeteria-based postings during Health Literacy Month and invited presentations. Subsequently, we conducted two rigorous organizational assessments and provided recommendations and strategies for change. This initiative had minimal funding, but nevertheless was successful because of the commitment of leaders at all levels of the organization. An evolving, learning process changed perspectives and practices over time.

Health Literacy Committee

Our first step in 2005 was to establish the Health Literacy Committee, composed of staff representing all areas of the institution, including the patient education, nursing, administration, outreach, and marketing divisions. The committee was very informal, with no budget. Members contributed time and their own resources. The committee included those who were already advocates for health literacy and those who were somewhat uncertain about the severity of the issue. We suspected that the overall perception among staff was that health literacy was not a major problem for our institution. We deemed it important for the committee membership to include and value skeptical voices.

The committee brought together findings from health literacy studies and articulated three primary goals:

1. Raise awareness of health literacy findings and provide professional development opportunities for staff
2. Initiate an ongoing assessment of the scope of the problem on an institutional level
3. Inform and guide change

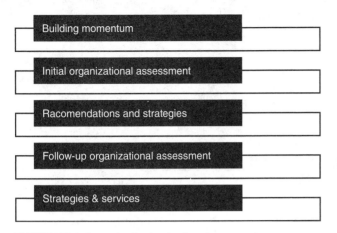

FIGURE 14A-1 Steps in the institutional approach.

Needs Assessment

Needs assessments can tap into felt needs (from the perspective of the audience) as well as into perceived needs (from the perspective of those seeing a problem). The needs assessment process and the dissemination of findings can also serve to bring heightened awareness of an issue previously not recognized.

The committee developed and administered a survey to assess the FCCC staff's knowledge and attitudes about health literacy. Survey results indicated that staff underestimated the extent of the problem at the national level and that half of the staff believed that few FCCC patients (fewer than 25%) would have low or limited health literacy. Survey results indicated a need for a broader systematic and institutional assessment. The committee provided national and local statistics along with survey results to raise awareness and as an argument for institutional attention to health literacy.

The committee also worked with FCCC's Office of Health Communications and Health Disparities (OHCHD), which addressed health disparities programs and research in the community and supported health literacy and patient education programs internally. This office, which was led and staffed by trained health educators, was building capacity to conduct health literacy evaluations of select patient education materials using best practice tools and approaches in health literacy. However, these activities did not, at the time, provide a formal process or known service. The findings indicated that many of the materials used within the institution were assessed at the 11th- to 12th-grade level. The health literacy literature indicated that this reading demand was far too high for the average U.S. adult. This evaluation, which focused on materials in active use, provided important data to share with those distributing the materials as well as

with organizational leadership. Once again, data provided an opportunity to raise awareness and provide an argument for action.

Awareness Raising

We recognized that to move forward, we would need funding for more foundational activities. Data gathered from the initial needs assessment and materials assessment results bolstered efforts to raise funds in support of health literacy activities. We secured some minimal funds through our patient navigation efforts with Pfizer, an organization then supporting health literacy education. We organized a series of health literacy presentations given by the Health Communications and Health Disparities Department (Fleisher and Raivitch). These presentations as well as other promotional activities (e.g., an ice cream social, articles in the internal newsletter, and materials in the cafeteria) were held in October during Health Literacy Awareness month. Collectively, these activities raised the dialogue and interest in health literacy.

Building Capacity

We applied for, and received, the Pfizer Visiting Health Literacy Scholar grant, which was instrumental to begin to build the capacity to address health literacy in a systematic approach and to provide credibility for these efforts. Often, this type of external validation and the opportunity to bring outside voices to the effort facilitate getting the attention of organizational leadership. The grant also provided an opportunity to structure a more in-depth visit that combined public talks, strategic meetings, and staff training.

We had the opportunity to bring in one of the case authors, Dr. Rima Rudd, a well-known health literacy expert, and one of her students at the time, Dr. Devorah Keller. This visit, in February 2008, included lectures on health literacy ("Helping Patients Through Complicated Medical Systems"; "Literacy Findings and Implications for Medicine"), a day-long training session on how to conduct an internal environmental assessment using *The Health Literacy Environment of Hospitals and Health Care Centers: Partners for Action: Making Your Healthcare Facility Literacy-Friendly*, and discussions with committee members and organizational leadership. Dr. Rudd also met and trained a team of FCCC's staff as well as staff from Temple Kidney Transplant, Geisinger Henry Cancer Center, and Mt. Nittany Medical Center on how to implement an environmental assessment.

More than 100 people, including FCCC staff, individuals from state and local departments of health, and educators and students from several neighboring universities, attended the general session; approximately 75 physicians and nurses attended the session for medical staff; and 30 people attended the assessment training. There were two components to the evaluation of this training. The first component consisted of a pre-test and a post-test, with the participants answering questions about their level of knowledge and confidence relating to health literacy and identifying barriers to health literacy. The second component comprised a series of three-month follow-up phone interviews. Findings from the pre- and post-tests showed a 50% increase from "not very knowledgeable" to "knowledgeable" or "very knowledgeable" about health literacy, and a 57% increase in the participants' knowledge of materials assessment. Prior to the training, most participants were unfamiliar with the SMOG and SAM readability tools. After the training, they felt able to use these tools, and there was an 86% increase in participants' self-reported ability to identify barriers to health literacy within their institutions. Activities and findings from the Health Literacy Assessment Team that was trained are discussed later in this report.

In addition, through funding from the Pennsylvania Department of Health, a two-day training seminar titled "Health Literacy and Plain Language: Skills for Clear Health Communication" was presented by Sue Stableford of the Health Literacy Institute of New England on June 25–26, 2008. The seminar, sponsored by FCCC's Office of Health Communications and Health Disparities, was held at the Pennsylvania College of Optometry and was attended by 23 people. The two-day training session, which was attended by both FCCC staff and staff of the Pennsylvania Department of Health, provided hands-on activities in writing in plain language and offered many helpful guidelines and resources for us to use as we moved forward with our health literacy initiatives at FCCC. In fact, many members of both the Fox Chase Health Literacy Committee and the Fox Chase Health Literacy Assessment team were in attendance. The training included hands-on exercises to identify key elements of plain language, lessons on the application of readability formulas, and practice in specific-plain language writing techniques. The training also included examples of layout design elements that enhance reading ease as well as issues in testing with the target audience. The two days provided many examples and discussions on each of these topics. All participants were provided with a workbook filled with materials as well as a long list of resources. An evaluation of the training was undertaken at the end of the second day in the form of a questionnaire; the evaluations were extremely positive.

Organizational Assessment

A Health Literacy Assessment Team was developed under the leadership of the Health Literacy Committee. The team met after the training and conducted the assessment over the next year. The group was split into two subteams, the print assessment team and the physical environment assessment team. Each team used the toolkit materials provided by Dr. Rudd to conduct its assessments.

The print assessment team was charged with reviewing materials produced by FCCC, including education materials, patient packets, result letters, informed consent forms, and promotional materials, and grading the readability levels of these materials. The SMOG formula was used to determine the reading grade level for the materials. Along with identifying the readability level, the team used a print communication rating system from the toolkit to rate each piece of material. The findings from this assessment (**TABLE 14A-1**) revealed that most materials produced and used by FCCC were written at a reading grade level above the average reading grade level of U.S. citizens.

The physical environment team was charged with conducting literacy environmental assessment exercises. This involved conducting "walkabouts" of the institution designed to identify potential health literacy–related barriers as teams attempted to navigate between locations in the facility. One exercise was conducted in February during the Pfizer Visiting Professorship on Health Literacy at FCCC by the workshop participants. In this activity, a non-FCCC employee was given a starting point and three assigned locations to find. The individual was asked to talk aloud about what they observed, signage (printed word and pictures), maps, personnel, overall atmosphere, and any cues or tools that help the visitor find target locations. A FCCC employee accompanied the observer and took notes.

The second exercise was conducted in the summer of 2008 by members of the FCCC Health Literacy Navigation Assessment Team. In most cases, exercises were performed by the members themselves. One member had a new employee to help her with the exercise. Each person made observations as described in the first exercises, paying particular attention to concerns discussed after the initial exercise. Results of both exercises revealed common themes (see **TABLE 14A-2**).

TABLE 14A-1 Results of Print Assessment

Name of material	Type of material	SNOG	Print communication rating
Patient Guide to Services Booklet	Patient/client orientation	12 grade level	75% - Continue to monitor and eliminate literacy-related barriers
Partners in Safety brochure	Patient/client orientation	11 grade level	80% - Continue to monitor and eliminate literacy-related barriers
Prevention Alert	Patient Education Material	15 grade level	66% - Augment efforts to eliminate literacy-related barriers
South Jersey health Cancer Services	Community Relations	16 grade level	51% - Augment efforts to eliminate literacy-related barriers
Understanding Brain Cancer partner e-newsletter	Community Relations	13 grade level	57% - Augment efforts to eliminate literacy-related barriers
Prevention Matters newsletter Winter/Spring 2008	Community Relations	13 grade level	74% - Continue to monitor and eliminate literacy-related barriers
Forms		**PMOSE/IKIRSCH**	
New Patient Assessment Form Ambulatory Care	Form patients fill out	Levels 3 - Moderate complexity range including Grade 12 equivalent to some education after high school	57% - Augment efforts to eliminate literacy-related barriers
Patient Registration Form	Forms patients fill out	Levels 4 - High complexity range including 15 years of schooling to college degree equivalent	63% - Augment efforts to eliminate literacy-related barriers

TABLE 14A-2 Results of Physical Environmental Assessment

Category	Comments	Suggestions
Signage	<ul><li>Largely unaware of color-coding system</li><li>Existing signs were sometimes not easy to see (too high, not at eye level)</li><li>Signs were not easy to read (small font size or use of italics)</li><li>Some areas did not have signs</li><li>No signs were observed in any other language other than English or Braille</li><li>No clear sign indicating Main Lobby</li><li>Wall maps were difficult to read</li><li>Maps at Info Desk were not available or difficult to read (copy quality poor)</li></ul>	<ul><li>Provide maps at entrances (wall-mounted and paper maps) including a key to color coding of signs</li><li>Have signs at eye level (hanging down from ceilings)</li><li>Avoid use of italics on signs</li><li>Have Braille available throughout more areas of the center</li><li>Consider Spanish or other language signage—at least a Welcome sign in other languages with a contact number for assistance for those who do not speak English</li></ul>

Category	Comments	Suggestions
Environment	■ Outpatient area chairs, fireplace, and bookcase made it feel cozy ■ Liked the use of texture and color on donor wall ■ Main Lobby noted to be warm, not cluttered, clean, well-lit with a nice, large colorful painting ■ Area from hospital to outpatient lab was light, clean throughout, no hospital smell ■ Liked the coffee smell ■ No benches were available for people to sit when navigating between locations, some of which were quite far apart ■ Clutter was noted next to Area B desk	
Navigation	■ Inconsistency noted in terminology/signage used by staff (e.g., Area A for Lab/Infusion Room Waiting Area) ■ Cancer Prevention Pavilion sign says Prevention Pavilion, Snack Bar/Terrace Café	■ Consider patient surveys to assess their navigation experiences
Staff/personnel	■ No doorman, concierge, or "Ask Me" person; visitors felt lost and confused ■ Several staff members were asked directions and were "great, friendly, and repeated directions" ■ Two staff persons who were unsure found another staff person to help ■ Others, including a security guard and a van driver, were not as helpful in terms of directions ■ Shuttle van did not have number on it and passed by too quickly (missed it twice) ■ Directions given by staff did not usually mention different buildings	■ Staff education (common terms for names of areas, use of color coding, how to direct people) ■ Have a "greeter" at all entrances

▶ Recommendations and Strategies

The results of the initial environmental assessment (See **TABLE 14A-3**) conducted at FCCC pointed to a need for a more comprehensive and systematic approach to addressing health literacy issues within the institution and resulted in a list of recommendations focused on resources, training, and new processes/approaches. Two departments (Office of Health Communications and Health Disparities & Patient Education) took on the primary responsibility of addressing these recommendations and leading the Health Literacy Committee.

Office of Health Communications and Health Disparities/Resource and Education Center Activities

The Office of Health Communications and Health Disparities has provided leadership to the Health Literacy Committee, developed a health literacy evaluation service (supporting both hospital and research), developed resource guides, and led subsequent organizational assessments.

Health Literacy Evaluation Service

Evaluation and revision of materials for increased readability service include using software designed to

TABLE 14A-3 Recommendations from the Initial Organizational Assessment

Resources and Training

1. Produce and disseminate a style guide for writing easy-to-read materials
2. Identify and disseminate other tools designed to assist in this process (i.e., *Health Literacy Resource Guide, A Practical Guide to Informed Consent, Health Literacy Innovations*, Readability PLUS, StyleWriter)
3. Build capacity by conducting plain-language trainings and in-service programs for both research and nonresearch personnel who are developing materials for patients, family members, participants, and the general public
4. Explore developing a health literacy training component to integrate into existing cultural competency efforts through Workforce Development

Procedures and Review

1. Consider implementing institutional readability guidelines for all consumer materials based on best practices and recognized standards (i.e., FCCC institutional review board [IRB] already requires informed consent documents to be written at the eighth-grade level)
2. Consider establishing a plain-language review process for all consumer materials, similar to those currently conducted by the Patient Education Committee and FCCC Forms Committee
3. Obtain professional plain-language review and editing assistance
4. Identify a cadre of volunteers to pilot test materials
5. Consider implementing changes to simplify and standardize the language on institutional signage and names of areas (e.g., outpatient versus ambulatory care)
6. Provide customer service training to standardize knowledge of changes and staff practices
7. Expand environmental assessment process to include areas not addressed in first two rounds of assessment: policies and protocols, technology, oral exchange
8. Conduct periodic reassessments of print communications and navigation
9. Health Literacy Environmental Assessment Teams could continue to serve this function
10. Interdisciplinary FCCC Health Literacy Committee should continue to act as an internal advisory committee to guide and contribute to the assessment process as well as to identify other opportunities for staff awareness and education

measure reading level as well as to identify problems with plain language. These services have been provided to various departments and in collaboration with several committees for a variety of materials, including patient education information, patient correspondence, consent forms, patient intake forms, and website content for access by FCCC patients as well as the public at large. Examples include the following:

- The FCCC Patient Bill of Rights (through work with the Patient Education Committee)
- Health History Questionnaire for the Thoracic Program (through work with the FCCC Forms Committee)
- Mobile Mammography result letters (through work with the Health Literacy Committee and Corporate and Community Outreach)
- Cancer content pages for the FCCC website (through work with the FCCC website team)
- Cancer websites for use by FCCC patients evaluated and compiled in a list by the Resource and Education Center

- The NCCN's Breast Cancer Patient Guidelines (through work with the Cancer Information Service)

In addition, readability evaluations and revisions were provided for research-based materials, including protocols, informed consent forms, study scripts, recruitment brochures, and websites and web-based tools to be used in connection with proposed and funded studies. Examples include the following:

- Plain-language evaluation and redesign of informed consent documents for use in *A Practical Guide to Informed Consent: Providing Simple and Effective Disclosure in Everyday Clinical Practice*. This guide was developed with a grant funded by the Robert Wood Johnson Foundation and in collaboration with Dr. Suzanne Miller's group and groups at Temple University and University of California at San Francisco.
- Print and web-based interventions for Dr. David Weinberg's *Two Delivery Channels to Improve Colorectal Cancer (CRC) Screening* and materials and

brochures for his Colon Cancer and Genetic and Environmental Risk Assessment (GERA) study.

- Identification and evaluation of websites, and plain-language revisions of content for web-based intervention for Dr. Mary Ropka's *Trusted Advisor for Cancer Health Decisions (TACH-D): Hereditary Cancer Decisions* web-based patient decision support intervention
- Evaluation of materials for the FCCC Prostate Risk Assessment Program's *Take Charge of Your Prostate Risk*
- Evaluation of materials for Dr. Suzanne Miller's TC3 study
- Evaluation of web-based tools for Dr. Catharine Wang's *Overcoming Barriers to Genetic Literacy Among Underserved Minorities*
- Plain-language evaluation and revisions of content for web-based intervention of Dr. Neal Meropol's Pre-ACT: Preparatory Education about Clinical Trials study

Health Literacy Resources

Two resource guides were used: *Resource Guide to Health Literacy* and *A Practical Guide to Informed Consents*. Both resource guides are available on FCCC's website.

Patient Education Committee

The Patient Education Program consists of an administrative assistant and a multidisciplinary committee with more than 35 members. The committee has been very responsive to principles related to health literacy when developing or reviewing the more than 100 Patient Information Sheets available in our Patient Education Resource Cart (PERC). Members strive to use plain language and aim for an eighth-grade or lower reading level when developing materials. Committee members work closely with other departments within the institution that develop or utilize information intended for patients, seeking to increase awareness of the need to consider literacy and readability

and to assist as needed. We have several kiosks that have patient education information available in Spanish and have recently put the translation site healthinfotranslations.org as a link on our PERC Online.

▶ Today

This 10-year initiative has made significant strides in building the institutional capacity to address health literacy both through patient education and research efforts, and has increased the awareness of the problem and changed the organizational culture. As an internal *grassroots effort*, it has taken tremendous dedication from a few committed individuals and departments that have stayed the course and built support with senior leadership. The Health Literacy initiative at FCCC is now an active effort with multiple components working together to effect changes for the benefit of the entire Fox Chase Cancer Center community.

References

1. Nutbeam D. The evolving concept of health literacy. *Soc Sci Med*. 2008;67(12):2072-2078.
2. Rudd RE, McCray AT, Nutbeam D. Health literacy and definitions of terms. In *Health Literacy in Context: International Perspectives*. Hauppauge, NY: Nova Sciences; 2012:13-32.
3. Bass SB, Gallo R, Crookes DM, Berger T, Fleisher L. *Your Resource Guide to Health Literacy*. Harrisburg, PA: Pennsylvania Department of Health; 2008.
4. Rudd R. Need action in health literacy. *J Health Psychol*. 2013;18(8):1004-1010.
5. U.S. Department of Health and Human Services, Office of Disease Prevention and Health Promotion. National Action Plan to Improve Health Literacy. 2010. https://health.gov/communication/initiatives/health-literacy-action-plan.asp. Accessed December 27, 2016.
6. Institute of Medicine. *Health Literacy: A Prescription to End Confusion*. Washington, DC: National Academies Press; 2004.
7. Brach C, Dreyer B, Schyve P, Hernandez L, Baur C, Lemerise A, Parker R. *Attributes of a Health Literate Organization*. Institute of Medicine Discussion Paper; January 2012.

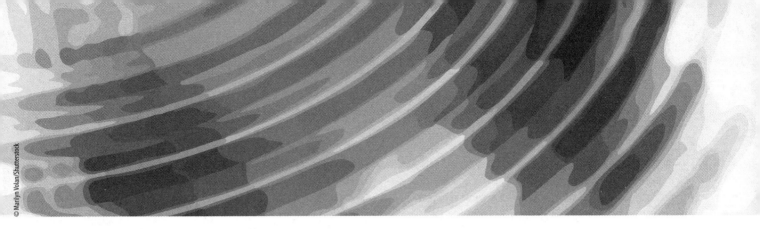

CHAPTER 15

Crisis and Emergency Risk Communication: A Primer

David W. Cragin and **Claudia Parvanta**

LEARNING OBJECTIVES

By the end of this chapter, the reader will be able to:

- Find up-to-date resources from the Centers for Disease Control and Prevention on how to handle an emergency situation.
- Explain the difference between risk and emergency risk communication, and recognize the challenges of both.
- Define risk assessment terms used by the Environmental Protection Agency.
- Use Hill's criteria to evaluate causality.
- Describe processes to undertake before, during, and after a public health emergency.
- Apply key theories to crafting emergency risk messages.
- Use tools for organizing a communication response:
  - An emergency communication plan
  - Message maps
  - Question-and-answer techniques
- Understand which factors affect how the public responds during an emergency.
- Follow basic guidance for presenting emergency risk communication to the public.
- Review how communications needed to change to confront the Ebola epidemic in Africa.

▶ Introduction

Attack

It has been nearly two decades since the world was shocked by the attacks on and destruction of the World Trade Center towers in New York; the attack on the Pentagon in Washington, D.C.; and the crash of a hijacked airplane in Pennsylvania on September 11, 2001. I (CP) and most of my colleagues in the Office of Communication at the Centers for Disease Control and Prevention (CDC) were watching the horrific events unfold on television, wondering if Atlanta would be a target. CDC medical staff were dispatched to New York, Washington, D.C., and Pennsylvania; CDC communication officers were sent to support the front lines of each "event," as we came to call an emergency situation. The rest of us did the backstopping, establishing a 24/7 workforce to anticipate questions and prepare answers for the media, prepare spokespersons, develop and clear materials, and communicate with a rightfully worried public.

Transformations

What we did not know then was how transformative this and subsequent events would be for the United States as a whole, and the CDC in particular. It was barely a month later when my (CP) boss, Vicki Freimuth, who held the senior communication position at the CDC, received a phone call telling her that a man working at American Media Inc. in Florida had been given a probable diagnosis of **anthrax**. I was sitting in her office at the time and did not understand the significance of that information. Unfortunately, we were about to learn much more than we ever wanted to know about anthrax—and about emergency risk communication on a national and international scale.

In the weeks and months that followed, CDC was transformed from an agency that rarely spoke directly to the public (preferring instead to work through state and local intermediaries), to one that made frequent appearance on the nightly news. Its entire view of preparing materials for the public also changed from scientists resisting having to "dumb it down," to understanding their roles as "subject matter experts" (SMEs) who were expected to team up with communication and health literacy professionals. The field epidemiologists also learned that when conducting investigations, people considered them to be "healthcare providers," and they upgraded their interpersonal communication skills accordingly. Training of media professionals in health departments and their journalist counterparts intensified.

Shortly after the anthrax case, personnel at the CDC had to deal with the emergence of severe acute respiratory syndrome (**SARS**) as a concern. Meanwhile, the agency began intensive preparations for pandemic flu and started developing strategies and materials for terrorist-induced public health emergencies, including use of smallpox as a weapon. These prevention efforts were mirrored across the United States through grants made to state, local, territorial, and tribal health departments and preparedness centers (academic partners). The National Public Health Information Coalition (NPHIC) was strengthened, and began coordinating a weekly briefing and conference call, as well as publishing toolkits and materials frequently. Efforts to reinforce emergency preparedness have been ongoing through Public Health Emergency Preparedness cooperative agreements.[a] As of this writing, the ability of communication officers working in health departments to mount a coordinated response for most emergencies should be excellent.

Outbreak

On a global basis, we cannot overestimate the amount of suffering that continues to occur due to conflict, drought, famine, and other disasters. The World Health Organization (WHO), CDC, and many emergency organizations (e.g., International Red Cross, Médecins Sans Frontières) assist in addressing these crises as they can. Even with the scope of these ongoing health challenges on a global scale, the 2014-2015 **Ebola** virus disease outbreak in West Africa stands out as the worst such public health emergency during modern times.[b] **BOX 15-1** provides an analysis of this outbreak as a "black swan event," as explained by K. Swain.

Again, the global health community was tested in its ability to deliver care to the sick and dying, and to prevent others from contracting the disease, in one of the poorest regions in the world. For an example of a perspective from the front lines of Ebola, see **BOX 15-2**. Sam Turay's experience differs from that of many brave and talented communication experts from CDC, WHO, and Médecins Sans Frontières who volunteered to help during the crisis in West Africa. **Appendix 15A** shares a full communication plan developed by the Ministry of Public Health in Liberia with the assistance of a CDC communication officer, Jana Telfer.[c]

Response

Emergencies and crises such as these scare most of us to death. But, in fact, it is possible to prepare for and practice what needs to be done to contain or minimize

---

a. http://www.cdc.gov/phpr/coopagreement.htm

b. http://www.who.int/mediacentre/factsheets/fs103/en/

c. Telfer was months away from retirement when she volunteered for the Liberia Ebola tour of duty. She returned safely to the United States.

BOX 15-1 Ebola: A Black Swan

The world was unprepared for the first global Ebola epidemic in 2014. The virus and its terrible *sequelae* were first discovered in 1976 near the Ebola River in the Democratic Republic of the Congo. Between 1976 and 2013, WHO reported 24 outbreaks involving 1716 cases. Mild, flu-like symptoms appear within 2 to 21 days of infection with Ebola virus. Symptoms progress to intense vomiting, diarrhea, rash, and internal and external bleeding. Prior to 2014, the outbreaks had a case fatality rate ranging from 25% to 90%.[1]

Patient Zero, a Guinean 2-year-old thought to have contracted the virus from a fruit bat, died in December 2013. By March 2014, the disease had flared in Guinea, Sierra Leone, and Liberia in West Africa, then crossed national borders and oceans through international travel. What began as a small outbreak provoked an international debate on global health security. The final toll, as reported by WHO in January 2016, included 28,601 suspected, probable, and confirmed cases; 15,215 laboratory-confirmed cases; and 11,300 deaths.[2]

In Liberia, the world's fifth-poorest nation and home to more than 4 million people, hundreds of international emergency and healthcare workers responded amid severe challenges. The infections spiked in June through October 2014, the height of the rainy season. Fifteen years of civil war had already destroyed the country's infrastructure. The Liberian tradition is to bury the dead wherever they were born, even if they must move the body for the funeral. Highly infectious Ebola corpses traveled across borders in pickup trucks and taxis, spreading the disease far and fast.

Major challenges in curbing the spread of Ebola in Liberia included insufficient beds for patients, no vaccine, and an outbreak in a highly-populated area near the borders of three countries, and with healthcare workers being among the most affected groups. Other challenges included low literacy levels, porous international borders, lack of capacity and coordination, and lack of risk communication framing in messages. (For more on problems with messaging during Ebola, see the discussion in Box 15-2.)

The Black Swan

The black swan theory was introduced by former Wall Street trader and risk analyst Nassim Nicholas Taleb in 2001, and popularized in his 2007 book *The Black Swan*.[3] A black swan is an event, positive or negative, that is improbable yet causes massive consequences. As a catastrophic "outlier" event, it is rare, unexpected, and disruptive, and defies conventional wisdom. Nothing in the past can convincingly point to its possibility. Like other black swans—such as the September 11 terrorist attacks, the Japanese attack on Pearl Harbor in 1941, and the creation of the Internet— the impact of the Ebola outbreak was extreme. Most black swans affect the global market as well. Society often engages in concocted rationalizations in hindsight, framing black swans as explainable and predictable, even though they are not.

Taleb regards most major scientific discoveries, historical events, and artistic accomplishments as "black swans" because they are undirected and unpredicted. His metaphor highlights the fragility of any thought system. A set of conclusions will unravel once any fundamental reasoning that follows from that underlying logic is disproved. Taleb argues that rather than try to predict the risk of black swan events using a normal distribution model, society should build robustness against the negative ones that do occur so as to reduce vulnerability and exposure to these events.

The Ebola epidemic emerged as a global "black swan" moment because it was a surprise, it had a major effect, and 40 years of relevant data about previous Ebola outbreaks were of little use in risk mitigation programs. Although the likelihood of Ebola becoming airborne appears small, that possibility cannot be ruled out. The odds of "catching Ebola" in the United States before 2014 were estimated at 1 in 13.3 million—or less likely than dying in a plane crash.[4] All scientists knew is that an outbreak in the United States would require an unprecedented and virtually uncontrolled outbreak in Africa. This black swan swam by in 2013.

References

1. World Health Organization. Fact sheet: Ebola virus disease. Updated August 2015. http://www.who.int /mediacentre/factsheets/fs103/en/

2. Centers for Disease Control and Prevention. 2014 Ebola Outbreak in West Africa- Case Counts: Countries with Former Widespread Transmission and Current, Established Control Measures. http://www.cdc.gov/vhf/ebola /outbreaks/2014-west-africa/case-counts.html. Accessed January 15, 2016.

3. Taleb NN. *The Black Swan: The Impact of the Highly Improbable.* London, UK: Penguin; 2007.

4. Doucleff M. What's my risk for catching Ebola? *Goats and Soda: Stories of Life in a Changing World.* October 2014. http://www.npr.org/sections/goatsandsoda/2014/10/23/358349882/an-answer-for-americans-who-ask-whats-my -risk-of-catching-ebola. Accessed January 15, 2016.

BOX 15-2 Behind Enemy Lines: A Perspective on Ebola from Sierra Leone

Samuel Dilito Turay

Forward

Samuel Dilito Turay earned his master's in public health degree (MPH) in the United States and returned to his native Sierra Leone as a policy analyst supporting the Ministry of Health and Sanitation in 2013. At that time, the last reported Ebola hemorrhagic fever case was a distant memory in the region. Little did Turay imagine he would go from analyzing statistical reports in the capital city to mobilizing his own nongovernmental organization (NGO) to deliver food and supplies to Ebola virus disease (EVD) victims and survivors in remote rural areas.

Hands for Life (HFL)—an NGO Turay created while still earning his MPH in Philadelphia—was meant to provide for primary healthcare needs in his native village of Kamakwie, Sierra Leone. Turay started Hands for Life with a handful of university faculty, fellow students, and friends from Sierra Leone living in the United States. During the height of the Ebola outbreak in Sierra Leone, Turay's supporters, including the U.S.-based Healing the Children (New Jersey affiliate), used Internet "crowd sourcing" to raise funds to support Hands for Life in its critical mission of caring for those behind the quarantine lines. Turay's story provides a valuable front-lines picture that is not a "research study," a "review of the literature," or the report of a visiting scientist. Turay and his Hands for Life staff placed themselves directly in harm's way to persuade rural families to follow directions concerning reporting of illness, treatment of the dead, sanitization, and other disease-ending, life-saving measures. This personal touch was necessary to gain the confidence of rural villagers who could not understand, or believe, the information coming over mass media. What Turay experienced and explains in the following feature represents painful lessons learned by a native of Sierra Leone who used his recent training in public health to help conquer the worst outbreak of Ebola in recorded history.

Claudia Parvanta

Background

The World Health Organization describes Ebola virus disease as "a severe and often fatal illness in humans transmitted to people from wild animals, and spread in the human population through human-to-human transmission with an average case fatality rate of around 50%. Case fatality rates have varied from 25% to 90% in past outbreaks. There is a 2 to 21 days incubation period for the individual infected with the virus to show symptoms and be [capable of infecting] others who come in contact with his/her bodily fluids."*

The most recent outbreak of this disease occurred in the West African countries of Guinea, Liberia, and Sierra Leone. Starting in Guinea (March 2014), the virus spread across the borders to Liberia (April 2014) and Sierra Leone (May 2014). This outbreak lasted the longest and caused the highest numbers of confirmed cases and deaths from Ebola virus in recorded history. Sierra Leone was declared Ebola-free in late 2015.

Stopping EVD in West Africa

Previously known as a disease of rural communities due to the nature of earlier outbreaks, Ebola virus disease (EVD) arrived in cities and towns in the affected countries this time around. It is not surprising that ending the outbreak proved to be more challenging without the natural die-off of the virus in less populated and remote villages. Many health workers in the affected countries consider EVD to be a "socio-medical" disease—that is, a disease requiring a combination of medical and social approaches to defeat it. Specifically, its elimination required (1) managing the symptoms of the disease, (2) changing deeply ingrained behaviors that contributed to the spread of EVD, and (3) providing psychosocial support to the infected families and communities.

Without the time necessary to build trust, both indigenous and international organizations asked citizens in the affected West African countries to violate some of their most cherished beliefs and practices in a desperate attempt to end the outbreak. A multimedia onslaught carried messages to the population calling for an understanding of the outbreak and the need for a behavior change. Health authorities used television, FM radio, billboards, newspapers, mobile public address systems, cell phones, and meetings to attempt to spread messages throughout the country.

"Our Town:" Explaining Ebola in Rural Sierra Leone

Hands for Life (HFL) worked in the rural communities of Makeni, located 137 kilometers from Freetown, and Kamakwie, located 92 more kilometers north of Freetown, and about 2-hour drive east of Guinea. In these towns, very few people can read in any language. Very few use FM radio, there is no television, and the majority of the population uses local dialects to communicate. Very few people understand Krio (a pidgin English), which is widely spoken in the towns and cities.

Adult males serve as the head of households and community institutions. They are the primary decision makers and opinion leaders, and can strongly influence what happens in the community—including what others may consider as personal and private, such as seeking health care. Women have the responsibility of providing care when a member of the family falls sick.

Initial Findings

Since multiple forms of media had been spreading information about Ebola for weeks by the time we started our work, we anticipated a good number of persons would be aware of, and practicing, the key behaviors such as frequent hand-washing, limited touching, and promptly informing healthcare workers about the illness and death of a family member or a member of the community. Instead, what we found was the following:

- Few people had received the communications sent through television, radio, or print media. If the messages were transmitted, they were not understood by the population, likely due to the language barriers or the inability to make sense of the information.
- Resistance to behavior change was still evident. The sick were still being kept or treated at home, and families were washing corpses and refusing to inform health authorities about sickness and deaths.
- A gap existed between the communicators and the receivers. The people had difficulty personalizing the messages, which reduced their determination to own and commit to the required actions.
- Misconceptions existed in the minds of people about the Ebola outbreak. Some blamed others and held them responsible for the initial outbreak (citing political gains, economic gains, and witchcraft as motivations for the perpetrators).
- Some could not understand the rationale for not providing direct care to sick family and community members (even when not infected with virus), why patients had to be taken away to treatment centers, and why black body bags should be for burial as opposed to white body bags. (In Sierra Leone, the color black is culturally associated with evil and bad luck and white with purity and good luck.)

What We Did: Intervention

Representatives from HFL embarked on a campaign using the interpersonal approach to reach out, educate, and support residents of these communities. We went house to house and met people in their yards, farms, the marketplace, and places of worship; in the street; when cooking and eating; and so on. HFL core staff recruited additional team members from the local communities. The inclusion of these personnel on the HFL team provided several advantages, including these individuals' better understanding of local traditions and dialects, and it enhanced the confidence and trust of the people. Team members could freely move about the community. We trained these community team members in delivery of the key messages, in personal safety, and in additional health communication skills.

At the start of every community engagement, HFL team members introduced themselves and the purpose of their visit. If they were at an individual home, they observed the premises for the presence and use of hand-washing supplies and noted whether people were touching or shaking hands. The team asked the residents questions to assess their awareness of Ebola information. Finally, they investigated the community's perceptions of the messages and their willingness to follow the directions. This assessment was then followed by a session of sharing messages and making attempts to answer questions. Importantly, residents were guided in decision making for the required behavior changes. We encourage dialogue as an opportunity for self-expression.

We worked through opinion leaders in the family and community to facilitate a behavior-change diffusion process. The dialogue process involved sharing messages using an empathy approach to portray the messages and required changes in behavior as not just for the immediate audience, but for all of us. We used words such as "we" and "us," as opposed to "you," "they," and "them." This helped us to engage in frank conversations. We repeatedly demonstrated the steps in hand washing to ensure clarity and confidence to continue the practice. We emphasized that the result of the behavior change would benefit the opinion leaders and everyone in the family and larger community—and eventually Ebola would be stopped. We used appropriate verbal and body language as well as appropriate cultural symbols to demonstrate concepts. We came back to reinforce the new behaviors. Finally, we provided material support, including soap, disinfectant, gloves, gowns, and food and cooking oil, which were not getting past quarantine lines in some areas.

Implications of Our Interventions

We found that residents displayed more understanding, trust, and confidence in the interventions after we discussed them than during our initial assessments. Perhaps the most important change was that communities became more receptive and tolerant of having outside health workers come in. They began reporting more cases of relatives, friends, and members of the community who fell sick to the appropriate authorities. They became more vigilant and responsible for the safety of their community. The arrival of a stranger (i.e., someone who may have left another area because of illness) was promptly reported to the authorities, as opposed to the earlier practice of hiding the individual. We found that families, community

(continues)

BOX 15-2 Behind Enemy Lines: A Perspective on Ebola from Sierra Leone *(continued)*

leaders, religious and social group leaders, and popular opinion leaders became more involved in spreading information about safe behaviors. While mass media could certainly reach greater numbers of people than we could going village to village, we believed we could make a change at a truly grassroots level. Without this kind of intervention, it is unknown how long the rural communities in which we worked would have resisted the changes necessary to end the Ebola outbreak.

Recommendations

- Since each form of media (mass media, mid-media, and interpersonal) can make a significant contribution to the communication process for behavior change, it is important that all three approaches are adequately utilized. While mass-media and mid-media messages can reach much wider audiences within a very short time, it is important for the interpersonal approach to be incorporated as early as possible. The interpersonal communication approach can reach and benefit individuals and communities who do not benefit from the mass-media and mid-media approaches due to lack of the ability to use them.
- Where the literacy and cognitive level of the audience is known or claimed to be low, the interpersonal approach will yield better results and should be used.

Sam Turay, MPH, worked in the Strategy and Policy Unit, Office of the Chief of Staff, State House, in Sierra Leone.

*http://www.who.int/mediacentre/factsheets/fs103/en/.

---

death and suffering. The impact of these major public health crises has been to stimulate an unprecedented development of emergency risk communication plans, tools, and strategies for dealing with the next "Big One," which is sure to come either with or without warning signs. CDC staff communication experts created material for what became known as **crisis and emergency risk communication (CERC)** with the help of crisis communication experts—in particular, Peter Sandman and Vincent Covello. It is not possible to disentangle the contributions of these experts, or their colleagues, including Baruch Fischoff, Paul Slovic, and Matthew Seeger, or CDC's partners at Prospect Associates and ORISE, from what became the CDC's approach to emergency risk communication. CDC's Barbara Reynolds has taken the lead in that area, doing training around the United States in CERC. The most recent version of the CERC manual is 462 pages long and includes a list of major contributors to it and previous versions.[1]

Following the same learning progression as CDC, this chapter discusses normal risk communication (RC) first, followed by emergency risk communication (ERC). Both approaches provide information to people so that they may protect themselves. Risk communication can be done by a toxicologist, by a healthcare provider, or through an online program. For CERC, the magnitude of the crisis, lack of warning, associated fear and suffering, and the need for speedy and accurate responses dramatically add to the communication challenge.

▶ A Basic Risk Framework[d]

Most health risk discussions concern **causality**, meaning "Does A (something) cause B (health condition)," or **risk**, meaning "If you are exposed to A, what is your likelihood of suffering B?" **BOX 15-3** provides some

---

BOX 15-3 Useful Definitions in Risk Communication

- **Hazard**: Any source of potential damage or harm or adverse outcome. For example, a substance (such as benzene), source of energy (e.g., electricity), process (e.g., crossing the street) or condition (e.g., wet floor).
- **Risk**: The chance or probability that a person will be harmed or experience an adverse outcome if exposed to the hazard.
- **Exposure**: Contact with a hazard. Exposure varies by the manner of exposure (breathing in, skin contact, whole body) and the quantity of time spent in an exposed condition.
- **Toxicity**: The intrinsic ability of a substance to cause adverse health effects.

U.S. Environmental Protection Agency's Risk Assessment Guidance for Superfund (RAGS). Washington, DC: Environmental Protection Agency; 1989.

---

d. Most of this section was prepared by David Cragin.

useful definitions and examples for distinguishing among key concepts in risk communication.

The distinctions in Box 15-3 are important. Toxicity is innate to a substance, whereas exposure, hazard, and risk are situation specific. For example, lead is toxic, but brief exposure to a block of lead is not hazardous and presents a very low health risk. By comparison, prolonged exposure to very fine, absorbable particles of lead is very hazardous and presents a high risk of poisoning. A small amount of ethanol dissolved in water presents no fire hazard, whereas pure ethanol is highly flammable. We all plug and unplug grounded electrical equipment routinely with little risk of electrocution, but ungrounded equipment and momentary inattention can result in a serious shock or electrocution.

Many experts in risk assessment rely on the criteria that Sir Austin Bradford Hill developed in the 1960s to demonstrate the causal association between tobacco and a specific disease (**TABLE 15-1**). According to Hill, "None of my nine viewpoints can bring indisputable evidence for or against the cause-and-effect hypothesis and none can be required *sine qua non*."[2] With that disclaimer, the more of these criteria that are satisfied by an event, the stronger the likelihood of causation.

TABLE 15-1 Important Considerations for Assessing Causality: Hill's Criteria

Label	Meaning	Rules of Evidence
1. Strength of association	What is the magnitude of relative risk?	The probability of a causal association increases as the summary relative risk estimate increases. Hill was suspicious of relative risks less than 2; others have set the limits higher. However, a relative risk of less than 2 does not rule out the possibility of causality.
2. Dose–response	Does a correlation exist between exposure and effect?	A regularly increasing relationship between dose and magnitude is indicative of a causal association. This works for bad things—for example, the greater your exposure to radiation, the worse your symptoms (usually). It also works for things that we are trying to measure in relation to behavior change—for example, if you are exposed to 10 prostate-specific antigen (PSA) screening tests for prostate cancers as opposed to 1, will your behavior be any different?
3. Consistency of response	How many times has this effect been reported in various populations under similar conditions?	The probability of a causal association increases as the proportion of studies with similar (e.g., positive) results increases.
4. Temporally correct association	Does the exposure precede the effect, or does the occurrence of the disease show the appropriate latency?	Exposure to a causal factor must precede the effect. This is an immutable requirement that is often ignored.
5. Specificity of the association	How specific is this effect? Do many things influence the effect?	For uncommon health effects (e.g., liver cancer), this evidence can be useful. For diseases with many causes, it is of little use.
6. Biological plausibility	Is the mechanism of action known or reasonably postulated?	See criterion 7.

(continues)

TABLE 15-1 Important Considerations for Assessing Causality: Hill's Criteria		(continued)
Label	**Meaning**	**Rules of Evidence**
7. Coherence	Does the cause–effect interpretation seriously conflict with generally known facts of the natural history and biology of the disease?	While a mechanism of action is not a requirement for determining causality, the finding of causality should not be biologically implausible. In contrast, a plausible mechanism of action or other supportive evidence increases the likelihood of a causal association.
8. Experimental evidence	Do laboratory animals show a similar effect?	As in criteria 6 and 7, findings in laboratory animals are supportive of a causal association. However, some chemicals that are notably carcinogenic to humans have tested negative in animal studies and vice versa.
9. Analogy	Do structurally similar chemicals cause similar effects?	For some classes of compounds, such as nitrosamines, structure–activity predictions can be supportive of a causal association. In contrast, materials such as organotins do not lend themselves to cross-class extrapolations.

Data from: Friis RH, Sellers TA. *Epidemiology for public health practice*. Gaithersburg, MD: Aspen; 1999; and U.S. Department of Health, Education, and Welfare, Public Health Service. *Smoking and health: Report of the Advisory Committee to the Surgeon General of the Public Health Service*. Washington, DC: Government Printing Office; 1964. PHS Publication No. 1103; and Hill AB. The environment and disease: association or causation? *Proc R Acad Med*. 1965; 295–300.

This vocabulary can be used to describe risk, hazards, toxicity, and exposure, as well as likelihood of causality, to other scientists. Later we will discuss why logic and clarity alone may be insufficient when communicating risk to the public. But before that, it is important to understand the logic underlying a risk assessment and the means by which it is presented.

Presenting Risk

The vast majority of people in the United States have never studied statistics, epidemiology, toxicology, or any of the other scientific disciplines that relate to risk assessment. Indeed, far too many of us have difficulty deciphering a train schedule or interpreting a food label, let alone understanding a "confidence interval." While a scientist may consider "less than a tenth of one part per million" of a toxic substance in drinking water to be absolutely safe, much of the public will hear this as "millions of parts" of something dangerous contaminating the water. Others hold the mistaken belief that "If you can't say zero, then it's not safe." Thus, part of the challenge in risk communication is translating fairly complex statistical concepts into pictures and language that can be broadly understood.

We have discussed health literacy and numeracy issues elsewhere. Health literacy guidance needs to be applied to all risk and emergency risk communication work. However, even clear language and visual aids are often not sufficient to give people an accurate appreciation of risk. The psychology of risk must also be taken into consideration.

The Psychology of Risk Perception

Researchers have been studying **risk perceptions** for decades. Through their work, a long list of characteristics that can affect the public perception of different kinds of hazards has been developed. Some factors that affect a person's perception of risk, such as immediate danger to oneself or one's family, are obvious; other factors are more obscure (**TABLE 15-2**).

Fischoff discusses the use of multidimensional scaling techniques to identify factors that position various hazards in people's minds. The most important seem to be "unknown" and "dread," which, Fischoff says, "capture the cognitive and emotional bases of people's concern, respectively.... When a third factor (dimension) emerges, it appears to reflect the scope of the threat, (or its) 'catastrophic potential.'"[3] These factors represent the biggest three for risk aversion. Bioterrorism, for example, can rank at the very top of all three of these scales.

While these factors clearly influence how the public will generally react to a risk assessment, one factor has been shown to modify their perception above

TABLE 15-2 Sources of Public Concern

Term	Explanation	Example
Benefit unclear	People are more concerned about hazardous activities that are perceived to have unclear benefits than about hazardous activities that are perceived to have clear benefits.	While all medications have potential side effects, taking a drug for prophylaxis (e.g. anti-malarials) causes more concern than taking a drug for a diagnosed illness.
Causation (attributability)	People are more concerned about risks that are perceived to be due to human actions than about risks that are perceived to be natural in origin.	Industrial accidental chemical exposure or terrorism, versus hurricanes or earthquakes.
Catastrophic potential	Fatalities and injuries that are grouped in time and space cause more concern than fatalities and injuries that are scattered or random in time and space.	Airplane crashes versus automobile accidents.
Children involved	Activities that are perceived as putting children specifically at risk cause more concern than activities not generally so perceived.	Kidnapping or online child endangerment versus adult disappearance or online exploitation of adults.
Controllability (voluntariness of exposure)	Risks that are perceived to be not under individuals' personal control engender more concern than risks that are perceived to be under their personal control.	Traveling as a passenger in an airplane or automobile versus driving an automobile. Smoking cigarettes versus secondhand smoke. Exposure to unlabeled food additives versus sunbathing.
Dread	The public is more concerned about risks that evoke a response of fear, terror, or anxiety than about risks that are more common and likely, but not especially dreaded.	Exposure to potential carcinogens from toxic waste dumps, nuclear radiation, or a terrorist attack versus car crashes, household accidents, or influenza.
Equity	People are more concerned about activities that are characterized by a perceived inequitable distribution of risks and benefits than about those characterized by a perceived equitable distribution of risks and benefits.	Distribution of antibiotics during the 2001 anthrax attack: Ciprofloxacin (first) to members of the U.S. Senate, amoxicillin (later) to postal workers.
Familiarity	People are more concerned about risks that are unfamiliar than about risks that are familiar.	Genetically modified food versus chlorine bleach.
Future generations	People are more concerned about activities that pose risks to future generations than about risks that are not perceived to pose risks to future generations.	Genetic effects due to exposure to radiation versus binge drinking. Smoking during pregnancy versus smoking as a single adult.

(continues)

TABLE 15-2 Sources of Public Concern		*(continued)*
Term	**Explanation**	**Example**
Identifiable victims	People are more concerned about risks to identifiable victims than about risks to statistical victims.	Astronauts or coal miners versus thousands of people killed in motor vehicle crashes. Individual soldiers versus U.S. forces in Iraq and Afghanistan.
Media attention	People are more concerned about risks that receive a lot of media attention versus those that receive little.	Airline crashes versus worksite accidents. Violent crimes versus domestic violence.
Understanding/uncertainty	Activities characterized by poorly understood exposure mechanisms or processes cause more concern than those that are seemingly well understood.	Nuclear radiation versus solar ultraviolet (UVA and UVB) radiation. Genetically modified food versus selective breeding or pollination in agriculture.

Modified from: McCallum D. Risk communication: A tool for behavior change. In: Becker, TE, David, SL, Saucy, G. *Reviewing the Behavioral Science Knowledge Base on Technology Transfer*. National Institute on Drug Abuse (NIDA) Research Monograph 155; 1995, Figure 1, pp. 70–71. Copyright: Public Domain, NIH. Downloaded from: http://www.nida.nih.gov/pdf/monographs/155.pdf, January 6, 2016.

all others—namely, the level of trust in the information source. Public health risk communicators often present information to people who do not trust them because they work for "the government." Sometimes, of course, they are trusted for precisely the same reason. Institutional or organizational trust is crucial to engaging the public in a frank discussion of the risks associated with a particular hazard. Personal physicians and the medical profession as a whole continue to maintain a level of credibility with the public not enjoyed by most other professions.[4]

▶ Presenting a Risk Assessment

Risk assessments in the health field have primarily examined environmental or toxicologic risk—that is, the risks of drugs, industrial chemicals, pollutants, food additives, and the like. In this section, we will walk through the parts of a typical risk assessment report.[5]

Note that some concepts, such as "dose–response," may not be relevant when assessing a non-environmental exposure.

Report Content

1. *Introduction:* Provide an overview of the risk question to give the reader context for the risk assessment. If there are two schools of thought on the issue, discuss them both upfront.

2. *Hazard identification* (and possibly benefit identification): Identify the agents(s) of concern (e.g., drugs, pesticides, pollutants) or other factors related to a risk. Hazard identification is the primary filtering step in the report. Every risk issue has many facets, but delving into unrelated or unimportant issues will detract from the focus of the report. The hazard identification step identifies only those hazards that are relevant to the risk assessment being conducted. Hazard identification is a judgment process.

  For example, when examining the potential cardiac benefits of low-dose aspirin tablets, potential patients need not be concerned that powdered aspirin can be an eye irritant. In contrast, when examining the hazards to workers who manufacture aspirin, the eye irritation potential of aspirin is relevant, while the potential for stomach irritation is much less salient. Similarly, although the needle used to give a vaccination is a "hazard," the hazard it presents is miniscule compared to that of illnesses for the recipient of the vaccine. For healthcare workers, needle sticks, particularly when working with patients with blood-borne infectious diseases, are more significant. Use the hazard identification step to eliminate insignificant hazards from further consideration.

A basic concept in risk assessment is that protecting people from the adverse effect that occurs at the lowest dose will protect them from the effects that occur at higher doses. Another aspect of hazard identification is determining the most important health effect in the time frame of interest. Are the health effects being assessed acute, subchronic, or chronic (or all three)? Which health endpoint is relevant for each time frame? For salt exposure to a population, chronic health effects are likely of interest. In contrast, acute effects might be of concern when addressing health effects for workers in salt processing plant. Cigarettes generally present subchronic and—more importantly—chronic risk. In contrast, most street drugs present acute and subchronic risks. Although infectious diseases often do not fit neatly into any single category, most present an acute or subchronic hazard.

Similarly, the benefit identification seeks to determine the primary benefits that may occur from a particular action. What are the health, financial, or other benefits relevant to the action that will be taken? Many risk assessments do not include a benefit analysis, so include this information only if it is relevant to the risk question.

3. *Exposure assessment*: Identify the human receptors (e.g., subpopulation groups) likely to be exposed to chemicals of concern. For assessing chemical risks, evaluate the receptors that are likely most sensitive to the effect you are assessing. That is, are the young or the old, pregnant women, or others most sensitive to the adverse effect or outcome in question? For example, Reye's syndrome—a severe systemic disorder related to aspirin administration in children—is relevant for infants but not for adults. When assessing the risk of inducing Reye's syndrome, children are identified as the receptors and the need to assess adult risks is discounted. This aspect of the discussion of adult versus infant sensitivity to aspirin may also be relevant in the introduction and hazard identification sections of the report. In contrast, when examining the risks associated with aspirin administration for prevention of stroke and myocardial infarction, infants would not be a relevant receptor.

4. *Dose–response assessment*: Describe the relationship between the magnitude of exposure (dose) and the risk (probability) of occurrence of adverse health effects (response) associated with the chemical(s) of concern.

5. *Risk characterization*: Integrate the results of the exposure assessment with the dose–response assessment to provide quantitative estimates of risk. This is often a very short section. It should have little or no commentary and should be presented in an objective format.

6. *Conclusions*: Include a summary of the findings of the preceding assessment.

7. *Uncertainty analysis*: Discuss uncertainties associated with the calculated exposures and potential health risks. Any aspects of the assessment that may have biased the results should be discussed here. For example, which elements of the risk assessment might have under- or over-estimated potential risks? Which factors are less certain or may have a bias?

8. *Risk management*: Discuss the potential actions that could be taken to mitigate risks identified in the report. Technically, this discussion is not part of a risk assessment, but it is often included.

The Written Document

Because the risk assessment is often both lengthy and detailed, the written report should begin with an executive summary. This much shorter, stand-alone document conveys the basic methodologies and findings addressed in the risk assessment. Many people will read only the executive summary, so it should provide an accurate synopsis of the report. The summary should include the following elements:

- Why the risk assessment was done
- How it was done (in general terms)
- Major conclusions

There is no need to reference other parts of the report or to provide detailed information about the methodology or data. Try to keep the executive summary to one page. While it comes first in a written report, most people prepare this summary last.

The written document should also include full citations for references cited in the report. A references section is preferable to citations within text because it is easier to read.

Oral Presentation

Presenting a risk assessment to a community requires good preparation, practice, and thick skin. The classic town meeting is held in an auditorium with a large number of seats. Speakers present information to the audience from a podium or stage. Usually, a series of specialists will explain what they know about the different facets of the investigation. This type of presentation might sound like it is a good idea, but it has numerous drawbacks. In fact, when asked how he runs an effective town meeting, the head of community affairs at one chemical company replied, "You don't. Town meetings don't work."

In the town meeting format, a few vocal individuals can completely dominate the discussion. Often these people are very angry individuals. Even if most of an audience supports the organization that is running the meeting, many will be unwilling to speak up against an extremely upset individual. In addition, the town meeting format presumes that everyone in the audience will arrive on time to hear all of the presentation and that the audience listens to every part. It also presumes that every audience member will be willing to speak up and voice his or her questions of concern. These assumptions may not be valid.

Poster Session

A more effective alternative is a poster session, similar to what presenters use at scientific meetings. In this type of presentation, the room is set up with posters around the periphery and an expert manning each one. This setup allows the audience members to meet the experts on a one-on-one basis and greatly facilitates questions and answers. An individual too shy to ask what he or she might perceive to be a "stupid" question in an open auditorium is much more likely to speak on an individual basis, particularly if the expert has made the effort to promote dialogue. In addition, poster sessions give experts a chance to solicit the opinions and feelings of large numbers of participants. The participants, in turn, get a chance to see the experts as people. **BOX 15-4** provides more information on poster sessions.

Depending on the situation, a hybrid town meeting/poster session may be appropriate. For example, it might facilitate discussions for the experts to give very concise upfront talks and then direct the audience to talk with them at each of their posters.

Remote Presentations

All efforts should be made to meet with the concerned community in person. Nevertheless, sometimes the best expert needs to be elsewhere and, therefore, cannot personally attend a meeting. There are few alternatives in such a situation.

Online discussion platforms are available (e.g., Facebook, LinkedIn). Some may feel these are too casual for the subject matter. In contrast, using a monitored discussion blog offers a way to respond to many questions from the public in an open and accountable

---

BOX 15-4   Conducting Poster Sessions for Risk Assessments

Poster sessions cater to both visual and auditory learners. Those who would like to read or view images to learn can do so; those who would prefer to talk with the expert can do so. Poster sessions offer excellent opportunities for blended learning. They also give the control to the audience—that is, individuals can decide which posters to visit and which information matters most to them.

Another strength of poster sessions is that they accommodate extremely busy individuals whose schedules do not allow them to spend an entire night in a town meeting. With a poster session, a participant can arrive at any time or leave at any time and not miss key information.

Poster sessions also offer the best possible forum to engage your worst critics in discussion. Conversely, these discussions can help you identify key allies in the community. For example, you may be able to identify a professor, a schoolteacher, or other highly respected member of the community who can contribute to the discussions.

The following steps can enhance the value of poster sessions:

1. Offer a handout at each poster.
2. Ensure that each expert has training in risk communication.
3. Assess the content of posters: Do they provide the appropriate level of detail? Are they too complex/too simplistic?
4. Provide a refreshment area, including some healthy snacks. Food promotes discussion, while also acknowledging that people may have come directly from work to attend the sessions and skipped their meal. Hunger makes people angry.

manner that could be used in conjunction with more direct means. During the Ebola crisis in 2014, when not offering a televised briefing with live journalist questions, the CDC used a monitored conference call system to hold briefings. Everyone could hear the questions and responses, but callers were activated to speak by the telephone operating system and could speak only one at a time. This proved to be an equitable, civilized, and time-efficient way to interact with the media, many of whom could not attend a meeting in person. This approach could be adapted for smaller communities as well.

Engaging the Public in Risk Assessment and Reporting

Social media, particularly applications that allow for geo-location, have become an important tool in identifying problem areas, such as high-crime locations in the United States or sources of pollution or infestation. **Appendix 15B** provides a case study from Sri Lanka on using mobile devices and applications to develop a greatly enhanced system to reduce the transmission of dengue, a mosquito-borne illness in the southern hemisphere. This kind of intervention would be equally useful for eliminating mosquitoes carrying Zika virus, which expanded as a mosquito-borne threat (chiefly to gestating infants) in late 2015.[e] As will become apparent in the next section, having health workers and the public already engaged as partners for one risk is a good way of preparing for an emergency.

▶ Emergency Risk Communication

Emergency risk communication (ERC), also called crisis and emergency risk communication (CERC), is a term the CDC coined to describe the process of communicating about risk with various publics during a complex emergency. It has been a key element in the CDC's cooperative agreements with state, local, territorial, and tribal health departments for health emergency preparedness. The CDC is careful to note that ERC/CERC is not "tactical communication," which involves communication among responders such as the military, police, fire, and other local emergency units.

The CDC and its partners have developed many resources to support ERC/CERC; these resources have been used extensively to develop this chapter,[f] which in no way represents everything you need to know about ERC/CERC. If you are working in a health department and need to have a professional level of competency in this domain, take advantage of additional information contained in the references mentioned.[g] Although we use ERC to refer to the generic activity and CERC when using CDC source material, the terms mean basically the same thing in this chapter.

What Distinguishes ERC from Routine Health Communication?

The first major difference between ERC and routine health communication is the characterization of the audiences. **FIGURE 15-1** shows the concentric nature of the audience segments associated with a disaster. Different audiences have different needs for information. We will describe the specifics—for example, what is meant by vicarious rehearsal—in more detail later.

Channels and Media Choices

As an interactive process, ERC needs to provide accurate, credible, and timely information to the many different population groups who need that information to make the best decisions possible during emergencies. Meeting this need means making important media choices and generating multiple forms of content at the right reading level, as well as specific versions for different cultural and linguistic audiences. Members of the public need to be able to call, go online, or ask someone in person about their concerns. These communication efforts need to be monitored to ensure that information is received, understood, and acted upon. While Figure 15-1 indicated audiences by their proximity to an event, **TABLE 15-3** identifies audiences based on potential media channels to reach them, communication products, and considerations beyond their primary information needs.

---

e. http://www.cdc.gov/zika/

f. https://emergency.cdc.gov/cerc/resources/index.asp

g. See also National Public Health Information Coalition's incident communication resource at https://www.nphic.org/nphicicsearch and Association of State and Territorial Officials' publications at http://www.astho.org/default.aspx.

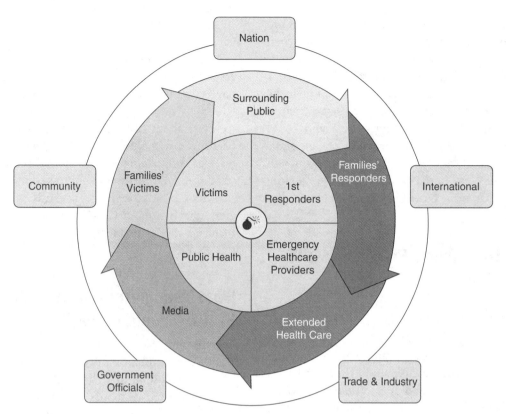

FIGURE 15-1 Audiences characterized by relationship to event.
Based on CERC, CDC.

Do Social Media Stand Out?

Instantly updated and widely used social media, particularly Twitter, have become a go-to channel in many emergency situations. As mentioned earlier, social media—like all emergency communication channels—are most effective when time is invested upfront to create a network of reliable social media partners. The official Twitter handle for CDC's Emergency Preparedness feed is @cdcemergency. **BOX 15-5** offers more tips on using social media for crisis communication.

TABLE 15-3 Audiences by Channels and Products

AUDIENCES				
Unaffected Public (General)	**Affected Communities**	**Public Health Professionals**	**Clinical Care/First Responders**	**Civic Leaders: Local, State, National**
Vicarious rehearsal readiness	Personal and family Safety Pet safety Property protection Interruption of normal activities Stigmatization	Personal safety Resources to accomplish response and recovery Treatment recommendations Media talking points	Personal safety Resources to accomplish response and recovery Treatment recommendations Media talking points	Quality of response and recovery Informing constituents Statutes and laws Opportunities for expressing concern Impact on trade, industry Media talking points

CONCERNS

AUDIENCES					
	Unaffected Public (General)	**Affected Communities**	**Public Health Professionals**	**Clinical Care/First Responders**	**Civic Leaders: Local, State, National**
CHANNELS	Agency website News media Public inquiry phone hotline TV/radio PSAs (optional)	On-site responders[1] State/local websites Local news Phone hotline (dedicated or general) TV/radio PSAs	Agency listserve Agency website Conference calls PHIN* Health alerts (HAN)[†] Webcasts EpiX[2] MMWR[3] Preparedness center sites (by state) As appropriate, clinical networks	Agency listservs Agency website Webcasts Conference calls Phone hotline Medical Association host sites PHIN Health alerts (HAN) Webcasts EpiX MMWR	Telebriefings Agency listserve Dedicated agency subsite HAN News media
Communication Products Typically Requiring Clearance During Emergency					
PRODUCTS	Responses to media questions (Q&As) Scripts for public information line PSA scripts, storyboards Fact sheets Backgrounders Website content	Spokesperson talking points (If not lead SME) Risk communication materials Informed consent documents Patient education sheets	Health alerts Fact sheets Information sheets for channel specific distribution	Triage guidelines Post-exposure Prophylaxis Diagnosis, treatment Short-term follow-up patient care Long-term follow-up	Talking points Website content
Other Communication Considerations					
ISSUES	Literacy level Language Disability requirements	Fear/outrage Spokespersons Media options Literacy level Language Disability requirements	PHIN, EpiX access Local area networks Level of BT communication preparedness	Computer/Internet access Needs for patient materials (literacy, language)	Federal, state policy Localized data

[1] Direct communication to on-site responders and clinical care team handled by Emergency Response Command and Subject Matter Experts (SMEs) according to role.

[2] EpiX has separate emergency clearance procedures—included as channel in table for audience.

[3] MMWR has separate emergency clearance procedures—included as channel in table and articulates tightly with others as source of cleared materials.

*PHIN http://www.cdc.gov/PHIN/

[†] HAN http://www2a.cdc.gov/HAN/Index.asp

Psychological Needs During a Disaster

Each emergency creates its own psychological wake. A university-trained health communicator should have some background in psychology, but this is likely not a match for the psychological needs and stresses that the population is experiencing. Having qualified psychologists as part of the response team would be ideal. It is not hard to imagine that people caught up in the throes of an emergency, such as an earthquake,

BOX 15-5 Using Social Media Before and During a Crisis

Social media have changed how crisis and risk information is handled prior to, during, and after a public health emergency. This information may take the form of text, audio, visual, or multimedia messages. Social media have affected every step in the process of handling crisis information, including how it is created, manipulated, processed, shared, and disseminated.

Developing relationships with audiences before a crisis occurs builds trust. In addition, using social media before a crisis can help promote preparedness and educate audiences about risks. Organizations need to be regular users of social media before a crisis. For the health communicator, it is important to establish social media relationships early. If not, social media users will go to other sources and groups with whom they already have relationships for information.

Following are some best practices for using social media for risk communication before a crisis.[1]

Best Practices for Social Media *Before* an Event

Determine how social media engagement will be used as part of the organization's risk and crisis management policies and approaches.

Every crisis communication plan should have a section on communicating with stakeholders and working with the media. Social media can be used to communicate directly with stakeholders and the media at the same time. More importantly, social media provide built-in channels through which stakeholders can communicate directly with organizations. Incorporating social media into the plan ensures that social media tools will be analyzed and tested before the crisis. It also requires regular updating of the communication plan as social media evolve.

Incorporate social media tools into environmental scanning procedures to listen to audience concerns.

One important aspect of social media is the opportunity provided, if this channel is used well, to listen to the concerns of the public and others who may be bearing risks. When users create and manage their own content, external and internal social media monitoring becomes even more critical. In addition, tracking issues through social media and reporting the results to the crisis management team can increase the potential that a crisis will be addressed sooner. It will also demonstrate to the team why social media need to be embraced in the crisis response.

Use social media in daily communication activities.

Individuals may have information that is crucial to handling the crisis, but they probably will not share that information if they do not trust the organization or know where to find it online. Do not wait until you are in the middle of a crisis to try using social media. To build partnerships and build trust, the discussion with members of the public should already be taking place. Internally, using social media such as wikis on day-to-day projects can streamline communication within the organization and increase efficiency.

Follow and share messages with credible sources.

Collaborating with trustworthy and supportive sources can enhance the credibility of the organization and increase its reach. By cross-posting and retweeting messages among partner organizations, a coalition of credible sources is established. Moreover, more individuals are reached through shared networks.

During a Crisis

While social media are important before a crisis occurs, the immediacy of social media is a particularly important feature during a crisis. In such a situation, public health emergency managers and communicators are challenged with the demand for delivering accurate information rapidly. Such communication must be done in a manner that can be altered and shared through diverse social media channels. The various forums discussed earlier can be expected to play a role during a crisis. The most immediate forms, such as Twitter and Facebook, will be prevalent in the earliest stages. For example, within one week of the 2010 earthquake in Haiti, "more than one in 10 Americans (13%)—including 24% of those younger than 30—reported that they'd gotten or shared information about the Haiti earthquake through Facebook, Twitter, or another social networking site."[2] Social media should also be accessible during a crisis from a multitude of digital handheld devices.

Highly mobile communication devices have created additional access to social media and are particularly useful for transmitting hazard and risk warnings to those members of the public who principally rely on these devices for news and communication. The rapidly evolving Commercial Mobile Alert System (CMAS) communicates alerts and warnings to handheld devices.[3] Mobile media are discussed in more detail later in this chapter.

With social media, all users have the potential to be watchdogs, citizen journalists, photo journalists, and caring or nosy neighbors who can constantly survey the world around them and share what they find online. Stakeholders on the ground of a crisis event are generally the ones with first-hand knowledge. They become key sources of information and facilitators of a broader understanding of the event. They may do the following:

- Provide information that is critical for situational awareness
- Distribute information
- Create content and visuals
- Assist in connecting people and information via social media

Although they may not intend to help CERC communicators, the information they provide inherently can do so.

Best Practices for Social Media *During* an Emergency Situation[4]

Join the conversation, help manage rumors by responding to misinformation, and determine the best channels to reach segmented audiences.
Health communicators can do more with social media than just track issues. It is essential that they interact with their audience to address misinformation and establish the organization as a credible source. Responding to posts demonstrates that the organization cares what stakeholders think. It also demonstrates that the organization is engaged and able to address their concerns. Reaching specific audiences with a key message is the foundation of targeted communication. In CERC, however, communicators often resort to standard mass-media push messages to reach everyone at once. Health communicators must still consider how those messages will be interpreted and who will not be reached by them. After all, those who face the greatest risks are often those with the least access to information. Determining the best communication channels for specific audiences online or in the community should be incorporated in communication plans.

Check all information for accuracy and respond honestly to questions.
Inaccurate information that is shared and retweeted, or passed on through other social media outlets, not only makes the organization look bad, but can also make the user who passes on the information look bad. It is easier simply to skip over a post that you do not want to address than it is to ignore a pointed question from the media. However, the public, like the media, will turn to other sources if the organization stonewalls on key issues. If you do not know the answer to a question, it is better to communicate the uncertainty of the situation and explain what you are doing to find out the answer than to answer incorrectly or not answer at all.

Recognize that the media are already using social media.
The crisis will likely be discussed through social media, and traditional media will be part of that discussion. If the organization is not engaged in this dialogue, the media will find other sources through social media to comment on the crisis. Thus, when it comes to being accessible to the media, not engaging in social media can have the same effect as not returning a reporter's call.

Remember that social media exchanges are interpersonal communication.
Social media allow for human interaction and some degree of emotional support, and have been shown to be important to stakeholders dealing with crises.[5] If communicators use social media to send out messages that come across as generic marketing blurbs, however, these messages will be seen as cold, callous, and impersonal—they will not encourage the relationship building and mending needed in a crisis. Organizations should be ready to pull messages, such as advertisements or campaigns, in case of a crisis. It took two days after the attacks on September 11, 2001, for advertisers in Times Square to change their billboards to messages of sorrow, charity, or patriotism. Two days is a lifetime online, especially as it relates to social media. Incorporating and responding to emotional appeals are ideal uses of social media; organizations must be ready to move to that message exchange channel in an instant.

Use social media as the primary tool for updates.
Organizations often promise to follow up with the media and public as soon as they have new information, but then wait to release that information until a press release can be drafted, refined, cleared, and sent out. Generally, such a message is posted to the organization's website after the release is published. Sometimes, organizations will wait until the next scheduled press conference to provide their updated information; this allows them to have a spokesperson deliver the information while also displaying the appropriate emotions. Using social media allows organizations to keep their promise of providing timely updates to the media and public.

Organizations have another option.
Organizations can use social media to provide updates on the crisis response and recovery. This practice allows them to humanize the response and continue to be a reliable source without requiring all the exact details and time needed to fill out a press release or hold another press conference.

(continues)

BOX 15-5   Using Social Media Before and During a Crisis   *(continued).*

Ask for help and provide direction.

Giving people something meaningful to do in response to a crisis helps them make sense of the situation. As partners in the crisis response, the members of public can provide essential information, especially if the event affects them directly. By providing that information, social media users are taking action. When an organization requests useful information via social media, it helps both the organization and the stakeholders who respond in managing the crisis. If individuals can take specific actions to reduce their risks or assist in the recovery efforts, social media are an ideal forum for reaching them with the directions needed. In fact, just by simply forwarding, cross-posting, or retweeting the directions, users are taking action.

Social Media Are Not the Solution to All Communication Problems

Social media represent a channel or tool that is characterized by technological advancements, rapid access to information, large numbers of users, low cost, and ease of use. The power to communicate, however, resides in the behaviors of the communicating organization and the content it produces—it is not inherent in the technology. The real value in communicating through social media comes from the quality of the content being disseminated. That content needs to explain the actions of the organization while demonstrating compassion and empathy for those affected by the crisis. Thus, using social media is not a best practice in CERC. Instead, social media are a tool that can assist practitioners in following best practices.

References

1.   Veil S, Buehner T, Palenchar MJ. A work-in-process literature review: incorporating social media in risk and crisis communication. *J Contingencies Crisis Manage.* 2011;19(2):110-122. http://onlinelibrary.wiley.com/doi/10.1111/j.1468-5973.2011.00639.x/pdf.

2.   Pew Research Center for the People and the Press. Haiti dominates public's consciousness: nearly half have donated or plan to give. January 20, 2010. http://people-press.org/report/580/haiti-earthquake.

3.   Penn D. Emergency alerts delivered to your phone: what our new PLAN means to you. In: *FEMA Blog.* Washington, DC: Federal Emergency Management Agency; May 13, 2011. http://blog.fema.gov/2011/05/emergency-alerts-delivered-to-your.html.

4.   Mazmanian A. Of hurricanes and hashtags: disaster relief in the social-media age. *National J.* June 3, 2012. http://www.nationaljournal.com/tech/of-hurricanes-and-hashtags-disaster-relief-in-the-social-media-age-20120603.

5.   Sutton J, Palen L, Shklovski I. Backchannels on the front lines: emergent uses of social media in the 2007 Southern California wildfires. In: Fiedrich F, Van de Walle B, eds. *Proceedings of the 5th International Information Systems for Crisis Response and Management (ISCRAM) Conference.* Washington, DC: May 5–7, 2008: 624-632, Session 7, Track 3. http://www.iscramliveorg/portal/node/2236%3Cbr%20/%3E..

Centers for Disease Control and Prevention. *Crisis Emerg Risk Commun.* 2014: 268-271.

hurricane, or terrorist attack, possibly stripped of their home, access to money, or even identity, would be fearful and anxious. Surrounding them are people either trying to help, or observing from a distance, but still concerned.

BOX 15-6 presents some key psychological variables that influence how people react during a crisis, according to the CDC.[6]

BOX 15-6   Psychological Reactions During a Crisis

It is important for the health communicator to understand that in crisis, people often manifest the following psychological reactions:

- Vicarious rehearsal
- Denial
- Stigmatization
- Fear and avoidance
- Withdrawal, hopelessness, and helplessness

Vicarious Rehearsal

Interestingly, experience has shown that people farther away (by distance or relationship) from the threat may exercise less reasonable reactions than those who are facing the crisis more directly. The communication age allows some people to vicariously participate in a crisis without risk and "try on" the courses of action presented to them. These "armchair" victims have the luxury of time to choose a course of action and may become hypercritical about the value of a recommendation. In some cases, they may reject the proposed course of action, choose another, or insist that they are also actually at risk and need the recommended remedy, such as a vaccination or a visit to an emergency room. In its most troublesome form, these "worried well" will heavily tax the recovery and response.

Denial

Members of the community will experience denial. Some people will respond to the crisis in the following ways:

- Avoid getting the warnings or action recommendations
- Become agitated or confused by the warning
- Believe the threat is not real
- Believe the threat does not apply to them

An individual experiencing denial may not take recommended steps to ensure his or her safety until the absolute last moment, sometimes when it is too late. This maladaptive crisis response is often associated with the sudden, deep feeling that the universe is no longer a rational and orderly system.

Stigmatization

In some instances, victims may be stigmatized by their communities and refused services or public access. Stigma is the negative characterization of an individual or group because of disease, behavior, or background (e.g., tuberculosis, people with piercings, ethnicity) that leads to fear, avoidance, and even violence on the part of others. Stigmatization will hamper community recovery and affect evacuation and relocation efforts. In a disease outbreak, for example, a community is more likely to separate from those perceived to be infected.

Fear and Avoidance

Fear in the affected population is an important consideration in the response to a crisis. The fear of the unknown or the fear of uncertainty may be the most debilitating of the psychological responses to disaster. With fear at the core, an individual may act in extreme, and sometimes irrational, ways to avoid the perceived or real threat.

Withdrawal, Hopelessness, and Helplessness

Some people can accept that the threat is real, but the threat looms so large that they believe that the situation is hopeless. They feel helpless to protect themselves and so, instead, they withdraw.

For more on the range of emotional reactions that a crisis can provoke, and ways to deal with these various emotions, see the following resource by Peter Sandman: *Beyond Panic Prevention: Addressing Emotion in Emergency Communication*, http://www.orau.gov/cdcynergy/erc/Content/activeinformation/resources/BeyondPanicPrevention.pdf.

The Psychology of a Crisis — How Knowing this Helps Communication. Available at http://www.orau.gov/cdcynergy/erc/content/activeinformation/essential_principles/EP-psychology.htm

▶ The Stages of Crisis and Emergency Risk Communication

Emergency risk communication starts when things are quiet. In a not too optimistic way, this is referred to as the pre-event phase. **FIGURE 15-2** shows the CERC life cycle for communication.

In reality, the actual event usually kicks off the cycle (unless we have been very well prepared). When things start quieting down, we examine what went right and wrong during what we call the post-event phase. We focus on pre-event planning in this text. During the first 48 hours of an event, it is useful to follow steps from a specific plan such as those outlined in the CDC's checklist (**BOX 15-7**).

As a junior person in a public health team, you will largely be following instructions during an actual emergency. During the post-event phase, you can gather and learn a lot about what went right and wrong and then make modifications in materials and plans for the next time, when the responsibility for the CERC plan and execution may be yours.

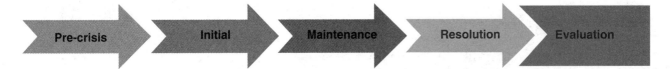

| Pre-crisis | Initial | Maintenance | Resolution | Evaluation |

- Be prepared.
- Foster alliances.
- Develop consensus recommendations.
- Text messages.

- Acknowledge the event with empathy.
- Explain and inform the public, in simplest forms, about the risk.
- Establish agency and spokesperson credibility.
- Provide emergency courses of action, including how and where to get more information.
- Commit to stakeholders and the public to continue communication.

- Help the public more accurately understand its own risks.
- Provide background and encompassing information to those who need it.
- Gain understanding and support for response and recovery plans.
- Listen to stakeholder and audience feedback, and correction misinformation.
- Explain emergency recommendations.
- Empower risk/benefit decision-making.

- Improve appropriate public response in future similar emergencies through education.
- Honestly examine problems and mishaps, and then reinforce what worked in the recovery and response efforts.
- Persuade the public to support public policy and resource allocation to the problem.
- Promote the activities and capabilities of the agency, including reinforcing its corporate identity, both internally and externally.

- Evaluate communication plan performance.
- Document lessons learned.
- Determine specific actions to improve crisis systems or the crisis plan.

FIGURE 15-2 Crisis and emergency risk communication (CERC) life cycle.

CDC, CERC Manual 2014 Edition: Figure 1-1, p.9.

BOX 15-7 CERC Checklist: First 48 Hours

Critical First Steps After Verification

Notification:

- Use your crisis plan's notification list. Make certain that your chain of command has been notified and they know you are involved.
- Ensure that your leadership is aware of the emergency, especially if awareness of the event comes from the media and not the emergency operations center. Let them know you are involved.
- Give leadership your first assessment of the emergency from a communication perspective and inform them of your next steps. Remember: Be first, be right, be credible.

Coordination:

- Contact your local, state, and federal partners now.
- Contact your Federal Bureau of Investigation (FBI) counterpart, if there is potential for criminal investigation.
- Secure a spokesperson as designated in the plan.
- Initiate alert notification and call in extra communication personnel, per the plan.
- Connect with the emergency operations center and make your presence known.

Media:

- Be first: Provide a statement that your agency is aware of the emergency and is involved in the response.
- Be right: Begin monitoring the media for misinformation that must be corrected.
- Be credible: Tell the media when and where to get updates from your agency.
- Give facts: Don't speculate. Ensure partners are saying the same thing.

The public:

- Trigger your public information toll-free number operation. Do this now if you anticipate that the public will seek reassurance or information directly from your organization. Adjust the hours of operation and the number of on-call managers as needed.

- Use your initial media statement as your first message.
- Ensure that your statement expresses empathy and acknowledges public concern about the uncertainty.
- Give the precleared facts you have and refer the public to other information sources as appropriate.
- Remind people that your agency has a process in place to mitigate the crisis.
- Start call monitoring to catch trends or rumors now.

Partners and stakeholders:

- Send a basic statement to partners and stakeholders to let them know you are thinking about them. Get them involved as needed.
- Use your prearranged notification systems, preferably email lists.
- Engage leadership to make important first phone calls, based on your plan. Have them reach partners and key stakeholders to let them know your organization is responding.
- Use the internal communication system (probably email) to notify employees that their agencies are involved in the response and updates will follow. Ask for their support.

Resources:

- Disseminate contact lists as appropriate.
- Conduct the crisis risk assessment and implement assignments and hours of operation accordingly.
- Stake out your preplanned place in the emergency operations center or adjoining area.

CDC, CERC Manual 2014 Edition: Checklist 4-1, pp:129-130.

Pre-event Planning

If you are not actively dealing with an emergency, you are in a pre-event phase, even if you are still mopping up (in post-event) from the last one. Ideally, you should feed everything you learned from the last emergency into your preparations for the next ones—thus, the pre-event phase blurs into the post-event phase.

While it might seem somewhat daunting, the CDC's Emergency Communication Checklist, shown in **TABLE 15-4**, summarizes everything you need to have ready to manage a communication response during a public health emergency. If you look carefully, you will see that the rest of the checklist is just the details in response to item 1.1, "Does your organization have an emergency response/crisis communication operational plan… ?" Unless the organization has already worked through most of this checklist, then the answer to this question is no.

Your objective during the pre-event phase is to imagine the unimaginable—the various disasters that could occur. These are listed under checklist item II, "Messages and Audiences in the Checklist." You also need to work out your logistical, partnership, resource, and personnel arrangements and commit them to printed (yes, old-fashioned paper) plans as well as online plans. You will want to create and pre-position (e.g., post electronically, distribute to partners, print out, make camera ready, record videos) content you would need in the first 48 hours of a disaster.

Who Is in Charge?

Much of the plan deals with coordination of plans, spokespersons, and public information officers, at all emergency response agencies, public health departments, and government offices that would be involved in an emergency. Ensuring such coordination is in place requires meetings and development of the following resources:

- Lists that are turned into listservs, phone-trees, Twitter groups, and any other form that can be used instantly to connect with one another. This should include after-hours (cell phone) contacts for all public information officers (PIOs) and supervisory officials.
- Memoranda of understanding that designate lines of authority, subject matter experts, spokespersons, clearance procedures, training and resource availabilities, and so on.
- Other elements needed to get the job done:
  - Training. While you have the time, train everyone in ERC principles. In particular, encourage SMEs and officials to become community or media spokespeople.
  - Resources. Have you identified space, facilities management (i.e., heat and light), equipment, and people who can operate an office, possibly on a 24/7 basis, if needed? What if that center needs to be set up far away from your present location? You might need to establish contracts with vendors (including local universities) for language translation, printing, photocopying, door-to-door dissemination, media monitoring, survey research, and other services on an as-needed basis.

TABLE 15-4 Emergency Risk Communication Checklist

Use this comprehensive checklist to help assess your organization's preparedness for responding to an emergency.

I. Planning, Research, Training, and Evaluation [Yes/No]

1.1 Does your organization have an emergency response/crisis communication operational plan for public information and media, partner, and stakeholder relations?

If yes, does the plan have the following elements: [Yes/No]

a. Designated line and staff responsibilities for the public information team?
b. Information verification and clearance/approval procedures?
c. Agreements on information release authorities (who releases what/when/how)?
d. Regional and local media contact list (including after-hours news desks)?
e. Procedures to coordinate with the public health organization response teams?
f. Designated spokespersons for public health issues in an emergency?
g. Public health organization emergency response team after-hours contact numbers?
h. Contact numbers for emergency information partners (e.g., governor's public affairs officer, local FBI public information special agent in charge, local or regional department of agriculture or veterinarian public information officers, Red Cross and other nongovernment organizations)?
i. Agreements/procedures to join the Joint Information Center (JIC) of the emergency operations center (if activated)?
j. Procedures to secure needed resources (space, equipment, people) to operate the public information operation during a public health emergency 24 hours a day/7 days a week, if needed?
k. Identified vehicles of information dissemination during a crisis to public, stakeholders, partners (e.g., e-mail list servs, broadcast fax, door-to-door leaflets, press releases)?

[Yes/No]

1.2 Have you coordinated your planning with the community or state emergency operation center?
1.3 Have you coordinated your planning with other response organizations or competitors?
1.4 Have designated spokespersons received media training and risk communication training?
1.5 Do the spokespersons understand emergency crisis/risk communication principles to build trust and credibility?

II. Message and Audiences [Yes/No]

2.1 Are any of the following types of incidents (disasters) likely to require intense public information, media, and partner communication responses by your organization:

a. Airborne infectious disease outbreak (e.g., pandemic influenza)?
b. Foodborne infectious disease outbreak (e.g., Listeria)?
c. Waterborne (Cryptosporidiosis)?
d. Vector borne (West Nile virus)?
e. Outbreak with potential to spread outside your region or to your region?
f. Unknown infectious agent?
g. Chemical or toxic material disaster?
h. Natural disasters?
i. Unknown infectious agent (international) with potential to spread to the United States?
j. Known infectious agent (international) with potential to spread to the United States?
k. Large-scale environmental crises?
l. Radiological event?
m. Terrorist event
   1. Biological (suspected or declared)?
   2. Chemical?
   3. Radiological?
   4. Mass explosion?
n. Site-specific emergencies
   1. Laboratory incident with laboratory worker?
   2. Laboratory incident/release of material in community?
   3. Death of employee/contractor/visitor while on campus/premises?
   4. Hostage event with/by employee/contractor on campus/premises?
   5. Bomb threat?
   6. Explosion/fire—destruction of property?
   7. Violent death of an employee/contractor or visitor on campus/premises?

[Yes/No]

2.2 Have you identified special populations (e.g., elderly, first language other than English, tribal communities, border populations)? List any specific sub-populations that need to be targeted with specific messages during a public health emergency related to your organization (e.g., tribal nations, persons with chronic respiratory illness, unvaccinated seniors).

2.3 Have you identified your organization's partners who should receive direct information and updates (not solely through the media) from your organization during a public health emergency?

2.4 Have you identified all stakeholder organizations or populations (groups or organizations that your believes have an active interest in monitoring activities—to whom you are most directly organization accountable, other than official

2.5 Have you planned ways to reach people according to their reactions to the incident (fight or flight)? Are messages,messengers, and methods of delivery sensitive to all types of audiences in your area of responsibility?

2.6 Are there mechanisms/resources in place to create messages for the media and public under severe time constraints, including methods to clear these messages within the emergency response operations of your organization (include cross clearance)?

2.7 Have you identified how you will perform media evaluation, content analysis, and public information call analysis in real time during an emergency to ensure adequate audience feedback?

[Yes/No]

2.8 Have you developed topic-specific pre-crisis materials for identified public health emergency issues, or identified sources of these materials if needed:
   a. Topic fact sheet (e.g., description of the disease, public health threat, treatment, etc.)?
   b. Public questions/answers (Q/As)?
   c. Partner questions/answers?
   d. Resource fact for media/public/partners to obtain additional information?
   e. Web access and links to information on the topic?
   f. Recommendations for affected populations?
   g. Background beta video (B-roll) for media use on the topic?
   h. List of subject matter experts outside your organization who would be effective validators to public/media regarding your activities during a public health emergency?

III. Messenger [Yes/No]

3.1 Have you identified public health spokespersons for media and public appearances during an emergency?

If yes, have you:
   a. Identified persons by position to act as spokespersons for multiple audiences (e.g., media spokesperson, community meeting speaker, etc.) and formats about public health issues during an emergency?
   b. Ensured that the spokespersons understand their communication roles and responsibilities and will incorporate them into their expected duties during the crisis?

IV. Methods of Delivery (Information Dissemination) and Resources [Yes/No]

4.1 Does your organization have go kits for public information officers who may have to abandon their normal place of operation during a public health emergency or join a JIC?

If yes, does the kit include: [Yes/No]
   a. A computer(s) capable of linking to the Internet/e-mail?
   b. A CD–ROM or disks containing the elements of the crisis communication plan (including media, public health, and organization contact lists, partner contact lists; information materials, etc.)?
   c. A cell phone or satellite phone, pager, wireless e-mail, etc.?
   d. A funding mechanism (credit card, etc.) that can be used to purchase operational resources as needed?
   e. Manuals and background information necessary to provide needed information to the public and media?
   f. Care and comfort items for the public information operations staff?

4.2 Have you identified the mechanisms that are or should be in place to ensure multiple channels of communication to multiple audiences during a public health emergency?

If yes, do they include: [Yes/No]
   a. Media channels (print, TV, radio, Web)?
   b. Websites?
   c. Phone banks?

(continues)

TABLE 15-4 Emergency Risk Communication Checklist   *(continued)*

    d. Town hall meetings?

    e. Listserv e-mail?

    f. Broadcast fax?

    g. Letters by mail?

    h. Subscription newsletters?

    i. Submissions to partner newsletters?

    j. Regular or special partner conference calls?

    k. Door-to-door canvassing?

4.3 Are contracts/agreements in place to post information to broadcast fax or e-mail systems?

4.4 Have locations for press conferences been designated and resourced?

V. Personnel [Yes/No]

  5.1 Have you identified employees, contractors, fellows, interns currently working for you or available to you in an emergency who have skills in the following areas:

    a. Public affairs specialist?

    b. Health communication specialist?

    c. Communication officer?

    d. Health education specialist?

    e. Training specialist?

    f. Writer/editor?

    g. Technical writer/editor?

    h. Audio/visual specialist?

    i. Internet/Web design specialist?

    j. Others who contribute to public/provider information?

  5.2 Have you identified who will provide the following expertise or execute these activities during a public health emergency (including backup):

Command and control: [Yes/No]

    a. Directs the work related to the release of information to the media, public, and partners?

    b. Activates the plan, based on careful assessment of the situation and the expected demands for information media, partners, and the public?

    c. Coordinates with horizontal communication partners, as outlined in the plan, to ensure that messages are consistent and within the scope of the organization's responsibility?

    d. Provides updates to organization's director, Emergency Operations Center (EOC) command and higher headquarters, as determined in the plan?

    e. Advises the director and chain of command regarding information to be released, based on the organization's role in the response?

    f. Ensures that risk communication principles are employed in all contact with media, public, and partner information release efforts?

    g. Advises incident-specific policy, science, and situation?

    h. Reviews and approves materials for release to media, public, and partners?

    i. Obtains required clearance of materials for release to media on policy or sensitive topic-related information not previously cleared?

    j. Determines the operational hours/days, and reassesses throughout the emergency response?

    k. Ensures resources are available (human, technical, and mechanical supplies)?

Media: [Yes/No]

    a. Assesses media needs and organizes mechanisms to fulfill media needs during the crisis (e.g., daily briefings in person, versus a Website update)?

    b. Triages the response to media requests and inquiries?

    c. Ensures that media inquiries are addressed as appropriate?

    d. Supports spokespersons?

    e. Develops and maintains media contact lists and call logs?

    f. Produces and distributes media advisories and press releases?

    g. Produces and distributes materials (e.g., fact sheets, B-roll)?

    h. Oversees media monitoring systems and reports (e.g., analyzing environment and trends to determine needed messages; determining what misinformation needs to be corrected; identifying concerns, interests, and needs arising from the crisis and the response)?

    i. Ensures that risk communication principles to build trust and credibility are incorporated into all public messagesdelivered through the media?

    j. Acts as member of the JIC of the field site team for media relations?

    k. Serves as liaison from the organization to the JIC and back?

Direct public information: [Yes/No]

    a. Manages the mechanisms to respond to public requests for information directly from the organization by telephone, in writing, or by e-mail?

    b. Oversees public information monitoring systems and reports (e.g., analyzing environment and trends to determine needed messages; determining what misinformation needs to be corrected; identifying concerns, interests, and needs arising from the crisis and the response)?

    c. Activates or participates in the telephone information line?

    d. Activates or participates in the public e-mail response system?

    e. Activates or participates in the public correspondence response system?

    f. Organizes and manages emergency response Websites and Web pages?

    g. Establishes and maintains links to other emergency response Websites?

Partner/stakeholder information: [Yes/No]

    a. Establishes communication protocols based on prearranged agreements with identified partners and stakeholders?

    b. Arranges regular partner briefings and updates?

    c. Solicits feedback and responds to partner information requests and inquiries?

    d. Oversees partner/stakeholder monitoring systems and reports (e.g., analyzing environment and trends to determine needed messages; determining what misinformation needs to be corrected; identifying concerns, interests, and needs arising from the crisis and the response)?

    e. Helps organize and facilitate official meetings to provide information and receive input from partners or stakeholders?

    f. Develops and maintains lists and call logs of legislators and special interest groups?

    g. Responds to legislator/special interest groups requests and inquiries?

Content and material for public health emergencies: [Yes/No]

    a. Develops and establishes mechanisms to rapidly receive information from the EOC regarding the public health emergency?

    b. Translates EOC situation reports and meeting notes into information appropriate for public and partner needs?

    c. Works with subject matter experts to create situation-specific fact sheets, Q/As, and updates?

    d. Compiles information on possible public health emergency topics for release when needed?

    e. Tests messages and materials for cultural and language requirements of special populations?

    f. Receives input from other communication team members regarding content and message needs?

    g. Uses analysis from media, public and partner monitoring systems, and reports (e.g., environmental and trend analysis to determine needed messages; what misinformation need to be corrected; and identify concerns, interests, and needs arising from the crisis and the response) to identify additional content requirements and materials development?

    h. Lists contracts/cooperative agreements/consultants currently available to support emergency public/private information dissemination?

VI. Suggestions to Consider about Resources [Yes/No]

Do you have space:

    a. To operate your communication teams outside the EOC? (You need a place to bring media on site, separate from the EOC.)

    b. To quickly train spokespersons?

    c. For team meetings?

    d. For equipment, exclusive for your use? (You cannot stand in line for the copier when media deadlines loom.)

(continues)

TABLE 15-4 Emergency Risk Communication Checklist   *(continued)*

Have you considered the following contracts and memoranda of agreement: [Yes/No]
- a. A contract with a media newswire?
- b. A contract with a radio newswire?
- c. A contract for writers or public relations personnel who can augment your staff?
- d. A contract for administrative support?
- e. A phone system/contractor to supply a phone menu that directs type of caller and level of information desired, including:
  - 1 General information about the threat?
  - 2 Tip line, listing particular actions people can take to protect themselves?
  - 3 Reassurance/counseling?
  - 4 Referral information for healthcare/medical facility workers?
  - 5 Referral information for epidemiologists or others to report cases?
  - 6 Lab/treatment protocols?
  - 7 Managers looking for policy statements for employees?

Do you have the following recommended equipment: [Yes/No]
- a. Fax machine (with a number that's pre-programmed for broadcast fax releases to media and partners)?
- b. Website capability 24/7? (You should attempt to have new information posted within 2 hours; some say within 10 minutes.)
- c. Computers (on local area networks [LANs] with e-mail listservs designated for partners and media)?
- d. Laptop computers?
- e. Printers for every computer?
- f. Copier (and backup)?
- g. Tables? (You will need a large number of tables.)
- h. Cell phones/pagers/personal digital devices and e-mail readers?
- i. Visible calendars, flow charts, bulletin boards, easels?
- j. Designated personal message board?
- k. Small refrigerator?
- l. Paper?
- m. Color copier?
- n. A/V equipment?
- o. Portable microphones?
- p. Podium?
- q. TVs with cable hookup?
- r. Video recording and playing capability?
- s. CD–ROMs or flash drives?
- t. Paper shredder?

Do you have the following recommended supplies: [Yes/No]
- a. Copier toner?
- b. Printer ink?
- c. Paper?
- d. Pens?
- e. Markers?
- f. Highlighters?
- g. Erasable markers?
- h. Shipping and postal supplies?
- i. Sticky note pads?
- j. Tape?
- k. Notebooks?
- l. Poster board?
- m. Standard press kit folders?
- n. Organized B-roll in media ready format (keep VHS copies around for meetings)?
- o. Formatted computer disks?
- p. Color-coded items (folders, inks, etc.)?

q. Baskets (to contain items you're not ready to throw away)?
r. Organizers to support your clearance and release system?
s. Expandable folders (alphabetized or days of the month)?
t. Staplers?
u. Paper punch?
v. Three-ring binders?
w. Organization's press kit or its logo on a sticker?
x. Colored copier paper (for door-to-door flyers)?
y. Paper clips (all sizes)?

CDC, CERC Manual 2014 Edition: Checklist 4-5, pp:136-147.

Message and Audience

The list in section 2.1 of the ERC Checklist is scary and thorough. Perhaps the only thing you might be able to cross off this list ahead of time are emergencies dealing with laboratories, if you are not responsible for that response. A good use for this list is as a basis for prioritizing your preparations. But how can you say that a terrorist event with a chemical agent is less important to prepare for than an airborne infectious disease outbreak? If the crisis involves, for example, a biological or chemical agent terrorist event, it is likely that the FBI and the CDC will take charge and you will basically follow their lead and use their materials. Many of the disasters included in the ERC Checklist are actually "routine" emergencies for public health departments, and most choose to focus on them first, when using their own resources. (If they have received money for terrorism preparation, the funding goes to support that effort.) You might also need to tailor your notification, operations, and other lists by type of incident. An attack with waterborne chemical agents, for example, will require different network partners (e.g., local water management officials) than an explosion at a fuel refinery.

ERC Checklist sections 2.2, 2.3, and 2.4 deal with finding and reaching specific populations. Many government offices, local Chambers of Commerce, or other organizations maintain websites that contain many community details. Many local organizations have formed networks of "block captains"—that is, people who will go door-to-door in the case of an emergency and tell their neighbors what do to. It will be very helpful to know the organizations that established and maintain this structure and to find a way to share materials with them.

The Community Assessment for Public Health Emergency Response (CASPER)[h] toolkit can help you link your program to U.S. Census Bureau mapping programs to identify needs and resources. Census data provide a rough estimate of the community needs in terms of overall population size, categorized by reported sex, race, religious affiliations, disabilities, language needs, and educational levels. Data on heating fuel, vehicle ownership, and phones are more relevant to other emergency planners, but completing a CASPR assessment is a good starting point for determining which religious organizations and community groups might need to be involved to plan appropriate meeting sites and identify partners to train.

A full list of all broadcast media is also generated as part of the ERC Checklist (the list in the example is truncated for space). Combining this information with information on businesses, schools, and any other potential stakeholder organizations, you would develop plans and lists, as was required in Section I, to have a rapid communication network ready in case of an emergency. You would then use these or more customized data to plan your materials in ERC Checklist section 2.8.

Topic-Specific Pre-crisis Materials

ERC Checklist section 2.8 lists some pre-crisis materials that you can prepare and have ready to go in the event of an emergency. As mentioned earlier, you should have both electronic and print copies of your materials. Print versions are needed in case the power is cut off or the Internet has been sabotaged, and you need to produce photocopies the old-fashioned way. Paper in a file folder is great preparation for this possibility, as are DVDs, flash drives, and other more permanent records of materials. You cannot count on having access to the Internet (or electricity) in an emergency!

---

h. http://emergency.cdc.gov/disasters/surveillance/pdf/casper_toolkit_version_2_0_508_compliant.pdf

The good news is that a good repository of fact sheets, Q&As (question-and-answer sets), clinical guidelines, and other information that you could use within the first 48 hours of a response is already available. The CDC has focused on this time period for the emergency response because it can be particularly chaotic. After this point, you will need to update the materials with what you have learned about the specific incident. To get out of the starting gate, however, a wealth of templates and topic-specific materials are available from the CDC and are ready to go.

Through a cooperative agreement with several schools of public health, the CDC developed sets of materials for specific populations across the United States, including American Indians, African Americans, Hispanics, and persons with lower literacy abilities in English. There are also multiple language translations (e.g., Spanish, Russian, Vietnamese, French) for many materials. Based on your community's needs, you would download these materials, print them out, and store them on flash drives so you have them readily available, wherever you might have to set up shop. **BOX 15-8** and **BOX 15-9** present a few sample materials from the CDC and *CDCynergy* ERC.

Message Maps

Particularly for planning oral presentations, some people find it very useful to prepare **message maps**. The CDC learned about message mapping for health emergencies from Vincent Covello.[7] Message maps organize complex information into units to help a speaker to focus on key points. They also are designed to automatically provide sound bites for the media. Messages are presented in three short sentences that convey three key messages in 27 words. (These limits were developed based on research showing that front-page media and broadcast stories usually carried three key messages in less than 9 seconds for broadcast media or 27 words for print.) While this approach predates Twitter, such compact emergency messages could be "tweeted."

Message maps should be written at a sixth-grade reading level. Each primary message may have a maximum of three supporting messages that can be used when and where appropriate to provide context for the issue being mapped.

BOX 15-10 shows the CDC's draft sample message maps for pandemic influenza. The Association of State and Territorial Health Officers also prepared message maps for Ebola virus disease, which can be accessed online.[i]

BOX 15-8 Message Examples For Emergency Communication

Message Template for the First Minutes for All Emergencies

The following suggested template could be used in the first minutes after a suspected terrorist incident when little is known.

1. Please pay close attention. This is an urgent health message from [your public health agency].
2. Officials [emergency, public health, etc.] believe there has been a serious incident [describe incident including time and location] in _____ area.
3. At this time, we do not know the cause or other details about the incident.
4. Local officials are investigating and will work with state and federal officials to provide updated information as soon as possible.
5. Stay informed and follow the instructions of health officials so you can protect yourself, your family, and your community against this public health threat.
6. [Give specific information about when and how the next update will be given.]

When more information is known, additional messages could be added about what is happening, the specific terrorist agent, the actions people should take to protect themselves and others, and where to go for more information. Because these messages were developed to be effective for a variety of scenarios, they will need to be adapted to the specific event.

Message Development Worksheet

Step 1: Determine the audience, message purpose, and delivery method by checking each that applies.

Audience:

- Relationship to event
- Demographics (age, language, education, culture)
- Level of outrage (based on risk principles)

---

i. http://www.astho.org/infectious-disease/top-questions-on-ebola-simple-answers-developed-by-astho/

Purpose of message:

- Give facts/update
- Rally to action
- Clarify event status
- Address rumors
- Satisfy media requests

Method of delivery:

- Print media release
- Web release
- Prominent spokesperson (e.g., a TV or in-person appearance)
- Radio
- Other (e.g., recorded phone message)

Step 2: Construct the message using the six basic emergency message components.

1. Expression of empathy:
2. Clarifying facts/call for action:

   Who:

   What:

   Where:

   When:

   Why:

   How:

3. What we do not know:
4. Process to get answers:
5. Statement of commitment:
6. Referrals:
7. Next scheduled update:

Step 3: Check your message for the following:

DOES YOUR MESSAGE USE…	YES	NO
Positive action steps?		
An honest/open tone?		
Applied risk communication principles?		
Test for clarity		
Simple words, short sentences?		

DOES YOUR MESSAGE AVOID…	YES	NO
Jargon?		
Judgmental phrases?		
Humor?		
Extreme speculation?		

(continues)

BOX 15-8 Message Examples For Emergency Communication *(continued)*

General Chemical Agent Exposure Content for an Extended Public Health Message

Health and Safety Information for the First Hours

Reading Grade Level: 8.2

Points:

1. What is happening?
2. What to do if you are near the release of the chemical—either in the immediate area or the surrounding area.
3. What to do if you have symptoms or think you have had contact with a chemical.
4. Can the illness caused by a chemical agent be spread from person to person?
5. What are the symptoms of contact with various chemical agents?
6. What to do if you are in a car that is in the immediate area of the release.
7. What to do if you are concerned about xxx [add name] chemical agent.
8. What is being done and how to get more information.

Note to users: Much initial health and safety information is identical for all chemical agents, except for symptoms. Specific symptoms are listed by category of agent. It will be necessary to carefully review and revise the messages during an actual event once the agent is confirmed.

What is happening?

- This is an urgent health message from the U.S. Department of Health and Human Services (HHS). Please pay careful attention to this message to protect your health and that of others.
- Public officials suspect that a chemical agent has been released in the xxx area or xxx building. [add information]
- xxx number [add information] of cases have been reported, with symptoms of [chemical agent]. These symptoms include: [list of symptoms].

Note to user: Give description of agent (e.g., colorless gas, odorless, or mild smell of garlic or almond), depending upon the agent.

- If the chemical was released in your building, follow instructions from emergency personnel. You should leave the building as quickly as possible.
- How people were exposed to this chemical or the full extent of the problem is unclear.
- Local, state, and federal officials, including HHS, FBI, and Homeland Security, are working together to find out more about this situation. Updates will be made as soon as officials know more.
- If you are near the xxx area [add information], protect yourself and your family by staying home or where you are and wait for further instructions.
- If you are not close to the xxx area [add information], stay where you are and avoid unnecessary travel until further instructions.
- We have challenges ahead, and we are working to find out more about this situation. By staying informed and following instructions from health officials, you can protect yourself, your family, and the community against this public health threat.
- For more information on chemical agents, go to the HHS website at www.hhs.gov, the Centers for Disease Control and Prevention's Chemical Emergencies website at https://emergency.cdc.gov/chemical/ or call the CDC Hotline at 1-800-CDC-INFO for the latest updates.
- This message contains additional information that can help protect your health and the health of others.

What to do if you are near the release of the chemical—either in the immediate area or the surrounding area

If you are outdoors, emergency personnel may ask you to leave the area or find shelter nearby. If you are told to go indoors or you are already inside a shelter, follow these instructions:

- *Go to the highest level of the building.* Find a room with as few windows and doors as possible.
- *Reduce air flow from outside to inside.* Close vents, air conditioning, fireplace dampers, and anything else that exposes the room to outside air.
- *Seal the room.* Use plastic and duct tape to close all openings, including windows, doors, vents, and electrical outlets. Even if you cannot seal all openings, follow the other instructions.

- *Eat only sealed, stored food and water.* Do not eat or drink anything that may have been exposed to the chemical.
- *Turn to the radio, television, or Internet news for updated health and safety announcements.* Announcements will be made about when it is safe to go outside.

What to do if you have symptoms or think you have had contact with a chemical

- Do not touch other people to prevent getting the chemical on them.
- Remove your outer layer of clothing.
- Do *not* remove clothes over your head. If necessary, cut clothes off.
- If possible, put clothes inside a bag and seal it. Put this sealed bag into another bag and seal again.
- Wash your hair and body thoroughly with soap and water right away.
- If eyes are burning or irritated, rinse with water for 10–15 minutes. Do not use soap in your eyes.
- After you have followed these instructions, call your doctor or local public health department right away at xxx-xxx-xxxx [add information]. They will tell you how and where to get more help.

Can the illness caused by a chemical agent be spread from person to person?

- The *illness* caused by a chemical agent *cannot* spread from person to person. It is *not* a contagious disease that can be spread by coughing or sneezing.
- People can spread the *chemical* via their their skin, clothing, hair or body fluids, such as vomit.
- Once exposed people take off their clothes and shower, most of the chemical will be removed and is much less likely to be spread by these people.

What are the symptoms of contact with various chemical agents?

Symptoms of contact with a blister agent:

- Contact with this type of chemical causes blistering on the skin and in the nose, mouth, and throat.
- After contact with a blister agent, symptoms may occur immediately or may take up to 24 hours to appear.
- First symptoms may include red, itchy, or painful skin, followed by blisters.
- Later symptoms may include pain or swelling in the eyes and lungs, tears in the eyes, and trouble breathing.

Symptoms of contact with a blood agent:

- Contact with this type of chemical deprives the blood and organs of oxygen.
- After contact with a blood agent, symptoms may occur immediately or may take up to 24 hours to appear.
- In general, symptoms may include rapid breathing, nausea, convulsions, and loss of consciousness.

Symptoms of contact with a nerve agent:

- Contact with this type of chemical can damage the nervous system and affect movement and breathing.
- After contact with a nerve agent, symptoms may appear immediately or up to 18 hours later.
- Symptoms include seizures, drooling, eye irritations, sweating or twitching, blurred vision, and muscle weakness.

Symptoms of contact with a choking agent:

- This type of chemical attacks the respiratory system and causes difficulty breathing.
- After contact with a choking agent, symptoms may occur immediately or may take 24 to 48 hours to appear.
- In general, symptoms may include coughing; burning in the eyes, nose, or throat; blurred vision; upset stomach; fluid in the lungs; and difficulty breathing.

Note to users: Officials might offer particular instructions for reducing exposure if people are in their cars. Following is a message for staying in the car and pulling over.

If you are in your car in xxx [add information] area, you can help prevent being exposed to the chemical by following these steps:

1. Pull over to the side of the road in a manner that will not block or interfere with the movement of emergency vehicles.
2. Temporarily turn off the engine and shut down any vents that draw in outside air, including those of the air conditioner. Running the engine and driving pull outside air into the car and could expose you to additional chemicals.
3. To minimize the amount of chemical you inhale, cover your mouth and nose with a cloth, such as a scarf or a handkerchief.
4. Listen for further instructions from emergency personnel on the scene or listen for news on the radio.

(continues)

BOX 15-8 Message Examples For Emergency Communication *(continued)*

What to do if you are concerned about xxx [add information] chemical agent

- It is natural to be concerned or afraid at a time like this. Staying informed and following instructions from public health officials will help you stay as safe and healthy as possible.
- Many chemical agents are commonly used in industry and household products. In this situation, [chemical agent] may have been released deliberately. We are not sure at this time if this is the case.
- If you are near the xxx area [add information], protect yourself and your loved ones by staying home or where you are and wait for further instructions from officials.
- If you are not close to the xxx [add information] area, stay where you are and avoid unnecessary travel until further notice.
- Stay informed by turning to the radio, television, or Internet news for updated health and safety announcements.

What is being done and how to get more information

- Federal, state, and local health officials are working together to find and treat people who have symptoms or who may have had contact with xxx [add information] chemical agent. They are also taking actions to prevent others from being exposed.
- Officials will share information and give more instructions as the situation develops and they learn more.
- Go to [insert local media information here] to hear the latest information from local officials.
- For more information on botulism, visit the HHS website at http:www.hhs.gov, the Centers for Disease Control and Prevention's Chemical Emergencies website at https://emergency.cdc.gov/chemical/, or call the CDC Hotline at 1-800-CDC-INFO for the latest information.

General Chemical Agent Short Message

Health and Safety Information for the First Hours

Reading Grade Level: 9.3

- This is an urgent health message from the U.S. Department of Health and Human Services.
- Public officials suspect that a chemical agent has been deliberately released in the xxx area or xxx building [add information].
- xxx [add information] number cases have been reported with symptoms of [chemical agent]. These symptoms include: [list of symptoms].

Note to users: Give description of agent (e.g., colorless gas, odorless or mild smell of garlic or almond), depending upon the agent.

- If you are outdoors in the xxx area [add information], emergency workers will ask you to leave the area or find shelter nearby.
- If you are indoors in the xxx area [add information], go to the highest level of the building and close windows, doors, and fireplace dampers. Turn off heating and cooling systems and close vents so that the room is not exposed to outside air.
- If the chemical was released in your building, follow instructions from emergency personnel.
- How people were exposed to this chemical or the full extent of the problem is unclear.
- Local, state, and federal officials, including HHS, FBI, and Homeland Security, are working together to find out more about this situation. Updates will be made as soon as officials know more.
- If you are near the xxx area [add information], protect yourself and your family by staying home or where you are and wait for further instructions.
- We have challenges ahead, and we are working to find out more about this situation. By staying informed and following instructions from health officials, you can protect yourself, your family, and the community against this public health threat.
- Go to [insert local media information here] to hear the latest information from local officials.
- For more information on chemical agents, go to the HHS website at www.hhs.gov, the Centers for Disease Control and Prevention's Chemical Emergencies website at https://emergency.cdc.gov/chemical/ or call the CDC Hotline at 1-800-CDC-INFO for the latest updates.

CDC, CERC Manual 2014 Edition: Message Template 3-1, pp: 74-75.

BOX 15-9 Anticipated Questions-and-Answers Worksheet

Use these worksheets to write anticipated questions about a specific event; then develop appropriate answers for the public and sound bites for the media.

Step 1: Review the following list of questions commonly asked by the media. The spokesperson should have answers to these questions prepared and change/update as necessary throughout the duration of the crisis:

Questions Commonly Asked by Media in a Crisis*

- What is your (spokesperson's) name and title?
- What effect will it have on production and employment?
- What happened? (Examples: How many people were injured or killed? How much property damage occurred?)
- Which safety measures were taken?
- When did it happen?
- Who is to blame?
- Where did it happen?
- Do you accept responsibility?
- What do you do there?
- Has this ever happened before?
- Who was involved?
- What do you have to say to the victims?
- Why did it happen? What was the cause?
- Is there danger now?
- What are you going to do about it?
- Will there be inconvenience to the public?
- Was anyone hurt or killed? What are their names?
- How much will it cost the organization?
- How much damage was caused?
- When will we find out more?

Step 2: Using the following Answer Development Model, draft answers for the public and sound bites for the news media in the space provided after the model. Then go back and check your draft answers against the model. Sound bites for the news media should be 8 seconds or less and framed for television, radio, or print media.

Answer Development Model

IN YOUR ANSWER/SOUND BITE, YOU SHOULD...	BY...
1. Express empathy and caring in your first statement	<ul><li>Using a personal story</li><li>Using the pronoun "I"</li><li>Transitioning to the conclusion</li></ul>
2. State a conclusion (key message)	<ul><li>Limiting the number of words (5–20)</li><li>Using positive words</li><li>Setting it apart with introductory words, pauses, inflections, and other spacers</li></ul>
3. Support the conclusion	<ul><li>At least two facts</li><li>An analogy</li><li>A personal story</li><li>A credible third party</li></ul>
4. Repeat the conclusion	<ul><li>Using exactly the same words as the first time</li></ul>
5. Include future action(s) to be taken	<ul><li>Listing specific next steps</li><li>Providing more information about</li><li>Contacts</li><li>Important phone numbers</li></ul>

*Covello VT. Risk perception and communication: Tools and techniques for communicating risk information. In: Department of the Environment (Ed.), *HMIP Seminar proceedings: Risk Perception and Communication*; Oakham, UK. 15-16 June 1995.

BOX 15-10 Sample Message Maps for Pandemic Flu

Pre-event Message Map

What is pandemic flu?

Pandemic flu is a worldwide flu outbreak.

- A new influenza virus causes the outbreak. Flu pandemics occurred three times in the last century.
- The flu spreads from person to person and is highly contagious.
- Pandemic flu is expected to have a high death rate.

Pandemic influenza is different from seasonal flu.

- Seasonal outbreaks of flu are caused by viruses that have already spread among people.
- Pandemic influenza is the development of a new virus that most people in the world have never been exposed and have no immunity.
- Vaccine will not be available initially. New vaccine production can take 3–6 months.

We are prepared to respond with a flu pandemic plan.

- Through a sentinel surveillance system, we track disease outbreaks. We receive early notification so that we may respond appropriately.
- In the event of a pandemic, our trained staff and partners would receive and distribute medications and vaccine at local mass-dispensing sites, as they become available.
- [Health Department name] will coordinate with hospitals and emergency care facilities to respond most efficiently to public needs.

Treatment Message Map: Pandemic Flu

What treatment is there for pandemic flu?

This is a new strain of flu. There would be no specific vaccine available.

- Researchers are currently trying to make a vaccine to protect humans against influenza strain [x and y].
- Vaccine will be distributed when made available.
- Watch the media for updates.

Antivirals or Tamiflu may be available.

- There are influenza antiviral drugs approved by the Food and Drug Administration (FDA) for the treatment and or relief of influenza symptoms.
- They will not keep someone from getting the flu.
- They can lessen symptoms if taken within 24 hours of becoming ill with the flu.

Those who are ill should remain at home.

- Drink plenty of fluids and rest.
- Use good respiratory hygiene (wash hands, cough into sleeve or tissue).
- Limit exposure to family members and friends.

Symptom Message Map: Pandemic Flu

What are the symptoms of pandemic flu?

Signs and symptoms of seasonal flu are well known.

- Symptoms include fever, headache, aches, and cough.
- Signs and symptoms appear approximately 2–5 days after exposure.
- Illness may last 1–2 weeks.

Signs and symptoms of pandemic flu may differ.

- Event specific sign or symptom 1
- Event specific sign or symptom 2
- Event specific sign or symptom 3

If you believe you have the (event-specific) flu, contact your healthcare provider right away.

- Receiving the proper health care early is important.
- You can call xxx 24/7 hotline for more information. The toll-free phone number is [1.xxx.xxxxxxx].

- Additional information is available on xxx website: www.xxx.com.

Event Message Map: Pandemic Flu

What should the public know about an outbreak of pandemic flu?

A worldwide outbreak of influenza virus has now reached [state].

- This flu is highly contagious and is spread by coughing and sneezing.
- Other states are reporting high mortality rates. Past influenza pandemics have led to high levels of illness, death, social disruption, and economic loss.
- Cases have been reported in ___ counties.

Vaccine supply is limited, and additional vaccine may not be available for 3–6 months.

- Since vaccine supply is limited, _____ will receive the flu shot first.
- Those not getting the vaccine early can do the following to reduce risk: avoid close contact with the sick, wash hands (use soap), quit smoking, and wash your hands before you touch your eyes, nose, or mouth.
- If you're sick, stay away from others, cover your mouth when sneezing or coughing, throw away used tissue, and sanitize household objects.

We want to reduce contact and slow the spread of disease.

- We may close schools and public gatherings for protection.
- ___ may be forced to ask for voluntary isolation of those who have been exposed for the duration of the incubation period of the disease.
- Those who are ill should remain isolated until the fever is gone.

Message Map Bullet Form. Available at ftp://ftp.cdc.gov/pub/phlpprep/Legal%20Preparedness%20for%20Pandemic%20Flu/7.0%20-%20Other%20Governmental%20Materials/Avian%20Flu%20Message%20Maps/Message%20Map%20Bullet%20Form.doc.

Some communication experts believe that message maps can be confining and make the speaker sound too rehearsed. They recommend that spokespersons keep a list of the key points available instead. Message maps probably work best when used to prepare materials ahead of time to ensure that the most important concepts are presented prominently, succinctly, and in simple language. Having more than 10 maps for a subject should also be avoided to prevent overload. Keep moving priority information to the top and shed the rest.

▶ Communicating During an Emergency

In an emergency, what you *cannot* do is wait until all the information is in to craft the perfect message. Getting to the audience early and establishing a trusting partnership will set the tone for how they hear and respond to what you say. And accuracy is crucial. CERC's motto puts it altogether, "Be first. Be right. Be credible." Your first communications need to let the audience know:

- You are aware of the emergency.
- You care about the people who were harmed and their loved ones.

- You are putting a response in place.
- Here is what you know now.
- This is how you know it.
- Here is what you do not know.
- This is why you do not know it.
- Here is what you are doing to learn more information about this problem.

You do not want to speculate about what you do not know, because the public will latch onto these guesses and expect them to be borne out. If they are not, then your credibility decreases. It is also critically important that experts agree on facts and speak with one voice. Inconsistent messages will increase anxiety and quickly diminish experts' credibility. Finally, and most importantly, the first words out of your mouth need to show your empathy and caring.

Seven Recommendations

The following recommendations, were selected by the CDC's Office of Communication as critical based on lessons learned in the wake of the anthrax crisis in 2003:[j]

- Be careful with risk comparisons.
- Do not over-reassure.
- Use sensitive syntax.
- Acknowledge uncertainty.

j. http://www.psandman.com/col/part1.htm

- Give people things to do.
- Stop trying to allay panic.
- Acknowledge people's fears.

BOX 15-11 summarizes Sandman's recommendations on these seven issues. It intersperses his words with those of the ERC *CDCynergy* authors.

▶ Conclusion

You may hope that you will never have to deal with a disease outbreak, a hurricane, a toxic chemical spill, a terrorist strike with a dirty bomb, a chemical attack, or bioterrorism. But if you work in public health, chances are you will need to deal with a crisis one day, even if it is "just" an outbreak of meningitis at an area college or

a toxic runoff from an upstream CAFO (concentrated animal feeding operation). For timely risk communication, public health departments need to keep their all-hazards preparations up-to-date, including having solid communication plans and draft materials ready to go.

While emergencies are never routine, the practiced expert risk communication response can be. You can become expert in ERC, just as you can learn to create effective health promotion campaigns to combat child obesity or prevent neural tube defects caused by a lack of folic acid. In fact, many of the emergency communication principles that have held up under crisis conditions are useful for effective health communication under less urgent circumstances.

BOX 15-11 Sandman's Communication Advice for Emergencies

The advice presented here was selected from 26 recommendations made by Peter Sandman to the CDC in the aftermath of the anthrax attacks. The full set of recommendations is available on his website, (http://www.psandman.com/col/part1.htm). It remains the most thoughtful work you can find on the subject.

Recommendation 1: Be Careful with Risk Comparisons

The true risk and the perceived risk can be quite different. The source of the risk can be as troubling as the degree of risk. People do not like injustice. If they perceive that the risk has been imposed on them, that they have been unfairly singled out to experience the risk, or that a fellow human being deliberately put them in the position to be exposed to the risk, they are likely to perceive the risk with more concern or outrage. Sandman cautions about risk comparisons by exploring both the true risk and the perception of that risk. He defines "hazard" as the seriousness of a risk from a technical perspective.

According to Sandman, "outrage" is the seriousness of the risk in *nontechnical* terms. Experts view risk in terms of hazard; the rest of us view it in terms of outrage. The risks we overestimate are high-outrage and low-hazard. The risks we underestimate are high-hazard and low-outrage.

When technical people try to explain that a high-outrage, low-hazard risk is not very serious, they normally compare it to a high-hazard, low-outrage risk. "This is less serious than that," the experts tell us, "so if you are comfortable with that, you ought to be comfortable with this." In hazard terms, the comparison is valid. But the audience is thinking in outrage terms, and viewed in outrage terms the comparison appears false. Although "this" is lower hazard than "that," it is still higher outrage.

Terrorism is high-outrage and (for most of us, so far) low-hazard. You cannot effectively compare it to a low-outrage, high-hazard risk, such as driving a car—which is voluntary, familiar, less dreaded, and mostly under our own control. Even naturally acquired anthrax fails to persuade as a basis for comparison. People are justifiably more angry and frightened about terrorist anthrax attacks than about other natural outbreaks, even if the number of people attacked is low.

A volatile risk comparison can work, but only if you are trying to inform the public's judgment, not coerce it. For example, if you are trying to inform the public about a risk, the most effective thing to do would be to bracket the risk: Bigger than "X," smaller than "Y." If you report only that the risk is smaller than "Y," your audience will feel that they are being coerced.

To use risks for comparison, they should be similar in the type and level of emotion they would generate. Here is a risk comparison that can work: "Research indicates that a person is 10 times more likely to be killed by a falling coconut than to be killed by a shark." In this case, the risks are both natural in origin, fairly distributed, exotic, and outside the control of the individual. Although being killed by a shark may cause greater terror or emotion, its comparison to being killed by a coconut helps the individual to see that he or she may be perceiving the risk as greater than it is. Most people have never considered their risk of dying by coconut.

Remember that all risks are not accepted equally. The following are examples:

- Voluntary versus involuntary
- Controlled personally versus controlled by others
- Familiar versus exotic
- Natural versus human-made
- Reversible versus permanent
- Statistical versus anecdotal
- Fairly versus unfairly distributed
- Affecting children versus affecting adults

If you use risk comparisons, be sure to tell people how confident you are. Acknowledge uncertainty, especially beforehand (i.e., when talking about future possible risks), but also in mid-crisis. The worst thing about a risk comparison is the implication that you actually know how big the risk is and, therefore, can compare it to another risk. For more on Sandman's argument against over-reassuring, see the section "Being Alarming Versus Being Reassuring … " in his article "Dilemmas in Emergency Communication."

Recommendation 2: Do Not Over-Reassure

Expect high outrage if an emergency event is catastrophic, unknowable, dreaded, unfamiliar, in someone else's control, morally relevant, and memorable. Too much reassurance can backfire. For example, when people are in outrage, reassurance can increase their outrage because their perception is that you are either not telling them the truth or you are not taking their concerns seriously. Instead, tell people how scary the situation is, even though the actual numbers are small, and watch them get calmer.

Even if reassurance worked (which it does not), it is important to remember that an over-reassured public is not your goal. You want people to be concerned, vigilant, and even hyper-vigilant at first. You want people to take reasonable precautions—to feel the fear, misery, and other emotions that the situation justifies.

During a crisis, if you must amend the estimate of damage or victims, it is better to have to amend down, not up. It is "less serious than we thought" is better tolerated by the public than "it is more serious than we thought."
Note: The recommendation to "not over-reassure" is considered controversial and is not universally accepted.

Recommendation 3: Sensitive Syntax: Put the Good News in Subordinate Clauses

The recommendation not to over-reassure does not mean that you should not give people reassuring information. Of course you should! But do not emphasize it. Especially do not emphasize that it is "reassuring," or you will trigger the other side of your audience's ambivalence.

One way to avoid this outcome is to use "sensitive syntax." Sensitive syntax means putting the good news in subordinate clauses, with the more alarming information in the main clause. Here is an example of using sensitive syntax: "Even though we have not seen a new anthrax case in X days (subordinate clause with good news), it is too soon to say we are out of the woods (main clause with cautioning news)." The main clause is how seriously you are taking the situation or how aggressively you are responding to every false alarm.

Recommendation 4: Acknowledge Uncertainty

Acknowledging uncertainty is most effective when the communicator both shows his or her distress and acknowledges the audience's distress: "How I wish I could give you a definite answer on that…" "It must be awful for people to hear how tentative and qualified we have to be, because there is still so much we do not know…" More information on acknowledging uncertainty can be found in "Yellow Flags: The Acid Test of Transparency" (http://www.psandman.com/col/yellow.htm) and in the section "Tentativeness vs Confidence…" of Sandman's article "Dilemmas in Emergency Communication."

Recommendation 5: Give People Things to Do

Action helps with fear, outrage, panic, and even denial. If you have things to do, you can tolerate more fear.

In an emergency, some actions communicated are directed at victims, persons exposed, or persons who have the potential to be exposed. However, those who do not need to take immediate action will be engaging in "vicarious rehearsal" regarding those recommendations and may need to substitute action of their own to ensure that they do not prematurely act on recommendations not meant for them. In an emergency, simple actions will give people back a sense of control and will help to keep them motivated to stay tuned to what is happening (versus denial, where they refuse to acknowledge the possible danger to themselves and others) and prepare them to act when directed to do so.

(continues)

BOX 15-11 Sandman's Communication Advice for Emergencies *(continued)*

When giving people something to do, give them a choice of actions matched to their level of concern. Give a range of responses: a minimum response, a maximum response, and a recommended middle response. For example, when giving a choice of actions for making drinking water safe, you could give the following range of responses:

Response Type	Example
Minimum response	"Use chlorine drops."
Maximum response	"Buy bottled water."
Recommended middle response	"We recommend boiling water for two minutes."

Another way of looking at this is a three-part action prescription:

1. You must do X.
2. You should do Y.
3. You can do Z.

This type of clarity is very important in helping people cope with emergencies.

Some of the "things to do" are different types of behaviors:

- Symbolic behaviors: things that do not really help externally, but help people to cope (attending a community vigil)
- Preparatory behaviors: things to do now that will minimize your risk if bad things happen
- Contingent/"if then" behaviors: things to do not now, but only if bad things happen (implementing a family disaster plan)

The section "Democracy and Individual Control vs. Expert Decision-Making" of Sandman's article "Dilemmas in Emergency Communication" provides further information on these issues.

Recommendation 6: Stop Trying to Allay Panic

Panic is much less common than we imagine. The literature on disaster communication is replete with unfulfilled expectations of panicking "publics." Actually, people nearly always behave extremely well in crisis.

The condition most conducive to panic is not bad news; it is double messages from those in authority. People are the likeliest to panic (though still not very likely) when they feel that they cannot trust what those in authority are telling them—when they feel misled or abandoned in dangerous territory. When authorities start hedging or hiding bad news to prevent panic, they are likely to exacerbate the risk of panic in the process.

Experience shows that in a true emergency (matter of life and death), people do respond exceptionally well. However, it also seems that the inverse is true: The further away the public is from the real danger (in place and time), the more likely they are to allow their emotions full range. This vicarious rehearsal ("How would I feel in an emergency? What would I do? Does this advice work for me?") can be overburdening in an emergency. Therefore, the communicator must recognize the differences among audiences. The person anticipating the "bad risk" is much more likely to respond inappropriately than the person "in the heat of the battle" who is primed to act on the information and does not have quite the same amount of time to mull it over.

The section "Planning for Denial and Misery vs. Planning for Panic" of Sandman's article "Dilemmas in Emergency Communication" provides further discussion of these issues.

Recommendation 7: Acknowledge People's Fears

When people are afraid, the worst thing to do is to pretend they are not. The second worst thing to do is to tell them they should not be afraid. Both responses leave people alone with their fears.

Even when their fear is unjustified, people do not respond well to being ignored, nor do they respond well to criticism, mockery, or statistics. When the fear has some basis, these approaches are even less effective. Instead, you can acknowledge people's fears even while giving them the information they need to put those fears into context. Giving people permission to be excessively alarmed about a terrorist threat, while still telling them why they need not worry, is far more likely to reassure them.

Adapted from Sandman P. ERC *CDCynergy*. http://www.psandman.com/col/part1.htm.

Wrap-Up

Chapter Questions

1. What is the difference between a hazard and a risk?
2. When someone asks you what the chances are from dying of a particular disease or calamity, how can you respond to that question?
3. How would you characterize "nanoparticles" in make-up and the potential harm they can do to our bodies in terms of how the public appraises hazards?
4. Which of the most common concerns in risk do you worry about the most?
5. What is the difference between how we think about audiences during routine health communication and during emergency risk communication?
6. What is the risk from stigmatization during an emergency?
7. Use the message template and draft an emergency message for the release of a toxic chemical on your campus.
8. Why is it not a good idea to tell everyone, "There's nothing to worry about"?
9. Why is the 2014 Ebola virus outbreak considered a black swan event?

References

1. Centers for Disease Control and Prevention. CDC crisis and emergency risk communication. 2014. http://emergency.cdc.gov/cerc/resources/pdf/cerc_2014edition.pdf. Accessed January 4, 2017.
2. Hill AB. The environment and disease: association or causation? *Proc R Soc Med*. 1965;58:295-300.
3. Fischhoff B. Risk perception and communication. In: Detels R, Beaglehole R, Lansang MA, Gulliford M, eds. *Oxford Textbook of Public Health*, 5th ed. Oxford, UK: Oxford University Press; 2009:940-952. Reprinted in Chater NK, ed. *Judgement and Decision Making*. London, UK: Sage.
4. Blendon RJ, Benson JM, Hero JO. Public trust in physicians: U.S. medicine in international perspective. *N Engl J Med*. 2014;371:1570-1572. doi: 10.1056/NEJMp1407373.
5. *U.S. Environmental Protection Agency's Risk Assessment Guidance for Superfund (RAGS)*. Washington, DC: Environmental Protection Agency; 1989. http://www.epa.gov/risk/. Accessed January 4, 2017.
6. Sandman PM. Beyond panic prevention: addressing emotion in emergency communication. http://www.orau.gov/cdcynergy/erc/Content/activeinformation/resources/BeyondPanicPrevention.pdf. Accessed January 4, 2017.
7. Covello VT. Risk communication and message mapping: a new tool for communicating effectively in public health emergencies and disasters. *J Emerg Manage*. 2006;4(3):25-40.

Appendix 15A

Liberia Ebola Response Strategic Communication Plan in 2014—Unoffical Draft

Jana Telfer

▶ Background

Liberia, along with four other West African nations, is combating the world's first Ebola epidemic. Different from previous Ebola outbreaks, this time the disease has spread from remote villages to major metropolitan areas. Lack of knowledge and understanding about Ebola and the actions people need to take to protect themselves have complicated efforts to halt the spread of the disease.

Ebola has become so widespread that it is beginning to affect the capacity for non-Ebola-related healthcare services as well as sectors in addition to health, such as the economic well-being, social protection, education, and border security. If the situation remains unchanged, the potential exists for still other critical pillars to be affected, such as food security, budget cuts, and reductions in development projects and programs. Until enough facilities and beds are available to turn the tide of the disease, communication is the nation's first line of defense. The way that government at every level as well as partners and the private sector communicate about Ebola has significant implications for supporting disease control, mitigating its consequences, and enhancing Liberia's ability to ensure a strong and robust recovery.

Public health officials know what to do to stop the spread of the virus, and numerous international organizations are lending their economic, technical, and physical support. Nonetheless, the steps required to end the epidemic will take time. During that period, significant expansion in communication through multiple channels, using multiple methods, is needed to help the people of Liberia understand, accept, and implement the measures needed to protect themselves, their families, and their communities.

The Ministry of Health and Social Welfare has a deep understanding of health promotion and social mobilization. The Ministry has identified and tested initial health protection messages as well as proven methods of deploying those messages to communities. However, resource limitations have hampered the ability to keep pace with the spread of the disease.

The Ministry of Information and Cultural Affairs has a sophisticated understanding of the channels and tools needed to transmit messages broadly throughout Liberia, a diverse country. The unrelenting advance of the virus calls for government to lead an integrated response, engaging multiple ministries and partners in a common cause: to support the restoration of health to people and the country alike.

A substantial research base exists in both health communication and crisis and emergency risk communication that can be practically applicable in this circumstance. Advancing the government's core capacity in integrated, practical application of research-based communication holds the promise of coalescing the population and providing measurable support to halt the progress of this epidemic, as well as strengthening governmental and community capacity for possible future events.

Communication is more than giving messages; it is a process with an outcome (e.g., ending an outbreak), which promotes dialogue among everyone involved in the response, beginning with affected community members. Effective listening can strengthen relationships, build trust, and enhance transparency. The real challenge for governments and institutions is incorporating the response to the information and knowledge obtained by implementing methods to listen and transform audience insights into appropriate actions. Effective, integrated communication can be a major contributor to national health security, thereby strengthening the government's ability to safeguard the health of its people.

This communication plan outlines goals, audiences, strategies, and tactics to support that end.

▶ Strategic Objectives

- Ensure consistency in government, partner, and private-sector communication related to Ebola, its effects, and the actions needed to control the spread
- Support a timely end to the epidemic by using communication methods to increase public confidence and acceptance of health protection strategies
- Enhance integrated communication among diverse government agencies and levels of government, especially in times of emergency
- Build community resilience for emergency situations

▶ Communication Objectives

- Support adoption of health protective measures by increasing awareness of accurate information about Ebola and how to prevent it
- Increase self-efficacy among the population at all levels and in all locations
- Enhance the ability of trusted intermediaries to share accurate health information
- Engage key internal and external partners with communication objectives and programs
- Build health literacy regarding Ebola and public health among community leaders and populations
- Promote alignment with activities undertaken by the government of Liberia and its international partners
- Engage community members to provide feedback to help improve the messages and strategies

TABLE 15A-1 Audiences

Internal	External
Primary	
Government	*Nongovernmental*
President and key staff	International partners ■ World Health Organization (WHO) ■ UNICEF ■ International Federation of Red Cross and Red Crescent Societies (IFRC) ■ Doctors Without Borders (MSF) ■ CDC ■ UN Mission in Liberia (UNMIL) ■ Africa Governance Initiative (AGI) ■ The Carter Center ■ U.S. military
Minister of Health and key deputies	News media ■ Radio stations, including community radio and UNMIL radio ■ National newspapers ■ International print and broadcast
Minister of Information and key deputies	Telecommunications companies
County and district health officials	Religious leaders ■ Imams ■ Christian leaders ■ Leadership associations/councils
National legislature	Traditional leaders

Secondary		
Employees of Ministry of Health and Social Welfare	Volunteers associated with Ministry of Health	
	Business associations	
Employees of Ministry of Information, Cultural Affairs, and Tourism	International business entities with interests in Liberia	
	■ Airlines	
Ministry of Internal Affairs	■ Engineering and construction	
	■ Import/export companies	
Ministry of Transportation	■ Contractors and infrastructure developers	
	■ Fuel distributors and shippers	
Ministry of Foreign Affairs		
Ministry of Finance		
Ministry of Agriculture	International NGOs with interest in Liberia	
Ministry of Defense and Police	International workers	
	■ Healthcare workers	
Ministry of Commerce and Industry	■ Workers from international industries	
	Airlines	

▶ Key Messages

The top-level messages are designed to serve as a strong foundation for the duration of the Ebola response. Sub-bullets may change as the initiative progresses; however, the main elements (those in bold type) should be strong enough to endure throughout the emergency response.

Research has demonstrated that messages constructed in nine-word triads are easier for both spokespersons and audiences to understand, recall, and repeat. Although the messages given here are not precisely nine words each, they are purposely spare. Messages in this plan incorporate tested information from the Ministry of Health and Social Welfare as well as international organizations. Messages are based on health and risk communication theory and research.

▶ Top-Level Messages

Together we can stop the spread of Ebola.

■ We know how to stop the spread of Ebola.
■ Stopping this epidemic is our top priority.
■ When we work together over time, more people can survive Ebola.

Stopping the Ebola epidemic will take time.

■ You can take steps to protect yourself and your family while new treatment centers are built.
■ We are building new Ebola treatment units as fast as we can. Until there is one close to you, keep sick people in their own area.
■ The sooner we can place most sick people in Ebola treatment units, Ebola care centers, or in their own area at home, the sooner the epidemic will slow down and stop.

Defeating Ebola demands that we make many temporary changes in our traditional practices.

■ Change is hard, but losing our loved ones to a disease that we can stop is even harder.
■ The spread of Ebola means we must change our traditional burial practices.
■ The sacrifices we make right now will help us stop the epidemic and return to our regular way of life sooner.

Every death from this disease is a loss to our entire nation.

■ Our hearts go out to every family that has lost someone to Ebola.

- Thousands of people from Liberia and around the world are working to stop the sickness from reaching anyone else.
- This time of hardship can bring us together and strengthen our nation for future generations.

▶ Health Messages (as of September 19, 2014)

Ebola is real, but you can survive it.

- Protect yourself by washing your hands often with soap and clean water or with chlorine water.
- Protect your family by knowing the signs and symptoms of Ebola.
- Protect your community by telling your community leader if someone you know is sick.

Everyone in Liberia plays a part in fighting Ebola.

- Do not touch the skin or body fluids of people who are sick with Ebola.
- Do not touch the skin or body fluids of people who have died from Ebola.
- Wash your hands with clean water and soap or chlorine water.

You can help stop Ebola.

- Know the signs and symptoms of Ebola.
- Tell your community leader if someone you know has symptoms.
- Call 4455 to report if someone has symptoms of Ebola.
- Do *not* run away or hide sick people. Only by telling someone about Ebola in your family can you get care as soon as it is available.

▶ Strategy

1. **Emphasize person-to-person communication methods. Establish a community-based network of trusted intermediaries.** *Extensive experience in outbreak, epidemic, and development communication shows that local leaders are pivotal in changing the course of events.* Provide county and district health officers, local leaders, traditional leaders, and respected community resources (e.g., teachers) with health and progress information they can share with others. Keep them informed of new developments. Capture, record, and share stories and images of local innovations and successes in fighting the disease. Where possible, arrange community meetings with national-level leaders to link government more closely with people.

2. **Use multiple channels and methods to layer consistent messages and information.** Identify key health protection messages. Use these messages in radio broadcasts, news releases, speeches, public service announcements (PSAs), posters, dramas, community education, text messaging, and social media. Use social media (e.g., text messaging) and local/traditional leaders to micro-target messages. Find the places where people gather most frequently and place information there.

3. **Share process information regularly to strengthen trust.** Use radio to share consistent information widely, quickly, and regularly. Provide regular (e.g., weekly) updates on actions taken to combat the disease. Incorporate local stories illustrating innovative ideas or successes. Report on actions of partners that have quantifiable measures. Use the Internet as a means of sharing progress information with international audiences.

4. **Increase self-efficacy through concise, consistent, actionable messages.** Identify key behaviors and reinforce them through multiple channels. Modify messages as surveillance indicates alterations may be needed. Ensure government and partner organizations are consistent in key messaging.

5. **Celebrate and share victories.** Create a series of stories from the Survivors Network and share these through multiple channels from worship services to text messages. Provide an easy method for community leaders and volunteer workers to share information and observations with county and national leaders. Report achievements widely.

▶ Methods

Risk Communication Frame

Acknowledge loss, change, hardship, and human impact of the epidemic. Emphasize anticipatory guidance, self-efficacy, and process information. Acknowledge what we know, what we do not know, and which steps are being taken to close the gap.

Internal Communication

Create a method of sharing data and information regularly and quickly across all government agencies at the national, county, and district levels. Utilize low-cost, visible means such as fact sheets posted in lunch rooms or stairwells.

Meetings

Conduct regular intragovernmental meetings among agencies affected by the epidemic to exchange updates on trends, share information, and harmonize messages. Continue regular meetings with partner groups to organize, track, and measure activities; identify trends; monitor results; and harmonize messages. As feasible, conduct regional, county, or district meetings with leadership and outreach personnel to provide for information gathering about local issues, identify message and other information needs, and achieve prompt awareness of issues or barriers. Share meeting summaries or reports in regular radio broadcasts or news briefings. Report progress against stated goals; acknowledge gaps or delays and explain steps being taken to remedy them.

Media Outreach

Provide regular, proactive media updates about actions completed by government addressing the epidemic. Develop and provide programming or public service announcements addressing the latest information needs as assessed by media tracking, call center input, and feedback from field personnel.

Advertising

Monitor information needs and adapt billboard, radio, and point-of-contact advertising (e.g., posters in gathering places) to reflect current message needs. Develop public service announcements and other relevant promotional materials from members of the Survivors Network, traditional leaders, government officials, healthcare workers, and others who serve as trusted messengers.

Social Media

Utilize text messaging to target or micro-target messaging to population groups. Use Facebook and other applicable social media (e.g., YouTube, Flickr, Twitter) to create more personalized communication at the institutional level, including photos from different parts of the country and stories from workers, survivors, and leaders. Consider naming an administrator from more than one agency or creating tabs for specific agencies.

Reports

Provide brief but regular reports to primary audiences documenting actions completed and progress realized since the last report. Include a section for cumulative information that may be shown in graphs, charts, or illustrations (e.g., growth in Ebola treatment unit [ETU] beds since the onset of the outbreak, survivors discharged).

Internet

Establish a website to aggregate Ebola action information for the benefit of not only citizens, but also international partners, reporters, and other governments.

▸ Tools

- **Key messages**
  - Shared broadly and regularly throughout government each time they are updated
  - Top-level messages
  - Health protection/promotion messages
- **Advertising collateral**
  - Point-of-service/contact placement
  - Billboards
  - Posters
  - Leaflets
- **Public service announcements**
  - Survivors Network members
  - Traditional leaders
  - Doctors or other healthcare workers
  - President or other government officials
  - DVDs for trainers and partners to play on computers
- **Fact sheet or flip book for leaders and influencers**
  - Data about actions and progress
  - Information updated as events/trends may indicate
- **Meeting plan**
  - Target dates for meetings with important groups (e.g., primary audiences)
  - Agenda template
  - Materials list to support sharing of consistent information
- **News releases**
  - Progress/action steps (e.g., shipments of materials from partners; actions such as training of large groups or launching of outreach efforts; opening of a new ETU or addition of beds)
  - Issues/challenges addressed
  - Feature stories on survivors or community action

- **Photos**
  - Community-level action
  - New Ebola treatment units
  - Survivors
  - Working "heroes" (e.g., healthcare workers, ambulance drivers, health officers)
- **Reports**
  - Charts or graphs showing growth in ETUs and ETU beds, Ebola care centers (ECCs), and so on
  - Charts of graphs showing persons trained in different functions (e.g., burial teams, teachers, general community health volunteers)
  - Number of calls to 4455
  - Time from call to 4455 to response
- **Speeches and presentations**
  - Scripts for brief speeches on topics related to the epidemic that can be delivered at association meetings
  - Slide set explaining Ebola 101
- **Social media**
  - Schedule for posting information
  - Templates for information sharing
- **Webpage content** (Elements listed here are possible, not required; decisions about content should be based on information gathered about messaging needs)

- Photo gallery showing people and communities in action
- Feature stories about workers, survivors, and communities
- Illustrated health protection/promotion information
- Graphs/charts showing progress over course of the epidemic (e.g., beds in ETUs, cases)
- Regular messages from senior officials

▶ Internal Tools

- Regular meetings with key stakeholder groups within participating ministries for coordination of activity toward milestones
- Graphs or charts showing progress posted regularly (e.g., weekly/biweekly) in gathering places (e.g., lunchrooms, stairwell landings)
- Q&A shared by supervisors or in handout when critical events occur that may generate public questions or news coverage
- Message from president or minister to employees recognizing their work, particularly at moments of significant progress (e.g., Ministry of Health and Social Welfare move to emergency operations center)

▶ Metrics

TABLE 15A-2 Increase Awareness of Factual Information About Ebola and How to Avoid Infection	
Measure 1	Uptake of accurate messages about Ebola
Rationale	Because much misinformation has spread during the first part of the epidemic, documented signs of use by primary and secondary audiences, news media, and others will indicate progress in public understanding.
Data source	Data are generated from Google, Bing, other applicable Internet search engines as well as analysis with available analytical tools.
Data frequency	Monthly analysis
Data validation	Comparison between data sources
Measure methodology	Number of mentions of key messages identified through an Internet search or other method that do not originate with government entities but rather from partners, media, or other sources

TABLE 15A-3 Increase Self-Efficacy Among the Population at All Levels and in All Locations

Measure 2	Evidence of adoption of top recommended health protection efforts
Rationale	Evidence suggests that information that allows people to evaluate risk and make rational choices for protecting themselves, their family, and their community has been effective in influencing behavior change.
Data source	Data are generated from field reports from health volunteers, teachers, county/district health officers, and others documenting both advances and issues/barriers.
Data frequency	Monthly analysis
Data validation	Comparison between data sources
Measure methodology	Number of reports documenting adoption of self-efficacy or behavior change measures (e.g., home hand washing stations, acceptance of altered burial practices)

TABLE 15A-4 Enhance the Ability of Trusted Intermediaries to Share Accurate Health Information

Measure 3	Documentation of national top-level or health protection messages shared locally
Rationale	Evidence indicates that participatory and community-based approaches promote faster adoption of public health behaviors that contribute to stopping outbreaks.
Data source	Data are generated from field reports from county/district health officials and questions from target population.
Data frequency	Monthly
Data validation	Comparison of data sources
Measure methodology	Number of questions that indicate lack of understanding of or alignment with messages; number of reports documenting implementation of information

TABLE 15A-5 Engage Key Internal and External Partners with Communication Objectives and Programs

Measure 4	Uptake and issuing of aligned and harmonized messages by partners outside Ministry of Health and Social Welfare and Ministry of Information and Cultural Affairs
Rationale	Participatory communication has been shown to strengthen public health responses by integrating the perspectives of local populations.
Data source	Monitoring of community radio, meeting notes, field reports
Data frequency	Monthly
Data validation	Comparison of data sources
Measure methodology	Number of messengers issuing harmonious messages; number of messages that are consistent with monthly top-priority issues

TABLE 15A-6   Build Health Literacy Regarding Ebola and Public Health Among Community Leaders and Populations

Measure 5	Adoption and integration of changes in practice and custom
Rationale	Education about disease transmission and prevention facts has not been shown to be sufficient to promote behavior change. Understanding context and observing role models have been shown to support behavior change.
Data source	Field reports of behavior change; questions coming to 4455 hotline
Data frequency	Monthly
Data validation	Comparison of data sources
Measure methodology	Nature of questions coming to 4455; number of districts reporting adoption of key health protection measures

TABLE 15A-7   Promote Alignment with Activities Undertaken by the Government of Liberia and Its International Partners

Measure 6	Uptake of Ministry of Health and Social Welfare and Ministry of Information and Cultural Affairs messages by media and international partners
Rationale	Public trust in leadership is foundational for controlling emergency situations.
Data source	News reports, Internet search, review of collateral materials
Data frequency	Monthly
Data validation	Comparison of data sources
Measure methodology	Number and frequency of government of Liberia–led messages appearing in news reports and partner bulletins

TABLE 15A-8   Engage Community Members to Provide Feedback on the Messages and Strategies

Measure 7	Establishment of dialogue mechanisms resulting in regular input from community and other audiences
Rationale	Dialogue with affected audiences promotes more effective response.
Data source	Reports of partners involved in social mobilization, focus group discussions, comparison of call center data with messages
Data frequency	Weekly
Data validation	Comparison of data sources to messages delivered and timing
Measure methodology	Degree and timing of community support/cooperation with interventions and field teams

Appendix 15B

Social Media System for Dengue Prevention in Sri Lanka

May O. Lwin, Santosh Vijaykumar, and **Karthikayen Jayasundar**

This case study describes the development, implementation, and evaluation of Mo-Buzz, a social media system designed to address the problem of dengue, a mosquito-borne disease that affects millions of people in tropical and subtropical regions.

▶ Problem Definition

Dengue presents a formidable global economic and disease burden, with approximately half of the world's population estimated to be at risk of infection.[1,2] Transmission of dengue has increased over the past decades, with outbreaks increasing in frequency, magnitude, and number of countries involved.[3,4] The impact of dengue has been measured in terms of both monetary value and public health metrics, such as disability-adjusted life-years (DALYs).[5,6]

The focus of our case study, Sri Lanka, reported nearly 40,000 dengue cases in 2014. This disease has been a national public health concern for at least the past few years, with more than 55% of such cases found to originate in the western province of Colombo.[7] Colombo is grappling with an exhausted dengue outbreak management system. The problem is characterized by manual mechanisms of conducting surveillance (such as identifying breeding sites), paper-based reporting of dengue cases to the hospitals, and coordinating with other epidemiologic staff to treat breeding sites.[8] Mapping of dengue hotspots during a dengue outbreak is done reactively as the outbreak unfolds, as opposed to using predictive models to come up with proactive mapping that can help both authorities and the public undertake preventive actions in advance. Furthermore, in a country that is boasting rapidly increasing rates of Internet and cellular service penetration, community education and outreach about dengue continues to be executed using outdated media channels such as pamphlets and brochures. These issues limit the capacity of public health institutions to persuade the public to practice healthy behaviors to protect themselves from dengue.

Sri Lanka has witnessed an unprecedented growth in the penetration of mobile services recently, and, at present, enjoys among the most affordable rates of mobile services across the world, with penetration rates higher than those in most developing countries.[9] However, dengue programs have yet to benefit from this technological trend, even as vast swathes of the Sri Lankan population become increasingly susceptible to this vector-borne disease.

▶ Needs Assessment

To assess the dengue-related informational and technological needs of the public health inspectors (PHIs) in Colombo, we conducted a series of in-depth interviews with them that would allow us to gain a nuanced, multifaceted perspective on the issues of greatest concern to them. The interviews were analyzed for themes such as problems faced by the PHIs that affect the efficacy of their work.

The PHIs mentioned several key challenges that they face, and corresponding solutions were developed by the research team:

- Filling in lengthy forms was an arduous task, taking long amounts of time and frequently resulting in error. The solution proposed by the team was to digitize the process, decreasing the time needed to complete reports and reducing the number of errors.
- Using a global positioning system (GPS) tag that was not accurate was also mentioned as a problem. The team proposed using a tablet-based GPS system with heightened sensitivity.

475

■ The manual transmission of photographic evidence was mentioned as being time consuming, and the photographs often got misplaced or damaged in the transfer process. The team suggested using a digital camera that can transmit the photo to an online database immediately.

■ The PHIs mentioned outdated educational materials as being a catalyst for poor public reception of their work. The team proposed a digital portal through which the PHIs can share information and updates on dengue as interactive multimedia and infographics with members of the public.

These challenges shaped the improvements that could be made to the present process undertaken by the PHIs. Hence, the team developed a mobile application, Mo-Buzz, to address the challenges faced by the PHIs, and the corresponding requirements to carry out their duties efficiently.[10] We developed two versions of Mo-Buzz: one for the PHIs and the other for the general public. In the following sections, we describe each of the systems and then present different types of evaluations conducted around this intervention.

▶ Mo-Buzz for PHIs

The Mo-Buzz system digitizes three main functions of PHIs and presents these capabilities on handheld mobile devices and web interfaces: (1) capturing, storing, and recording visual, textual, and geographical information from patient visits and house/area inspections; (2) staying updated on dengue spread patterns in the Colombo region on a real-time basis; and (3) providing dengue education to the public in an engaging format that will retain their attention and interest.

Digital Surveillance

The digital surveillance component allows the PHI to capture clients' information on a digitized Dengue Investigation Form (DIF) form that is easy to use, and includes alerts in case the PHI has missed filling out certain fields. Additionally, the DIFs are automatically linked to Google Maps, thus enhancing every individual DIF with accurate geographical coordinates that can be reviewed by the authorities. This component also allows the PHI to capture photographs of breeding sites, which are automatically geo-tagged, and share them with all relevant authorities in the chain of command to view and take necessary action (such as fogging and pest control).

Digitized Dengue Monitoring and Mapping

The Mo-Buzz system offers a live real-time dengue map that is updated as and when PHIs submit DIFs to the system. This component also automatically draws information from the geo-tagged breeding site reports and represents this information visually in a map format so that the Ministry of Health (MOH) and its respective PHIs can plan their prevention activities accordingly.

Digitized Dengue Education

To increase engagement between the PHIs and their clients, the Mo-Buzz system offers a tablet-based health education component. The first version of the health educational module includes digitized versions of the Colombo Municipal Council's (CMC) dengue education materials, which the PHI presents to the clients and complements with verbal explanations of dengue prevention concepts.

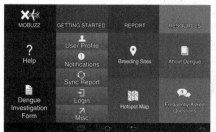
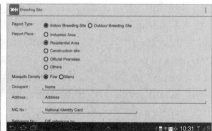
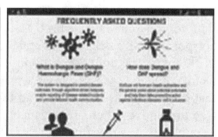

FIGURE 15B-1 Mo-Buzz for PHIs.

Courtesy of Mo-Buzz

Thus, it can be seen that Mo-Buzz was developed to address all the issues raised by the PHIs during the formative needs-assessment interviews that were conducted.

Process Evaluation of Mo-Buzz for the PHIs

In the latter part of 2015, a process evaluation was conducted to ascertain the effectiveness of Mo-Buzz through detailed interviews with 16 PHIs. The key findings from these interviews were as follows:

- Mo-Buzz significantly reduced the amount of time required to fill out forms, but the forms should allow for the PHI to enter the age of the patient in years and months, and not just in years.
- The GPS feature was extremely accurate, with minor glitches occurring infrequently.
- The predictive surveillance component of Mo-Buzz was useful for the PHIs, but they were unsure about releasing the information to the public, lest there be an outbreak of panic.
- The educational materials were useful, but could be improved in terms of interactivity, and could be further updated in terms of content.
- The built-in camera needs to be of better quality, and there needs to be flash, as most of the dengue breeding hotspots are in areas with poor lighting.

The interviews conducted are leading to further development of the application, and will result in an eventual update in capabilities.

Mo-Buzz for the General Public

The general public version of Mo-Buzz integrated three components: predictive surveillance, civic engagement, and health communication.

Predictive Surveillance

The predictive surveillance component helps to predict dengue outbreaks using an algorithm and computer simulation that is based on historic and current, dengue-related data. The predictions are made available to public health authorities and the general public in the form of hotspot geographical information system (GIS)–based maps, on their Android smartphones and/or tablet devices. The purpose is to forewarn these stakeholders of dengue outbreaks so as to facilitate quicker and more efficient resource planning among public health authorities, and to persuade the general public to practice personal protective behaviors that might reduce their risk.

Civic Engagement

The civic engagement component is built on the concept of crowd sourcing. Traditionally, communication about public health issues has been top-down, from health authorities to the general public. Disease surveillance during a public health outbreak has been the sole preserve of epidemiologic departments. We endeavored to create a two-way communication platform that could help public health departments obtain real-time intelligence about disease spread and risk factors from the general public in a manner that could facilitate rapid response with minimal delay. Mo-Buzz allows the general public to report dengue symptoms and post pictures of potential dengue mosquito breeding sites. Such reports and postings are automatically geo-tagged and sent to the health authorities with a click of a button, thereby stimulating the first stage of response by health authorities.

Health Communication

The health communication component comprises two sub-modules. The static module consists of educational materials about dengue pertaining to dengue transmission, symptoms, prevention, and treatment. The dynamic module refers to geographically targeted alerts (based on predictions in the hotspot maps) and messaging that is customized to the kind of report sent by the user. A more detailed elucidation of the rationale and description of the three components of Mo-Buzz is available elsewhere.[11]

Receptivity Assessment

We conducted formative research among the general public in Colombo, Sri Lanka, to assess the potential receptivity to such a system and seek answers to two overarching questions:

- RQ1: What is the level of potential acceptance of Mo-Buzz among the general population in Colombo, Sri Lanka?
- RQ2: In the context of Mo-Buzz, what are the demographic differences in dengue-related threat and response perceptions among the general population in Colombo?[11]

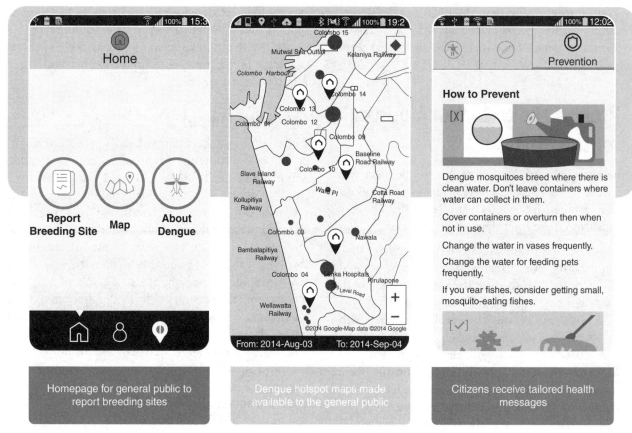

FIGURE 15B-2 Mo-Buzz for the general public.

Courtesy of Mo-Buzz

Theoretical Approach

The needs assessment was guided by protection motivation theory (PMT), which suggests that individuals' intention to perform a behavior is intrinsically driven by the need to protect themselves from the health threat under consideration.[12] PMT's fundamental argument supports the facilitation of behavioral change by appealing to an individual's fear through the magnitude of harm depicted, the probability of the event's occurrence, and the efficacy of the protective response.[13] The underlying principles of PMT are situated appropriately within the three components of Mo-Buzz, which highlight the existing and oncoming threat of dengue and provide a protective response to deal with this threat using the civic engagement and health education components.

Methodology

We conducted a cross-sectional survey among the target population for our application—in other words, individuals with access to smartphones and Internet connectivity. The survey examined perceived severity, perceived susceptibility, perceived response efficacy, perceived self-efficacy and intention-to-use among 513 individuals. We adopted a convenience sampling approach by utilizing the auspices of our collaborators to approach those sites where we were most likely to find substantial numbers of smartphone users. Our study sites included the official premises of Sri Lanka's national television channel, the official headquarters of a national bank and a national telecommunications provider, the telecommunications provider's outlets in two malls in the city, and one higher education institution.

Findings

The overall receptivity to the system was high, with a score of more than 4.00 on a 5-point scale. Participants belonging to younger, better-educated, and higher-income groups reported significantly better perceptions of the efficaciousness of the system, were confident in their ability to use the system, and planned to use it in the future. PMT variables contributed significantly to regression models predicting intention-to-use. We concluded that a social media–based system for dengue prevention will be positively received among Colombo residents and a targeted, strategic health communication effort to raise dengue-related threat perceptions will be needed to encourage greater adoption and use of the system.

▶ Baseline Evaluation

The receptivity assessment revealed that the application, if made available, would be positively accepted by the general public. Encouraged by these findings, we soft-launched the application in 2015 and conducted a baseline evaluation surrounding this event.[14] The purpose of this evaluation was to understand the contextual considerations that influence people's participation in such a system and the ways in which we could use this understanding of the underlying behavioral dynamics to shape future health intervention design. The baseline study was driven by three questions:

- RQ1: How strong is the intention to use Mo-Buzz at baseline and how does it differ by demographic variables (gender, age, education, and income)?
- RQ2: To what extent do perceptions related to individual, organizational, and social factors surrounding the use of Mo-Buzz differ by demographic variables?
- RQ3: What are the main individual, organizational, and social factors that influence intention to use Mo-Buzz and what is the extent of their influence?

Theoretical Approach

We investigated Mo-Buzz through the theoretical lens of behavioral change related to technology adoption. The classical technology acceptance model (TAM) offered perceived usefulness (PU) and perceived ease-of-use (PEOU) as determinants of perceived intention-to-use (PI) for the technology.[15] Scientific evidence was synthesized on TAM and proposed that individual differences, system characteristics, social influence, and facilitating conditions influence PU and PEOU.[16] When applied to Mo-Buzz, the modified TAM enables the examination of the extent to which potential users in a city with high mobile phone penetration, such as Colombo, would find Mo-Buzz useful and easy-to-use.[17]

At the individual level, we drew from PMT to assess whether perceived severity of and susceptibility to dengue in the users' city affected perceived usefulness.[18] In terms of facilitating conditions, we examined whether users' beliefs about the ability of the CMC to respond effectively (perceived organizational efficacy) to breeding site reports, and their trust in the CMC (institutional trust), shaped attitudes toward the technology. From a social influence standpoint, we examined whether cultural dimensions (individualism versus collectivism) interact with PU to influence behavioral intention. According to Hofstede, these dimensions allow for the assessment of how personal needs and goals are prioritized against those of the group/clan/organization.[19] In this case, users would be more inclined to report breeding sites and share health educational content if they believed doing so would protect the members of their social network and communities from dengue.

Methodology

We assessed responses to questions via in-person pen-and-paper surveys of mobile phone users in Colombo. Using a snowball sampling approach, respondents were recruited through mass emails and word-of-mouth by students and staff from University of Colombo, People's Bank, Mobitel, and Rupavahini Corporation. After small groups of 10 to 15 participants were invited to a meeting room in their respective premises, research staff briefed them on the study's purpose and sought informed consent. The three functionalities of Mo-Buzz were subsequently illustrated and explained using demonstrations with mobile devices. Research staff allowed those participants with further questions or doubts to briefly use the application on one of three mobile devices (two tablets, one mobile phone) and experience it for themselves. Following this introduction to the application, participants were requested to respond to a 30-minute survey questionnaire.

Findings

Descriptive analysis revealed high perceived ease-of-use, perceived usefulness, and intention-to-use among participants. Analysis of variance (ANOVA) indicated that participants in the 31–40 age group reported the highest PEOU, whereas the oldest group reported high perceived institutional efficacy and collectivistic tendencies. Significant differences ($p < 0.05$ level) were also found by education and income. Regression analysis demonstrated that PU, behavioral control, institutional efficacy, and collectivism were significant predictors of PI. We concluded that despite high overall PI, future adoption and use of Mo-Buzz will be shaped by a complex mix of factors at different levels of the public health ecology.

▶ Conclusion

This case study presented a novel intervention where social media were used not only for disseminating persuasive health messages but also for strengthening the health services infrastructure and creating real-time linkages between the general public and health authorities. The initial acceptance of the proposed system was positive. Future adoption and sustained use, however, will be driven by a complex set of variables at different levels of the social ecosystem. Consistent with previous research, we foresee that participation in passive (viewing hotspot maps) and active (reporting dengue hotspot) activities might be driven by different kinds of variables.[20]

To boost participation in the Mo-Buzz system, we are now in the process of launching a communication campaign to create greater awareness and uptake of the application. Future work will focus on expanding the capabilities of Mo-Buzz to address other health problems in Sri Lanka and around the region, and integrating its capabilities with the larger e-health information architecture in the region. Mobile and social media interventions, such as Mo-Buzz, are poised to play a greater role in shaping risk perceptions and managing seasonal and sporadic outbreaks of infectious diseases in Asia and around the world.

References

1. Brady OJ, Gething PW, Bhatt S, et al. Refining the global spatial limits of dengue virus transmission by evidence-based consensus. *PLoS Negl Trop Dis.* 2012;6(8):e1760.
2. Bhatt S, Gething PW, Brady OJ, et al. The global distribution and burden of dengue. *Nature.* 2012;496(7446):504-507.
3. Gubler DJ. Dengue and dengue hemorrhagic fever. *Clin Microbiol Rev.* 1998;11(3):480-496.
4. World Health Organization (WHO). *Dengue: Guidelines for Diagnosis, Treatment, Prevention and Control* (160). Geneva, Switzerland: Special Programme for Research and Training in Tropical Diseases, Department of Control of Neglected Tropical Diseases, WHO; 2009.
5. Murray CJ. Quantifying the burden of disease: the technical basis for disability-adjusted life years. *Bull WHO.* 1994;72(3):429.
6. Murray CJ, Vos T, Lozano R, et al. Disability-adjusted life years (DALYs) for 291 diseases and injuries in 21 regions, 1990–2010: a systematic analysis for the Global Burden of Disease Study 2010. *Lancet.* 2013;380(9859):2197-2223.
7. Ministry of Defense. Disease surveillance: trends. 2015. http://www.epid.gov.lk/web/index.php?option=com_casesanddeaths&Itemid=448&lang=en#. Accessed May 6, 2015.
8. Hettiarachchi K, Jeewandara S, Munasinghe A, Perera S. More dengue victims: staff shortage, ignorance of people, poor garbage management to blame. *Sunday Times (Sri Lanka).* June 9, 2013.
9. International Telecommunications Union. ITU statistical market overview: Sri Lanka. 2013. http://www.itu.int/net/newsroom/GSR/2012/reports/stats_sri_lanka.aspx. Accessed May 10, 2013.
10. Lwin MO, Santosh V, Fernando ON, et al. A 21st century approach to tackling dengue: crowdsourced surveillance, predictive mapping & tailored communication. *Acta Tropica.* 2013;130:100-107.
11. Lwin MO. Vijaykumar S, Foo S, et al. Social media-based civic engagement solutions for dengue prevention in Sri Lanka: results of receptivity assessment. *Health Educ Res.* 2015:cyv065.
12. Rogers R W. A protection motivation theory of fear appeals and attitude change. *J Psychol.* 1975;91(1):93-114.
13. Milne S, Orbell S, Sheeran P. Combining motivational and volitional interventions to promote exercise participation: protection motivation theory and implementation intentions. *Br J Health Psychol.* 2002;7(2):163-184.
14. Lwin MO, Vijaykumar S, Lim G, Fernando ON, Rathnayake VS, Foo S. Baseline evaluation of a participatory mobile health intervention for dengue prevention in Sri Lanka. *Health Educ Behav.* 2015. doi: 10.1177/1090198115604623.
15. Davis FD. Perceived usefulness, perceived ease of use, and user acceptance of information technology. *MIS Qtly.* 1989;13:319-340.
16. Venkatesh V, Bala H. Technology acceptance model 3 and a research agenda on interventions. *Decision Sci.* 2008;39:273-315.
17. International Telecommunications Union. ITU statistical market overview: Sri Lanka. 2015. http://www.itu.int/net/newsroom/GSR/2012/reports/stats_sri_lanka.aspx. Accessed January 4, 2017.
18. Rogers RW, Prentice-Dunn S. Protection motivation theory. In: Gochman DS, ed. *Handbook of Behavioral Research: Personal and Social Determinants.* New York, NY: Plenum; 1997:113-132.
19. Hofstede G. Cultural dimensions in management and planning. *Asia Pac J Manage.* 1984;1:81-99.
20. Vijaykumar S, Wray RJ, Buskirk T, et al. Youth, new media, and HIV/AIDS: determinants of participation in an online health social movement. *Cyberpsychol Behav Soc Network.* 2014;17(7):488-495. doi: 10.1089/cyber.2013.0124.

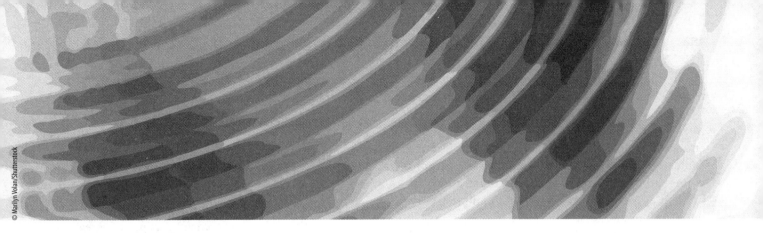

CHAPTER 16

Health Communication in Resource-Poor Countries

Carmen Cronin and **Suruchi Sood**

LEARNING OBJECTIVES

By the end of this chapter, the reader will be able to:

- Explain the historical trajectory of health communication in low-income countries.
- Identify interpersonal, community-led, and mediated communication approaches utilized in public health interventions.
- Describe the role of interactive communication technologies in international health communication.
- Understand the value of using multiple communication approaches to improve individual and societal health practices.
- Understand how communication can be used as both a means and an end to address public health issues.

▶ Introduction

Designing, implementing, and assessing the effectiveness of health communication programs in developing country settings can be challenging, especially given that these contexts are often characterized by a paucity of resources (human, technical, monetary, and infrastructural) and a multitude of basic human survival needs. This point is emphasized by the 10/90 gap popularized by the Global Forum for Health Research,[1] which indicates that less than 10% of the world's resources for health research are applied to the health problems of low- and middle-income countries, where more than 90% of the world's preventable deaths occur. This chapter highlights the extent to which health research related to the needs of low- and middle-income countries is grossly under-resourced.

The resource gap is also manifested as a lack of applied research and interventions related to international health communication. For example, a recent review of mass-media campaigns to change health behaviors noted that, with the exception of campaigns on birth rate reduction and child survival, much of the evidence on the effectiveness of such campaigns was generated from high-income countries, where most campaigns are implemented and where there is substantially greater research capacity.[2] Data and experience from such campaigns may not fit seamlessly into health communication interventions in resource-poor countries.

In this chapter, first we see how international health communication is related to the Millennium Development Goals and the global burden of disease. Next, we explain the intersection of communication and international health, situating it within the larger context of communication for development and providing information on health communication theory and applied international health communication interventions and research.

The third section of this chapter examines various communication approaches and provides examples of specific applications in low-resource countries. The final section discusses the utility of using multiple approaches (interpersonal, community-led, and mediated) to address public health issues across different levels of the social ecological model.

▸ Overview of International Health Communication

The Millennium Development Goals

In 2000, 189 United Nations member states adopted the Millennium Declaration, which outlined eight internationally agreed-upon Millennium Development Goals (MDGs) to tackle extreme poverty (**TABLE 16-1**).[3]

As a framework, the MDGs address the multidimensionality of poverty by focusing on income, hunger, disease, lack of adequate shelter, and exclusion. In so doing, they seek to create opportunities for prosperity, health, safety, and empowerment. The MDGs then go a step further by attempting to create environments of change through the promotion of gender equity, access to education, and environmental sustainability.

The Global Burden of Disease

As the World Health Organization (WHO) points out, the MDGs and health are inextricably linked.[3] Good health is fundamental to the achievement of the MDGs, and the MDGs themselves seek to improve

health around the world. Much progress has been made in the last 15 years[4]:

- Poverty rates have been halved.
- Deaths from malaria and tuberculosis have been significantly reduced.
- More than 2.3 billion people now have access to safe water sources.
- Primary school enrollment disparities by gender are narrowing, and women are playing an increasingly active role in politics.
- The creation of nationally owned development strategies, programs, and policies tailored to the specific needs of each country has been a critical factor in achieving these goals and one aided in large part by unprecedented levels of international collaboration.

Evidence of progress has not been evenly distributed around the world, and in some cases, progress has slowed.[4] While substantial gains have been made in reducing child undernutrition, present efforts in this area are flagging. Chronic undernutrition continues to affect one in four children younger than age 5 years. Child mortality has dropped by approximately 50%, a remarkable accomplishment, and maternal mortality has declined by approximately 45%—yet preventable communicable diseases remain the main causes of both child and maternal mortality. Antiretroviral therapy for human immunodeficiency virus (HIV)-infected individuals is proving to be successful, but coverage needs to be expanded to reach even more infected individuals. Vast improvements in sanitation have been made, but 1 billion individuals continue to practice open defecation. Finally, more efforts are needed to curb major threats to environmental sustainability.

The MDGs demonstrate that global collaboration is possible and can be used for poverty eradication. It is true that some goals had not been met by the 2015 time frame and that some improvements, despite global efforts, have been undermined by natural disasters, climate, food and economic crises, and political instability. Nevertheless, the MDGs have created a platform for future collaboration and action to be planned and implemented.

History of Health Communication in Resource-Poor Countries

The academic discipline of communication first made an appearance within universities in the United States after World War II and has undergone exponential growth since then. Paradigmatic shifts have been seen in the literature on communication, with it most recently being conceptualized as a tool for motivating individual and social change. Rimon[5] characterized international health communication as passing

---

TABLE 16-1 Millennium Development Goals

1. Eradicate extreme poverty and hunger
2. Achieve universal primary education
3. Promote gender equality and empower women
4. Improve maternal health
5. Reduce child mortality
6. Combat HIV/AIDS, malaria, and other diseases
7. Ensure environmental sustainability
8. Develop a global partnership for development

Millennium Development Goals. World Health Organization. http://www.who.int/topics/millennium_development_goals/about/en/ (n.d.). Accessed March 27, 2015.

through four distinct eras (**FIGURE 16-1**),[5-7] evolving over time from a medical- and supply-oriented model to one that is integrative and focuses on individuals and communities as producers of their own health.

The field of development health communication has continued to evolve since Rimon first outlined these eras. In general, it has moved from a top-down strategic behavior-change model to a horizontal, participatory convergent era based on facilitating the creation of an enabling environmental design that lays the foundation for and sustains social change.

In the international health arena, "developing country" is a value-laden term, with those opposed to this terminology arguing that it assumes all countries aspire for Western-style growth and development. Even while using the terms "developed" and "developing" in its classification of countries and geographical regions, the United Nations' Statistics Division clarifies this usage: "The designations 'developed' and 'developing' are intended for statistical convenience and do not necessarily express a judgment about the stage reached by a particular country or area in the development process."[8]

The Intersection of Communication and International Health

Health Communication for Development

The overarching field of health communication for development consists of four main pillars: health, governance, sustainability, and interactive communication technologies. Health is a crucial aspect of wider development strategies, and many development issues promoting public health focus on the role of communication to bring about long-term, sustainable change. In the current era, communication strategies are more frequently being incorporated into health development projects to reach community members, key influencers, decision makers, public health personnel, and healthcare providers. Health communication seeks to create environments supportive of positive health behaviors by fostering discussion and debate at various levels of society, implementing public policies that promote positive social norms and behaviors, and providing broader access to health information, which in turn enables individuals to make informed decisions about their health. The creation of such supportive environments can help set the stage for sustained improvement in health-related practices. It is no surprise, then, that health communication has become a vital tool in the achievement of the MDGs.[9]

Theoretical Underpinnings of International Health Communication

Communication is an inherent component of how people go about their daily lives. It shapes people's relationships; informs their attitudes, beliefs, and perceptions about the world around them; and ultimately

---

Clinic Era

The Clinic Era was marked by the mantra "Build it and they will come," and was based on the medical model that if services existed, then people would find their way to them (Rogers, 1973).

Field Era

The Field Era emphasized the use of outreach workers, community-based distribution, and information, education, and communication (IEC) products (Rogers, 1973).

Social Marketing Era

The Social Marketing Era borrowed from commercial marketing strategies of brand promotion to generate demand and improvement in supply chain mechanics to improve access to services. This era was characterized by the idea that consumers will buy products they want at subsidized prices (Rimon, 2001).

Strategic Behavior Change Communication Era

The Strategic Behavior Change Communication Era uses behavior change models and theories as the foundation for interventions and emphasizes the need to influence social norms and policy environments to facilitate both individual and social change (Figueroa, Kincaid, Rani, Lewis, 2002).

FIGURE 16-1 The Four Eras of Health Communication

Sources: Rogers EM. *Communication Strategies for Family Planning*. New York: The Free Press; 1973; Rimon JG. *Behavior Change Communication in Public Health*. In Beyond Dialogue: Moving Toward Convergence. Presented at the United Nations Roundtable on Development Communication: Managua, Nicaragua; 2001.; Figueroa ME, Kincaid DL, Rani M, Lewis G. *Communication for social change: An integrated model for measuring the process and its outcomes*. (Communication for Social Change Working Paper Series No. 1). 2002. Baltimore, MD: Rockefeller and Johns Hopkins University, Center for Communication Programs.

plays a role in people's behaviors and social norms. As Piotrow, Kincaid, Rimon, and Rinehart state: "[T]he issue is no longer whether health communication can influence behavior. Now the issue is how to sharpen our understanding of communication to do a better job."[10]

Beyond working with the social ecological model (see the work of Uri Bronfenbrenner[11] and previously mentioned theorists), Kincaid, Delate, Storey, and Figueroa argue that health communication programs take on a dialogic function by promoting a conversation between researchers/interventionists and community members.[12] From an evaluation perspective, this conceptualization is especially useful. Formative research and pre-testing can be envisioned as an opportunity to converse with community members about issues of importance, as well as to address programmatic and messaging components of future interventions. Process evaluation maintains this dialogue by gauging the proportion of the target population being reached and by determining who is being reached (and who is not). Finally, impact evaluation measures the proportion of the target population that adopts the promoted health behaviors, as well as informs the improvement of future iterations of the program.

This dialogic function of health communication programs illustrates how a set of communication activities can bring about improvements in health outcomes. But it is also worth considering how communication itself can be a desired outcome. Communicative action, as defined by Jürgen Habermas,[135] occurs when private citizens work together to reach a common understanding or consensus about a situation through deliberative process, reasoned arguments, and cooperation. In this sense, communicative action stands in contrast to strategic or instrumental action, which is goal-oriented and self-serving. Public participation, information sharing, and dialogue are pillars of communicative action that allow new ideas and innovations to be integrated into a society's way of life and create opportunities for social change.[14] These forms of discourse can take place in various public spheres—for example, the interpersonal, small-group, community, and policy levels. Public participation, information sharing, and dialogue exemplify this idea that communicating, in and of itself, can signal change and is not limited to being understood solely as a conduit for individual and social change. Moreover, the dialogic roots of communicative action inherently foment community connectedness, which can be linked to increased social capital such as strengthened social networks.[14]

▶ Health Communication Campaigns in Developing Countries

While the effectiveness of health communication campaigns is contested, there is ample literature supporting the necessary role that sustained health promotion and social marketing programs play in promoting large-scale change in health-related behaviors. In a systematic review of health communication campaigns in developing countries, Sood, Shefner-Rogers, and Skinner found that few campaigns referred to theoretical or conceptual frameworks to guide campaign development and implementation.[15] The authors lamented the slow pace at which the field of health communication is moving when it comes to developing and embracing more holistic theories of health behavior and social change that recognize the degree to which individuals are embedded within dynamic social systems.[16]

On a more positive note, Sood, Shefner-Rogers, and Skinner found that the campaigns included in their review often leveraged multiple strategic approaches, combining mass-media messages with community mobilization, interpersonal approaches, and interactive and mobile technologies.[15] In fact, these authors argue that the traditional conceptualization of campaigns as large-scale, mass-media efforts should be reexamined, as data from the review indicate a shift toward small-scale community-based communication efforts as the norm in developing countries. These findings underscore the need for a more evidence-based, strategic approach to designing, implementing, and evaluating health communication campaigns so as to advance the field of health communication and meaningfully contribute to global health efforts.

Communication Approaches

It is important to understand the different kinds of communication approaches that practitioners have at their disposal to improve health outcomes. This section provides a brief overview of the various communication approaches, as well as examples of how each communication approach has been applied in a real-world setting.

Interpersonal Communication Approaches

Interpersonal communication involves more than the simple transmission of information and ideas between two or more individuals. According to Braithwaite and Baxter, interpersonal communication is how individuals "negotiate meaning, identity, and relationships through person-to-person communication."[17] Communication is invariably laden with verbal and nonverbal messages, cues, signs, and symbols such as body language, mannerisms, tone of voice, and eye contact, all of which convey meaning and are subject to interpretation. Social and cultural traditions, conventions, and norms influence and shape the types of interactions individuals have, as well as dictate who interacts with whom. For example, within certain religiously conservative Muslim populations, women are prohibited from being alone with a male who is not a family member, including a male doctor. Therefore, many religiously conservative Muslim women will seek care only from female health providers. Similarly, religiously conservative Muslim men may be reluctant to receive care from a female physician.[18]

Gender, age, social status, sexual orientation, and power can also alter the dynamics of interactions. In some cultures, patients do not think they can ask providers questions, as this practice can be misconstrued as questioning the provider's authority. This is especially true if the patient comes from a lower class/caste or if the patient does not speak the provider's language natively, as is often the case with immigrant, refugee, and migratory populations. Individuals who identify as LGBTQ (lesbian/gay/bisexual/transgender/questioning) may be less likely to seek care for fear of being judged, stigmatized, or outright refused care.

More often than not, interactions are influenced by a combination of factors. Gender and power, for instance, intersect when it comes to condom use: In patriarchal societies, women may feel unable to demand that condoms be used during sex, even if they wish to protect themselves, because men are seen as the decision makers and women are supposed to be submissive.

Four major types of dyadic interactions exist: patient–provider, spousal/partner, parent–child, and peer education. Patient–provider interactions comprise the face-to-face communication that occurs between healthcare providers (e.g., doctors, nurses, midwives, skilled birth attendants, community health workers) and patients. Good patient–provider communication is fundamental to high-quality health care. Health providers must treat patients with respect and provide patients with sufficient information in an understandable manner so that they may make informed decisions about their health.[19]

Spousal or partner communication is especially critical in the context of family planning and reproductive health, as communicating allows partners to discuss beliefs, attitudes, opinions, expectations, aspirations, and even information about marriage, fertility, and contraceptive use. The *Let's Talk* program implemented in Nepal described later in this section offers an example of such communication.

Parent–child communication is important because children often model their own actions after the actions of their parents. Children who feel they are heard, understood, and respected by their parents are more likely to do the same with others and their future children. Parents who use violence to discipline their children instead of communicating their discontent are more likely to desensitize their children toward violence, so that those children become more likely to use violence in the future. For an overview of the effectiveness of communication for development to address violence against children, see **BOX 16-1**.[20]

BOX 16-1   Using Social and Behavior Change Approaches to Address Violence Against Children

In 2012, the Communication for Development (C4D) and Child Protection sections at UNICEF Headquarters in New York commissioned a global systematic review to determine the effectiveness of social and behavior change approaches to address violence against children (VaC). The global systematic review included 302 manuscripts (peer-reviewed and gray literature) retrieved from six search engines and published between 2000 and 2013. The findings revealed that few interventions are guided by conceptual models, use SMART (Specific, Measurable, Attainable, Relevant, Time-based) or SPICED* (Subjective, Participatory, Interpreted, Cross-checked, Empowering, Diverse) and disaggregated criteria to write program and communication objectives, segment audiences, or leverage multiple channels to reach intended audiences. Furthermore, there is a paucity of robust and rigorous evaluation data, especially from low- and middle-income countries. Finally, there is a serious underutilization of participatory research methods for any and all types of evaluation.

The number of manuscripts related to the use of C4D approaches to address VaC has steadily increased each year since 2000. Of the 302 manuscripts that were coded, 44% discussed an intervention implemented in a developing country, which speaks to the geographic robustness of this review. Roughly half of the interventions reviewed did not explicitly reference a conceptual model to underpin the interventions. In those that did, the authors typically cited individual or cognitive conceptual models, and a majority of the reports focused on the

(continues)

BOX 16-1   Using Social and Behavior Change Approaches to Address Violence Against Children   *(continued)*

individual level of change. Few program objectives utilized SMART or SPICED criteria to write program objectives or focused on positive changes that individuals could undertake to promote behavior and social change. All of the C4D objectives were written in "cognitive" terms, with no reference to addressing affective and behavioral domains. Most interventions did not report segmenting audiences into primary, secondary, or tertiary groups. Interventions commonly used more than one approach to meet stated objectives, with interpersonal communication and training being the dominant approaches. However, nearly two-thirds of interventions did not select multiple channels to meet the needs of their diverse and segmented audiences. New technologies and mobile forms of communication were used to a lesser degree, although cross-tabulations with the year of publication showed a growing reliance on new technologies.

The paucity of robust and rigorous monitoring and evaluation underscores the need to invest more heavily in research, especially in low- and middle-income countries. Few manuscripts included in this review described formative research or process evaluations, whereas significantly more manuscripts reported on impact evaluations. Qualitative observational data were a commonly utilized evaluation methodology. Unfortunately, relying solely on this type of data makes a weak case for C4D attribution to program outcomes. Overall, the authors of this review found a serious underutilization of participatory research methods for any and all types of evaluations.

In summary, it is essential to expand outcome evaluation studies so as to enhance our understanding of global best practices, which in turn need to be contextualized based on what works at a local level to address VaC. Future research and practice should consider the following overall recommendations:

1. Specifically address children within other forms of violence
2. Explore linkages among different forms of VaC
3. Examine VaC along a spectrum
4. Contextualize violence both as a cause and as an outcome
5. Broaden conceptualizations of C4D approaches that involve any form of communication/communicative action
6. Clarify the direct and indirect linkages between stated program outcomes and communication objectives and messages
7. Reconfigure program and communication objectives of VaC interventions
8. Move beyond individually focused knowledge, attitudes, and practices by addressing social, emotional, and behavioral competencies
9. Embrace the social ecological model for behavior and social change
10. Move beyond a place-based approach to a norms-based approach to incorporate innovative communication channels and tackle the culture of violence
11. Start early and continue into adulthood
12. Segment audiences by gender and address gender-specific needs and differences
13. Scale up promising interventions
14. Position VaC as a "global" issue through qualitative and quantitative measurement
15. Enhance investment in research

*"SPICED" criteria from Roche, CJR. *Impact Assessment for Development Agencies: Learning to Value Change*. 1999, Great Britain, Oxfam. http://policy-practice.oxfam.org.uk/publications /impact-assessment-for-development-agencies-learning-to-value-change-122808

Sood S, Cronin C. *C4D Approaches to Address Violence Against Children: A Systematic Review*. New York: UNICEF; 2015.

Peer education is an approach in which lay individuals are trained with specific health information and then go out in their communities to share that information with others who have similar backgrounds or life experiences. As an example of a peer education component (described later in this section), the *For a Happy Life* program in Albania seeks to increase the use of modern contraceptive methods.

Beyond these four dyads, one must not forget that individuals often turn to family, friends, teachers, community leaders, and other trusted individuals for information or support especially when confronted with difficult situations such as a cancer diagnosis or a positive HIV test. Not only is it important to understand to whom individuals talk, but also what they talk to them about. Understanding social networks provides insight into who the key influencers are in a given community and who is best positioned to disseminate health messages to the intended audience. More open communication can, in turn, serve to strengthen and expand social networks. This is especially true for taboo topics: Breaking the silence and initiating conversations is a critical first step toward destigmatizing and addressing taboo issues.

Initiatives leveraging interpersonal communication must carefully consider both the words used to convey health promotion messages and the words used to address program participants. Similarly, programs must strive to establish trust and two-way communication. Programs must also consider ways in which they can empower individuals to voice their needs and demands. It is for these reasons that interpersonal communication is an essential component of behavior and social change programs.

Let's Talk: Improving Sexual Health Communication Between Women and Men in Nepal.

In Nepal, health information has traditionally been passed along among women through kinship channels or close female friends.[21] Men and women in Nepal do not discuss sexual health, not even with their own spouse. With the onset of rapid urbanization, however, more and more women are being isolated from their families and consequently are turning to close female friends and media sources for knowledge and advice on sexual health.

In 2008, the *Let's Talk* intervention was designed to increase communication about sexual health between women, within mother-in-law and daughter-in-law relationships, and with men (e.g., male friends, brothers, intimate partners/spouses) and to change norms around communication.[21] In addition, the intervention sought to dispel myths and misconceptions about HIV and sexually transmitted infections (STIs) through an educational component. The intervention was pilot-tested between February and May 2008 with a sample of urban Nepali women.

The information-motivation-behavioral skills (IMB) model of HIV risk prevention guided the development of the *Let's Talk* intervention.[22] The IMB model provides a conceptual framework to understand complex health behaviors. It pays special attention to how information, motivation, and behavioral disease prevention skills can predict preventive behaviors such as condom use. The authors chose this model for the intervention specifically because of the intervention's objectives of increasing knowledge, promoting communication, and teaching communication skills so that Nepali women could have more control of their sexual health. Based on formative research, the intervention consisted of three 2-hour group sessions to allow for open discussion about sexual communication, HIV and STI prevention information, proper condom use, general discussion, and role-playing activities.[23] These sessions were held one week apart—giving participants enough time to talk with other women without forgetting the information learned.

The findings revealed that the participants started having more open conversations with other women and men about sex. Participants reported feeling less shame about sex and sexuality and greater comfort discussing sex after the intervention.[21] The findings of the pilot study are promising and demonstrate that *Let's Talk* can potentially fill a gap in sexual health education in Nepal. A formal implementation of the intervention and a robust evaluation are warranted.

For a Happy Life: Promoting Family Planning in Albania.

Albania has the lowest rate of modern contraceptive method (MCM) use in Europe. According to the 2008 Demographic and Health Survey (DHS), only 11% of Albanians use MCM. The dominant family planning method is withdrawal (58%),[24] and use rates for male condoms (4%), female sterilization (3%), and the pill (2%) are all very low. The low use of MCM may be explained in part by the low contraceptive knowledge among both males and females of reproductive age. A survey administered in 2005 to individuals of reproductive age in three prefectures revealed that 40% of respondents had never heard of injectable contraception and 60% had never heard of an intrauterine device.[25]

To this end, Communication for Change (C-Change) funded by U.S. Agency for International Development (USAID) developed a national mass-media campaign and a peer education program with the goal of creating an enabling environment for the discussion, selection, and use of MCM among sexually active young adults, while also reducing the reliance on traditional methods. The objectives of the interventions were threefold: (1) to increase awareness of MCM, (2) to improve attitudes toward MCM, and (3) to increase uptake and use among young adults attending universities in Tirana, Vlorë, and Elbasan.[25]

In addition to a national mass-media campaign entitled *For a Happy Life*, an intensive peer education program was established with university students, both male and female. The peer education program trained university students living in the dormitories on family planning, interpersonal communication, and negotiating skills. The peer educators were tasked with starting and guiding discussions on MCM and serving as resources for young men and women about MCM. In total, the program trained 174 peer educators. Within the first three months of the program, 4148 students in Tirana and 573 students in Vlorë received information from or communicated with a peer educator.[25]

An evaluation of the program found that exposure to the peer education program significantly affected use of MCM. Those students who were exposed to the peer education program were 1.9 times more likely to report current use of an MCM as compared to those who were not exposed the program. Those exposed to the peer education program were 2.3 times more likely to identify three or more forms of MCM. Those exposed to both the national campaign and the peer education program were 8 times more likely to identify multiple forms of MCM.[25]

Community-Level Approaches

Community-level approaches have played a key role in international health development since the introduction of organized interventions beginning in the 1950s and 1960s. Major international meetings that have influenced the public health agenda in recent decades include those known as Alma Ata, the Ottawa Chapter for Health Promotion, and the Jakarta Declaration. At all of these meetings, the use of community-led communication approaches for improving health was strongly recommended. In turn, governments, nongovernmental organizations (NGOs), and donor agencies have used an array of community-level approaches in an attempt to diffuse new preventive treatments, promote family planning, combat malaria, encourage child immunization, and promote many other life-saving innovations. In recent years, such approaches have been central to efforts to curb the spread of HIV/AIDS.

Whereas the use of community-level approaches is rapidly expanding in health and social development programs in developing countries, empirical evidence of the effectiveness of these community-level approaches is surprisingly scarce. In part, this paucity can be explained by the fact that outcomes for community-led interventions are difficult to define. For some, simply carrying out the planned set of communication activities is sufficient to claim victory. More prosaically, to measure effectiveness, one needs to examine one of two outcomes: social change or health behaviors among the population in question. Wallerstein presents a sequence of events for the causal pathway that connects community-led approaches, social change, and health outcomes.[26] The assumption underlying some community-led approaches is that social change is an end unto itself, such that programs that promote social change, via participation, community capacity, empowerment, and social capital are expected to inevitably trigger changes in knowledge, attitudes, and self-efficacy and to lead to the specific desired health behaviors or health status change. For other programs, community-led approaches represent a means to an end: changing health behaviors to improve health status. Whereas community-led approaches assume these causal pathways, surprisingly few programs include both social change and health outcomes in assessing program effectiveness.

The elements that generally define a community-level approach include participatory processes that engage individuals to raise awareness and bring about social change. These approaches rely on the power of individuals, their connections, and resources to generate change. The collaborative, bottom-up orientation of community-level approaches seeks to include key individuals at other levels of society, such as government workers, policy makers, or other stakeholders who may be able to help find solutions to community-specific problems. At the core of community-level approaches are dialogue, participation, and self-reliance.[27] Minga Perú (described later in this section) illustrates these dimensions of community-led approaches.

Community-level approaches may include a range of actions including, but not limited to, holding a protest, organizing public forums such as community meetings, and holding community events to promote an issue. Community organizing and social mobilization are typically a part of community-led approaches and have a higher potential for sustainability. The Social Mobilization Network example from India (presented later in this section) illustrates a practical application of social mobilization.

Proponents of community-led approaches often tout the value of this approach in bringing meaningful and sustainable change among the members of a community or a network of communities in a given geographical area. Detractors of community-led approaches criticize this class of interventions as being very labor intensive, with few of these approaches "going to scale." Despite the criticism, national prevention programs and international donor agencies are increasingly incorporating community-led approaches into their communication/prevention strategies as part of large-scale (often national-level) programs.

Minga Perú: Using *Promotoras* to Foster Community Well-being. Minga Perú is a nonprofit, community-based communication for social change organization that addresses issues of social justice, human rights and dignity, health, gender equity, and protection of natural resources. Founded in 1988, it works primarily with rural communities of the

Peruvian Amazon and other countries in Latin America and the Caribbean. *Minga* (meaning "collaborative community work") forms the central tenet of the organization's mission and philosophy. All of this organization's programs collaborate with local communities to find and build upon local assets and strengths to devise sustainable solutions to community issues.[28]

The mainstay of Minga Perú is the radio program, *Bienvenida Salud* ("Welcome to Health"). This radio program consists of 30-minutes episode that are aired three times a week, once in the morning and again in the evening. The episodes are based on listener letters and to date have covered a range of health and social issues such as domestic violence, HIV/AIDS, gender equality, human rights, and conservation, all of which have been framed and approached from a community health perspective.[29] It is perhaps because of this truly collaborative approach, which fosters two-way communication, that traditionally private issues such as reproductive health and domestic violence are able to "enter the public domain via *Bienvenida Salud*."[30] By taking this approach, the radio program becomes a "mediated space in which population planning and gender-based development discourse can be contested, reworked, and negotiated."[30]

Minga Perú also has a network of *promotoras*, or lay community members, who provide outreach and leadership on health issues to supplement the radio program. The *promotoras* reinforce radio messages and disseminate information they learned in their training within the community. In this capacity, the *promotoras* serve as accessible resources for community members to ask questions and seek help on a range of topics. Each *promotora* works closely with 8 to 20 women who form part of Minga Perú's women's network to develop scripts for the radio program and training materials. Another key element of the *promotoras* component is how women become *promotoras* (**FIGURE 16-2**). Listeners of the radio program write letters nominating girls and women from the community, and through an election process, two *promotoras* per village are selected. This nomination process enables the community to select individuals whom they trust and who are invested in improving the health and well-being of the community. By engaging and involving women to be *promotoras* or to work alongside the *promotoras*, Minga Perú promotes women's rights, reconciliation, and harmony, all of which contribute to improving community well-being.[29]

Sengupta and Elias contextualize the work Minga Perú does within participatory development theorizing.[29] Participatory development advocates for a people-centered, bottom-up approach to development

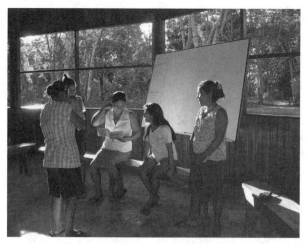

FIGURE 16-2 *Promotoras* from Minga Perú at a Participatory Skit Workshop

Courtesy of Ami Sengupta

in which all individuals are recognized as human beings, rather than being perceived as objects. Such an approach is firmly rooted in the idea that one size does not fit all, and programs need to be culturally tailored to fit the local context. Similarly, the participatory development paradigm calls for practitioners to look beyond economic and basic health needs to address social change and other dimensions of development such as human dignity.[31] As mentioned earlier in the chapter, over time, the communication for development field has placed increased importance on community participation, accepting and embracing multiple social-cultural worldviews and voices. Minga Perú's work empowers women by giving them opportunities to foster community well-being as *promotoras*, as well as giving community members a voice in dictating the issues covered in the radio program. In these ways, Minga Perú's work also embraces postcolonial feminist theories in its acknowledgment of the validity of the lived experiences and local knowledge systems of the Peruvian women. In so doing, it exemplifies the benefits of promoting a community-led, broader, holistic understanding of health.

The Social Mobilization Network for Polio Eradication. The World Health Assembly launched the Global Polio Eradication Initiative in 1988. Experts around the world acknowledged that polio eradication would be challenging in India given the size and diversity of its population. By 2006, four countries remained polio endemic—Afghanistan, India, Nigeria, and Pakistan. Cases of polio had been steadily declining in India thanks in large part to the "Pulse Polio" program, which included twice-yearly National Immunization Day campaigns and supplementary immunization activities. However, a spike in cases in the states of Uttar Pradesh and Bihar in India underscored the need for strengthened and innovative approaches to reach children in these vulnerable and high-risk states.

Established by the CORE Group network, UNICEF, and local nongovernmental organizations in India, the Social Mobilization Network (SMNet) was created with the goal of improving access and reducing family and community resistance to polio vaccination. SMNet contributed to the achievement of the following program objectives: addressing parental concerns, understanding vaccination refusals, creating trust between polio eradication personnel and local residents, tracking missed children, and identifying missed subpopulations.[32] The CORE group and UNICEF trained thousands of social mobilization field workers who worked at various levels: community, block, district, state and district, and regional and national. While all of the social mobilizers played different and important roles that contributed to the effectiveness of SMNet, the community mobilization coordinators were by and large the linchpins of the initiative.

The community mobilization coordinators (CMCs) were women from high-risk communities who received a small stipend to track pregnancies and immunizations in an assigned block of 400 to 500 households. The CMCs kept detailed community maps tracking pregnancies and immunizations of children younger than age 5 and promoted polio campaign efforts. During household visits, the CMCs promoted child immunization, hygiene, and sanitation; raised awareness about the importance of routine immunization and polio eradication; and tracked missed children and ensured they got vaccinations. The CMCs built trust and reduced resistance to vaccination by reaching out and working with community, religious, and cultural leaders, as well as other key informants.[32]

The CMCs also began involving children in community mobilization efforts. At first, children were engaged to encourage their families to vaccinate siblings. Later, groups of children known as *bulawwa tolies* ("calling teams") paraded around communities prior to polio campaigns promoting the health benefits of polio vaccination and encouraging community members to vaccinate their children.[32] In response to community demands for broader health initiatives, SMNet developed a range of creative behavior-change activities and materials to promote vaccination awareness and safety, household hygiene, sanitation, home diarrheal-disease control, and breastfeeding.

Analysis of immunization coverage data in India shows that SMNet has contributed to increases in oral polio vaccine (OPV) coverage in high-resistance communities. In fact, communities with CMCs had substantially higher proportions of OPV-vaccinated children at vaccination booths than communities without CMCs. Moreover, the SMNet strengthened partnerships among local NGOs, government, and multilateral agencies, and ultimately had a high return on investment.[32]

Mediated Communication

Mediated communication disseminates health messages through communication platforms such as television, film, radio, billboards, print, computers, and telephones. In contrast to face-to-face communication, these forms of communication can reach large populations at once. Mediated communication can be leveraged in the form of mass-media campaigns. These campaigns can be long or short in duration, and can either stand alone or be one of many program components.

In mass-media campaigns, exposure to messages typically occurs passively. In other words, individuals are exposed to a message through their daily consumption of media. For example, an individual might tune into a TV show and, during the commercial breaks, see a public service announcement about tobacco use. Another individual, while driving to work, might read a billboard with information on the warning signs of a stroke or spot an advertisement promoting HIV testing while flipping through the pages of a magazine.

Wakefield, Loken, and Hornik's systematic review of the use of mass-media campaigns to change various health-risk behaviors found that mass-media campaigns can directly or indirectly produce positive changes or prevent negative changes.[2] Success appears to be linked to the nature of the target behavior, with campaigns directed at changing episodic behaviors (e.g., cancer screening or vaccination) having more success as compared to those targeting ongoing behaviors (e.g., physical activity or food choices). Mass-media campaigns also seem to be more successful when coupled with other interventions. Similarly, the availability and access to services combined with supportive policies are critical if health-risk behaviors are to be curtailed.

The *Scrutinize* campaign from South Africa represents a real-world example of a mass-media campaign to prevent HIV among youth. Individuals can also actively seek out information through planned long-term health communication campaigns. Later in the chapter we discuss one successful mediated approach, entertainment-education.

Scrutinize: A Youth HIV Prevention Campaign in South Africa.

The *Scrutinize* campaign was a year-long youth HIV prevention campaign launched in South Africa. Formative research undertaken to design the campaign revealed that the rate of increase in HIV prevalence was leveling off. However, HIV prevalence remained too high among youth ages 15 to 32 years and disproportionately affected young women. The data revealed that condom use declined among those with multiple partners when their relationships stabilized. Moreover, many South Africans did not make the connection between HIV risk and the number of sexual partners. Based on this formative research, five campaign objectives were identified: (1) increase awareness of HIV infection risk due to multiple and concurrent sexual partners; (2) delay the initiation of sexual activity among young people; (3) reduce the number of multiple and concurrent partners; (4) promote correct and consistent condom use; and (5) increase the number of people who test for HIV on a regular basis.[12]

The driving force of the *Scrutinize* campaign was seven animerts (i.e., short, animated commercials). Energetic, funny, and chock full of colloquial language, these commercials were created to resonate with youth and drew inspiration from shows such as *The Simpsons* and *South Park*.[33] The commercials featured two characters—Victor and Virginia Scrutinize—and a ninja who personified HIV. The commercials dramatized how HIV could penetrate sexual networks in a way that visually and verbally underscored the risky nature of HIV. However, instead of telling audience members what to do (as HIV campaigns have traditionally done), the animerts encouraged audience members to reflect upon or *scrutinize* their own behavior. Aside from the animerts, the campaign utilized a range of communication activities and channels to disseminate campaign messages including posters, entertainment-education, social media, community outreach, and workshops to facilitate interpersonal communication.

Two theories influenced the design of the campaign: the theory of reasoned action and planned behavior and the extended parallel process model.[34-36] The primary campaign slogan "Eliminate the Element of Surprise—Scrutinize" contains a cognitive and emotional appeal, as well as a call to action. The payoff line—"Flip HIV to H.I. Victory"—strove to counter the fatalism surrounding HIV and reinforce the perceived efficacy of prevention behavior.[12]

Results from the theory-driven impact evaluation revealed that the TV campaign had statistically significant impacts on condom use, talking to one's friends and sexual partners about HIV testing, getting tested for HIV, and knowledge about the increased risk from having multiple sex partners.[12] In addition, the Undercover HIV animert had an unexpected positive effect on attitudes about multiple sexual partners among young men and those who thought that they were not at risk of getting infected. The impact evaluation also found a relatively high level of cost-effectiveness for the Undercover HIV animert. The strength and success of this campaign can be attributed to strong formative research to understand the population health needs and campaign audience, use of multiple communication approaches to reach and engage youth, strong partnerships and support, and evaluation driven by theory and methods.[33]

Interactive Communication Technologies

New information technologies can deliver a vast array of services, aid capacity-building efforts, empower communities, and connect individuals, as well as different social groups. For these reasons, interactive communication technologies (ICTs) have played a critical role in achieving the MDGs. While the literature is replete with creative examples of programs leveraging ICTs, it is important to recognize that ICTs—including mobile health (mHealth)—are not "silver bullets." That is, by themselves ICTs cannot guarantee sustainable behavior and social change. Rather, they must be integrated within multilevel programs that harness multiple communication approaches. The use of ICTs requires uninterrupted electricity and power, as well as technical and logistical support to function. Even when these supplies and services are guaranteed, one must also consider literacy barriers as well as socio-economic, gender, and power constraints with regard to access to electronic devices.

In a systematic review of mHealth interventions for behavior change communication, Gurman, Rubin, and Roess found that while the majority of mobile phone users live in developing countries, most interventions have been implemented in the developed world.[37] These authors agree that mHealth is a promising tool to foster behavior change, but conclude that there is a need for more robust evaluations to truly understand their effectiveness. **TABLE 16-2** lists the recommendations put forth by Gurman, Rubin and Roess.[37]

The *Liga Inan* ("Mobile Moms") Project: Timor-Leste's First mHealth Project.

Timor-Leste has one of the highest fertility rates and maternal

TABLE 16-2 Recommendations for Designing mHealth Interventions

- Understand your audience
- Target and tailor the content to your audience
- Use two-way communication
- Time the communication appropriately
- Minimize costs
- Ensure privacy
- Conduct long-term evaluation

Data from: Gurman TA, Rubin SE, Roess AA. Effectiveness of mHealth behavior change communication interventions in developing countries: A systematic review of the literature. J Health Commun, 2012; 17: 82-104.

mortality rates in Southeast Asia, according to the 2009 demographic and health survey (DHS).[38] Most women give birth at home (78%), and only 30% of births are delivered by a skilled birth attendant such as a doctor, midwife, or nurse. Contact with midwives is limited to prenatal care visits, which does not allow for the repetition and reinforcement of health messages that are most likely to produce behavior change. In addition, many Timorese women live in rural or remote locations, which further disconnects them from healthcare providers and services.

The goal of the *Liga Inan* program is to reduce maternal and neonatal morbidity and mortality by improving health and care-seeking behaviors of pregnant women. To support the program's objective of increasing the utilization of quality skilled care before, during, and after delivery, *Liga Inan* uses mobile phones to connect pregnant women and midwives. Baseline data supported this choice of communication channel: 69% of women in Manufahi and 67% in Ainaro (the project districts) reported that they have a mobile phone in the house.[39] In some cases, family members share a phone. However, 70% of women in Manufahi and 95% of women in Ainaro reported that one or more of the household phones belonged solely to them. Mobile phone use itself was also high in these two districts. More than 72% of women reported sending a text message once a day or more, and 97% reported that they had signal coverage either in the home or within a 5-minute walk. Text messages were requested in Tetum (the local language) by 98% of women. These data suggest that mobile phones are a prevalent and viable communication channel with the potential to foster two-way communication between mothers and midwives to improve maternal and newborn health.

In the *Liga Inan* program, an automated service enables the Ministry of Health to disseminate important gestation-specific maternal health messages to mothers. The messages were selected from the Mobile Alliance for Maternal Action (MAMA) database and cover prenatal care, nutrition, the importance of delivering under the care of a midwife, danger signs during pregnancy, delivery, postpartum care for both mother and child, and newborn care. These topics were selected based on the baseline data. The original messages were translated into Tetum, edited to fit the 160-character limit of a text message, and crafted as cues to action.[40]

Message pretesting was conducted with pregnant women from the two districts to assess the readability, comprehension, and acceptability of the messages. Feedback indicated that much of the information was new to the women, which in conjunction with feedback from a stakeholder meeting and a review of the literature, suggested the need for messages to be disseminated twice a week instead of once a week as originally planned. In addition, pretesting revealed the need to include messages discussing traditional practices around birth that may have harmful consequences. For example, many women in Timor-Leste practice the postpartum tradition of *tuur ahi* (literally "sitting fire") in which a new mother and baby are sequestered in a home for weeks next to an open fire, which is believed to have beneficial healing effects. A message was developed conveying the harmful effects of smoke on newborns and advising mothers to stay a protective distance away from the smoke.[40]

Midwives use their clients' mobile phones to enroll pregnant women into the *Liga Inan* program during the first prenatal care visit. Midwives also receive text reminders when a woman is nearing her due date. These reminders prompt midwives to call the pregnant woman to check in with her, discuss her health and plans for the delivery, and review warning signs that the mother should look for. After delivery, the midwife can use the phone to continue to monitor the health of both the mother and her child. In addition, midwives may use the mobile phones to alert women of other health initiatives happening in the area, such as vaccination campaigns or health fairs. On the flip side, mothers have a direct line to the midwives and can reach out to them at any point in time during pregnancy, birth, and the postpartum period with any questions or concerns they may have. This two-way line of communication empowers women to take control of their health, and enables them to establish rapport with the midwife and feel supported during pregnancy.

It is still too early to ascertain the impact that *Liga Inan* has had. Preliminary data, however, are promising. In one district in 2012, the average number of births attended by a skilled provider during a month was 38, and the average number of institutional deliveries was 27. In the first full month of the program in the same district, there were 56 births attended by a skilled provider and 38 institutional births.[41] These numbers, despite being early data, are encouraging, and it is hoped that such improvements will continue to be seen across the island. Further, women describe positive experiences with the program, with 94% saying they are satisfied with the program and 96% reporting the program is easy to access.[41] Results also indicate that women find the messages easy to understand, are retaining the messages' content, and are discussing the messages with other women.

At the same time, it is important to consider some limitations related to inconsistent program reach. Women recall receiving only 47% of messages sent in the last month. This low rate could be a sign of one or more of the following problems: recall bias, service provider issues leading to failed message delivery, limited mobile phone coverage, mobile phones being turned off, user error such as deletion of a message before reading it, literacy challenges, the message not being received by the mother because another family member has the phone, or other issues.[41]

While the results of *Liga Inan* are encouraging and its use of mHealth technology is exciting, it is important to consider other communication mechanisms that might potentially enrich the program and address some of the challenges associated with using mobile phones. Using multiple communication approaches, for example, could help expand the program's reach to include women without mobile phones and, perhaps more importantly, those pregnant women who do not seek prenatal care at all.

Entertainment-Education: An Integrated Approach

Over the past 25 years entertainment-education (EE) has emerged as an effective health communication strategy that combines or embeds educational messages into entertainment programs and popular culture to bring about social and behavior change. EE's roots trace back to oral traditions spanning hundreds, if not thousands, of years.[42] However, the conscious use of this technique as primarily a media strategy emerged in the early 1990s. One of the earliest studied examples of EE is the television program *Simplemente Maria*, which aired in Peru in 1969; it inspired viewers to sign up for adult literacy and sewing classes after watching the female protagonist on television

do the same.[43] Over time, EE has evolved to include a variety of forms: radio, music, theater, television, folk media, as well as emerging media, and combinations of media, such as the well-known South African program *Soul City*[44] (described later in this section). In addition, EE has emerged as a way to address health disparities, address the role of affect and narratives in promoting behavior and social change, and expand dialogue within as well as over and above an EE intervention framework.[45-47]

Public health and communication practitioners have been studying "how" EE works. Bandura's social learning theory was used to provide early understanding of EE, through the process of observational learning.[48] In this process, an individual audience member copies positive role-model characters by repeating their behaviors in his or her daily life in the hopes of being rewarded.[49] Scholars today, however, agree that how EE works is actually far more complex. Some argue that in addition to promoting direct behavior change, the impact of EE programs is amplified through mediating variables. Researchers have explored the direct impact of EE on variables such as audience involvement, efficacy, and interpersonal communication, which in turn result in behavior and social changes being promoted by the EE programs.[50,51] As the understanding of the complex processes through which EE interventions have their impact grows, increasing attention is paid to concepts of social consequences and normative influence.[52,53] As such, current EE interventions reflect a focus on communities and social norms in mediated explanations of EE.[54]

***Kyunki... Jeena Issi Ka Naam Hai* ("Because... That's What Life Is").** In a country as diverse as India, it is often a challenge to create effective communication that promotes social and behavioral change. Poor health indicators such as mortality in children younger than age 5, maternal mortality, malnutrition among children, lack of appropriate immunization, and the spread of HIV/AIDS increase the vulnerability of women and children, in particular. Nearly 153 million households in India own TV sets, and it is estimated that TV programming reaches more than 45% of the rural population in India, making it by far the most widespread form of communication.[55] Launched on World Health Day, April 7, 2008, and broadcast until the end of 2011, the soap opera *Kyunki... Jeena Issi Ka Naam Hai* ("Because... That's What Life Is") was a Hindi entertainment-education program that broadcast more than 500 episodes on Doordarshan, the national TV service.

The show was created and produced by UNICEF, with research partners Johns Hopkins University Center for Communication Programs (JHUCCP) and a local research agency, Centre for Media Studies (CMS). Government of India ministries such as National Rural Health Mission (NRHM) and National AIDS Control Organization (NACO) funded the show.[56]

The educational aspects of *Kyunki…* were based on UNICEF's Facts for Life (FFL; **TABLE 16-3**).[57] FFL provides critical messages and information for mothers and caregivers to use in changing behaviors and practices that can save the lives of children and help them develop and grow to their full potential. FFL is a repository of factual information on 14 key issues that can be tailored for various communication tools and approaches. The communication of FFL messages was situated within the child rights and systems strengthening contexts, which were priorities for both the government of India and UNICEF.

Kyunki… was a quintessential soap opera, a form of entertainment that is very popular in India. It took place in a rural setting, with its characters reflecting the large majority of Indians who reside in rural areas. The show was based in the fictional village of Rajpura and revolved around six main protagonists. Nurse bhen-ji (Savita), the city-bred auxiliary nurse-midwife (ANM), dreamed of making Rajpura an ideal village. Savita was assisted by an Aagnawadi worker (Shabnam), a victim of domestic violence who chose to live life on her own terms, and a young widow (Kamla) who over time became the village "Accredited Social Health Activist" (a government-recognized position).

TABLE 16-3   Facts for Life

Facts for Life provides important information and messages covering these issues:

- Timing births
- Safe motherhood and newborn health
- Child development and early learning
- Breastfeeding
- Nutrition and growth
- Immunization
- Diarrhea
- Coughs, colds, and more serious illnesses
- Hygiene
- Malaria
- HIV and AIDS
- Child protection
- Injury prevention
- Emergencies: preparedness and response

Facts for Life (4th Ed.). UNICEF. http://www.factsforlifeglobal.org/index.html. Accessed April 2015.

The final female protagonist was a female Sarpanch (Phoolwati), an elected figurehead who is highly successful. The male protagonist was the friendly primary school teacher (Master-ji), who ran a one-room school. The final protagonist was an inquisitive and vivacious girl (Meena).[54]

Research, monitoring, and evaluation played a vital role in content development. To better understand the impact of *Kyunki…*, UNICEF, in partnership with JHUCCP and a local research agency Center for Media Studies (CMS), put multiple research processes in place. A vigorous concurrent-monitoring framework was established that provided rapid audience assessment and content analysis to provide qualitative feedback. Neilson TAM (Television Audience Meter) is one of the main sources of data on viewership and audience engagement for television content. To assess *Kyunki…*'s popularity in comparison with other TV shows, weekly TAM ratings were analyzed. In early 2008, before the broadcast of the show began, a baseline survey was conducted with 10,000 respondents from 6 Hindi-speaking states. This research provided information on existing knowledge levels, attitudes, and perceptions of its viewers. Subsequently, a midterm survey in 2009 and an end-of-show survey in 2011 were conducted to assess the impact of the show.

Evaluation results indicated that *Kyunki…* elicited high levels of exposure, message, and story recall. In addition, according to Sood et al., *Kyunki…* illustrates the relative effectiveness of the FFL initiative as a whole, but also highlights the need to move beyond the awareness-generation model to design entertainment-education that is instrumental in changing attitudes, efficacy perceptions, and social norms.[54]

Tsha Tsha. *Tsha Tsha* is an entertainment-education television drama series that aired in South Africa in Xhosa from 2003 to 2004. The drama followed several youth on their journey into adulthood as they struggled with creating relationships, questioning their own identity, and dealing with HIV/AIDS. The drama was set in a fictional, small rural town, unlike most programs in South Africa. This setting allowed for the exploration of themes such as youth marginalization, as well as personal and social transformation in the context of community life. Moreover, evaluation data found that the rural setting appealed to both rural and urban residents.[58] One of the main features of the drama was ballroom dancing—hence the title's play on the Cuban dance, cha cha. Ballroom dancing was the thread that brought the characters together and connected the episodes; it provided a backdrop to explore intimacy, respect, and relationships.

Instead of relying upon didactic messages, *Tsha Tsha* promoted lessons that revolved around processes of self-reflection and weighing choices and consequences before acting. The storyline emphasized the complexity of problems and the need to think creatively to figure out effective solutions. The psychological depth of the characters played a critical role in ensuring they were relatable to the audience at both emotional and intellectual levels. In fact, data from the evaluation revealed that viewers attributed their development of several problem-solving skills to scenarios that played out in the drama.[58] The program promoted the development of individual- and community-level self-efficacy and empathy, aspired to make youth reflect upon problems they faced and come up with creative solutions, and inspired them to become active agents of change in their own communities. More specifically, the program addressed HIV/AIDS prevention, caring for dying or sick parents, facing the possibility of being HIV positive and dealing with a positive status, relationships and sexuality, life skills and problem solving, HIV-related stigma, challenges with avoiding HIV-risk behaviors, and sexual violence.

The evaluation of *Tsha Tsha* also revealed that knowledge and general awareness of HIV/AIDS increased among viewers. The show's strong, positive images of young people dealing with a positive HIV status was realistic and compellingly depicted the difficulties of living openly with HIV and sharing that information with others. As a result, viewers were more likely to have positive attitudes about HIV/AIDS, people living with HIV/AIDs, and HIV-preventive behaviors such as abstinence, staying faithful to one partner, and using a condom. In addition, *Tsha Tsha* was seen as providing positive role models for women as well as positive examples of male–female relationships. Several participants even remarked that they discussed the program as it aired and after it aired, although the fact that it aired on Fridays meant that viewers could not discuss it the next day at work or at school. In sum, the realism of *Tsha Tsha* allowed it to make an impression that started and shaped conversations on HIV/AIDS.[58]

▶ When More Is Better: Using a Transmedia Approach

Health communication is a long-term process. It is crucial that the interventions follow some key steps to achieve success. According to the report *Communication for Better Health*, which was published by Johns

Hopkins University Center for Communication Programs, both experience and evidence from around the world have highlighted several common characteristics of successful health communication programs, which can be categorized into five subgroups, as shown in **TABLE 16-4**.[59]

These guidelines clearly showcase the importance of communication efforts to address health issues by cutting across the various levels of the social ecological model and to promote change across multiple levels. To be effective, communication programs must be based on a thorough understanding (obtained through causal and audience analysis) of the problem to be addressed. Well-considered health communication must be designed to reach multiple audiences (primary, secondary, and tertiary). To meet the objectives of promoting long-term, sustainable, and scalable change across the social ecological domains and addressing the needs of multiple audiences, it is critical that the health communication be designed in ways that holistically address public health problems. Such holistic design is, by default, participatory in nature and based on a thorough understanding of the situation and the needs and strengths of the potential audiences. The implementation of such multiple-level and multiple-audience programs requires the utilization of several communication channels, so as to meet the preferences of different audiences. The following examples illustrate the use of multilevel approaches.

TABLE 16-4 Common Characteristics of Successful Health Communication Programs

- *Goals and objectives*: Setting SMART objectives and planning for scaling up
- *Theories*: Using communication as well as behavior and social change theories by emphasizing positive benefits of change
- *Research and evaluation*: Audience research for program design, pretesting materials, monitoring and evaluation for program revision, and justifying future investments
- *Participation*: Community involvement and local capacity building
- *Audience characteristics*: Using multiple channels to ensure widespread exposure, audience segmentation, and tailoring of messages to audience subgroups

Data from: Salem RM, Bernstein J, Sullivan TM, Lande R. *"Communication for better health"* Population Reports, Series J, No. 56. Baltimore: INFO Project, Johns Hopkins Bloomberg School of Public Health; 2008.

SIAGA Campaign

Indonesia's SIAGA (alert) initiative aimed to prevent maternal mortality related to complications of pregnancy and delivery. SIAGA—an acronym standing for SIap (ready), Antar (take, transport), and jaGA (stand by or guard)—began in 1998 under a United Nations Population Fund program implemented in conjunction with the Ministry for Women's Empowerment and Johns Hopkins Bloomberg School of Public Health/Center for Communication Programs (CCP). The original mass-media campaign—Suami SIAGA—focused only on husbands and their role in preparing for delivery.[60] The evaluation results from Suami SIAGA were impressive. Therefore, shortly after the UNFP project ended, the five-year Maternal and Neonatal Health (MNH) Program expanded and continued the program through support from USAID.

Whereas the concept of community involvement in maternal health was historically strong in Indonesia, interventions did not necessarily reflect the community needs and strengths. Indonesia's emerging democracy expanded community involvement from a centrally driven, message-dissemination network to a model engaging the community through the emerging civil society and NGOs. In a country such as Indonesia, where the reach of television and radio extends to far-flung islands and remote villages, mass media play an important role in instigating social change. The MNH Program incorporated a variety of complementary multimedia and community activities to support its objectives. The impact evaluation of Suami SIAGA (alert husband) in 2000 and the baseline assessment in six West Java districts in 2000–2001 provided insights and recommendations for the development of the subsequent Warga SIAGA (alert citizen) and Bidan SIAGA (alert midwife) campaigns. A local advertising agency assisted in specific message development and pretesting, while MNH stakeholders, including the Indonesian Midwives Association (IBI) and the Ministry of Health at the district and provincial levels, provided technical expertise. Launched between 1999 and 2002, each phase of the SIAGA campaign shared a common look but had distinctive goals and approaches. Popular Indonesian singer Iis Dahlia served as the spokesperson through all phases of the SIAGA campaign.[61]

For each of the intended audiences, the program identified a set of behaviors that make a person *SIAGA*. Suami SIAGA focused on promoting the husband's involvement in pregnancy, preparation for delivery, and any potential emergency. Warga SIAGA encouraged individual citizens to be alert and prepared for delivery by doing their part in arranging for transport,

funds, a blood donor, and recognizing danger signs. Bidan SIAGA promoted the midwife as a skilled and friendly provider who is prepared to help throughout the pregnancy. As a result of these components, SIAGA became the brand name for safe motherhood in Indonesia.

To ensure that women and families sought skilled providers at the time of birth, a grassroots participatory process led to the creation of 55 Desa SIAGAs, or alert villages, which established all four components of the Desa SIAGA system: pregnancy notification to a midwife, emergency fund plans, transportation, and blood donation mechanisms. Village facilitators played a central role in organizing birth preparedness and complication readiness actions within their communities. Strong political commitment from diverse stakeholders supported the community actions through the White Ribbon Alliance movement, while communication campaigns helped raise community awareness.[61]

Overall, the SIAGA campaign had a powerful impact on the intended audiences. Evaluation results indicate that almost three-fourths of the respondents exposed to the campaign agreed that the SIAGA information was relevant and they were able to apply it to their lives. Some 62% of respondents were exposed to the overall SIAGA campaign, measured in terms of exposure to either Bidan, Warga, or Desa SIAGA. Additionally, the fairly high level of interpersonal communication regarding SIAGA messages reported by 51% of respondents indicates that SIAGA sparked interest and discussion among the respondents' social networks. Researchers found clear differences in knowledge and practices pertaining to birth preparedness and complication readiness among respondents before and after the campaign, as well as among unexposed and exposed respondent groups at follow-up, across all key indicators.

These results indicate that the SIAGA campaign played an important role in making Indonesian women, their husbands, and their communities more prepared for complications during pregnancy and delivery. The MNH Program successfully engaged villages in preparing for obstetric emergencies and helped make motherhood safer.[62,63]

Soul City

The Soul City Institute for Health and Development Communication is a South African NGO that utilizes mass media (specifically, entertainment-education), social mobilization, and advocacy to improve the quality of life and health of South Africans.[44] Its programs are predicated on the idea that human rights are fundamental to health and development, and as such Soul City actively promotes citizen participation and social justice at the individual, community, and societal levels. Soul City's initiatives are all evidence-based programs that are crafted to effect meaningful change by creating an enabling environment, mobilizing collective action, strengthening services, developing skills and agency, and influencing healthy public policies. To date, Soul City programs have addressed a range of issues: HIV/AIDS and youth sexuality, tobacco, tuberculosis, interpersonal violence, domestic violence, sexual harassment, hypertension, parenting, youth life skills, small business development, and even personal finance.

Soul City 4 consisted of a 13-part prime-time television drama, a 45-part radio drama in nine languages, and three full-color information booklets that dealt with violence against women (specifically domestic violence and sexual harassment), AIDS (including youth sexuality and date rape), small business development and personal savings, and hypertension.[64] *Soul City 4* also forged a partnership with the National Network on Violence Against Women to connect individuals affected by domestic violence with support services. In so doing, Soul City intended to establish a mechanism by which individuals and communities could take action in the face of domestic violence and sexual harassment, and more effectively create an environment to support change.[65]

An evaluation of the program found that audience members identified with the series' characters and situations, which facilitated self-reflection. Exposure to *Soul City 4* was associated with increased knowledge and awareness of violence against women and the risks of hypertension. It also improved personal attitudes and beliefs, sparked interpersonal communication, and changed social norms related to domestic violence, HIV/AIDS, and youth sexuality. Importantly, these positive effects resulted in intentions to initiate positive behavior change.[64] Moreover, through the partnership between Soul City and the National Network on Violence Against Women, *Soul City 4* helped shift the debate on domestic violence and sexual harassment at the national level, while also addressing the community and individual domains. In fact, this program helped push South Africa's implementation of its Domestic Violence Act.[65]

Soul City's approach addresses multiple domains of the social ecological model and utilizes a range of complementary approaches—a blend that enables it to bring about social change. *Soul City 4*, in particular, was able to shift community norms and stimulate community dialogue and debate using media advocacy, community

mobilization, and entertainment-education with regard to HIV/AIDs and youth sexuality and domestic violence. This mix of approaches and channels also enabled public debates at community and national levels, which in turn put pressure on policy makers to address domestic violence. As a result, *Soul City 4* was effective (and also cost-effective at face value) in bringing about social change at three levels.[64] Moreover, the evaluation findings for this program demonstrate the value of using a social ecological model to guide behavior social change programs.[65]

Ndukaka: *Changing Norms Around Female Genital Mutilation*

Female genital mutilation (FGM) is a traditional practice involving the partial or full removal of external female genitalia (see **BOX 16-2** for the four classifications of FGM[66]). It is practiced in 29 African and Middle Eastern countries,[67] albeit with prevalence rates varying dramatically within and across countries.

In Nigeria, approximately 30 million females have experienced FGM.[68] The southern regions of the country have the highest prevalence of FGM, according to the 2003 DHS.[66] The social, psychological, and health consequences of FGM are numerous even for the least invasive forms of the practice.

Ndukaka (Igbo for "health is better than wealth") is a communication program that aimed to eliminate the practice of FGM in Enugu State, Nigeria, by combining community mobilization, advocacy, and mass-media approaches. *Ndukaka*'s primary objective was to decrease the number of families that practiced

---

BOX 16-2 Types of Female Genital Mutilation

FGM varies in its degree of invasiveness. The following describes in detail what each procedure entails:

- Type I, commonly referred to as "Sunna circumcision" involves the removal of part or all of the clitoris.
- Type II involves the excision of the clitoris and part of the labia minora.
- Type III involves the removal of the clitoris, labia minora, and partial excision of the labia majora.
- Type IV, also known as "Pharaonic circumcision," involves the removal of the clitoris and the labia minora, as well as the sewing together of the labia majora leaving a small opening for urine and menstrual blood to pass.

Data from: Toubia N. Female circumcision as a public health issue. *N Engl J Med*, 1993; 331(11): 712-716.

FGM.[68] The program objective was supported by five communication objectives: (1) to change relevant knowledge, attitudes, and behavioral intentions related to FGM; (2) to raise awareness of possible negative effects of FGM; (3) to increase community dialogue about the practice; (4) to address the cultural and socioeconomic factors reinforcing the practice; and (5) to mobilize community members to abandon the practice and advocate in favor of its elimination among their peers.

The program was based on the need to reach individuals and mobilize entire communities so that new, positive norms could be established. Given the sensitivity of the topic, the program utilized a nonconfrontational approach. It employed multiple strategic communication approaches (community mobilization, advocacy, and mass media) and communication channels (film, radio call-in shows, newspapers, community events, and public forums) to reach parents, teachers, law enforcement personnel, key influencers, and policy makers.

The community mobilization component was the driving force behind the program. These efforts drew upon the community action cycle (CAC), a community-driven process embodying community capacity building and mobilization for behavior and social change.[27] The CAC process consists of six phases: (1) prepare to mobilize, (2) organize the community for action, (3) explore the health issue and set priorities, (4) plan together, (5) act together, and (6) evaluate together.[69,70] As a bottom-up approach, this model draws on Paulo Freire's work on dialogue, praxis, and critical consciousness. Community participation by those most affected by the health issue, social outcomes, and ongoing dialogues are fundamental components of the CAC; together, they promote self-reliance and sustainability of the desired outcome.

In Nigeria, the Women's Action Research Organization (WARO) led the CAC process at the hamlet level by assisting women's groups and other groups of community members to identify health priorities. WARO carried out capacity-building efforts by teaching local community members about community mobilization and leading technical sessions where FGM and other issues could be discussed and analyzed. Community members and groups developed action plans including activities to eliminate FGM with assistance from WARO. Activities included health seminars, peer health education sessions, and meetings with both traditional leaders and local government entities to disseminate information about FGM and gain support for the elimination of this practice. Community groups held viewings of the documentary *Uncut:*

Playing with Life (produced by Communicating for Change). Groups also undertook advocacy visits to traditional leaders, held anti-FGM discussions during annual festivities, and organized networking meetings for local partners.

At the state level, the National Association of Women Journalists implemented radio call-in shows, established regular newspaper columns, and organized public forums on FGM. The radio call-in shows allowed community members to provide input and weigh in on the anti-FGM discussion, ask questions, and even get feedback from the radio hosts and guest speakers. Radio's wide reach and its audio format were powerful conduits for disseminating information to both literate and illiterate populations in the country. In fact, data from the program's evaluation found radio to be the primary source of exposure to program messages.[68] In contrast, the regular newspaper columns led to more limited participation and input by the public. Nevertheless, they consistently publicized local program activities and positioned FGM as a practice to be debated and discussed at the state government level, and even brought about social action through policy reform. Finally, the participatory and interactive nature of public forums created a space to disseminate program messages on FGM, foster local ownership of the anti-FGM movement, and catalyze community mobilization.

Community mobilization, mass-media campaigns, and advocacy allowed the program to influence multiple sectors and levels, which helped disseminate program messages to the different key audiences while also reaching a broader population.[70] These three components successfully created an enabling environment for change. The mass-media component motivated individuals to participate in community events and worked toward building a critical mass in support of the abandonment of FGM (a concept drawn straight from social convention theory). Similarly, the use of community groups and even community celebrations helped integrate the *Ndukaka* program into existing social structures. Not only does such integration "stimulate and fuse citizen energies, interest, and resources into a collective response for change," but this local ownership of the change process also promoted sustainability and reduced the need for external catalysts.[70]

A number of unintended positive consequences also occurred that underscored the effectiveness of the program. Community mobilization led to public support for the elimination of FGM by several traditional leaders. One leader publicly denounced FGM and played a pivotal role in the passage of a health bill on elimination of FGM.[72] Finally, women involved in the CAC process became "empowered advocates and change agents" on health issues and FGM, referring to themselves as "*Ndukaka* Women."[72] These women have the potential to mobilize communities in other areas, thereby sustaining change beyond the program's formal time frame.

▶ Conclusion

This chapter has provided an overview of the historical trajectory of health communication efforts in developing countries, which have evolved from a top-down "build it and they will come" approach to a dynamic and dialogic process inspiring individual and social change. Theorizing about health communication has shifted from traditional individual behavior change models to more holistic social ecological frameworks that examine the causal effects of communication within and across levels—for example, individuals, family, community, society, and policy. On the one hand, research on international health communication is relatively sparse, especially when studying developing country contexts. On the other hand, there is contradictory information on the effectiveness of health communication in achieving individual and social change. Entertainment-education in developing countries stands out in this regard. The challenge and future directions for EE lie in ensuring adoption of innovative design, implementation, and evaluation processes that put participation front and center.

Interpersonal, community-led, and mediated health communication approaches have mostly been successful in achieving their intended communication objectives, while ICTs offer great promise, although their use must be tempered with a clear understanding of issues of access and use. This chapter supports the value of using multiple communication approaches to address complex individual and social change issues. Communication is both a science and an art, which can foster broad national development objectives. International health communication can be conceptualized both as a mediating factor that contributes to change and as an outcome that sustains change by converting innovations in individual and social behaviors into normative practices.

Wrap-Up

Chapter Questions

1. What are the four eras of health communication in resource-poor countries?
2. What are the Millennium Development Goals, and how have they affected the global burden of disease?
3. What are some factors that can influence interpersonal communication?
4. How can community-level approaches be used to promote health?
5. What are some of the characteristics of mediated communication?
6. Why are ICTs not a "silver bullet" for addressing health issues?
7. What are the benefits of multiple communication approaches to promote individual and social change?

References

1. Global Health Forum. 2012. http://www.globalforum health.org/about/1090-gap/. Accessed March 2015.
2. Wakefield MA, Loken B, Hornik RC. Use of mass media campaigns to change health behavior. *Lancet.* 2010;376:1261-71.
3. Millennium Development Goals. World Health Organization. http://www.who.int/topics/millennium_development_goals/about/en/. Accessed March 27, 2015.
4. United Nations. *The Millennium Development Goals Report 2014.* Geneva, Switzerland: United Nations; 2014.
5. Rimon JG. Behavior change communication in public health. In *Beyond Dialogue: Moving Toward Convergence.* Presented at the United Nations Roundtable on Development Communication; Managua, Nicaragua; 2001.
6. Rogers EM. *Communication Strategies for Family Planning.* New York, NY: Free Press; 1973.
7. Figueroa ME, Kincaid DL, Rani M, Lewis G. *Communication for Social Change: An Integrated Model for Measuring the Process and Its Outcomes.* Communication for Social Change Working Paper Series No. 1. Baltimore, MD: Rockefeller and Johns Hopkins University, Center for Communication Programs; 2002.
8. United Nations, Statistics Division. http://unstats.un.org/unsd/methods/m49/m49.htm. Accessed November 2012.
9. World Congress on Communication for Development. *Communication for Development Making a Difference.*

White Paper. Section 3.2. Rome, Italy: Communication for Development in Health; 2006.

10. Piotrow PT, Kincaid DL, Rimon II JG, Rinehart, W. *Health Communication: Lessons from Family Planning and Reproductive Health*. Westport, CT: Praeger; 1997.

11. Bronfenbrenner U. *The Ecology of Human Development: Experiments by Nature and Design*. Cambridge, MA: Harvard University Press; 1979.

12. Kincaid DL, Delate R, Storey JD, Figueroa ME. Closing the gaps in practice and in theory: Evaluation of the *Scrutinize* HIV Campaign in South Africa. In: Rice RE, Atkin CK, eds. *Public Communication Campaigns*. Los Angeles, CA: Sage; 2013:305-319.

13. Habermas J. *The Theory of Communicative Action, Vol. 2: A Critique of Functionalist Reason*. Boston, MA: Beacon Press; 1987.

14. Jacobson TL, Storey JD. Development communication and participation: Applying Habermas to a case study of population programs in Nepal. *Commun Theor*. 2004;14(2):99-121.

15. Sood S, Shefner-Rogers C, Skinner J. Health communication campaigns in developing countries. *J Creativ Commun*. 2014;9(1):67-84.

16. Storey D, Figueroa ME. Towards a global theory of health behavior and social change. In: Obregon R, Waisbord S. eds. *The Handbook for Global Health Communication*. Hoboken, NJ: Wiley Blackwell; 2012:70-94.

17. Braithwaite DO, Baxter LA. Introduction: meta-theory and theory in interpersonal communication research. In: Baxter LA, Braithwaite DO, eds. *Engaging Theories in Interpersonal Communication: Multiple Perspectives*. Thousand Oaks, CA: Sage; 2008:1-18.

18. Padela AI, Rodriguez del Pozo P. Muslim patients and cross-gender interactions in medicine: an Islamic bioethical perspective. *J Med Ethics*. 2011;37(1):40-44.

19. Rudy S, Tabbutt-Henry J, Schaefer L, McQuide, P. Improving client-provider interaction. *Population Reports*. 2003;31(4). INFO Project: Center for Communication Programs, Johns Hopkins Bloomberg School of Public Health.

20. Sood S, Cronin C. *C4D Approaches to Address Violence Against Children: A Systematic Review*. New York, NY: UNICEF; 2015.

21. Harman JJ, Kaufman MR, Khati Shrestha D. Evaluation of the "Let's Talk" safer sex intervention in Nepal. *J Health Commun Int Perspect*. 2014;19:970-979.

22. Fisher JD, Fisher WA. Changing AIDS-risk behavior. *Psychol Bull*. 1992;111(3):455-474.

23. Kaufman MR, Harman JJ, Khati Shrestha D. Let's Talk About Sex: development of a sexual health program for Nepali women. *AIDS Educ Prev*. 2012;24(4):327-338.

24. Institute of Statistics, Institute of Public Health [Albania], ICF Macro. *Albania Demographic and Health Survey 2008–09*. Tirana, Albania: Institute of Statistics, Institute of Public Health, and ICF Macro; 2010.

25. Zazo A, Dragoti E, Karaj T, Volle J. *Albania Family Planning: Improving Access to and Use of Modern Contraceptive Methods Among Young Men and Women*. Washington DC: C-Change; 2011.

26. Wallerstein N. What is the evidence on effectiveness of empowerment to improve health? World Health Organization; 2006. http://www.euro.who.int/__data/assets/pdf_file/0010/74656/E88086.pdf. Accessed April 2014.

27. Shiavo R. *Health Communication: From Theory to Practice* (2nd ed.). San Francisco, CA: Jossey-Bass; 2014.

28. Minga Peru. http://mingaperu.org/. Accessed April 2014.

29. Sengupta A, Elias E. Women's health and healing in the Peruvian Amazon Minga Peru's participatory communication approach. In: Obregon R, Waisbord S, eds. *The Handbook of Global Health Communication*. Maklem, MA: John Wiley & Sons; 2012:488-506.

30. McKinley MA, Jensen LO. In our own voices: reproductive health radio programming in the Peruvian Amazon. *Crit Stud Media Commun*. 2003;20(2):180-203.

31. Rist G. *The History of Development: From Western Origins to Global Faith*. P. Camiller, trans. New York, NY: St. Martin's Press; 1997.

32. Coates EA, Waisbord S, Awale J, Solomon R, Dey R. Successful polio eradication in Uttar Pradesh, India: the pivotal contribution of the Social Mobilization Network, an NGO/UNICEF collaboration. *Glob Health Sci Pract*. 2013;1(1):68-83.

33. Spina A. *The Scrutinize Campaign: A Youth HIV Prevention Campaign Addressing Multiple and Concurrent Partnerships*. Arlington, VA: USAID AIDS Support and Technical Assistance Resources, AIDSTAR-One Task Order 1; 2009.

34. Fishbein M, Ajzen I. *Belief, Attitude, Intention and Behavior: An Introduction to Theory and Research*. Reading, MA: Addison-Wesley; 1975.

35. Ajzen I. The theory of planned behavior. *Organ Behav Hum Dec*. 1991;50:179-211.

36. Witte K. Putting the fear back into fear appeals: the extended parallel process model. *Commun Monogr*. 1992;59:329-349.

37. Gurman TA, Rubin SE, Roess AA. Effectiveness of mHealth behavior change communication interventions in developing countries: a systematic review of the literature. *J Health Commun*. 2012;17:82-104.

38. Institute of Statistics Directorate (NSD) [Timor-Leste], Ministry of Finance [Timor-Leste], ICF Macro. *Timor-Leste Demographic and Health Survey 2009–10*. Dili, Timor-Leste: NSD and ICF Macro; 2010.

39. Health Alliance International. *Maternal and Newborn Health and Mobile Phone Utilization in Manufahi and Ainaro districts: Baseline Survey of Knowledge, Practices, and Coverage Survey for the Mobile Moms/Liga Inan Program Extended Report September 2012*. Seattle, WA: Health Alliance International; 2012.

40. Health Alliance International. *Spotlight May 2013: The Lina Inan Project Timor-Leste*. Seattle, WA: Health Allicance International; May 2013. http://www.ligainan.org/media/Liga-Inan-case-study.pdf. Accessed January 10, 2017.

41. Health Alliance International. *Liga Inan Program Preliminary Results: Follow-up Phone Calls with Enrolled Women from Sub-district Same. August 2013*. Seattle, WA: Health Alliance International; 2013.

42. Singhal A, Rogers EM. The status of entertainment-education worldwide. In: Singhal A, Cody MJ, Rogers EM, Sabido M, eds. *Entertainment-Education and Social Change*. Mahwah, NJ: Lawrence Erlbaum Associates; 2004:3-20.

43. Singhal A, Obregon R, Rogers, EM. Reconstructing the story of *Simplemente Maria*, the most popular telenovela in Latin America of all time. *Int Commun Gaz*. 1995;54:1-15.

44. Soul City. http://www.soulcity.org.za/. Accessed November 2014.

45. Moyer-Gusé E. Toward a theory of entertainment persuasion: explaining the persuasive effects of entertainment-education messages. *Commun Theor.* 2008;18:407-425.

46. Moyer-Gusé E, Nabi RL. Explaining the effects of narrative in an entertainment television program: overcoming resistance to persuasion. *Hum Commun Res.* 2010;36:26-52.

47. Storey D, Sood S. Increasing equity, affirming the power of narrative and expanding dialogue: the evolution of entertainment-education over two decades. *Crit Arts.* 2013;27(1):9-35.

48. Bandura A. *Social Learning Theory.* Englewood Cliffs, NJ: Prentice Hall; 1977.

49. Sood S, Menard T, Witte K. The theory behind entertainment-education. In: Singhal A, Cody MJ, Rogers EM, Sabido M. eds. *Entertainment-Education and Social Change.* Mahwah, NJ: Lawrence Erlbaum Associates; 2004:117-149.

50. Papa MJ, Singhal A, Law S, et al. Entertainment-education and social change: an analysis of parasocial interaction, social learning, collective efficacy, and paradoxical communication. *J Health Commun.* 2000;50(4):31-55.

51. Sood S. Audience involvement and entertainment-education. *Commun Theor.* 2002;12(2):153-172.

52. Fishbein M, Yzer MC. Using theory to design effective health behavior interventions. *Commun Theor.* 2003;13(2):164-183.

53. Rimal R. Modeling the relationship between descriptive norms and behaviors: a test and extension of the theory of normative social behavior. *Health Commun.* 2008;23:103-116.

54. Sood S, Riley AH, Mazumdar PD, Chowdary N, Malhotra A. From awareness-generation to changing norms: implications for entertainment-education. *Cases Public Health Commun Market.*; 2015;8:3-26.

55. Indian readership survey. http://mruc.net/sites/default/files/irs_2013_topline_findings.pdf. Accessed 2013.

56. UNICEF. An entertainment-education initiative on television: a glimpse into the production process. 2014. https://www.comminit.com/files/kyunkiprodbook_final.pdf. Accessed April 2015.

57. UNICEF. *Facts for Life* (4th ed.). http://www.factsforlifeglobal.org/index.html. Accessed April 2015.

58. Kelly K, Parker W, Hajiyiannis H, Natlabati P, Kincaid, DL, Do M. Tsha: *Key Findings of the Evaluation of Episodes 1-26.* South Africa: CADRE; 2005.

59. Salem RM, Bernstein J, Sullivan TM, Lande R. *Communication for Better Health. Population Reports,* Series J, No. 56. Baltimore, MD: INFO Project, Johns Hopkins Bloomberg School of Public Health; 2008.

60. Shefner-Rogers C, Sood S. Involving husbands in safe motherhood: effects of the "Suami SIAGA" campaign in Indonesia. *J Health Commun.* 2004;9(3):233-258.

61. Mobilizing for Impact. Indonesia's SIAGA campaign promotes shared responsibility. 2004. http://ccp.jhu.edu/documents/Mobilizing%20for%20Impact-Indonesia%20SIAGA%20campaign%20promotes%20Shared%20Responsibility.pdf Accessed April 2015.

62. Sood S, Sengupta M, Shefner-Rogers C, Palmer A. Impact of the SIAGA maternal and neonatal communication campaign on knowledge of danger signs and birth preparedness in West Java, Indonesia. *J Health Mass Commun.* 2009; 1 (1-2): 40-57.

63. Sood S, Chandra U, Palmer A, Molyneux I. *Measuring the Effects of the SIAGA Campaign in Indonesia with Population Based Survey Results.* Baltimore, MD: JHPIEGO; 2004. http://pdf.usaid.gov/pdf_docs/PNADA613.pdf. Accessed April 2015.

64. Soul City. Soul City 4: *Theory and Impact (Synopsis).* South Africa: Soul City Institute; 2001. http://www.soulcity.org.za/research/evaluations/series/soul-city/soul-city-series-4/theory-and-impact. Accessed April 2015.

65. Usdin S, Scheepers E, Goldstein S, Japhet G. Achieving social change on gender-based violence: a report on the impact evaluation of Soul City's fourth series. *Soc Sci Med.* 2005;61:2434-2445.

66. Toubia N. Female circumcision as a public health issue. *N Engl J Med.* 1993;331(11):712-716.

67. World Health Organization. *Eliminating Female Genital Mutilation: An Interagency Statement.* Geneva, Switzerland: World Health Organization; 2008.

68. Babalola S, Brasington A, Agbasimalo A, Helland A, Nwanguma E, Onah N. Impact of a communication programme on female genital cutting in eastern Nigeria. *Trop Med Int Health.* 2006;11(10):1594-1603.

69. Howard-Grabman L, Snetro G. *How to Mobilize Communities for Health and Social Change: A Field Guide.* Baltimore, MD: Johns Hopkins Bloomberg School of Public Health, Center for Communication Programs; 2003.

70. Tsuyuki K. Community mobilization and empowerment around postabortion care in Bolivia. *Post Abortion Care in Action.* 2005;7.

71. Bracht N, Rice RE. Community partnership strategies in health campaigns. In: Rice RE, Atkin CK, eds. *Public Communication Campaigns.* Los Angeles, CA: Sage; 2013:289-304.

72. Helland A, Babalola S. Strategic communication changes norms, intentions related to FGC in Nigeria. *Communication Impact!* 2005;18.

Glossary and Common Abbreviations

Many of the words used in health communication and informatics have "real-world" meanings that are somewhat different from their meanings in the healthcare context. The definitions in this glossary are based on *our* jargon. Unless otherwise indicated, these definitions are adapted from *CDCynergy*, the NCI "Pink Book," or other resources in the public domain such as those created by the U.S. Department of Health and Human Services (DHHS) or Environmental Protection Agency (EPA). If a definition refers to a specific organization (e.g., the Advertising Council), the definition usually comes from that organization's website. Definitions marked with an *come from the American Marketing Association's online dictionary (http://www.marketingpower.com /layouts/Dictionary.aspx).

A

Acculturation 1. The learning of the behaviors and morals of a culture other than the one in which the individual was raised. For example, acculturation is the process by which a recent immigrant to the United States learns the American way of life. 2. The process by which people in one culture or subculture learn to understand and adapt to the norms, values, lifestyles, and behaviors of people in another culture or subculture.*

ACME Framework ACME (Activities, Context, Motivation, Enabling Technology) is a model that organizes the major principles of health campaign design, implementation, and evaluation. ACME also explicates the relationships and linkages between the varying principles. Insights from ACME include the following: The choice of audience segment(s) to focus on in a campaign affects all other campaign design choices, including message strategy and channel/component options.

Action theory A theory that guides the development of health promotion interventions by spelling out concepts that can be translated into program messages and strategies. Action theory is different from causal theory, in that causal theory helps you understand the contributing factors to a health problem, while action theory guides what you do about the problem. Also referred to as change theory or theory of action.

Activities Methods used within a channel to deliver a message. The activity of holding training classes to help seniors start their own walking clubs is an example of using a community channel.

Address A unique identifier for a computer or online site, usually a URL (uniform resource locator) for a website, which is marked with an at symbol (@) for an email address. An address is how your computer finds a location on the information superhighway.*

Adopters The people who take up a new behavior. Rogers classified responders into five groups according to the sequence of their adopting the change: (1) innovators (the first 2-5%); (2) early adopters (the next 10-15%); (3) early majority (the next 35%); (4) late majority (the next 35%); (5) laggards (the final 5-10%).

Advertisement Any announcement or persuasive message placed in mass media via paid or donated time or space by an identified individual, company, or organization.*

Advertising Council A nonprofit organization devoted to development and placement of public service media in the United States. Its legacy includes the following campaigns: Smokey the Bear's "Only you can prevent forest fires," the "Tearful Indian" campaign against pollution, the crash-test dummies for motor safety, "A Mind Is a Terrible a Thing to Waste," (for the United Negro College Fund), and more recently, "Buzzed Driving Is Drunk Driving." Website: http://www.adcouncil.org.

Advocacy Any attempt to influence public opinion and attitudes that directly affect people's lives. An individual can act on his or her own to advocate for a particular cause or belief, or may be part of a highly organized network of individuals joined by a common cause. Media advocacy amplifies an issue so that it is heard. Advocacy attempts to bring an issue up to a decision-making level, be it for one school, a community, or an elected official.

Affect 1. The feelings a person has toward an attitude object such as a brand, advertisement, salesperson, or something else. Affect is growing in importance in attempts to understand and predict consumer behavior. 2. The affective response itself, including emotions, specific feelings, and moods that vary in level of intensity and arousal.*

Anthrax A serious infectious disease caused by gram-positive, rod-shaped bacteria known as *Bacillus anthracis*. Rarely, people contract anthrax through contact with infected animals or contaminated animal products. Anthrax spores can remain infectious for years, and have been used as a weapon.

Anthropology The study of humans, past and present. To understand the full sweep and complexity of cultures across all of human history, anthropology draws upon knowledge from the social and biological sciences as well as the humanities and physical sciences.[1] Anthropologists use ethnographic methods to understand the deep cultural meaning of human behavior in a specific context, be it spatial or temporal.

Appeal A message quality that can be tailored to one's target audience(s); the motivation within the target audience that a message strives to encourage or ignite (e.g., appeal to love of family, appeal to the desire to be accepted by peer group, fear appeal).

App Short for application; typically, a program on a cell phone or computer that enables the user to perform a certain function or access information.

Ask Me 3 A patient education program designed to promote communication between healthcare providers and patients so as to improve health outcomes. The program encourages patients to understand the answers to three questions: "What is my main problem?", "What do I need to do?", and "Why is it important for me to do this?" It is maintained by the National Patient Safety Foundation.[2]

Association 1. Statistically, an observed relationship or statistical dependence between two or more events, characteristics, or variables. Association is broader than correlation and not equal to causality. 2. A type of organization.

Association of Schools and Programs of Public Health (ASPPH) The organization that represents the Council on Education for Public Health (CEPH)-accredited schools of public health located in North America. ASPPH promotes the efforts of schools of public health to improve the health of every person through education, research, and policy. Based upon the belief that "you're only as healthy as the world you live in," ASPPH works with stakeholders to develop solutions to the most pressing health concerns and provides access to the ongoing initiatives of the schools of public health. Website: http://www.aspph.org/.

ATSDR U.S Agency for Toxic Substances and Disease Registry (part of U.S. Department of Health and Human Services).

Attitude An individual's predisposition toward an object, person, or group, which influences his or her response to be either positive or negative, favorable or unfavorable.

Attribute (product attribute) The characteristics by which products are identified and differentiated. Product attributes usually comprise features, functions, benefits, and uses. These characteristics are not equivalent to the *benefits* of the product, which are perceived by the consumer.

Audience The people (or person) to whom communication(s) are directed. See also *primary audience, secondary audience*, and *target audience*.

Audience profile A formal description of the characteristics of the people who make up a target audience. Some typical characteristics useful in describing segments include media habits (magazines, TV, newspaper, radio, and Internet), family size, residential location, education, income, lifestyle preferences, leisure activities, religious and political beliefs, level of acculturation, ethnicity, ancestral heritage, consumer purchases, and psychographics.

Audience segment(s) A group of people who are enough alike on a set of predictors that one can develop program elements and communication activities that will likely be equally successful with all members of the segment, be it a school, a community, or an elected official.

Audience segmentation Division of a large group of people into smaller, more homogeneous groupings based on shared characteristics. Used to tailor messages and improve communication.

Average quarter-hour (AQH) persons The average number of persons listening to a particular station for at least 5 minutes during a 15-minute period.

B

Baby boomers Children born during the period from the end of World War II (1946) through the early 1960s (1964), when the number of births increased significantly, resulting in a population surge. An "echo boom" began in 1975 when the baby boomers began to have their own children. (See *Generation Y* and *Millennials*.) In between the "Boomers" and Generation Y is the group referred to as Generation X.

Backgrounder A relatively short document or oral presentation of essential information designed to help an audience understand or take action on a policy or issue.

Bandwidth The amount of information (text, images, video, sound) that can be sent through an Internet connection, expressed in bits per second (bps). A full page of text is approximately 16,000 bits. A fast modem can move approximately 15,000 bits in 1 second. Transfer of full-motion full-screen video requires approximately 1-10 million bps, depending on resolution and compression.*

Banner ad A graphical Internet advertising tool. Users click on the graphic to be taken to another website. The term "banner ad" refers to a specific size of image, measuring 468 pixels wide and 60 pixels tall (i.e., 468 × 60), but it is also used as a generic description of all graphical ad formats on the Internet. *

Barriers Hindrances to the desired change, which may be factors external or internal to audience members themselves (e.g., lack of proper healthcare facilities or the belief that fate causes illness and is inescapable).

Baseline study The collection and analysis of data regarding a target audience or situation prior to implementation of an intervention. Generally, baseline data are collected to provide a point of comparison for an evaluation.

Behave framework A simple and widely used framework for describing an audience, a behavioral change, a motivation, and a mechanism for change; it was developed by the Academy for Educational Development (AED).

Behavior The overt act(s) or action(s) of an individual or group, which can be directly observed.

Behavior change theory A theory based on research and experience that are used to systematically explain and/or predict behavior. Theories show relationships between concepts or variables, such as attitudes, beliefs, personal characteristics, and social and environmental factors, called constructs.

Behavioral belief Expectancies about positive or negative outcomes related to performing a behavior. Behavioral beliefs lead to formation of attitudes.

Behavioral lever The crucial, rate-limiting step in a complex behavior that makes it impossible for a person to perform a desired behavior or, alternatively, a facilitating step (or resource acquired) that allows the remaining steps to follow in sequence without further thought.

Belief A term that encompasses knowledge, opinion, or faith. Also the perceived association between two concepts. A belief can also be synonymous with knowledge or meaning because all of these terms refer to consumers' interpretations of important concepts. Unlike an attitude, a belief is always emotionally or motivationally neutral.*

Beneficiary The person or group of people who would benefit most directly from an intervention. Sometimes the audience and the beneficiary are the same. Sometimes others are asked to act on behalf of a third-party beneficiary, as when mothers are asked to adopt behaviors that benefit their children.

Benefit The value provided to a customer by a product feature. It is the consumer's perceptions that define a benefit.

Best practices A loosely defined term that refers to interventions or strategies that have been evaluated and found to be effective in more than one trial. When sufficient evidence exists of adequate quality, these solutions are referred to as evidence-based interventions. The term "best practices" indicates that less high-quality evaluation data are available, but the practice is recommended based on its cost, ease of use, or other criteria.

Bioethics The branch of ethics, philosophy, and social commentary that discusses the life sciences and their potential impact on our society. A set of principles or guidelines that are based on bioethics can articulate and assess ethical and moral dilemmas.

Bioterrorism The deliberate use of viruses, bacteria, or other biological agents by those wishing to cause illness or death in people, animals, or plants, thereby causing widespread fear, panic, and terror.

Blog Short for "Web log"; a hybrid form of Internet communication that combines a column, diary, and directory. It comprises a frequently updated collection of short articles on various subjects with links to further resources.

Bounce-back cards Preprinted, preaddressed, prepaid postcards distributed with program materials. Recipients are asked to respond to a few simple questions about the materials and then return the postcards by mail.

Branding Like a cattleman's mark, a brand symbolizes "ownership" of a product. When communications are branded, it usually means they carry the same iconography, color palette, logo, slogans, or other identifying marks to indicate their source. The term "brand" has also taken on the meaning of a reputation, or even a promise made to a consumer who associates a level of quality with a particular brand.[3]

BRFSS Behavioral Risk Factor Surveillance System; a surveillance system managed by the Centers for Disease Control and Prevention that assesses and tracks health behavior, risk behavior, and health status in the population through state-based phone interviews.

Broadcast quality The media industries' standards for material that can be aired. Technical format and content are both aspects of broadcast quality. Publicity submissions that are not broadcast quality generally will not be used.*

B-roll Videotaped footage that is not included in the final edited version of a video news release (VNR). B-roll is given to television stations along with the VNR to give the stations the option of putting together their own versions of the story, giving more time to aspects that a station feels will be of particular interest to its viewers.*

C

Case-control study A study that involves collecting data, often through surveys, about past exposures among a population with some type of health issue (e.g., "cases" with a disease or condition), and comparing these data with similar data collected from a comparable control group without the disease or condition.

Case study An epidemiologic description used in the classroom that is based on real-life outbreaks and public health problems. Each case study usually begins with the recognition of the problem and proceeds to slowly reveal more information about the problem. Periodic open-ended questions are used to highlight important aspects of the investigation and provoke discussion and exchange of ideas among classroom participants.

Causal theory A theory that describes the factors that influence a behavior or situation and identifies why a problem exists. Causal theory guides the search for modifiable factors such as knowledge, attitudes, self-efficacy, social support, or lack of resources. Also referred to as problem theory, explanatory theory, or theory of the problem.

Causality A relationship that answers the question, "Does A (thing) cause B (disease)?" Bradford Hill's nine criteria of causality have been widely used and adapted since 1965 in epidemiologic research.

CDC See *Centers for Disease Control and Prevention*.

CDCynergy A software tool developed at the Centers for Disease Control and Prevention (CDC) designed to help program planners develop and implement health communication programs. Website: http://www.cdc.gov/healthmarketing/cdcynergy/.

Centers for Disease Control and Prevention (CDC) The U.S. government agency dedicated to protecting health and promoting quality of life through the prevention and control of disease, injury, and disability. CDC is an operational unit of the U.S. Department of Health and Human Services.

Central-location intercept interviews A method used for pre-testing messages and materials. It involves "intercepting" potential intended audience members at a highly trafficked location (such as a shopping mall), asking them a few questions to see if they fit the intended audience's characteristics, showing them the messages or materials, and then administering a questionnaire of predominantly closed-ended questions. Because respondents form a convenience sample, the results cannot be projected to the population. Also called mall intercept interviews.

CERC Crisis and emergency risk communication. A term coined by the CDC that describes the process of communicating about risk with various publics during a complex emergency. It has been a key element in the CDC's cooperative agreements with state, local, territorial and tribal health departments for health emergency preparedness. See also *ERC*.

Channel The conduit or route of information delivery (e.g., interpersonal, small group, mass media).

Clear Communication Index A research-based tool to help health communicators develop and evaluate public communication materials.

Click-through rate The ratio of number of clicks on a specific link to the number of viewers of an online website page.

Clinical preventive services Services that can prevent disease or detect disease early, when treatment is more effective. These services include screenings for chronic conditions, immunizations for diseases such as influenza and pneumonia, and counseling about personal health behaviors.

Clinician–patient communication (CPC) The face-to-face communication between healthcare providers and their patients.

Cochrane Reviews Systematic reviews of the scientific literature that typically examine the effects of interventions for prevention, treatment, and rehabilitation in a healthcare setting, which are designed to facilitate the decision making of doctors, patients, policy makers, and others in the healthcare arena. Most of these reviews are based on randomized controlled trials, but other types of evidence may also be considered, if appropriate. Reviews are published in the Cochrane Library, by the Cochrane Collaboration, which is a global network of volunteers. Website: http://community.cochrane.org/cochrane-reviews.

Cognitive interviews A popular method for evaluating survey questions that offers a detailed depiction of meanings and processes used by respondents to answer questions.

Cohort studies Studies of a group of individuals for whom data are collected prospectively (i.e., going forward) or for whom historical data of some type exist (i.e., retrospective or looking backward). Data are examined for changes over time, such as whether there are changes in one subgroup exposed to some sort of "treatment," or stimulus, (e.g., a chemical in an occupational environment) compared with an unexposed subgroup.

Communication How people use messages to generate meanings within and across various contexts, cultures, channels, and media.[4]

Communication theory A theory that explores how messages are created, transmitted, received, and assimilated. When applied to public health problems, the central question that a theory of communication seeks to answer is, "How do communication processes contribute to, or discourage, behavior change?"

Community A group of persons joined together for a common purpose, be it geographical, social, or cultural, or because they share and want to discuss an illness, a condition, or a hobby. Such a group can exist in real space and time, or in virtual settings using communication channels, such as the Internet. In public health, the term "community" usually refers to participation in, and/or ownership and management of, an intervention by geographically local residents.

Community-Based Organization (CBO) An organization that offers services at a community level and usually, but not always, does so without a profit motive. CBOs often serve a larger geographic area than one neighborhood.

Community Guide The *Guide to Community Preventive Services*; a free resource offering systematic reviews that answer these questions: Which program and policy interventions have been proven effective? Are there effective interventions that are right for my community? What might effective interventions cost, and what is the likely return on investment? Reviews are prepared by the Task Force on Community Preventive Services, an independent body of researchers and practitioners supported by the CDC. Website: http://www.thecommunityguide.org/index.html.

Community of Inquiry (CoI) framework A collaborative learning experience developed by using a combination of social, cognitive, and teaching elements. It has roots in the work of 19th-century philosopher C. S. Pierce, who said that truth is what the community of observers ultimately come to believe.

Community-led approaches Communication strategies that address public health issues across the community level of the ecological model.

Competence The observable (measurable) characteristics of a skill or ability.

Competency A standardized requirement for an individual to properly perform a specific task.

Competition In social marketing, what the intended user is doing now, or using now, instead of the behavior or product promoted to improve the user's health. Sometimes this is just using brand X over brand Y; at other times, it is using a rock as a hammer, or teeth as scissors, or sugary soda in place of low-fat milk.

Comprehension The degree to which transmitted messages are understood; it can be estimated qualitatively ("low comprehension") or measured quantitatively (30% comprehension).

Comprehensive e-health research framework A framework that defines different stages of e-health programs and then applies evaluation theories to each of these stages to develop a comprehensive evaluation tool.

Comprehensive report A type of research synthesis on a health topic developed by a variety of different organizations or groups, performed for various purposes, and using different ways to synthesize and interpret the scientific literature. These documents are sometimes developed by expert panels or working groups, and may conclude with clinical, policy, or other guidelines or recommendations for individuals, organizations, or policy makers.

Concept An idea that can be communicated symbolically or artistically for discussion, sometimes referring to something whole or something new.

Concept testing The process of exposing representatives of the target audience to creative interpretations of ideas on which you might base your message. This process usually requires qualitative research, such as focus groups.

Confirmation bias Interpretation of messages so that they confirm what we already believe (e.g., "He only hears what he wants to hear").

Consensus (scientific) Agreement by a body of scientists about the best or optimal strategy in a particular situation for which definitive data are not available; it may be based on a meta-analysis, independent studies, or other forms of comparative research.

Consumer Traditionally, the ultimate user or consumer of goods, ideas, and services, but may also include the buyer or decision maker. A mother buying cereal for consumption by a small child is often called the consumer, even though she may not be the ultimate user of the product.*

Consumer-generated media (CGM) Websites that are created using Web 2.0 technologies (such as blogs, wikis, and social networking sites) and that often use their membership to generate at least a portion of the site's content. Also referred to as user-generated content (UGC) or user-created content (UCC).

Control belief The belief of an individual that he or she has some measure of control over his or her life and especially health issues; a positive factor in improving health behavior. See also *self-efficacy*.

Convenience sample A collection of respondents/participants in research studies who are typical of the target audience and are easily accessible. No attempt is made to collect a probability sample, and convenience samples are not statistically representative of the entire population being studied. Therefore, findings from studies using convenience samples are not generalizable.

Core elements The essential drivers of behavior change that must be preserved despite any adaptation of the model to fit local needs.

Correlational studies Studies that seek to determine whether a correlation between variables exists. Variables that have similar patterns of temporal and spatial occurrence are said to be associated; the degree of association is quantified by the correlation coefficient, r, whose value ranges from -1.0 to 1.0. Since a causal relation between two variables always results in a correlation coefficient significantly distant from zero, lack of correlation implies lack of causation. Unfortunately, the reverse is not true; variable correlation may be due to external factors affecting both variables. For example, sales of salt and snow shovels are seasonal, so they are correlated but not causally related.

Creative brief A document that includes information that will be needed by a creative team to develop concepts and messages. The brief contains information about the primary target audience as well as settings, channels, and activities for reaching the members of that audience. Promising message variables and thoughts on which materials will be needed are included. Secondary audiences are also profiled.

Credibility A quality that contributes to the ability of a messenger to be trusted by the recipient of the message. Components of credibility include whether the message source is considered trustworthy, believable, reputable, competent, and knowledgeable.

Cross-sectional studies Studies that involve collecting data from subjects at one time, the most typical cross-sectional study being a survey. The major drawback of this type of study design is that data are collected on potential exposures and outcomes at the same time, making it difficult to determine if exposures actually *preceded* the potential outcomes of interest.

Culturally and linguistically appropriate services A term developed to provide a commonunderstanding and consistent definition of culturally and linguistically appropriatehealthcare services. Such services were proposed as one means to correct inequities in theprovision of health services and to make healthcare systems more responsive to the needs of all clients.

Culture The acquired knowledge people use to interpret experience and generate behavior (James Spradley). Culturally constructed phenomena are any experiences that we shape by our perceptions, values, attitudes, and beliefs. We take many things for granted as "natural" that are actually cultural constructions, such as definitions of sickness and health.

Customer journey A series of orbits that a customer engages in when considering, evaluating, advocating for, or purchasing a specific product.

D

Data mining Also called data or knowledge discovery; the process of analyzing data from different perspectives and summarizing them into useful information—that is, information that can be used to increase revenue, cuts costs, or both.[5]

Delivery (assessment) The functioning of components of program implementation; it includes assessment of whether materials are being distributed to the right people and in the correct quantities, the extent to which program activities are being carried out as planned and modified if needed, and other measures of how and how well the program is working. Sometimes referred to as process evaluation.

Delphi method A small-group research technique that seeks a consensus among experts through sequential rounds of data collection and reduction.

Demographics Individual descriptors such as sex, age, ethnicity, income, or education that can be collected from a target audience; they can be useful for defining the target audience and understanding how to communicate more effectively with the target audience.

Deontological principles Ethical or moral principles that can be used to guide behavior (e.g., the golden rule, do the right thing, do the least harm, respect the individual).

Description In journalism, providing the basic facts of who, what, where, and when. Answering "why" and "how" questions often gets into explanation or interpretation.

Diffusion of innovations A theory developed by E. Rogers that addresses change in a group (e.g., a classroom, an organization, or a community) rather than an individual over time. According to this theory, new ideas (or innovations) are spread within the group via different communication channels within social systems over a specific time period. Also see *adopters*.

Direct costs That part of the budget which contributes directly to a program's outputs; includes personnel costs (salary and benefits) as well as "out-of-pocket" costs associated with products and services not obtained through a salaried employee.

Document literacy The ability to understand text presented in tables, forms, graphs, or other structured formats. Contrasts with the ability to understand "prose," which is text written in sentences and paragraphs.

Doer/non-doer analysis Formative research technique that involves identifying individuals performing a desirable behavior, and finding out how and why they are doing it. These "doers" are compared to individuals not performing the behavior, to see if their experiences can be promoted to the others to inspire them to also adopt the behavior. The anthropological concept behind this marketing term is "positive deviance."[4]

Downstream intervention An intervention that attempts to modify conditions for individuals at the narrowest or latest point of entry in the ecological model.

Downstream stories A term used in social or health policy to describe influencing community dynamics, or facilitating individual behavior change as a point of intervention. (See also *upstream intervention*.) Also refers to a story about a project that is complete for advocacy purposes.

E

Earned media Usually mass-media coverage of a story that is earned through public service methods. While no money changes hands between the sponsor and the media broadcast company, there is usually an agency that develops and helps place the story either for a fee or *pro bono*.

Ebola Also known as Ebola virus disease (EVD) or Ebola hemorrhagic fever; a severe and often fatal disease in humans. The time interval from infection with the virus to onset of symptoms is 2 to 21 days. Humans are not infectious until they develop symptoms. First symptoms are the sudden onset of fever fatigue, muscle pain, headache, and sore throat. This is followed by vomiting, diarrhea, rash, symptoms of impaired kidney and liver function, and, in some cases, both internal and external bleeding.

Ecologic studies Studies that typically seek to correlate or compare two types of population-level data. While they can be valuable for generating hypotheses (e.g., smoking prevalence tends to be higher in areas where populations have lower socioeconomic status), they can produce misleading results because data correlation does not mean causation.

Ecological model A public health model that assumes health and well-being are affected by *interactions* among multiple determinants, including biology, behavior, and the environment. Interactions unfold over the life course of individuals, families, and communities. An ecological *approach* to health is one in which multiple strategies are developed to impact determinants of health relevant to the desired health outcomes.

Ecology The study of the relations among living species and their physical and biotic environments, particularly adaptations to environments through the mechanisms of various systems.

EEG See *electroencephalography*.

Effectiveness The ability of an intervention to produce the desired beneficial effect in a real-world setting (in contrast to *efficacy*); usually refers to the performance of a drug taken by patients in a nonconstrained situation.

Effects evaluation A measure of the extent to which a program accomplished its stated goals and objectives. Also called impact, outcome, or summative evaluation.

Efficacy The ability of an intervention to produce the desired beneficial effect in expert hands and under ideal circumstances; usually refers to the performance of a drug in a controlled trial.

eHealth "The intersection of medical informatics, public health and business, referring to health services and information delivered or enhanced through the Internet and related technologies. In a broader sense, the term characterizes not only a technical development, but also a state-of-mind, a way of thinking, an attitude, and a commitment for networked, global thinking, to improve health care locally, regionally, and worldwide by using information and communication technology."[6]

Elaboration likelihood model (ELM) A model that suggests if people are already engaged in an issue, they will pay more attention to new information about this issue. If not engaged, communicators will need to use peripheral stimuli to grab the attention of an audience.

Electroencephalography (EEG) A diagnostic method (or research tool) that measures the electrical charge generated when neurons are activated in the brain. By placing electrodes on a person's scalp, the electrical signals can be detected and amplified for analysis. Different brain waves measure different brain processes.

Enabling factors Part of PRECEDE analysis. These factors are largely structural, such as the availability of resources, time, or skills that allow someone to perform a behavior.

Engage/inform/persuade paradigm A health communication model that begins by recognizing three main goals—to attract and involve members of the target audience, to provide accurate and accessible health information, and to encourage knowledgeable, healthy behavior—and evaluates the effectiveness of communication programs by measuring the extent to which these goals are attained.

Engaging content Content that encourages the recipient to be interested, interact, and get involved.

Entertainment-education The process of purposely designing and implementing a media message to both entertain and educate… [and] a communication strategy to bring about behavioral and social change.

Environmental Protection Agency (EPA) The federal agency formed in 1970 that protects human health and the environment by regulating and enforcing laws passed by Congress. Website: http://www3.epa.gov/.

EPA See *Environmental Protection Agency*.

ERC Emergency risk communication; the process of communicating about hazards and risks during an emergency. It involves three stages: planning, implementation, and follow-up evaluation. See also *CERC*.

Ethnography 1. A type of study conducted by cultural anthropologists, who investigate a group of people and their life-ways. 2. The published study.

Ethnolinguistic techniques Analytical techniques derived from anthropology that focus on the meaning and categorization of words. They are most often used to understand domains of cultural understanding such as about health, child care, and diet, so as to develop culturally appropriate recommendations.

Evaluation Assessment of an intervention that compares what was expected to what was observed. Types of evaluation include formative, delivery/implementation, cost/benefit, exposure/reach, effects, and theory-based evaluation.

Evidence-based intervention An intervention that has been tested in several different settings and has demonstrated both efficacy and effectiveness.

Executive summary An overview of a project, evaluation, or research findings, which is generally presented at the beginning of a report and which highlights such issues as which activities took place, why a study was conducted, how it was carried out, and what the results and recommendations are.

Experimental study A study in which the researchers "expose" some group of subjects (e.g., people or animals) to some type of intervention, and then compare their results with the results for a group of unexposed subjects that is generally similar to the exposed population.

Expert review Examination and critique of program plans or materials by selected people who are knowledgeable in a relevant content area.

Exposure Contact by a person or animal with a chemical or physical agent.

Exposure (media) The extent to which a message was disseminated (e.g., how many members of the target audience encountered the message); a part of process evaluation. This type of evaluation does not measure whether audience members paid attention to the message or whether they understood, believed, or were motivated by it.

Extended parallel process model (EPPM) A model based on the explanatory mechanism of Leventhal's parallel process model (PPM) with Roger's protection motivation theory (PMT) focusing on what makes fear appeals work. Specifically, the EPPM utilizes the PMT linkages among perceived levels of severity, susceptibility, response efficacy, and self-efficacy that lead to message acceptance and, ultimately, attitude, intention, and behavior changes.

External validity One criterion by which an experiment is evaluated; the extent—that is, which populations and settings—to which the observed experimental effect can be generalized.

Eye tracking technology Use of a head-mounted camera and computer screens designed for this purpose to detect and measure eye movements and gaze fixation as a person looks at an image (moving or still) or text. The innate response to imminent danger or arousal causes the pupils to dilate and the blink rate to change. These parameters can be measured photographically and can be used to measure reading ease as well as a subject's interest in an image, video, or text.

F

FCC See *Federal Communications Commission*.

FDA See *Food and Drug Administration*.

Fear A mental state that motivates problem-solving behavior if the intuitive "fight or flight" options are available. If these options are not available, it motivates other defense mechanisms such as denial or suppression, which are antithetical to rational decision making.

Fear appeal Messaging that attempts to elicit a response from the target audience by using fear as a motivator (e.g., fear of injury, illness, loss of a loved one). Fear appeals were once very popular before their negative consequences were fully understood.

Federal Communications Commission (FCC) An independent U.S. government agency, overseen by Congress, that regulates interstate and international communications by radio, television, wire, satellite, and cable in all 50 states, the District of Columbia, and U.S. territories. The FCC is the United States' primary authority for communications laws, regulations, and technological innovation. Website: https://www.fcc.gov/.

Fidelity monitoring Continuous tracking of a program's implementation throughout its course to ensure the program is implemented in accordance with the core components of the original program model.

Flesch-Kincaid (F-K) Readability Test Developed for the Navy and used by the Army to assess training manuals in the 1970s, the F-K formula uses a weighted combination of the number of syllables, words, and sentences in a passage to estimate reading grade level from fifth grade through college (or reading ease, with different weighting parameters).

Focus group A formative research technique that convenes a small group of people (usually 8-10) who share certain characteristics for a discussion of selected topics. This discussion generally follows a prepared guide and is led by a trained moderator. Focus groups provide creative themes and user language. The qualitative results may be extremely useful, even though they are not necessarily representative of a larger audience, and even if the sample is not large enough to draw statistical conclusions from its data.

Folic acid A B-vitamin that is essential to human health. It is required for the body to make DNA and RNA, the blueprints for development of all cells. Folic acid is especially vital to a developing embryo because rapid cell division occurs early in fetal development. Consuming folic acid before conception and through the first month of pregnancy will prevent 50% to 75% of all neural tube defects from occurring.

Food and Drug Administration The federal agency created by the Pure Food and Drug Act of 1906, which has the power to set standards for foods and food additives, to establish tolerances for deleterious substances and pesticides in foods, and to prohibit the sale of adulterated and misbranded foods, drugs, cosmetics, and devices. All new drugs must be submitted to the FDA for approval, and applications must be supported by extensive laboratory testing indicating efficacy and safety. Website: http://www.fda.gov/.

Formative research The information-gathering activities conducted prior to developing a health communication strategy; these activities include measurement of the extent to which concepts, messages, materials, activities, and channels meet researchers' expectations with the target audience.

Fotonovela From the Spanish *foto* (= photo) + *novela* (= short novel). Fotonovelas are typically soap opera-like stories told through the use of photos of characters, with their thoughts or conversations written in "balloons" or in captions, as in comic books. This medium is very popular in role model approaches.

Framing Use of words (or sometimes images) to put a message or a data point in a desired context. For example, if your chances of winning the lottery are 1 in 1 million, a positive frame states that 1 person out of 1 million will be a big winner; a negative frame states that 999,999 people out of 1 million will lose. Different frames lead people to draw different conclusions, even when the same data are being discussed.

Framing bias Phrasing of questions or answers in a way that, while technically accurate, leads people to interpret information incorrectly.

Free listing A formative research technique in which a respondent is asked to list all examples of a particular kind of thing that they know about. For example, the researcher might ask for a list of "appropriate foods for young children," "the most important qualities in a man," or "flu-like symptoms." The researcher records these items, usually onto separate index cards.

Functional magnetic resonance imaging (fMRI) An imaging technique that measures changes in blood flow in regions of the brain by means of the increased magnetic resonance of oxygenated blood in contrast to non-oxygenated blood. This technique provides high-resolution, three-dimensional images of brain activity, including its response to different products, stimuli, or situations.

G

Gain-framed messages Messages that are designed to emphasize the advantages of performing a desired behavior.

Galvanic skin response An electrical measure of reduced skin resistance indicative of perspiration triggered by sympathetic nervous system activity related to emotion.

Gatekeepers People who have a reputation, or perceived responsibility, for upholding standards in a community; they can help support a behavior change goal if they agree with it, or prevent its adoption if they disagree. Popular clergy members, business leaders, and healthcare providers are often community gatekeepers, and it is wise to seek their input when planning an intervention.

Generalizable finding A study result from which you can make reliable inferences about a larger population of people, places, or settings similar to those included in the study sample; a finding for which all criteria for external validity have been satisfied.

Generation X Children born following the "baby boom." See also *baby boomers*.

Generation Y Children of the baby boomers; also known as Millennials. See also *baby boomers*.

Gestalt From the German *gestalt*, meaning "form or shape"; an overall impression or wholeness, with the added meaning that the whole is greater than the sum of the parts. The *gestalt effect* refers to the process whereby the brain takes in incomplete sensory data and, based on prior experience, completes it to form a perceived object; this effect is the basis for many optical illusions and some of the differences in audience perception and observer bias.

Gray literature Unpublished reports (e.g., not published in scientific journals), whose development is usually undertaken for government agencies; they are not peer reviewed but often accurate and authoritative. Such reports are commonly available on program websites or through agency resources.

GRP Gross rating point; one percentage point of a specified target audience. The total GRPs for a campaign is calculated by multiplying the reach by the average frequency, and measures the advertising weight delivered by the various media within a given time period; it is the sum of ratings from many different spots and may be more than 100% of the total target audience.*

H

Hazard The real qualitative possibility of an adverse event occurring under a specific set of conditions. Generally, hazard = danger. See also *toxicity* and *risk*.

Headline The top component of a newspaper, magazine, or online article, or a print advertisement, that is meant to attract the reader's attention and provide a very brief summary of the information.

Health A state of complete physical, mental, and social well-being, and not merely the absence of disease or infirmity.[7]

Health 2.0 The use of social software and its ability to promote collaboration among patients, their caregivers, medical professionals, and other stakeholders in health.

Health behavior An action performed by an individual that can negatively or positively affect his or her health (e.g., smoking, exercising).

Health Belief Model (HBM) A model that was first developed to explain individual public health behaviors, such as participation in free tuberculosis screening programs. In the HBM, individual beliefs—specifically, about perceived susceptibility, perceived severity, perceived benefits of interventions, perceived costs of interventions, cues to activate behavior change, and perceived ability to act (self-efficacy)—motivate or discourage health behaviors.

Health communication The study and use of communication strategies to inform and influence individual and community decisions that enhance health. See also *public health communication*.

Health literacy The ability to understand and use complex health information.

Health-related quality of life (HRQoL) A broad multidimensional concept that usually includes self-reported measures of physical and mental health.

Healthcare environment The milieu in which health care takes place, including facilities, lighting, ambient sound, personnel, finance, scheduling and access, communication channels, education, family, and cultural care.

Healthy People 2020 (HP2020) The key U.S. government strategy for monitoring public health activities, which measures progress in population health through large trends, such as increased life expectancy and decreased chronic disease prevalence.

Heuristic A simplified "rule of thumb" by which decisions are made.*

Hierarchy of effects (HOE) model A model developed by McGuire, in which a "source" sends information out to a "receiver." This process leads to the lower-level effects of exposure, attention, interest, and comprehension, as well as a higher-order set of effects including acquisition of skills, changes in attitude, short-term retention of information, long-term retention of information, decision making, one-time performance of a behavior, reinforcement of the behavior, and maintenance of the behavior indefinitely through complex life changes.

HTML Hypertext Markup Language; a coding language used to create documents for use on the web. HTML resembles old-fashioned typesetting code, where markup tags surround a block of text (e.g., <html>, <title>Title Text </title>) that indicate how it should appear. Importantly, HTML allows "hyperlinking" of text to another location or file on the Internet.*

I

ICA See *International Communication Association*.

Image Consumers' perception of a product, institution, brand, business, or person, which may or may not correspond with "reality" or "actuality." For marketing purposes, the "image of what is" may be more important than "what actually is."*

Immediate outcomes Results of program activities that occur and can be measured directly after completion of the activity.

Impact The ultimate effect of the program on the problem or condition that the program or activity was supposed to address.

Impact evaluation Generally an assessment of health results, and not behavioral change. See also *effects evaluation*.

Impression A single view or display of an advertisement. Ad reports list total impressions per ad, which comprises the number of times an ad was served by the search engine when searchers entered the keywords (or viewed a content page containing the keywords). Also called media impression.*

IMR See *infant mortality rate*.

Inbound marketing A marketing approach that brings customers/clients/patients in by attracting attention, fostering interest, and improving accessibility.

Incentives Motivating factors that increase the likelihood that a desired health behavior will be demonstrated.

In-depth interviews A qualitative research method involving a one-on-one discussion between an interviewer and a respondent about selected topics. The structure and interviewing style are more flexible than that in surveys using a questionnaire.

Indirect costs Also called "overhead"; the expenses that an agency must pay simply to exist, but that are not tied directly to creating a program's outputs. Examples usually include office space, environmental management (e.g., heat, air conditioning, water, custodial services), and depreciation of equipment. Indirect costs are usually calculated as a percentage of direct costs.

Infant mortality rate The number of deaths of children younger than one year of age per 1000 live births in the same year. IMR = 1000 × infant deaths / live births.[8]

Informatics "The effective organization, analysis, management, and use of information."[9]

Information processing theory The mental processes by which consumers interpret information from the environment to make it meaningful and integrate that information to make decisions; a communication theory that focuses on how the mind receives, stores, retrieves, and uses information, addressing, for example, the mental processes by which consumers interpret and integrate information and use it in decision making.

Informed consent The means by which a researcher provides information to potential participants about a study (especially about potential risks involved) and those participants' ability to agree to participate in the study based on this information. Studies involving human subjects need to be reviewed by institutional review boards (IRB) for this purpose ("IRB approval").

In-kind contributions In the nonprofit world in which public health often operates, organizations' time, space, use of equipment, and other in-house resources. These resources, considered inputs to a project's budget, are used to produce program outputs but are not factored into the direct or indirect costs of the budget. Some donors may expect to see a match made of their investment through direct financial funds, in-kind resources, or additional donations.

Inoculation theory A theory that explains how people may resist unwanted persuasion attemptsby preparing counterarguments in advance.

Integrative model (IM) An evolved version of Ajzen and Fishbein's theory of reasoned action (TRA). The most important assumption of the IM is that the best predictor of behavior is *intention* to perform the behavior. Thus, this model focuses on the antecedents, or predictors, of an individual's intention to perform (or not perform) a behavior.

Intention A cognitive plan to perform a behavior or action ("I intend to go shopping later"), created through a choice/decision process that focuses on beliefs about the consequences of the action.*

Intercept interview A survey in which respondents are intercepted on the street, at an event, in a shopping mall, or in another public space.

Intermediate outcomes Results or outcomes of program activities that must occur prior to the final outcome in order to produce the final outcome.

International Communication Association (ICA) An academic association for scholars interested in the study, teaching, and application of all aspects of human and mediated communication. ICA began more than 50 years ago as a small association of U.S. researchers and now has more than 4500 members in 80 countries (https://www.icahdq.org/).

Interpersonal channel A communication channel that involves dissemination of messages through one-on-one communication (e.g., mentor to student, friend to friend, pharmacist or doctor to patient).

Interrupted time-series study Long-term serial observations of a population, interrupted by a health intervention and continued thereafter; such a study can be used to estimate the effect of an intervention on absolute values of a group of observations and to see the effect on trends or rate of change in the data.

Interval scale A scale marked by equal intervals, a yard stick, for example. The distance (interval) between two values in one region of the scale meaningfully represents the same distance between two values in another region of the scale (e.g., length, temperature, age).[8]

Involvement The degree of personal relevance a consumer perceives a product, brand, object, or behavior to have. High-involvement products are seen as having important personal consequences or as useful for achieving important personal goals for the consumer. Low-involvement products are not linked to important consequences or goals.*

J

JIC See *Joint Information Center*.

Joint Information Center (JIC) Either a physical or "virtual" operation in which public information staff representing all agencies and organizations involved in incident management activities coordinate and disseminate official, timely, accurate, easy-to-understand, and consistent information to the public. The National Incident Management System (NIMS) includes procedures that specify the responsibilities and operations of a JIC. State and local emergency response departments and agencies should be familiar with NIMS procedures and have plans in place for establishing or operating within a JIC.[10]

Joke Something that some people find funny. Humor must be used cautiously in health communication because people vary so greatly in what they find funny. Also, what seems funny in a small group may be interpreted very differently by the audience of a large media campaign. Use humor at your own risk, and at the risk of message misinterpretation.

JPEG Joint Photographic Experts Group; a compressed graphics format, newer than GIF, that displays photographs and graphic images with many colors and is easy to download. Also called JPG; both JPEG and JPG are pronounced "jay peg."

K

Key informants Persons or organizations whose opinions can be seen as representative of a community or target audience because of their experience or expertise with the target audience.

Keyword stuffing The act of adding extra keyword terms into the HTML or tags of a webpage beyond those needed represent the content and for the sole purpose of attracting viewers.*

L

Landing pages Those pages on a website on which visitors arrive from somewhere else (e.g., an ad, a link). Within the realm of marketing and advertising, landing pages are used to generate further action by a visitor, either "clicking through" to another part of the website or gathering data by means of a form.[11]

Latent need Something that you did not realize you needed; a marketing concept that refers to stimulating desire in a consumer for a product.

Leading causes of death This usually refers to the top 10 causes of death in a population, such as a state, country, or age group. In 2013, the leading causes of death in the United States were, in descending order: heart disease, cancer, chronic lung disease, accidents, stroke, dementia, diabetes, influenza/pneumonia, kidney disease, and suicide.

Leading health indicators A subset of *Healthy People 2020* objectives that have been selected to communicate high-priority health issues and the actions that can be taken to address them.

LEP See *limited English proficiency*.

Life expectancy The number of years a person is expected to live. The average for all U.S. residents in 2013 was 78.8 years.

Likert-type scales Three- to ten-point numerical rating scales used in surveys to quantify subjective feelings or judgments. A 3-point scale might be a good choice for a simple yes/no/unsure question. Five-point bipolar scales are widely used because reproducible test-retest values can often be obtained: 5 = strongly agree, 4 = agree, 3 = neither agree or disagree, 2 = disagree, 1 = strongly disagree. Ten-point scales are typically used for serial rating of pain intensity: "How bad is your pain on a scale of 1 to 10?"

Limited English proficiency (LEP) Inability to speak English well enough to understand instructions or questions; often (incorrectly) used to refer to people, rather than to their abilities.

Literacy The ability to use printed and written information to function in society, to achieve one's goals, and to develop one's knowledge and potential; an individual's ability to make sense of information in any form in which it is presented. While it was once sufficient to sign your name to be considered literate, this term has since acquired the larger meaning of social competence.

Living-room language Use of commonplace words and analogies to explain phenomena that are outside most persons' experience.

Logic model A visual design of how a problem will be solved through an intervention, depicting the structured flow of inputs, outputs, outcomes, and goals attained.

Long-term outcomes Permanent changes in status, environment, or behavior. Sometimes the term *impact* is used for long-term outcome changes in a population, such as a decreasing death rate.

Loss-framed messages Messages designed to emphasize the negative outcome of performing a desired behavior. Deciding whether to frame messages for gain, or for loss, can be difficult.

M

Macro plan A preliminary plan that includes the analysis of the problem, including its ecological setting, the affected populations, the core intervention strategy, and any additional research necessary to understand those persons who are affected by the problem and/or with whom you plan to communicate.

Market research The systematic gathering, recording, and analyzing of data with respect to a particular market, where "market" refers to a specific customer group in a specific geographic area.*

Materials Tangible products, using a medium, that contain the message to be delivered to the target audience (e.g., a brochure, a public service announcement video recoding, or a script for an oral presentation).

Maven A Yiddish word meaning "expert." Gladwell uses this term to describe an opinion leader in *The Tipping Point*.

Media (*sing*. medium) Any material or format used to convey a message. In health communication, predominantly print, electronic, audio, or visual media are used. Sometimes used to refer to broadcast journalism.

Media advocacy Using the mass media strategically to advance a social or policy initiative. It often involves staging events that the news media cover, including protest gatherings, release of a report or survey, or other gatherings of people who seem concerned about an issue; it may also involve use of public service announcements. In the political arena, media advocacy has become the predominant strategy, including purchased advertising.

Media alert Rapid communication to media newsrooms, usually about an upcoming event of public interest, typically in a one-page format that contains the who, what, when, where, and why of the event and contact details for more information.

Media kit A package for journalists that includes items for print or broadcast, such as press releases, contact information, camera-ready copies of print materials, video and audio formats, and a backgrounder with more in-depth information.

Media literacy "An informed, critical understanding of the mass media. It involves examining the techniques, technologies and institutions involved in media production; being able to critically analyze media messages; and recognizing the role audiences play in making meaning from those messages."[12] Improving media literacy is a health communication strategy that has been used effectively with, for example, middle school students to enable them to evaluate tobacco, food, and other advertising directed toward them as consumers.

Media relations The management of communication between an organization and its publics, primarily through the news media. In a large organization, a large group may release information to the news as well as respond to media and online questions.

Media scanning Examining media, including radio, TV, print, and Internet (search engine data, social media) sources, for signs of activity concerning a particular area of interest, a health issue, or related interventions.

Media tracking Monitoring of radio, television, and print media over a specified period, for a specific topic or message. Data gathered through these efforts can be analyzed for content or trends in amount in coverage.

Mediated communication A health communication strategy that disseminates health messages through communication platforms that can reach large populations at once, such as television, film, radio, billboards, print, computers, and telephones.

Mediators A type of third variable that helps to answer the questions how, why, or through which process, and that allows for understanding of mechanisms through which the independent (or predictor) variable affects the dependent (or outcome) variable.

Message The memorable, explanatory words or images that convey an idea; in health communication, the literal words or images that communicate what you want people to know, feel, or do.

Message map A visual framework used to organize a body of information into simple, short talking points. Message maps have been predominantly used in emergency risk communication. A typical map is directed to a specific audience (e.g., the public, emergency victims), and answers one question with a maximum of three key messages. The map provides a handy reference for a spokesperson: Multiple spokespersons can work from the same message map to ensure the rapid dissemination of consistent and core messages, and using maps minimizes the chance of a speaker saying something inap-

propriate or omitting something that should have been said. A printed message map allows spokespersons to check off the talking points as they are covered, which helps to prevent omissions of key facts or misstatements that could provoke misunderstandings, controversy, or outrage.[13]

Meta-analysis A study in which a researcher analyzes a body of published results on a specific topic. Using a set of well-defined rules for selecting studies and data sources, statistical approaches are used to pool data from multiple studies on the same topic and calculate a summary measure estimating the level of association between two variables. Meta-analyses extend the value of review articles, which may offer no pooled quantitative data. They are being increasingly used as the basis for evidence-based recommendations.

Meta-message is that part of a communication message that is not stated explicitly. It may encompass what you are "trying to say," but also refers to unexpected, even contradictory interpretations related to the receiver's personal or environmental expectations or biases.

Midstream stories Descriptions of the progress of a program already in place. Policy makers usually want to hear how funds are being used and what early results indicate about effectiveness.

Millennial generation Children born between 1982 and 2000; also known as Generation Y (following Generation X) or the "echo baby boom."

Mixed methods A research design that combines quantitative and qualitative methods, which may be sequenced or done simultaneously and triangulated.

Moderator A type of third variable that affects the magnitude and direction of change between the independent (or predictor) variable and the dependent (or outcome) variable, and that can answer such questions as when or for whom does this intervention work.

Moderator's guide A set of questions, probes, and discussion points used by a focus group moderator to help him or her facilitate the group. A guide can also contain reminders of which questions are most important to the research to help the moderator use discussion time effectively.

Morbidity Rate of disease, infirmity, or disability; often expressed as the number of cases per 1000 individuals per year.

Morbidity and Mortality Weekly Report (MMWR) Catchy title of the Centers for Disease Control and Prevention's weekly release of epidemiologic findings, special studies, or recommendations pertaining to disease and death in the United States or globally.

Mortality Rate of death, often expressed as the number of deaths per 1000 individuals per year.

N

NAALS National Assessment of Adult Literacy Survey.

National Cancer Institute (NCI) The federal government's principal agency for cancer research and training, which was established under the National Cancer Institute Act of 1937; it is a Center within the National Institutes of Health, and an operating agency within the U.S. Department of Health and Human Services. NCI oversees the National Cancer Program. Over the years, legislative amendments have maintained the NCI's authority and responsibilities and added new information dissemination mandates, as well as a requirement to assess the incorporation of state-of-the-art cancer treatments into clinical practice.[14]

National Public Health Information Coalition (NPHIC) A Centers for Disease Control and Prevention-affiliate organization whose members represent a variety of public health communication specialties, including public information and public affairs, risk communication, health promotion and marketing, community relations, social media, and communication research and evaluation.

Neuro-marketing Marketing research that uses methods and data derived from neuroscience such as electroencephalography, functional magnetic resonance imaging, and galvanic skin response, among others, to predict audience response to media and messages. See also *neuroscience*.

Neuroscience The study of the nervous system, which includes the brain, the spinal cord, and networks of sensory nerve cells (neurons) throughout the body. Neuroscientists use tools ranging from computers to special dyes to examine molecules, nerve cells, networks, brain systems, and behavior. From these studies, they learn how the nervous system develops and functions normally and what goes wrong in neurologic disorders.[15]

News peg The main point of a news release that justifies (to the media) the value of using the story. A news peg generally links the story to current events or concerns. It may be used for only a few hours or a few days, but the main news peg is timeliness.

Nielsen The self-described "world's leading marketing and media information company." Nielsen measures and analyzes how people interact with digital platforms, traditional media, and in-store environments, locally as well as globally. It has long been known for estimating the size of television audiences, with "Nielsen ratings" determining which shows stay on the air or are discontinued.

Nominal scale Classification into unordered qualitative categories (e.g., race, religion, country of birth).[8]

Normative beliefs Perceptions about what others are doing or thinking about a health behavior or issue; part of the integrative model, along with behavioral beliefs and control beliefs. Effective health communication interventions need to consider, and may need to address, these antecedent beliefs.

Numeracy The ability to think and express oneself quantitatively. In reference to health literacy, it encompasses the knowledge and skills required to estimate quantities from food labels, use a glucometer or thermometer correctly, measure medicine doses, or perform any other mathematical operation necessary for non-health professionals to manage their own or a loved one's health care or wellness.

O

Objective The desired result to be achieved by a specific time, such as for a health program or communication campaign. In health communication, an objective is more specific than a program goal. SMART objectives are specific, measurable, actionable, relevant (or realistic), and time bound.

Observational study A study in which individuals are observed in a natural setting with minimal observer interaction (e.g., observing shoppers in a grocery store to see if they are reading posted nutritional charts).

Op-ed An opinion editorial that consists of a statement or short essay submitted to a new editor (e.g., at a newspaper) by an individual or representative of an organization. Historically, these pieces were printed in a newspaper on the page opposite the editorial page—hence the name "op-ed."

Open-ended questions Questions that are worded to avoid prompting, and that encourage an individual to respond freely in his or her own words.

Opinion leader The most influential member of a group; the one to whom others turn for advice and information, and who wields greater personal influence on the attitudes, opinions, and behavior of others.*

Ordinal scale Classification into ordered qualitative categories (e.g., a Likert scale from strongly disagree to strongly agree, or from 1 to 5). While there is a distinct order $(3 > 2 > 1)$, there is no measured distance between the possible values of the categories.[16]

Outcome The degree to which objectives are reached in a program; can be a behavior change or acquisition of an antecedent state (i.e., change in knowledge.)

Output The end product of an effort, such as a report written, personnel trained, immunizations delivered, and so on.

P

Page view A request to load a single HTML page from a website; often used as a measure of website traffic.

Partners Individuals or organizations/agencies that contribute to the efforts initiated by a leader or head organization/agency. Partners can have a variety of roles (e.g., contribute research data, share evaluation experience, help to spread the health message).

Past medical history (PMH) A dated list of prior medical care, hospitalizations, treatments, and diagnoses obtained as part of the medical history (Hx), typically obtained during a patient visit. Other parts of the classical medical history are as follows: CC = chief complaint; HPI = history of present illness; PMH = past medical history; ROS = review of systems (sometimes SR = system review, referring to detailed questioning about each of the body systems); Meds = present medications; SH = social history (e.g., drug use, occupation, marital status, travel, pets); FH = family history. While this sequence is useful for preparing a medical report, it should not be used as an outline for obtaining the history but rather applied later in the process to supplement the narrative history.

Patient-centered health communication A style of communication in which the clinician or caretaker is responsive to patient needs and incorporates the patient's perspective and experiences in care planning and decision making.

Patient-centered medical home (PCMH) A cooperative healthcare setting that focuses on the patient, facilitates partnerships between healthcare facilities, individual patients and their personal physicians and, when appropriate, the patient's family. Electronic sharing of health-related information is a key feature.

Patient–provider communication (interaction) (PPC) The interpersonal, often face-to-face communication between a healthcare provider and a patient.

People and places model of social change Maibach's model, which asks, "What about the people, and what about the places, needs to be happening for those people (and those places) to be healthy?" Forces that affect people at the individual, social network, community, or population level are referred to as "people fields of influence"; those that are linked inextricably to location, at a local level, or a higher administrative level (state, nation, world), are referred to as "place fields of influence."

Performance objective An intervention mapping term that defines exactly what you hope the recipient of an intervention will do.

Peripheral cue A symbolic reference valued by the intended user of content that does not deal directly with the subject matter, but rather is used to capture attention.

Peripheral route to persuasion A key component of the elaboration likelihood model. In the peripheral route, the consumer does not focus on the central message in an ad (or other material), but rather on other stimuli such as attractive or well-known celebrities or popular music. The presence of these other stimuli may change the consumer's beliefs and attitudes about the information or product.*

Personal health record (PHR) A document containing information about an individual's health that is compiled and maintained by that individual. It differs from the medical record, which contains information about an individual's health compiled and maintained by a healthcare provider.[17] The PHR may be maintained in print or in an online form.

Personal medical record See *personal health record.*

Persuasion Convincing someone to perform a desires behavior. In health communication, also referred to as "behavior change communication."

PESO model A model originating in public relations; refers to Paid, Earned, Shared, and Owned media channels or content.

Pile sorting A rapid technique for organizing cards or other visual indicators into groups of like and unlike, often used in ethnography to explore categories and relationships of items according to another person's worldview. Also called card sorting.

Pilot test A trial of a marketing package or health communication intervention in its entirety in a limited location. Results are used to fix problems before a large-scale launch, or to make a "go/no go" decision.

Pink Book Nickname for the National Cancer Institute's publication *Making Health Communication Programs Work,* because the original printed cover was bright pink.

PIO See *public information officer.*

Point-of-purchase (POP) Promotional materials placed at the immediate area where a consumer will select an item, or complete a purchase (e.g., in retail store), which are designed to attract consumer interest or call attention to a special offer.

Policy communication Research, analysis, and reporting activities designed to inform decision makers about a specific issue.

Policy maker Anyone who makes a decision that affects others; in this text, chiefly elected officials (e.g., city council members, state legislators, U.S. representatives and senators) or key appointed staff members in organizations.

Poll An inquiry into public opinion conducted by interviewing a sample or panel of people, and usually designed to be representative of the population. Examples include the Harvard Opinion Research Program,[18] Quinnipiac University polls on social and political phenomena, and Gallup[19] and Harris Interactive[20] polls.

Portal A website featuring a suite of commonly used services, serving as a starting point and frequent gateway to the web (web portal) or a niche topic (vertical portal).*

Positive deviance An anthropological approach that is based on the identification of successful behaviors or practices of the most successful members of a group (the positive deviants) in an area or population that is largely unhealthy or unsuccessful at negotiating the environment. This is an excellent first step in promoting successful behavior in the group as a whole and is the basis of the doer/non-doer model.

Practice strategy In intervention mapping, the way that a theory-based method is delivered in an intervention (see *theory-based methods*). An example of a practice strategy is the use entertainment-education (a method informed by social cognitive theory) to deliver role modeling messages.

Precaution adoption process model (PAPM) A stage-based model that predicts how an individual will adopt or refuse a risk-reduction intervention. The stages are (1) unaware of the issue, (2) aware of the issue, (3) deciding what to do, (4) planning to act, (5) deciding not to act, (6) acting, and (7) maintenance.[21] The PAPM is very similar to the Transtheoretical Model, apart from having a stage of deciding not to act entirely.

PRECEDE-PROCEED model Developed by Green, Kreuter, and associates in the 1970s, a model that works backward from a desired state of health and quality of life, and asks what about the environment, behavior, individual motivation, or administrative policy is necessary to create that healthy state.[22] PRECEDE stands for Predisposing, Reinforcing, Enabling Constructs in Educational/ Environmental Diagnosis and Evaluation; PROCEED stands for Policy, Regulatory, and Organizational Constructs in Educational and Environmental Development. PRECEDE-PROCEED has nine steps: (1) social assessment, (2) epidemiologic assessment, (3) behavioral and environmental assessment, (4) educational and ecological assessment, (5) administrative and policy assessment, (6) implementation, (7) process evaluation, (8) impact evaluation, and (9) outcome evaluation.

Predisposing factors The group of factors included in the educational diagnosis stage of the PRECEDE model; existing beliefs, attitudes, and values (e.g., cultural or ethical norms) that influence whether a person will adopt a behavior. See also *enabling factors* and *reinforcing factors*.

Press release An outreach document prepared for news outlets and designed to make reporters aware of an issue or topic.

Pretesting A type of formative research that involves systematically gathering target audience reactions to messages and materials before those messages and materials are produced in final form.

Primary audience The group of people most affected by a problem, and usually the individuals whose attitude, knowledge, intent, or behavior you hope to change. See also *audience segmentation*.

Propensity score/propensity score mapping (PSM) The use of statistical methods (e.g., logistic regression) to estimate the likelihood of subjects falling into a treatment group based solely on known preexisting factors. Propensity scores are used to reduce the confounding effect of prior factors when comparing treatment and control groups; they can be helpful when randomized control trials are too small to include blocks for each relevant factor.[23]

Prose literacy The ability to read simple, ordinary, or complex sentences and paragraphs; part of the National Assessment of Adult Literacy Survey (NAALS) scoring of adult literacy.

Prospect theory A theory developed by Tversky and Kahneman, which posits that people make decisions based on the potential of loss or gain rather than the probable outcome. The prospect of loss carries more weight than that of gain. Often people will take risks to avoid a loss, but avoid taking a risk for a possible gain, i.e., people are risk averse unless there is something to lose.

PSA See *public service announcement*.

Public domain Any information or media that are not under copyright to any person or entity. These materials and text can be reproduced and used without obtaining permission from the producer or paying fees or royalties. Unless specifically stated otherwise, items produced by the U.S. federal government, or employees of the federal government, are in the public domain.

Public health communication An integrated cycle of health data collection, interpretation, and communication to support public health objectives.

Public health informatics The systematic application of information and computer science and technology to public health practice, research, and learning.

Public information officer (PIO) The lead communications person for an organization or agency who is responsible for engaging with the media and other publics.

Public relations The methods and activities employed in persuading the public to understand and regard favorably a person, business, or institution.

Public service announcement (PSA) A form of advertising that is typically aired or published without charge by the host channel; can be in print, audio, or video form.

Q

Qualitative research Investigation that collects information from individuals or groups in greater depth, or in more nuanced ways, than quantitative methods allow. In mixed methods work, it is commonly used to generate hypotheses for quantitative research studies. After a quantitative research study is completed, a qualitative method is often used to help explain findings. Focus groups, in-depth personal interviews, and "Photovoice" are commonly performed types of qualitative research.

Quality of life A sense of well-being about a person's or society's way of life and lifestyle, often estimated by social indicators. Major factors that influence quality of life include income, wealth, safety, recreation facilities, education, health, aesthetics and leisure time.*

Quantitative literacy The ability read, understand, and use numbers and calculations in activities of daily living.

Quantitative research A research design that counts, measures, and statistically analyzes items from a defined collection (data set). In communication, quantitative research is often conducting using surveys to obtain responses to closed-ended questions on knowledge, attitudes, beliefs, and behaviors.

Quasi-experimental A research design that assigns individuals to receive an intervention or remain unexposed, but without random assignment. Pre- and post-intervention assessments are often made. This design is used when it is impossible to do random assignment.

R

Random sample A sample of respondents in which every individual in a defined population has a known chance of being included in the sample.

Randomized controlled trial (RCT) A type of study in which research participants are randomly assigned to be either exposed to a program intervention(intervention group) or not exposed (control group). The same series of tests are performed (or questions asked) before and after the intervention to facilitate comparison. Pre/post group differences are analyzed statistically to detect changes related to the intervention. The RCTs is considered to be the "gold standard" research method.

Rank order Placing a series of values in an ordered list, typically from lowest to highest; used as a nonparametric approach (e.g., Spearman's rank-order correlation) to measure correlation between two ranked variables when conditions for "standard" (e.g., Pearson's product moment) correlation are not met.

Readability testing Applying a formula to written materials to predict the approximate reading grade level that a person must have achieved to understand the material.

REALM Rapid Estimate of Adult Literacy in Medicine; a widely used tool for estimating health literacy. See also *TOFHLA*.

RE-AIM A framework for Assessing Reach, Effectiveness, Adoption, Implementation, and Maintenance of an intervention; developed by Glasgow while at Kaiser Permanente.

Recall The extent to which respondents remember seeing or hearing a message that was shown in a competitive media environment; usually centers on main idea or copy recall. See also *unaided recall*.

Recurring costs Those costs for planning, implementing, and evaluating health communication efforts that occur at regular intervals (e.g., salaries, utility bills).

Reducing complexity An important step in improving health literacy, medication adherence, and access to health care.

Reinforcing factors A set of factors in the PRECEDE model that encourage or discourage adoption of a behavior; they include family and community approval or discouragement.

Resources (Inputs) The first consideration in the logic model of health communication, followed by activities, outputs, outcomes, and impact.

Risk The *quantitative* likelihood of an adverse event occurring under a specific set of conditions; a function of probability. See also *hazard* and *toxicity*.

Risk perception Individual beliefs about the level of health risk associated with a particular behavior, exposure, or treatment.

Rothschild's behavioral management model A model contrasting perceived costs and benefits against education, marketing, and law as influencing behaviors.

Rough A mock-up of a print advertising layout or an early version of a television storyboard prepared by art directors and copywriters to help them visualize the advertising idea and discuss it with others in the advertising agency, and sometimes with clients.

RSS Rich Site Summary or Really Simple Syndication; an Extensible Markup Language (XML) format for distributing news headlines on the web. Also known as syndication.*

Run-of-press (ROP) The positioning of ads anywhere within the pages of a newspaper or magazine as the staff of the publication prepares the various pages for printing. In contrast, advertisers pay premium prices so that ads will be placed in specific locations in a magazine or newspaper.*

S

SARS Severe acute respiratory syndrome.

Saturation 1. A message's ability to gain wide coverage and high frequency, which enables it to achieve the maximum impact. 2. In qualitative research, the point in data collection at which no new information is uncovered about a specific topic.

Science A body of knowledge learned through systemic study using agreed-upon methodologies by others in the same field, and which attempts to discover generalized truths about phenomena using hypotheses and deductions.

Screener An instrument containing short-answer questions used in the recruitment process for research methods such as focus groups and central location intercept interviews. Interviewees' answers to the questions determine who is and who is not eligible to participate in the research.

Search engine optimization (SEO) The organization of website content to include items that will result in higher page placement by automatic Internet search algorithms (e.g., Google, Yahoo, DuckDuckGo).

Secondary audience A group(s) of individuals who can help reach or influence the intended audience segment (primary audience). These audience(s) should be identified through profiles created for the primary audience(s). See also *audience segmentation*.

Secondary research A research method that obtains, synthesizes, and analyzes existing data related to the problem or population.

Selective exposure Limiting media exposure to channels that offer information and opinions with which an individual agrees.

Self-administered questionnaires Forms designed to be completed by the respondent without assistance; they can be distributed by mail, distributed in person, or programmed into a computer enabling respondents to enter answers electronically.

SEO See *search engine optimization*.

Setting A location or environment where the target audience can be reached with a communication effort (e.g., a grocery store where audience members can be reached with educational pamphlets).

Share The percentage of those listening to radio in a geographic area who are listening to a particular radio station. [AQH persons to a station / AQH persons to all stations] × 100 = Share (%).

Sigma encoding A process in which an electronic device is attached to each video of a public service announcement (PSA) sent to a television station. When the PSA is aired, a signal is sent to a central location where records are kept on when, where, and how often the PSA appears.

Small-group channel A communication channel in which messages are disseminated at the small-group level (e.g., meetings on health topics, cooking demonstrations).

SMART objectives See *objectives.*

SMOG Index Simple Measure of Gobbledegook; an index of readability developed by H. McLaughlin in England in 1969. See also the Fog Index[24] and the Flesch Formula.[25]

Smokefree.gov A website that provides free, accurate information and assistance to help individuals quit smoking and stay tobacco-free; it is sponsored by the Centers for Disease Control and Prevention.

Social cognitive theory (SCT) Developed by Bandura, a theory that hypothesizes individual behavior is the result of constant interaction between the external environment and internal psychosocial characteristics and perceptions; this idea has been dubbed reciprocal determinism. SCT includes numerous constructs, such as self-efficacy, which have migrated into other theories as well.

Social marketing "The design, implementation and control of programs aimed at increasing the acceptability of a social idea, practice *[or product]* in 1 or more groups of target adopters. The process actively involves the target population who voluntarily exchange their time and attention for help in meeting their needs as they perceive them."[26] In this context, "social marketing" does *not* refer to the use of social media, or social causes, to promote commercial products and services—though such use in common in other contexts.

Socio-cultural competence The ability to understand and relate to behavioral patterns that are determined in part by membership in racial, ethnic, and social groups. This term is used to emphasize the major role of social factors (e.g., age, income, education, living circumstances) in successful patient–provider communication. (Cultural competence should have the same meaning but often is limited to gender, ethnic, and nationality issues by common usage.)

SOCO form A news briefing preparation form that asks for the single overriding communication objective (SOCO) in one sentence, a few sentences, and a paragraph. Originated by the CDC's Division of Media Relations for authors publishing in CDC's *Morbidity and Mortality Weekly Report.*

Source credibility The perceived trustworthiness of a source of scientific information assessed along two dimensions: (1) individual scientists and their respective institutions, and (2) the publication or publisher of the information. The credibility of individual researchers is based on their prior research, their reputation within their field among other scientists, and the institution where they work.

Stages of Change Model A model based on specific thought and action stages through which individuals move when modifying or adopting a new behavior. See also *Transtheoretical Model.*

Strategy A systematic plan of action that leads to accomplishment of a goal; it may encompass several activities.

Stratify To arrange the population at large into subpopulation groups that can be targeted for an intervention; a technique often used in data analysis to compare outcomes by groups.

Style A message quality that can be tailored to the target audience(s); it includes such issues as presenting cartoon figures versus detailed graphs, or using flowery, embellished text versus short, pithy text.

Suitability assessment of materials A tool that rates how difficult it is to read words and understand their meaning based on criteria such as content, literacy demand, graphics and layout, learning stimulation and motivation, and cultural appropriateness.

Summative evaluation In time-limited interventions, an assessment of a program's impact on measurable outcomes, such as behavior change or associated health measures. See also *effects evaluation.*

Surgeon General's Report (SGR) The Surgeon General serves as the United States' top health communicator by providing Americans with the best scientific information available on how to improve their health and reduce the risk of illness and injury. Official publications of the Office of the Surgeon General include the SGR, Calls to Action, and other documents. SGRs tend to be thorough (and therefore lengthy) summaries of scientific findings, and may provide policy recommendations; they often set a course of action for the U.S. Public Health Service.

Surveillance systems Data collection systems established at national, state, and local levels to record and monitor events or assess trends in health statistics.

Survivorship care planning Identifying and prioritizing cancer survivorship needs with a goal of advancing cancer survivorship public health efforts.

Sustainability Meeting the needs of the present generation without compromising the ability of future generations to meet their own needs.

SWOTE analysis A plan developed in the 1960s for assessing a program's internal strengths and weaknesses and its external opportunities and threats (SWOT). In this text, we have added an "E" for ethical assessment.

Systematic review A review of scientific studies on a specific topic using pre-defined rules to select studies for inclusion or exclusion; it identifies relevant studies, assesses their quality, and summarizes the evidence.

T

Tailored health communication (tailoring) Custom fitting a health communication material or message to an individual, or group of individuals, needs based on information about that individual or individuals. It is often based on theoretical constructs such as readiness stage, health beliefs, and self-efficacy; demographic factors; factors specific to a health behavior or condition; and name(s) or other personal information deemed relevant to the intervention.

Talking points Prepared notes used by a speaker to guide his or her presentation.

Target audience In health communication, the person or persons who are the intended recipients of specific messages. These people often share critical features in common, such as demographic factors, risk behaviors, or roles to play in enabling or facilitating change for others.

Targeted health communication The use of demographic, cultural, or other group references in the communication media or channel strategy to reach specific audiences. For example, MTV and BET cable television networks are often used to target communication messages to reach youth and African American audiences, respectively. Church-based outreach to promote breast cancer screening among older African American women is another targeted channel strategy. Billboards and print advertising frequently feature models of recognizable ethnicities, sex, and age to appeal to target market segments. (In the past, this practice was often called "tailoring," until truly individualized communication became feasible through the Internet and informatics applications.)

Teach-back A way to make check to see if a healthcare provider explained information clearly to an individual in a clinical setting; asking patients (or family members) to explain—in their own words—what they need to know or do, in a caring way (not as a test or quiz).

Tertiary audience A group that affects the behavior of an intermediate audience, which in turn may affect a primary audience, e.g., for a desired behavior change. The "public at large" is often considered a tertiary audience in communications directed to patients (as primary audiences) and providers or caregivers (as secondary audiences).

Test market The geographically limited area in which a new or modified product, service, or promotion is tested, usually with all strategy elements in place. Test marketing is usually the last step in a "fail early, fail small" strategy before taking an intervention to scale. See also *pilot test*.

Theater testing A research method in which a large group of people (60-100, and sometimes as many as 300) are gathered in a theater-style setting to view and respond to audiovisual materials such as newly commercials or public service announcements. Alternative audiovisual materials that are not being tested are also shown to provide realism and to see how memorable the test materials are by comparison.

Theoretical constructs Discrete concepts or elements that build a theory. They can stand alone (much like atomic elements), but they are most effective when used in relation with the other elements (or constructs) of the entire theory. (Water is to theory as hydrogen and oxygen are to constructs.)

Theory-informed method An intervention mapping term that describes translation of a behavior change theory into an action. An example is the use of "vicarious learning" (learning from another's experience) to promote constructs from social cognitive theory. A practice strategy delivers this method in an intervention.

Theory of Reasoned Action (TRA) A theory that states individual performance of a given behavior is primarily determined by a person's intention to perform that behavior.[27,28] This intention is determined by two major factors: the person's attitude toward the behavior (i.e., beliefs about the outcomes of the behavior and the value of these outcomes) and the influence of the person's social environment or subjective norm (i.e., beliefs about what other people think the person should do, as well as the person's motivation to comply with the opinions of others).

Time-series study A study in which pre- and post-intervention measures are collected multiple times from members of the intended audience. Evaluators use the pre-intervention data points toproject what would have happened without the intervention and then compare theprojection to what did happen using the post-intervention data points.

TOFHLA Test of Functional Health Literacy in Adults; a widely used tool for estimating health literacy. See also *REALM*.

Tone A message quality referring to the manner of expression along chiefly emotional lines (e.g., a fatherly tone, an alarming tone, a friendly tone).

Total budget The sum of direct and indirect costs, including in-kind contributions and other donations.

Toxicity The intrinsic ability of a substance to cause adverse health effects. For example, lead is a toxic substance for humans, but brief exposure to a block of lead is not hazardous and presents a very low health risk. Chronic ingestion (through paint chips) or inhalation of lead (gasoline prior to removal of lead) is very hazardous and presents a high risk of anemia and brain damage.

Trademark A distinctive symbol, picture, or word(s) that identify a specific product or service; it is obtained through registration with the U.S. Patent and Trademark Office.

Traffic The number of visitors a website receives, measured by examination of web logs* and often by use of a proprietary program such as Google-based Adsense.

Transactional model of communication A graphic representation used to clarify the collaborative and ongoing message exchange between individuals, or an individual and a group of individuals.[29] A communicator encodes (e.g., puts thoughts into words and gestures), then transmits the message via a channel (e.g., speaking, email, text message) to the other communicator, who then decodes the message (e.g., take the words and apply meaning to them). The message may encounter noise (e.g., any physical, psychological, or physiological distraction or interference), which could prevent the message from being received or fully understood as the sender intended.*

Transtheoretical Model (TTM) A model developed by Prochaska and Di Clemente, in which individuals move through a specific process when deciding whether to change, and then actually change, their behavior.[30] This model includes five stages: precontemplation, contemplation, preparation, action, and maintenance.

Trialability A marketing term reflecting the extent to which a product can be tried and tested by the consumer (e.g., free samples in supermarkets, airplane toiletries, small-size products).

Twitter "A real-time short messaging service that works over multiple networks and devices" and is connected to the web.

U

UGC User-generated content. See *consumer-generated content*.

Unaided recall In survey research, when the respondent states a fact, name, or message without prompting from the researcher (e.g., a list is not read); considered the strongest form of message recall.

Unique selling proposition/point (USP) An approach to developing an advertising message that concentrates on the uniquely differentiating characteristic of the product that is both important to the customer and a unique strength of the advertised products when compared to competing products.* It emphasizes benefits over costs.

Upstream intervention An intervention that is directed at the source of a problem, the broadest or earliest point of entry.

Upstream story A type of success story that highlights a project that is needed or just developing.

URL Uniform resource locator; the location of a resource on the Internet. This term is often used interchangeably with "domain" and "web address."

Usability testing A research step in the design and launch of a website where users evaluate the ease of use of the website's navigation, layout, and other attributes.*

User-centered design A structured product development method that involves users throughout all stages of materials and message development. Involving users ensures that products and information are more likely to meet their needs and preferences.

Uses and gratifications theory A theory that suggests media users play an active role in choosing and using the media, take an active part in the communication process, and are goal-oriented in their media use. A media user is posited to seek out the media source that best fulfills their needs. Uses and gratifications theory assumes that users have alternative choices to satisfy their needs.[31]

USP 1. United States Pharmacopeia; a nongovernmental, official public standards–setting authority for prescription and over-the-counter medicines and other healthcare products manufactured or sold in the United States. It also sets widely recognized standards for food ingredients and dietary supplements. 2. The University of the Sciences in Philadelphia; a private university with a programmatic emphasis on health and science. Formerly the Philadelphia College of Pharmacy and Science. 3. See *unique selling proposition*.

Utilitarianism The theory that decisions should be judged by their consequences. The goal is to maximize the net utility for all parties involved in a decision.

V

Value 1. The perception that benefits outweigh costs; 2. Belief(s) widely shared by members of a culture about what is desirable or good (thrift, free speech, or honesty) and what is undesirable or bad (arson, bigotry, or deceit). 3. Within the behavior change context, values are the important, enduring ideals or beliefs that guide behavior within a culture or for a specific person. If an individual accepts a value, it can become a major influence on his or her behavior.

Value proposition The sum total of benefits a customer is promised to receive in return for the associated payment or other value transfer.*

Video news release (VNR) A publicity device designed to look and sound like a television news story. The publicist prepares a 60- to 90-second news release on video, which can then be used by television stations as is or after further editing.*

Viral marketing A marketing strategy that facilitates and encourages people to pass along a message through social networks; it is nicknamed "viral" because it relies on a small number of people being initially exposed to a message who then pass it along to others, like a virus or disease. "Buzz marketing" is term used more often now.

W

Web 2.0 The second generation of Internet-based services, which include tools that let people collaborate and share information online, such as social networking sites, wikis, communication tools, and folksonomies.*

Website A collection of interconnected electronic "pages" available on the Internet through a specific URL and used to provide information about a company, organization, cause, or individual.*

Widget 1. A live update on a website, webpage, or desktop; it contains personalized, neatly organized content or applications selected by its user. 2. An old-school marketing term meaning the thing you are trying to sell—your product.

Wiki (from the Hawaiian *Wiki*, quick or fast) 1. A web application that allows users to add content, as on an Internet forum and allows anyone to edit the content. Also, the collaborative software used to create such a website.*

Word-of-mouth (WOM) communication Originally, the passing of information from person to person by oral communication. Now, also includes sharing information, positive or negative, about products or promotions through a social network. Viral or buzz marketing can be seen to either stimulate genuine WOM or create artificial WOM.

Worldview How people perceive their level of control over their own lives, and how they think power and wealth are distributed. Examples include fatalism, individualism, egalitarianism, and respect and trust for authority.

X

XML Extensible Markup Language; a data delivery language.

Z

Zapping (zipping) Using a remote control to change television stations when commercials appear, or to fast-forward through advertisements on video recordings. Both commercial advertisers and developers of public service announcements must take this behavior into account.

Zika According to the Centers for Disease Control and Prevention, "[a virus] that is spread to people primarily through the bite of an infected *Aedes* species mosquito. The most common symptoms of Zika are fever, rash, joint pain, and conjunctivitis. The illness is usually mild, with symptoms lasting for several days to a week. People usually don't get sick enough to go to the hospital, and they very rarely die of Zika."[32] In 2016, Zika was being considered as a causal factor in microcephaly (a birth defect in which the brain does not fully develop and the related small head size of the infant).

Zine A magazine that is published digitally on the Internet, rather than on paper. Some are mainstream, whereas others appeal to a very small niche of readers.

ZIP code A geographical classification system developed by the U.S. government for mail distribution consisting of a 5 + 4 scheme. The first 5 digits—which indicate state, county, and post office—are not very useful for targeted, demographic marketing because they cover wide areas; the plus-4 code provides a smaller, normally more economically cohesive unit.

References

1. http://www.aaanet.org/about/WhatisAnthropology.cfm
2. https://npsf.site-ym.com/?page=askme3
3. According to Judd Harner (judd@juddbranding.com), "True brands are rare. They are consistent across a full customer journey; consistently delivered over time; driven by an authentic mission (not manufactured—the Internet outs pretenders); emotionally compelling and rewarding; distinctive relative to their competitors".
4. PD Hearth: http://www.positivedeviance.org
5. http://www.anderson.ucla.edu/faculty/jason.frand/teacher/technologies/palace/datamining.htm
6. Eysenbach G. What is eHealth? *J Med Internet Res.* 2001;3(2):e20.
7. Preamble to the Constitution of the World Health Organization as adopted by the International Health Conference, New York, 19-22 June, 1946; signed on 22 July 1946 by the representatives of 61 States (Official Records of the World Health Organization, no. 2, p. 100) and entered into force on 7 April 1948. http://www.who.int/about/definition/en/print.html. Accessed January 10, 2017.
8. Last JM. *Dictionary of Epidemiology* (3rd ed.). New York, NY: Oxford University Press; 1995.
9. https://www.icahdq.org/
10. http://www.fbcoem.org/external/content/document/1528/257624/1/JICBestPractices.pdf
11. See http://unbounce.com for particularly useful definitions of Internet marketing tools.
12. Shepherd R. Why teach media literacy. *Teach Magazine.* October/November 1993. Toronto, ON: Quadrant Educational Media Services.
13. http://www.epa.gov/nhsrc/news/news040207.html
14. http://www.cancer.gov/aboutnci/overview/mission
15. http:///www.sfn.org
16. http://www.fda.gov/
17. http://www.nlm.nih.gov/medlineplus/personalmedical records.html
18. http://www.hsph.harvard.edu/horp/
19. http://www.gallup.com/home.aspx
20. http://www.harrispollonline.com/
21. Weinstein ND, Sandman PM. A model of the precaution adoption process: evidence from home radon testing. *Health Psychol.* 1992;11(3):170.
22. Green LW, Kreuter MW. *Health Promotion Planning: An Educational and Ecological Approach* (3rd ed.). New York, NY: McGraw-Hill; 1999.
23. Rosenbaum PR, Rubin DB. The central role of the propensity score in observational studies for causal effects. *Biometrika.* 1983;70:41-55.
24. Gunning, R. *The Technique of Clear Writing.* New York, NY: McGraw-Hill; 1952.
25. Flesch R. A new readability yardstick. *J Applied Psychol.* 1948;32(3):221-233.
26. LeFebvre C, Flora J. Social marketing and public health intervention. *Health Educ Qtly.* 1998;15:299-315.
27. Ajzen I, Fishbein M. *Understanding Attitudes and Predicting Social Behavior.* Englewood Cliffs, NJ: Prentice-Hall; 1980.
28. Fishbein M, Ajzen I. *Belief, Attitude, Intention, and Behavior.* Reading, MA: Addison-Wesley; 1975.
29. https://www.natcom.org/discipline/
30. Prochaska JO, & Di Clemente CC. Stage and processes of self-change of smoking: Toward an Integrative Model of Change. *Consult Clin Psychol.* 1983;51(3):390-395.
31. http://www.uky.edu/~drlane/capstone/mass/uses.htm
32. http://www.cdc.gov/zika/disease-qa.html

Index

Note: "Page numbers followed by b, f, or t indicate material in boxes, figures, or tables, respectively."

A

Academy for Communication in Healthcare (AACH), 14
advocacy
  audience questions, 145
  community-based prevention marketing (CBPM), 142
  data collections, 145
  Florida Prevention Research Center (PRC), 141
  media related tools, 145, 146b–149b
  new media advocacy, 142
  report cards, 145
  traditional media advocacy, 143
Affordable Care Act (ACA), 305
Agency for Health Research Quality (AHRQ), 13
Agency for Healthcare Research and Quality (AHRQ), 27, 161
AIDS Healthcare Foundation (AHF), 301
All-terrain Vehicles (ATVs). *See* ATV safety
Annenberg National Health Communication Survey (ANHCS), 238
anthrax, 428
Association for Measurement and Evaluation of Communication (AMEC), 266, 355
Association of Schools of Public Health (ASPH), 10
Association of State and Territorial Health Officials (ASTHO), 35
ATV safety, 44
  adolescent ATV riders, 66
  ATV crashes, 66
  develop intervention, 70–72
  implement plan, 73–74
  plan evaluation, 72–73
  plan intervention, 69–70
  problem statement, 65–67
audience, channel, message, and evaluation (ACME), 40
audience segments, 232–233

B

behavior change communication. *See* theories, models, and practice strategies
behavior change theory
  diffusion of innovations, 183
  elaboration likelihood model, 183
  health belief model, 180
  health communication/education, 68
  integrative model, 182
  on life expectancy, 5f
  precaution adoption process model, 182
  social cognitive theory, 180–182
  transtheoretical model, 180
behavioral beliefs, 183
behavioral determinants, 6b
Behavioral Risk Factor Surveillance Survey (BRFSS), 5, 19, 239
behavioral targeting, 199, 205
Breast Cancer and the Environment Research Program (BCERP), 111

C

cancer prevention care
  cancer control continuum
    detection and diagnosis, 411
    palliative care, 412
    prevention, 410–411
    survivorship, 412–413
    treatment decisions, 411
  cancer information landscape
    internet, 413
    peer groups, 414
    social media, 414
    television, 413–414
  in clinical settings
    complexity, 415
    health literacy, 415
    patient-centered care, 414–415
  goals, 410
  health literacy in
    assessments, 420
    awareness raising, 420
    building capacity, 420–421
    committee, 419
    evaluation service, 423–425
    organizational assessment, 421–423
    patient education committee, 425
    resources, 425
  information and communication, 410
  LIVESTRONG for survivors, 416
  preventing cervical cancer, 415
  shared treatment decisions, 415–416
CDC Clear Communication Index (CCI), 169
  National Violent Death Reporting System (NVDRS), 169–170
  Thimerosal, 171–172
Centers for Disease Control and Prevention (CDC)
  concepts developed for, 327b–329b
Certified Health Education Specialist (CHES), 10
Children's Health Insurance Program (CHIP), 305
Chlamydia in North Carolina County
  data presentation, 95
  development and implementation, 96
  outcome evaluation, 96
  planning, 93–94
  replicable informatics, 94–95
Cholera and Other Vibrio Illness Surveillance System (COVIS), 36
clinician-patient communication (CPC)
  acute *vs.* chronic, 393
  barriers to communication, 392b
  clinical skills, 396
  clinician-patient encounter
    anamnesis, 398
    environment, body and mind, 397–398
    listening, 398
    physical examination, 400
    progressive dialogue, 400
    respect, 397
    review and summation, 400
    story, 399

clinician-patient communication (CPC)
(*Continued*)
communication skills, 396
communicative process, 395
external issues, 397
levels, 395
modes, 395–396
tools, 396–397
conceptual framework, 392, 392f
electronic health record (EHR), 391
environmental distractions, 394, 394f
gender-based communication, 396
health *vs.* disease, 393
individual patients, 391
interpreters, 401
mind *vs.* body, 393
mutual understanding, 394
past medical history (PMH), 399
patient-centered health communication, 399
patient-centered medical home
(PCMH), 403, 403b–404b
peer-based communications, 396
power-based doctor–patient interaction, 396
prospects, 403–404
public *vs.* private, 393
review of symptoms (ROS), 399
sociocultural competence, 396
barriers, 394
dichotomies, 393
goals, 394
soul of communication, 393b
special cases
dying patient, 402–403
informed consent, 402
language barriers, 400–402
spoken communication, 395
subconscious, 395
talking *vs.* listening, 393
teach-back technique, 400, 401b
unspoken communication, 395
communication intervention
budget
direct costs, 350
indirect costs, 350
in-kind contributions, 350
total budget, 350
content pre-testing
group/individual, 335–336
higher-tech pre-testing, 341
questions, 336, 336b–337b
creative brief, 321
to concept, 326
elements of, 322–326
folic acid campaign, 323b–324b
materials designed, 330
messages, 326
pre-testing, 322
tobacco control, 324b–326b
creative concepts

CDC/folic acid campaign,
327b–328b
former smokers campaign,
329b–330b
gatekeepers, 330
pre-test, 330
effect size, 320
higher-tech pre-testing
EEGs and fMRI, 342, 345b
eye tracking, 342
galvanic skin response, 342
physiological effects testing,
341–342
pupil dilation, 342
usability testing, 341
implementation plan, 355
market research online communities
(MROCs), 335
media channels
communication strategies,
334b–335b
content management and strategy,
332–333
content-focused components,
332–333
cost-effectiveness, 334
people-focused components, 333
production value, 333
reach and scalability, 333
sustainability, 333–334
media package testing
in-situ testing, 346
pilot testing, 346
test marketing, 346
planning tools
e-cigarette use, 320–321
RE-AIM, 316, 316b–319b
SMART objectives, 319–321
timeline, 353362, 356b–357b
Tobacco Free Alachua (TFA), 320
work plan, timetable, and budget
budget, 350–353, 351b–353b
international partners, 346–347
measurement and evaluation,
353–355, 358b–359b
partner assets worksheet, 347t–349t
partner roles, 346
partnering in US, 347
planning tool, 354b
timeline, 353
communication planning framework
approaches to, 40–41
CDCynergy, 40–41, 41b
behavioral management model, 50f
dissemination and publication plan, 43
ecological model, 41, 42t
evaluation plan, 43
health communication plan, 41–43
implementation, 43
importance of, 39
information, 49

latent need, 52
logic model
activities, 54
business tool (*See* SWOT analysis)
immediate outcomes, 55
long-term outcomes, 55
outcomes, 55
outputs, 55
partnership
audience-oriented approach, 52
benefits and barriers, 53b
plan, 43
problem-solving, 52
task-oriented, 52
persuasion, 49
planning
behavior management model, 50
communication strategy, 48–49
ecological framework, 44–47
educational approaches, 50–51
evidence-based intervention, 47
policy approaches, 51
primary audience, 47–48
social marketing, 51–52
program management (*See* logic
model)
programs, 43–44
Smoke Free Alachua, 44
strategic health communication plan, 41
strategic thinking
opportunities and threats, 62
strengths and weaknesses, 61
sustainability, 52
SWOT analysis, 55–60, 57b–58b
bioethics, 60b
deontological (duty-based)
principles, 59
ethical dimensions, 57
opportunities, 56–57
strengths, 55–56
threats, 57
utilitarianism, 57
weaknesses, 56
Tips From Former Smokers (Tips),
43–44
communications team. *See* New Jersey
Academy of Family Physicians
(NJAFP)
control beliefs
county health rankings, 23–25, 24f
creative brief, 321–332
crisis and emergency risk communication
(CERC)
anthrax, 428
causality, 432
dose–response assessment, 437
emergency communications
seven recommendations, 461–462,
462b–464b
emergency risk communication (ERC),
439–445

hazard identification, 436–437
outbreak
    "black swan event," 429b
    Ebola virus disease, 428
Pentagon attack, 427–428
presenting a risk assessment
    oral presentation, 438
    public in, 439
    remote presentations, 438–439
    report content, 436–437
    written document, 437
presenting risk, 434
response, 428, 432
risk assessment, presenting, 436–439
risk characterization, 437
risk framework
    causality, 432–434, 433t–434t
    risk communication, 432b
risk management, 437
risk perception, 434–436
stages of
    CERC checklist, 446b–447b
    CERC life cycle for communication,
        446f
    message and audience, 453
    message maps, 454, 461, 461b–462b
    pre-crisis materials, 453–454
    pre-event planning, 447–453
transformations, 428
Customer Journey Mapping (CJM),
    233–234

D

data communication
    data presentation
        bar chart, 87f
        dashboards represent, 88
        data metaphors, text (words), 85–86
        data table, 87f
        extensive details, 85
        line graph, 88f
        narrative, 85
        pie charts, 88
        visual data presentation (See visual
            displays)
        visualizing health project, 86
    integration
        communication and implementa-
            tion plan, 85
    people and numbers
        numeracy, 82
        tendencies and biases, 82–83
    presenting public health numbers,
        85–91
    principles, 83
        audience analysis, 83
        contextual information, 84
        data integration, 85
        data overload, 84

ethical responsibility, 83
familiar data, 84
framing effects, 84
gain-framed messages, 84
implementation plan, 85
probability data, 84
risk estimates, 85
unfamiliar terms, 84
public health data systems
    data finding, 78
    disease outbreak, 79b–80b
    surveillance systems, 77–78, 78b
    websites for, 81t
single overarching communication
    objective (SOCO), 83
visual displays
    audience understanding, 86
    infographics, 88–90
    visual modalities, 86–88
visualizing data project, 90f
dengue prevention, social media
    assessment, 475–476
    baseline evaluation, 479–480
    civic engagement, 477
    digitized dengue education, 476–477
    disability-adjusted life-years (DALYs),
        475
    Mo-buzz for PHIs, 476–477
    Mo-Buzz system, 476
    monitoring and mapping, 476
    predictive surveillance, 477
    problem definition, 475
    protection motivation theory (PMT),
        478
    public health inspectors (PHIs), 475
Department of Health and Human
    Services (DHHS), 2, 13
diffusion of innovations (DI), 183–184
disease and death
    environmental disease, 18
    health care, 18
downstream interventions, 6
drinking water laws, 18

E

Ebola Response Strategic
    Communication Plan
    advertising, 471
    internal communication, 471
    internal tools, 472
    meeting plan, 471
    metrics, 472–474
    news releases, 471
    public service announcements, 471
    risk communication frame, 470
    tools, 471–472
    top-level messages, 469–470
ecological model, 4, 4f
    applying theory, 193

health communication, 41
electroencephalographic (EEG), 342
emergency risk communication (ERC).
    See crisis and emergency risk
    communication (CERC)
    channels and media choices, 439,
        440t–441t
    psychological needs, 441, 444,
        444b–445b
    social media, 440, 442b–444b
    vs. routine health communication,
        439–440
Emerging Infections Network (EIN), 36
entertainment education (EE), 194,
    197–198
European Association for
    Communication in Healthcare
    (EACH), 14
Extended Parallel Process Model
    (EPPM), 192

F

Food and Drug Administration (FDA),
    14, 27
formative research
    analyzing information, 224–225
    data mining, 238–239
    diagnostic role play (DRP), 246
    ethnolinguistic techniques, 247–248
    focus group discussions (FGDs),
        246–247
    in-depth interviews, 246
    intercept interviews, 247
    market research, 225
        online communities, 248
    message framing
        assessments, 253
        environmental scan, 252–253
        grabbing frame, 256–258
        health promotion, 258–259
        media scan, 253
        message development, 254
        online surveys participants, 256
        online surveys results, 256
        phone-based, 255–256
        protection theme, 260
        supporting statements, 262–263
        theoretical basis, 251–252
        working together theme, 261
    online qualitative research, 248
    online surveys, 241, 243–244
    PD research, 229
    Pew Research Center, 241, 243
    PhotoVoice investigation, 244–246
    positive deviance approach, 228–232,
        229b–231b
    research processes
        audience profiles, 233b
        audience segments, 232–233

formative research (*Continued*)
  customer journey mapping, 233–234, 235b–236b
  doer/non-doer analysis, 228–232, 229b–231b
  energy balance attitudes and behaviors, 232f
  insurance purchase journey map, 237f
  marketing, 225–226
  organized framework, 225–226
  personas, 232–233
  positive deviance approach, 228–232, 229b–231b
  social marketing, 226–228, 226b–228b
  research tools
    HIV-Positive Patients' Perceptions, 242b
    interviews, 239
    perceptual mapping, 241, 241b–242
    qualitative methods, 244–248
    quantitative methods, 238–244, 238f
    survey administration, 241
    surveys, 239–244
    verbal probing, 240–241
  reviewing information, 224–225
  scope of, 223–225
  SHARE framework, 224, 225f
framing bias, 184
framing message, 184
functional magnetic resonance imaging (fMRI), 342

G

gain-framed, 184
Galvanic Skin Response (GSR), 342
GreenBook Research Industry Trends Report (GRIT), 234

H

Haemophilus influenzae type b vaccine (Hib), 34
hand washing behaviors, campaign, 361–367
health
  communication intervention, 6
  definition of, 2
  rankings, 23–25
Health and Human Services (HHS), 13
health behaviors, 25
Health Belief Model (HBM), 19, 180
Health Communication Capacity Collaborative (HC3), 214
health determinants data
  physical environment, 27
  social and economic factors, 26
health disparities, 23

health indicators
  health disparities, 23
  Healthy People 2020, 22t
Health Information National Trends Survey (HINTS), 239
health information technology, 13–14
health literacy
  American Academy of Pediatrics (AAP), 159
  assessing
    clinical practice, 164
      measuring instruments, 162–163
      universal precautions toolkit, 164
    case study – smokefree.gov, 173–174
  in clinical practice, 164
  components
    determinants, 154
    types of literacy, 153
    U.S. Department of Education, 153–155
  conceptual framework,
  culturally and linguistically appropriate services (CLAS), 157
  determinants of
    communication skills, 155–156
    context, 157–158
    healthcare complexities, 158–160
    informed consent, 160
    knowledge, 156
    language and culture, 156
    local language proficiency, 157
  developing/assessing materials
    clear communication index, 165–166
    key principles, 164–165
    suitability assessment of materials, 165–166
  document literacy, 153
  eHealth Literacy Scale (eHEALS), 163
  electronic health record (EHR) programs, 160
  Flesch-Kincaid grade level readability test, 165
  Health Literacy Skills Instrument (HLSI), 163
  Health Literacy Tool Shed, 163–164
  healthcare environment, 166
  human learning and development, 152–153
  Institute of Medicine (IOM), 160
  integrated model of, 152F
  limited English proficiency (LEP), 157
  literacy, 152
  modeling, 152
  national policy
    Clear Communication Index (CCI), 161
    Healthy People 2020, 161, 162b
    National Action Plan, 161–162, 162b
    patient protection, 161
    The Patient Protection and Affordable Care Act (ACA), 161

    Plain Writing Act of 2010, 164
    Newest Vital Sign (NVS), 163
    numeracy, 153
    Numeracy Understanding in Medicine Instrument (NUMi), 163
    PIAAC proficiency levels, 154t–155t, 155f
    Program for the International Assessment of Adult Competencies (PIAAC), 153
    prose literacy, 153
    quantitative literacy (QL), 153
    Rapid Estimate of Adult Literacy in Medicine (REALM), 163
    SMOG (simple measure of Gobbledygook), 166
    suitability assessment of materials (SAM), 165
    Test of Functional Health Literacy in Adults (TOFHLA), 163
    universal precautions toolkit, 164
    Women, Infants, and Children (WIC) program, 159
healthcare, 27
healthcare-associated infections (HCAIs), 270
health-related quality of life (HRQoL), 25
Healthy People 2020 (HP 2020), 2, 21, 23, 22t
  goals of, 4–5
    health indicators, 2
  objectives, 3b
  Patient Protection and Affordable Care Act, 161
hierarchy of effects (HOE), 6
high sensation seekers (HSS), 219
Hispanic health communications, ACA
  demographic analyses, 306
  evaluation and improvement, 310
  health insurance literacy, 306–307
  implementing, 308
  messages and materials, 307–308
HIV testing rates, radio power impact, 302–303
  Los Angeles, 301
  New York City, 302
HIV/AIDS medical care, 301
Hollywood, Health, and Society (HH&S) program, 197
Hornik, Robert, 5
HPV vaccine. *See* human papillomavirus (HPV) vaccine
human papillomavirus (HPV) vaccine, 184

I

infectious disease
  antibiotic medications, 37
  emerging infectious disease(EID)

bacterial resistance, 37
 communicating about, 36–37
 impacting factors of, 36t
 sources of, 36
morbidity and mortality weekly report, 34
vaccines
 benefits, 35
 childhood vaccination, 33
 communication resources, 35–36
 national immunization survey, 34
 preventable diseases, 33–34
 safety basics, 35
information-building approach. *See* scaffolding
Institute of Medicine (IOM), 36, 99
International Agency for Research on Cancer (IARC), 107
International Communication Association (ICA), 14

K

Kenya hand washing campaign
 behavior change, 362
 campaign goals,361–362
 description and methodology, 364–365
 development of, 362
 evaluation, 366–367
 formative research, 362–363
 implementation, 366
 materials used, 365–366
 objectives, 363–364
 problem definition, 361
Klaiman, T, 232

L

leading health indicators, 2
life expectancy (LE), 5
 behavioral changes on, 5f
loss-framed, 184
low sensation seekers (LSS), 219
low sensation value (LSV), 219

M

Marmot, Michael, 19
measles-containing vaccine (MCV), 34
media
 broadcast media channels
  print media/magazines, 268
  radio, 268
  television, 268
 CDC's best practice
  Facebook, 294–295, 285b–286b
  Twitter, 287b–288b
 channel selection
  customer journey (CJ), 269–270

customer journey life cycle, 271f
  management framework, 270
  PESO model, 272, 272f
  Theory-Informed Media Selection (TIMS), 269
 content management and strategy, 332–333
 cross-channel, 290
 earned media, 270–271
 information, search for, 272
  news, 272–273
  website or blog, 272–275
 media richness theory, 269
 news, 272–273, 273f
 Nielsen's analysis, 266, 267t
 owned media, 272
 paid media, 270
 production and dissemination factors, 333–334
 radio personalities, 268
 shared media, 271
 social media
  cell phone texting, 277–283
  demographic breakdown, 276
  Facebook, 284
  leading network, 276
  in public health communication, 288–289
  social networking sites, 284–287
  tools, 276–277
  Twitter, 287–288
 social networking sites
  Facebook, 284–285
  Twitter, 287
 texting
  emergency communication and health promotion, 286–292
 texting and health agencies, 277–283
 transmedia storytelling, 290, 290b–292b
 in United States
  sources, 266
 Uses and Gratifications Theory (UGT), 269
 vehicles, 266
 virtual reality technology, 290, 292b–293b
 website/blog
  click-through, 274
  content marketing, 274–275
  inbound marketing, 274
  landing pages, 274
  search engine, 273–274
Mediamark Research & Intelligence (MRI), 268
meducation. *See* National Institutes of Health (NIH)
message sensation seeking, 193
message sensation value (MSV), 193, 219
Morbidity and Mortality Weekly Report (MMWR), 34

N

National Academy of Medicine. *See* Institute of Medicine
National Academy of Sciences Institute of Medicine (NAS/IOM), 14
National Antimicrobial Resistance Monitoring System (NARMS), 37
National Cancer Institute (NCI), 13, 25, 224
National Commission for Health Education Credentialing (NCHEC), 10
National Communication Association (NCA), 2, 14
National Electronic Disease Surveillance System (NEDSS), 34
National Health and Nutrition Examination Survey (NHANES), 25
National Health Interview Survey (NHIS), 25
National Immunization Survey, 34
National Institutes of Health (NIH), 13, 402
National Notifiable Diseases Surveillance System (NNDSS), 78b
National Public Health Information Coalition (NPHIC), 12–13, 13b
National Syndromic Surveillance Program (NSSP), 78b
National Vital Statistics System (NVSS), 78b
New Jersey Academy of Family Physicians (NJAFP), 111
normative beliefs, 183
North Carolina Department of Public Health (NCDPH), 94
North Carolina Electronic Disease Surveillance System (NC EDSS) data, 94

O

occupational safety laws, 18
Office of Behavioral and Social Science Research (OBSSR), 215
Office of Disease Prevention and Health Promotion (ODPHP), 13
Office of the National Coordinator (ONC), 13

P

Patient Centered Outcomes Research Institute (PCORI), 224
patient education, research to
 breast cancer
  communication plan, 114–115
  communication team, 111–112, 112t

patient education, research to
(*Continued*)
concept brochure, 118f–119f
focus group, 115–116
materials, 119–120
message strategies, 113–114
Breast Cancer and the Environment
Research Program (BCERP), 111
new jersey academy of family physicians (NJAFP), 111
nominal group technique process
(NGT), 112
pelvic inflammatory disease (PID), 94
perceived message sensation value scale
(PMSV), 219
perceived normative pressure
See normative beliefs
Pew Research Center, 27, 241, 266, 268,
286
mail-based surveys, 243
media vehicle, 266
policy communication
advocacy, 123–124
citizens, public policy, 124
advocacy, organizations, 126,
127b–128b
elections, 124
lobbying, advocacy, and policy,
126–127
PAC (*See* political action committees (PACs))
political action committees (PACs),
124
super PACs, 124–125
Internal Revenue Service (IRS), 125
policy brief, 141
policy presentation, 138
media scanning, 140
online tools, 140
polling surveys, 140
strategic policy
audience, 131
delivering message, 136–138
direct policy communication, 129
individual spokespersons,
134b–136b
legal government processes,
129b–130b
messenger, 133
metrics, 138, 137b–140b
policy making stages, 132
state legislators, 132b, 132t
population health
causes of death, 19f, 26f
communication challenges
chronic disease, 30
perception *vs.* reality, 29–30
risk perception, 29
County Health Rankings, 24f, 25
evolution of
CDC (*See* Centers for Disease Control and Prevention (CDC))

clinical preventive services, 18
environmental disease, 18
health care, 18, 27
health determinants, 21b
health risk behaviors, 18–19
lifestyle, 18–19
social determinants, 19–20
health indicators, 21–23
health ranking, 23–24
safe drinking water information
system, 27
sources of information
determinants data, 25
evidence-based policies, 28–29
health care, 27
media, 29
outcomes data, 25–26
physical environment, 27
reports, 27
social and economic factors, 27
systematic reviews, 28
Whitehall Studies, 19–20, 20b
practice strategy, 194
program evaluation
health communication, 369–371
health communication program,
369–371
in context, 369–371
public health activities. *See Healthy People
2020* (HP 2020)
public health communication
as career, 8–9
causes of death, 17–18, 17–29
communication, 2
skills, 9t–10t
transactional model of, 2
competencies in, 9–10, 11t–12t
credentialing, 10–12
ecological model, 4, 41
foundation, 6
health communication interventions,
6–7
advertising, 6–7
customer journey, 7, 8b
health-promoting behavior, 7
incubators, 13–14
population health model, 5–6
public health, 2
social media, 289
public health services, 9f

Q

quality-adjusted life expectancy (QALE), 5

R

RE-AIM planning tool, 316–319
research factors
representativeness and causality, 98–99

study design, 98
research syntheses, 99–100
Rosling, Hans, 29

S

Satcher, David, Dr., 19–20
scaffolding, 152
science and research
assessing quality
information sources, 101–102
interpretation, 103–104
processing information, 103–104
research factors, 98–99
scientific consensus, 99–101
case study
from article, 106–107,
comprehensive scientific report,
107–109
interpreting science, 109
communication fundamentals
advice/recommendations, 104
content, 104
context, 105
description, 104
explanation and interpretation, 104
overload, 105
comprehensive report, 99
cross-sectional studies, 98
evidence-based research reviews,
99–100
experimental studies, 98
meta-analyses, 99
patient education
(*See* patient education, research to)
scientific information, 102
culture, 103
health, interest in, 102–103
scientific knowledge, 102–103
trust and belief, 103
worldview, 103
scientific studies, 99
SGR (*See* surgeon general report (SGR))
surgeon general report (SGR), 107–109
preventing tobacco use, 107b
scientific report, 107
website materials, 108
systematic reviews, 99
scientific consensus
meta-analyses, 100
research syntheses, 99–100
severe acute respiratory syndrome
(SARS), 36
sexually transmitted disease (STD), 274
short message service (SMS), 277
single overriding communication
objective (SOCO), 105
SMART, 319–320
social cognitive theory (SCT), 180–182
social marketing, 51–52, 205–213,
226–228

social media
  case study – smokefree.gov, 173
  digital channels and tools, 276
  engagement, 48–49
  function and use, tools, 277
  networking sites, 284–288
  new media advocacy, 142
  in public health communication, 288–290
  tools, 277–283
Society for Public Health Education (SOPHE), 14
Stages of Change (SOC) Model, 180
Substance Abuse and Mental Health Services Administration (SAMHSA), 14
sudden infant death syndrome (SIDS), 50
Surveillance, Epidemiology and End Results (SEER), 25

T

telephone-based surveillance system. *See* Behavioral Risk Factor Surveillance System (BRFSS)
texting. *See* short message service (SMS)
theory, models, and practice strategies
  behavioral change, 177–178, 208b–213b
  CDC HIV risk assessment tool, 205f
  communication studies
    extended parallel process model, 192
    inoculation theory, 185–192
    media richness theory, 193–194
    message framing, 184–185
    message sensation value and sensation seeking, 193

contemplation stage, 180
in health communication
  behavior change theory, 180–184
  sources of, 178–179
  value of, 178
individualized communications, 205
message sensation value
  audience targeting, 219
  evaluating messages, 220
  programmatic research, 221
  theory-based message design, 219
  MIYO, communication tool, 199–203
practice strategies
  behavioral targeting, 199, 204
  demographic targeting, 198–199
  elaboration likelihood model, 198
  entertainment education (EE), 194–198
  intervention mapping, 194
  participatory approach, 194
  practice strategy, 194
  tailoring, 205
  theory-based methods, 194
pre-conceptional health, 199
precontemplation, 180
social marketing
  audience segmentation, 206
  behavior, 206
  benefits, barriers, and competition, 213–214
  competition, 213–214
  cost, 213
  customer orientation, 206
  economic concept, 213
  immutable laws of, 206–208
  partner-based segmentation, 206
  resources, 214

tobacco prevention, 208b–209b
Theory of Planned Behavior (TPB), 67, 362
theory-based methods, 194
transactional model of communication, 2
Transtheoretical Model (TTM), 185. *See* Stages of Change (SOC) Model
2020 health indicators, 22t

U

United States Agency for International Development (USAID), 246
upstream interventions, 6
U.S. Agency for International Development (USAID), 14
U.S. Department of Agriculture (USDA), 14
uses and gratifications theory (UGT), 193

V

vaccine benefits and safety, 35
vaccine-preventable diseases, 33–35
visualizing data project, 89f–90f

W

Wiio, Osmo A., 2

Y

Youth Risk Behavior Surveillance System (YRBSS), 239